PAEDIATRIC CLINICAL EXAMINATION

A Santhosh Kumar, MD, MNAMS, DPed
Professor in Paediatrics, Azeezia Medical College, Kollam
Former, Prof and Head, Department of Paediatrics
Govt Medical College and SAT Hospital
Thiruvananthapuram, Kerala, India

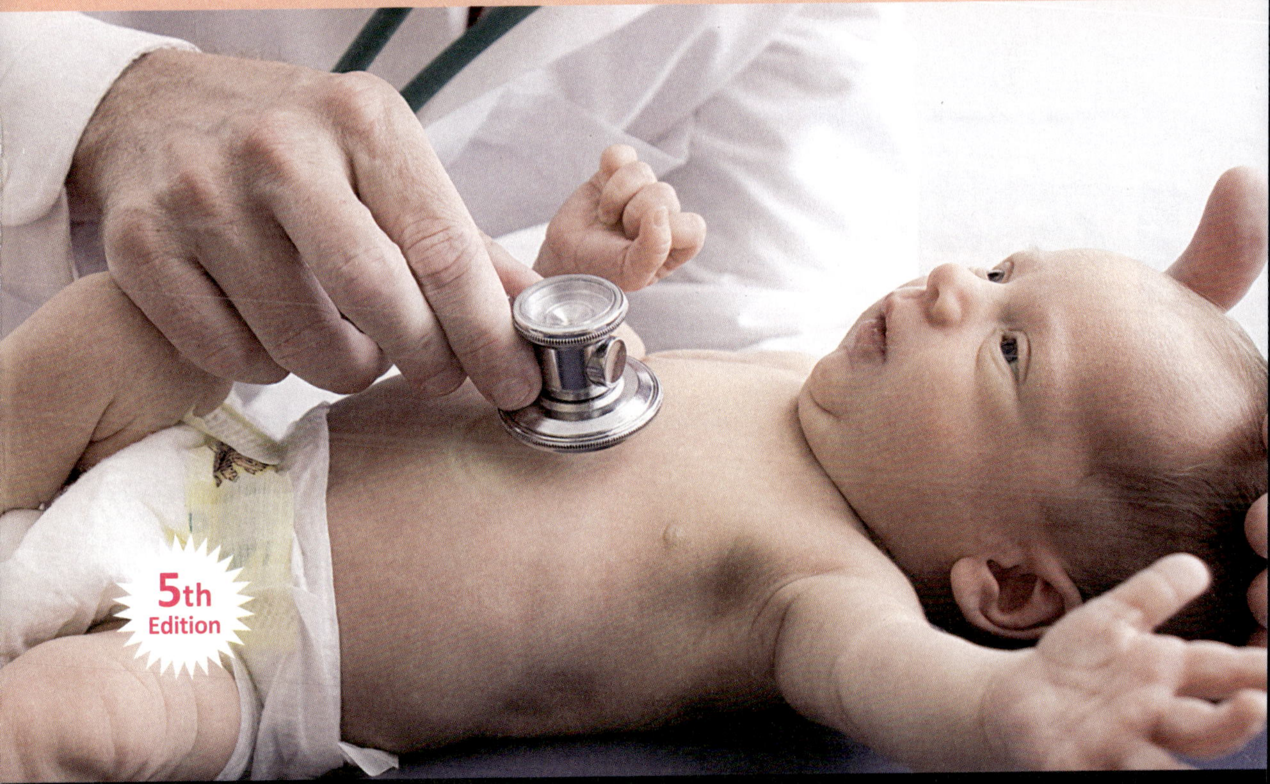

Paras Medical Publisher
Hyderabad ▪ New Delhi, India

PAEDIATRIC CLINICAL EXAMINATION

PARAS

Explore the New Possibilities

Paras Medical Publisher
5-1-473, First Floor, Putlibowli
Hyderabad—500001, Telangana, India
parasmedpub@hotmail.com

Branch Office: 2/25, Grd. Floor
Daryaganj, Ansari Road,
New Delhi-110 002, India

1/ed 2004; Reprints 2005, 2007
2008; 2/ed 2008; 3/ed 2011
4/ed 2014, Reprint 2015, Reprint 2017
5/ed 2018, Reprint 2019, Reprint 2021
Revised reprint 2022, Reprint 2023,
Revised 1st reprint 2025, 2nd Reprint 2025
3rd Reprint 2026

ISBN: 978-81-8191-494-1

Note: Medicine is an ever-changing science. As new research and clinical experience broaden our knowledge, changes in the diagnosis and treatment occur. The authors and the publisher of this work have checked with sources believed to be reliable in their efforts to provide information that is complete and generally in accord with the standards accepted at the time of publication. Exhaustive efforts have been made to ensure accuracy and correctness of contents of the book at the time of going to press. However, in view of possibility of human error or changes in medical science, the author, publisher or any other person who has been involved in preparation of this work accepts no responsibility for any errors or omissions or results obtained from use of information given in the book. Every effort has been made to put reference to tables and figures. If any table and figure has been taken from a source, which has not been quoted it is an oversight and will be corrected at the earliest possible opportunity. The authors have made every effort to trace the copyright holders for borrowed material. If they have inadvertently overlooked any, they will be pleased to make the necessary arrangements at the first opportunity. This book is being published with the understanding that the material provided by the author(s) is original. This book is for sale in India only and cannot be exported without the permission of the publisher in writing. Any disputes and legal matters to be settled under Hyderabad jurisdiction only. *Printed in Hyderabad, India.*

PREFACE

Welcome to the fifth edition of "***Paediatric Clinical Examination***." With the mushrooming of numerous medical colleges throughout India, the relevance of this book has increased tremendously. The present day curious phenomenon is that medical colleges with heavy patient load has no time to teach and medical colleges with not enough patients have enough time to teach. In both scenarios, the student is the loser, either by not getting guidance as to how to do clinical examination of the available patients or not having patients at all to master clinical methods. The only way out is a heavily illustrated book showing the physical examination with proper explanations. And this book provides exactly that.

An additional bonus is that all clinical case scenarios that figure in university examinations have been covered separately, immediately after the chapter of physical examination of that system. Each case sheet formats carries all the necessary and pertinent points to be noted while taking the history and performing the physical examination. This has been a radical change from the conventional books on physical examination, which is undoubtedly going to benefit the students both in graduate and postgraduate training. The section on clinical examination of newborn is specially designed for the postgraduate student.

This book has image galleries with short discussions, which will be thought provoking and would encourage the students to read further in depth from other sources. The visual treat provided in this book covers all the common entities and even the clinical rarities. So much so, there may not be any clinical entity the reader of this book may not be familiar with. This will definitely help them to gain confidence in clinical case discussions and ultimately their success in examinations.

Many changes and remodelling of medical education have taken place, with the emphasis shifting to entrance examinations and skill stations. Still the most important core skills the medical students have to master remain the same: history taking and physical examination to arrive at a plausible diagnosis. It is a matter of grave concern that clinical skills are dying out as a natural consequence of increasingly relying on investigations. As always I reiterate that no amount of book reading will ever substitute for bedside acquisition of clinical skills, because the patient is always the best teacher. This book is designed as a carry along companion for such a patient examination, to make the student proficient in the basic skills of history taking, clinical examination, differential diagnosis of signs and symptoms and discussion of clinical cases during examination.

The manner in which the previous editions have been received by the students and medical teachers has overwhelmed me and exceeded all my expectations. I hope students will take this edition also to their hearts in the same way and also hope that I am able to instill in them a desire to take up this wonderful branch of medicine.

A Santhosh Kumar

ACKNOWLEDGEMENTS

My heartfelt thanks to...

Dr Gibby Koshy

Dr S Pradeep Babu

Dr Anand Srinivasan

Dr Sheela Nampoothiri

Dr Shahanaz Ahmed

Mr Divyesh Kothari, Paras Medical Publisher, Hyderabad for his continued enthusiasm and support throughout the preparation of this book.

CONTENTS

LIST OF SKILLS AS PER CBME

CBME mandates that a student acquires specified skills to pass the examination. Ref: Competency-Based Medical Education Curriculum (CBME) Regulations, 2023 (No. U. 1 4021 1812023-UGMEB) released by National Medical Commission on 1st August 2023.

This book contains all the practical skills required to be mastered during the curriculum. Listed below are the important skills to be acquired with the page number in this book where it is discussed.

Students are advised to use the images in this book to make learning easier

Skill: Elicitation of History

Format for history: **p 1**

Elicitation of history (General): **p 30–38**

Elicitation of history related to specific signs and symptoms: Chapter 8, **p 151–178**

Elicitation of history related to specific system illnesses:

- Nervous system: **p 250**
- Cardiovascular system: **p 328**
- Respiratory system: **p 370**
- Gastro intestinal system: **p 406**
- Hematological system: **p 424, 429**
- Genitourinary system: **p 439**
- Endocrinology: **p 446**
- Rheumatology: **p 457, 470**

Skill: Measurement of anthropometric parameters, plotting in growth charts and its interpretation: p 44–60

Skills required is not just the measurement, but include plotting and interpretation in WHO/IAP growth charts. The students must practice plotting the measured values in the chart. The student is expected to find out BMI, mid parental height etc as part of interpretation (either from charts or by calculation). The student is expected to know the normal expected ages of eruption of teeth (**p 51**).

Skill: Assessment of mile stones of development: p 60–65

The assessment includes both the history of achievements of mile stones plus the student making the child perform the achieved mile stones. The student must be able to comment whether the development is appropriate for age or is there any delay. If there is a delay, whether its global delay or limited to one domain of development. Compare the development mile stones of a given child with the expected development of a normal child and find out any deviation from normal in any domain of development. The student is expected to know the difference between growth and development and also the factors affecting normal growth and development.

Skill: Assessment of stages of sexual development of adolescents: p 51

Skill: Assessment and classification of the nutrition status of children and recognition of deviations from normal; and classification of undernutrition p 44–48

Skill: Elicitation of diet history by 24 hr recall from mother/informant and find out the Calorie and protein input using the knowledge of nutrient contents

of common food items (p 66) and compare with the recommended daily nutrient intakes (p 67) and comment on the adequacy of dietary intake and insufficiencies if any.

Note: The student must note that the nutrition recommendations of their institute/hospital may vary slightly from ICMR recommendations and hence the student is advised to be familiar with the recommendations followed in their hospitals also. This is because in areas where people are consuming cereal-based diet with no pulses or animal protein, the protein requirements from diet may be as high as 1 g/kg per day.
Know various causes of Failure to thrive. **p 174**
Know various causes of Short stature. **p 175**
The student is advised to read from theory books the grading as per IMNCI

Skill: Write an appropriate diet for a healthy child of given age:
First write down the calorie and protein requirement for the expected weight of the given child. Then write down a diet such that it provides the calculated requirements. Also see that the diet contains micronutrients as well (calcium, vitamins etc). **p 66–67**

Skill: Plan an appropriate diet for a child with common diseases like glomerulonephritis.
Refer under individual conditions in this book.

Skill: To give nutrition counseling for a child with failure to thrive.
Identify dietary deficiencies of nutrients and counsel regarding food items to be included to close the nutritional gap. **P 66–67**
The student may read about mother and Child Protection card (MCP card)

Skill: To elicit focused history to find out the etiology of obesity, investigations and management.
p 453

Skill: Elicitation of history physical examination and knowledge on causes and classification of short stature. p 175, 449

Skill: Identification and management of deficiencies of vitamin A (p 488, 492), B complex (p 390-391), C (p 567), D (p 72, 490, 567).

Skill: Counsel on national immunization program (p 33).
The student is expected to visit immunization clinic and familiarize with the techniques of ID, SC, IM injections

Skill: Interpretation of Mantoux reaction.
Fig 24.84 A, **P 527**

Skill: Identify severe acute malnutrition; discuss the clinical features, diagnosis, management and counseling of parents. p 68, 487

Skill: Elicitation of history, clinical signs and management of diarrhea. p 158, 414

Skill: Elicit history and do a clinical examination of a normal newborn. p 10

Skill: Assessment of a preterm/LBW baby. p 21

Skill: Assessment of a newborn baby with jaundice p 26

Skill: Demonstration of Moro reflex. p 15

Skill: Interpretation of X rays & CTs. p 555

Skill: Clinical case discussion
Clinical examination of children with specific diseases followed by discussion of the case. Skills assessed include elicitation of relevant history, physical examination, interpretation of physical findings, formulation of a plausible diagnosis correlating history and physical findings, knowledge

to offer a few differential diagnoses, investigations, treatment, and counseling on prognosis.

Nutrition:

- Severe acute malnutrition **P 68, 487**
- Obesity **p 453**
- Anemia: Chapter 19

Genetic:

- Down syndrome. **p 146, 507**
- Turner syndrome. **p 148, 518**
- Draw and interpret pedigree chart. **p 36**
- Nervous system cases: Chapter 11
- Cardiovascular system cases: Chapter 14
- Respiratory system cases: Chapter 16
- Gastro intestinal system cases: Chapter 18
- Hematology cases: Chapter 19
- Kidney and urinary tract cases: Chapter 20
- Endocrinology cases: Chapter 21
- Rheumatology/collagen vascular cases: Chapter 23
- OSCE spotters: Chapter 24
- X rays and CT for examination: Chapter 25

The student is advised to acquire the following skills by interpreting lab data of their patients in the wards and interacting with the parents.

Skill to obtain informed consent for a procedure.

Skills to interpret lab data:

Interpretation of CBC, LFT, RFT, iron panel in iron deficiency anemia, urine exam etc. blood sugar report and A1C in diabetes.

Skill to counsel the parents of a child with:

1. Failure to thrive child
2. Developmental delay
3. SAM/MAM
4. Chronic systemic illnesses
5. Child getting discharged after common illnesses, like asthma, ADD, acute glomerulonephritis, Nephrotic syndrome, hepatitis etc
6. Terminally ill child

The student is required to visit the immunization clinic and understand the components of safe vaccine practices, observe the handling and storing of different vaccines documentation of the immunization in the immunization record. Also they must observe the health care provider educate and counsel the parents for immunization (age at which different vaccines are given, the schedule and expected side effects. They must observe the administration of different vaccines. They must observe the infection control measures being practiced and appropriate handling of the sharps. In skill lab the student shall practice the correct administration of different vaccines in a mannequin.

Demonstration of common pediatric procedures and instruments (to be practiced in skill labe): IV cannulation, intraosseous line, NG tube insertion, bone marrow aspiration/bone marrow biopsy, lumbar puncture, liver biopsy etc.

Neonatal resuscitation: The student is advised to read newborn topics from *Manual of Newborn Care*, A Santhosh Kumar, Paras Medical Publisher. After reading, the student may practice in mannequin in skill lab.

Basic/advanced life support need be practiced in skill lab.

CHAPTER 1

Paediatric Case Sheet

Personal Data

- Patient's name :
- Age :
- Sex :
- Address :
- Informant :
- Date of examination and date of admission to hospital (optional):

More details on personal data on p 27.

I. HISTORY

1. Presenting complaints : (p 30)
2. History of the present illness : (p 30)
3. History of past illnesses : (p 30)
4. Antenatal, natal & postnatal history: (p 31)
5. Immunization history : (p 32)
6. Development history : (p 34)
7. Dietary history : (p 34)
8. Family and socioeconomic history : (p 35, 38)

Always start the interaction by introducing yourself to the child/parent; be polite, diplomatic and tactful; you must be flexible in scheme of examination depending on the child's attitude; sticking on to a rigid scheme of examination as you have been trained, can be counterproductive in examination setting. After finishing the history, make a list of problems and then organize it appropriately so that the most relevant/current issues are presented first to the examiner followed by the others in the order of relevance to the patient at hand.

Organizing a systematic summary of complaints and relevant history at this stage will help the student to decide the probable diagnosis and thus decide which system to be examined first. Postgraduate examiners expect such a summary from the candidate (either after history or after history and general examination). The summary must include positive and relevant negative findings elicited in history and general examination.

After completing the physical examination, if the diagnosis reached at is very different from what was assumed after history, then the candidate must go back to the history again. There could be some additional history unelicited that could have led the student to the accurate diagnosis.

> **Note**
>
> The **MAIN** additional history/general examination points in paediatric case sheet compared to adult case sheet are:
>
> - **M**ilestones of development
> - **A**nthropometry
> - **I**mmunization
> - **N**utrition
>
> In MBBS examination, of the two cases that are usually allotted, one case will be ear marked to assess the candidate's proficiency in the areas of "MAIN" and hence its importance.

II. GENERAL EXAMINATION

1. General Comment

Is the child sick looking, tachypnoeic/dyspnoeic? Comment on the build and nourishment.

2. Vital Signs (Compare with the normal values for age)

- Pulse rate, respiratory rate, blood pressure and temperature (p 40).

3. Assessment of Growth (Anthropometry or Measurements)

- Weight (p 44)
- Height (including upper segment–lower segment ratio) (p 46, 48)
- Head circumference (p 48)
- Chest circumference (if relevant) (p 49)
- Mid-arm circumference (if relevant) (p 50)
- Arm span (if relevant) (p 50)

4. Assessment of Development (p 60)

In cases of developmental retardation, the student is required to assess the development by examination rather than depending totally on history. For example, in addition to getting a reliable history, the student may test if the child can perform specified tasks (e.g., pick up a pellet from floor). If the case at hand is not the one with retarded development, this step can be skipped. See 180° flip at p 256.

5. Head to Foot Examination (Hand to head and Head to Toe) Examination (p 42)

History and general examination are discussed in some detail in Ch. 3. For dysmorphism and musculoskeletal system, it is always advantageous to proceed from hand to head and then head to foot examination. In addition, the child should be inspected in front profile, side profile and back. Do not forget to notice any abnormality of skin. Ask the child to walk and inspect the gait (see p 183). In fact, the vital signs also may be looked for during this hand to head to foot examination, but mentioned as a separate heading as given in the case sheet format when the case is presented to the examiner. Findings of front, side and back profile inspections can be incorporated into the head to foot examination rather than mentioning it as a separate profile heading (follow your teachers protocol). (p-144) for profile appraisal.

III. EXAMINATION OF SYSTEMS

One or more systems may have to be examined depending on the complaints and history.

CENTRAL NERVOUS SYSTEM

1. Higher Functions

It is easy to remember when arranged in alphabetic order.

- **A**ppearance
- **B**ehaviour
- **C**onsciousness level
- **D**elusions (only in relevant cases)
- **E**motional state (e.g., emotional lability in chorea)
- **G**ait (some authorities discuss gait under motor system)
- **H**allucinations (only in relevant cases)
- **I**ntelligence
- **M**emory
- **O**rientation in time and place
- **S**peech
- **S**leep

2. Cranial Nerves

I	Sensory Test each nostril separately
II	Sensory Acuity of vision Field of vision Colour vision Fundus
III,	Motor Ptosis

contd.

IV & VI	Nystagmus Strabismus (also ask for diplopia in history) Movements of eye ball Pupils (size, symmetry, direct/consensual reflex, accommodation reflex)
V	Motor (masseter, pterygoids, temporalis) Sensory (sensation over the face; also ask for blunting of sensations in history) Corneal reflex may be elicited now or along with examination for reflexes
VII	Motor (also ask about history of deviation of angle of mouth, hyperacusis, leaking of food and saliva from the mouth) Sensory (taste over anterior 2/3rd of tongue) Secretomotor (salivation/lacrimation) Need not mention if specific complaints are not there
VIII	Sensory Vestibular (ask about history of vertigo) Hearing (watch test/Rinne's test/Weber's test; mention if there is tinnitus)
IX, X	Motor (movements of soft palate; also ask the history of dysphagia and dysarthria) Gag reflex Sensory (taste sensation of posterior 1/3rd of tongue; not to be tested routinely)
XI	Motor Test trapezius and sternomastoid
XII	Motor Look for wasting, fasciculations Test protrusion of tongue and its lateral movements (also ask for history of dysarthria)

3. Motor System

Bulk of muscles: Wasting/hypertrophy/pseudohypertrophy. In pseudohypertrophy, the hypertrophied muscles are weak.

Tone: Normal/hypo/hypertonia. If hypertonic, assess if it is spasticity or rigidity.

Power: Grade the power. Make a note of posture of the limbs at rest, as it may give a clue to the weakness. For example, if one lower limb remains externally rotated while in supine position, it could mean that limb is weak.

Coordination of movements: Finger-nose test, past pointing, dysdiadochokinesia, heel-knee test, rebound phenomenon, tandem walking, gait, etc. Alternatively, one may mention these tests under a separate heading of cerebellar signs.

Involuntary movements: Tremor, chorea, athetosis, fasciculations, flapping tremor, tics, etc.

1

4. Reflexes

Superficial Reflexes

- Corneal
- Conjunctival
- Abdominal
- Cremasteric
- Plantar
- Anal (need not be elicited routinely)

Deep Tendon Reflexes

- Jaw jerk
- Biceps
- Triceps
- Supinator
- Knee
- Ankle
- Clonus, if any (ankle, patellar)

If the reflexes are not elicitable, examine after reinforcement (Jendrassik manoeuvre). When reflexes are exaggerated, look for ankle/patellar clonus.

Organic/Autonomic Reflexes

- Bowel and bladder habits (from history). Loss of sweating in affected parts. History of dizziness on standing could mean postural hypotension and hence look for standing and supine BP.

Primitive Reflexes

- In relevant cases (see p 233).

5. Sensory System

Lateral Column Sensations

- Touch (light touch, e.g., touch with cotton wool)
- Pain (use sterile blunt pin)
- Temperature (cold & warm)

Posterior Column Sensations

- Vibration
- Joint position sense
- Pressure touch

Cortical Sensations

- Tactile localization, two-point discrimination, stereognosis, graphaesthesia and sensory inattention.

6. Cerebellar Signs

It may be mentioned under the heading of tests of muscle coordination or under a separate heading of cerebellar signs (the student may follow the protocol of his teacher). A separate heading is justified in a case of cerebellar dysfunction, because the tests of cerebellar function include assessment of gait, speech, nystagmus and muscle tone in addition to coordination of movements.

7. Signs of Meningeal Irritation

- Neck stiffness (p 226)
- Kernig's sign
- Brudzinski's sign

8. Skull, Spine, Peripheral Nerves

- Crack pot sign
- Cranial bruit/carotid bruit
- Transillumination of skull (only in young infants)
- Look for vertebral defects, dermal sinus, tuft of hair, gibbus, etc. Percussion tenderness over the spine.
- Thickening of peripheral nerves

CARDIOVASCULAR SYSTEM

The usual symptoms related to cardiovascular system are exertional dyspnoea, oedema, easy fatiguability, joint pain, chest pain, palpitation, syncope, etc.

1. General

Pulse (rate, rhythm, volume, character, radio-femoral delay): Palpate all peripheral pulses. Mention pulse deficit, if any.

Blood Pressure (all four limbs when indicated)

JVP (mention, the height of JVP, the waves seen and hepatojugular reflux)
In case of aortic regurgitation and endocarditis, look for related peripheral signs. In rheumatic fever, look for joint swellings, rashes, chorea and subcutaneous nodules.

2. Inspection of Precordium

- Shape of precordium
- Apex beat
- Visible pulsation over the precordium (usual areas are the second space on the left side, suprasternal area, parasternal area, epigastrium and the neck)
- Dilated veins
- Any scars

3. Palpation

- Apex beat (location, nature)
- Other pulsations/thrills
- Left parasternal heave
- Palpable events in the second space

4. Percussion

- Locate the upper border of liver dullness
- Cardiac borders (use light percussion only)
- Determine whether the pulmonary area is resonant or dull

5. Auscultation

Auscultate area by area:

- Heart sounds: Concentrate on S_1, S_2, muffling/ accentuation, splitting of sounds.
- Murmurs: If a murmur is detected, comment on its timing, character, pitch, area where it is best heard, conduction, and changes with manoeuvres like exercise, posture, etc.
- Additional sounds: Look for additional sounds like S_3, S_4, opening snap, clicks, pericardial rub, etc.

RESPIRATORY SYSTEM

The usual symptoms related to respiratory system are cough, dyspnoea, wheezing, chest pain, haemoptysis, abdominal pain (muscle pain due to cough or referred pain of pneumonia), post-tussive vomiting, halitosis, etc.

1. Upper Respiratory Tract

- Nose: Discharge, bleeds, ala nasi working or not, deviations of nasal septum, nasal mucosa (congested and hypertrophied in allergy), etc
- Paranasal sinuses: Tenderness
- Throat: Tonsils and pharynx
- Ear: Discharge. Other details of ear are discussed in general examination.

2. Inspection

- Respiration: Respiratory rate, rhythm (regular or not), character (is it predominantly abdominal or thoracic); are the ala nasi and other accessory muscles of respiration active during breathing or not.
- Trachea: Position of trachea, is it central or shifted to one side as is evident by the Trail's sign.
- Apex: Its location is to be mentioned if visible.
- Shape of chest: Comment whether it is bilaterally symmetrical or not. Look for kyphosis/ scoliosis/kyphoscoliosis and pectus excavatum /carinatum. Look for any drooping of shoulder, hollowing (at the infraclavicular area), flattening/bulging. Bulging of intercostal spaces must be looked for.
- Movement of chest: Observe to see if it is bilaterally symmetrical. Any indrawing of lower chest wall.
- Dilated veins or pulsations.

3. Palpation

- Position of trachea, is there any shift?
- Position of apex beat, is there any shift? (indicating shift of mediastinum)
- Expansion of chest with inspiration, is it symmetrical bilaterally? If not, try to document the differential expansion, although it is likely to be far from accurate
- Vocal fremitus, in different areas
- Palpable rhonchi, crepitations or rub
- Tenderness

1

4. Percussion

- If any abnormality is detected, describe it by areas. If dullness is detected, look for a higher level in axilla and shifting dullness.
- Cardiac dullness (use light percussion)
- Upper border of liver dullness (confirm by tidal percussion)
- Percuss Traube's space

5. Auscultation

- Intensity of breath sounds: If the breath sounds are normal in character (vesicular), is it of normal intensity or reduced intensity?
- Type of breath sounds: If there is a bronchial breathing, describe it by areas.
- Adventitious sounds: Crackle, wheeze or pleural rub. Look for post-tussive crepitations if crepitations are not readily obvious.
- Vocal resonance: Comment if it is normal, decreased or increased. Is there any whispering pectoriloquy or aegophony?
- Coin sound if indicated (rarely done these days)

- Succussion splash, when hydropneumothorax is suspected.

GASTROINTESTINAL SYSTEM

1. Upper GIT

- Lips: Cheilitis, angular stomatitis, fissuring, pigmentation, vesicles (herpes), etc.
- Gum: Gingivitis, bleeding, hypertrophy, etc.
- Teeth: Number of teeth (permanent or milk teeth or both), hygiene, discolouration, caries, fluorosis, etc.
- Tongue: Dry (dehydration), jaundice (look at the undersurface), cyanosis, thrush, desquamation (e.g., geographic tongue), redness, papillae, etc.
- Oral mucosa: Ulcers, bleeds, pigmentation (e.g., Peutz-Jeghers syndrome, Addison, etc).
- Palate: Cleft, movement of soft palate.
- Tonsils: Normal or hypertrophied, inflamed, or not.
- Pharynx: Inflamed, pharyngeal tonsils (small nodules in the pharyngeal wall).

2. Inspection

- Shape of abdomen: Is it normal, distended or has any localized bulges.
- Movement with respiration: Type of respiratory movement and whether all parts of abdomen are moving symmetrically.
- Skin over the abdomen: May look shiny in ascites; may have scars of surgeries.
- Dilated veins, and if present, find the direction of flow in them.
- Umbilicus: Normal/everted/transversely stretched.
- Visible pulsation, peristalsis or visible mass.
- Flanks: Whether flanks appear full or not.
- Examine the hernial orifices and external genitalia.

3. Palpation

- Feel of abdomen: Softness, guarding, etc.
- Look for any area of warmth or tenderness.
- Organomegaly: Liver, spleen, kidney; rarely urinary bladder, gall bladder or other masses may be palpable. If found, describe in detail. See p 396 for sequence of palation.
- Tenderness of the renal angles.
- Rectal examination (not to be done routinely).

4. Percussion

- Percussion over the enlarged organs. Find out the liver span.
- Shifting dullness (if ascites is present).
- Fluid thrill (it may be discussed as part of palpation or percussion).
- Puddle sign for minimal fluid (only if indicated).
- Dullness of the renal angles.

5. Auscultation

- Bowel sounds: Normal/increased or decreased.
- Bruit: Especially over the renal artery/over the enlarged organs.
- Rub: Extremely unusual to find splenic or hepatic rub.

IV. DISCUSSION

Discussion of the case must start with a summary of relevant history and physical examination findings that is properly arranged and structured to lead on to a specific diagnosis. If properly structured, the diagnosis that can be arrived at by the student and the examiner cannot be different and this makes the discussion part non-conflicting. The student must now proceed to offer a diagnosis and possible differential diagnosis citing reasons for and against each diagnosis. The next part of discussion will be the laboratory investigations needed for the case and how to prioritize them for the particular case at hand. The discussion of management of the child comes next. There will be further discussions on the expected complications and how to tackle them. Lastly, the candidate is required to counsel the parents regarding the prognosis and also address all their apprehensions regarding their child's illness.

Essential Equipments the Student Must Carry in Examination Hall

Stethoscope (paediatric), knee hammer, torch, measuring tape, tuning fork (128 and 256/512 Hz) and tools for development assessment (see p 60).

The examination centre usually provides weighing machine, height measuring tape pasted to the wall or stadiometer, infantometer, thermometer, BP apparatus, tongue depressor, auroscope (otoscope), ophthalmoscope, etc.

USEFUL TIPS AND ADVICES FOR CANDIDATES APPEARING FOR EXAMINATION

1. Ask parents what the examiners looked for when they examined the child, or what the treating unit doctors examined for. At times it may help you realize that you have forgotten to look for something important.
2. Underline or box the relevant positive and negative points.
3. If the examiner pursues with a question that you cannot answer, most probably it means this is pertaining to something basic, which you ought to know. So just steady your mind and think what basic fact you have wronged. When you are back to the wall, then it is best to admit that you do not know rather than going for wild guesses. Hopefully the examiner will go to the next area of questions and answers of which you might know.
4. Short case assesses a candidate on his speed and accuracy of handling a case, which are essential in out-patient setting. Long case mandates a good case sheet writing skill and comprehensive examination: i.e., the long case assesses a candidate in his proficiency in handling the in-patients. Emphasis is both on method of physical examination as well as sensible interpretation of signs elicited in relation to the patient at hand. The student must be confident while presenting his case to the examiner. However, he should not overstep the boundary; he should not argue (but only discuss) with the examiner even if the examiner is wrong. The future doctor is supposed to be trained in discussion, not argument. All practicing doctors will come across situations where you are correct and patient is wrong, but still you are not supposed to be arrogant with the patient. Since examination is the assessment of future practitioners, arguments and arrogance will be negatively marked.
5. You need not get the correct diagnosis to pass. In fact, a correct diagnosis will not get you past the pass mark if that diagnosis does not fit in with your history and physical findings.
6. Failure: 50% is because of inadequacy of teaching programs or teachers themselves. Reading texts and reproducing it faithfully is not teaching. Teaching involves the teacher himself learning the subject properly and then assimilating it and reproducing it in such a way that it becomes understandable to majority of students. Teaching is an art by itself and in addition requires lot of preparation and dedication to teaching. The present day teachers have no time for such preparations in their struggle to earn. Teaching programs can fail if you are posted to areas, which are in no way useful to you in your examination or future practice. Another reason for failure of teaching programs is inadequate teaching material; e.g., not enough variety of patients. This problem can partly be compensated by books like this one.
7. Difficulty in responding to examiner's questions: Setting apart the lack of fluency of English, the other reason is that you have not practiced enough responding to questions. Thought block is common for many candidates and only way to get rid of it is to prepare

well (so that you are confident that you can perform) and practice case presentation over and over again in front of abrasive teachers so that in due course of time you will become mentally tough.

8. Succumbing to stage fright: Solution is again more and more of practice sessions in front of terrorizing examiners! Do not shy away from them during your training.
9. Do not take drugs like propranolol to get rid of your anxiety.

   Propranolol will make you respond damn cool despite your making an array of mistakes; a scenario that will ensure failure in examination; because a doctor should at least feel worried if he commits mistakes. Then only he will make conscious efforts to correct himself later on. In addition, propranolol may cause hypoglycaemia, another most unwanted thing for the examination candidate.
10. Reading from the case sheet without even looking at the examiner is a bad habit. There is nothing wrong in looking at the case sheet for the necessary details, but whenever possible face the examiner and talk.
11. During the discussion the student should vary his pace and style as per the mood and body language conveyed by the examiner.

CHAPTER 2

Examination of Newborn

The following is the format for newborn examination:

1. **Name**: To be mentioned as baby of....... (mother's name)
2. **DOB**: (Time of birth if baby is less than 72 hrs of age)
3. **EDC**: (Especially for preterm)
4. **Age in days** (hours if less than 72 hrs)
5. **Sex**:
6. **Gestation as per LMP**:
7. **Weight**: (AGA/SGA/LGA)
8. **Maternal age**:
9. **GPLA** (gravida, para, live births and abortions):
   Sample statement: Baby of....... , a .... gestation age baby boy/girl, now .... day/ hours old, born to a.......year old, G...P... A...L...mother, non-consanguinous/ consanguinous marriage, parents residing at ....Baby was born on....... at.......pm/am, at ....Hospital/home, mother's LMP was on ....And EDD was.....
10. **Presenting complaint**
    Some examples are icterus, feeding difficulty, seizures, bowel/bladder problems, "looking sick," etc. Generally, there will be no presenting complaints and the examination candidate is given a specific task, like assess the gestational age of this baby; assess and comment on the icterus of this baby; counsel the mother on feeding of this preterm baby, etc.
    Sample statement: Presently, the baby is in the NICU/mother's room for routine newborn care/jaundice/preterm care/any other complaint.
11. **Antenatal history**
    - 1st trimester: Maternal age, years since marriage (infertility treatment or not), registered pregnancy or not. Any pre-existing illnesses. Pregnancy detected at which month; whether folic acid was started and if so, when. Total number of antenatal visits, 1st trimester ultrasound, hyperemesis, if present. Any fever/rash during first trimester, any history of drug intake/accidental radiation exposure, any vaginal bleeding/spotting (threatened abortion).
    - 2nd trimester: Iron, calcium started or not. Injection tetanus toxoid 2 doses, any hypertension or diabetes, oligamnios/polyhydramnios, when was quickening felt.
    - 3rd trimester: Any hypertension/diabetes, antepartum bleeding. Any drug intake, viral illnesses, weight gain during pregnancy, oligo- or polyhydramnios/anaemia/smoking, decreased fetal movements.
12. **Mother's obstetric and medical history, if relevant**
    Previous child's neonatal history, if relevant.
13. **Delivery details** (normal/assisted, vertex/ breech, colour of liquor if known, etc)
    - Premature labour/PPROM (>18 hrs), UTI/ fever, foul smelling liquor, maternal fever (risk for early onset sepsis), abdominal (uterine) tenderness.
      Colour of liquor, duration of labour, mode of delivery (indication for LSCS), need for resuscitation and immediate neonatal events, if any.

- Feeding, passage of urine and meconium, treatment (if any), immunization.

14. **Postnatal history**: Cried/not after birth, whether needed NICU admission (indication). When was initial feed given, did the baby suck, when was initial meconium/urine passed. Acute NICU care needed – oxygen/ventilation, IV fluids, phototerapy, antibiotics, etc. Present clinical behaviour – feeding/suck, urine/stool, tone/activity. Present medications/interventions, if any. Breast feeding - duration, frequency, adequacy (sleeping between feeds, urine output, let down reflex, weight monitoring). If top feeds – dilution, frequency, hygiene, bottle/spoon.
15. **Immunization history**: BCG/polio/hepatitis B.
16. **Family history** as relevant. Any hereditary/major illnesses. Recurrent blood transfusions, jaundice, tuberculosis. Neonatal deaths in family (inborn errors of metabolism), development problems, etc.
17. **Socioeconomic history** – Education and income in brief.
18. **General comment** (wash and warm the hands before examination)
19. **Posture and activity**: Term baby has universal flexion (good tone of flexors). Extremely premature baby of 28 weeks or less will have no appreciable flexor tone, both upper and lower limbs remain extended.

HISTORY & CLINICAL EXAMINATION OF NEWBORN

Examination is best done ½–1 hr after feeds.

1. Vitals

- Colour: Term baby is pale pink, the extreme premature ones are very red.

  Peripheral cyanosis may be acceptable as normal as long as it disappears by proper warming/clothing. Central cyanosis indicates cyanotic heart disease or respiratory distress or CNS depression. Localized cyanosis may be there due to local pressure during delivery. Pale baby may mean significant anaemia or circulatory shock.

  Icterus: Must be examined in good day light (take the baby to the window). Skin may be blanched by gentle thumb pressure and immediately after taking off the thumb, the blanched area is looked for icterus. The areas to look for jaundice is forehead, sternum, abdominal wall, thigh, legs and sole. See pg 27.
- Temperature: 36.5–37.5°C is normal. Baby is said to be in cold stress if temperature is 36–36.5°C. Baby is hypothermic if temperature is below 36°C. Feel the temperature over the anterior abdominal wall and compare with the extremity temperature. Cold extremities may be because of peripheral vasoconstriction due to exposure to cold or peripheral vasoconstriction in early shock to maintain systemic blood pressure.
- Respiratory rate: 40–60 per min is the normal rate. Periodic breathing with a pause of a few seconds is perfectly normal for newborn. In apnea of prematurity, there is cessation of breathing of over 20 sec or bradycardia/cyanosis. Respiration is almost entirely diaphragmatic.
- Heart rate: It is easier to document heart rate rather than pulse rate. Feel all peripheral pulses while the baby is quiet. 120–140 per min is the normal rate.
- Capillary filling time: Tested by pressing over the forehead or sternum for 5 sec and releasing. Colour returns instantaneously in normal babies; 3 sec or more is abnormal.
- Blood pressure need not be routinely taken by the candidate; flush method is inaccurate.

2. General Behavior

Comment on alertness, tone, movements and activity.

3. Gestational Age Assessment

Physical and neurological criteria must be scored and plotted to find the exact gestational age.

Expanded Ballard score (full score is not needed, rough estimation is enough) or Dubowitz scoring system are useful. However, for a rapid assessment during examination, one may use physical criteria, consisting of ear recoil, breast nodule, skin texture, external genitalia and sole creases (Table 2.2, p 21).

Gestational age by last menstrual period:

- A baby delivered at <37 completed weeks of gestation is preterm baby.
- A baby delivered at >42 weeks is post term baby.
- A baby delivered between 34–36 weeks + 6 days is late preterm.

Anthropometry

- Weight: Ideally, baby must be weighed naked in electronic weighing scale with 5 g accuracy. The examination candidate may suggest that the weight of the baby is taken with clothes and then the weight of clothes must be subtracted. This will be impressive because the candidate's concern of baby's well-being will be positively taken by the examiners.
- Length: Infantometer is used to measure (Fig. 4.5, p 46). 47–50 cm is normal for a term baby.
- OFC (head circumference): 33–35 cm is normal.
- CC (chest circumference) measured at the level of nipples.
- Ponderal index =

$$\frac{\text{Weight (in gm)}}{\text{(Length)}^3\text{(in cm}^3\text{)}} \times 100$$

(See Chart 2.1 & 2.2)

Head to Foot Examination

- Dysmorphism
- Skull (anterior and posterior fontanels, caput, cephalhaematoma, etc). Normal PF will admit just tip of little finger. PF closes by 6–8 weeks. Overlapping of cranial bones at suture lines in the newborn is mostly due to moulding during delivery. Transillumination of skull may be considered if there is hydrocephalus (test is positive in hydranencephaly; see p 227).
- Face: If there is any obvious dysmorphism, evaluate each part in detail.
- Eyes: Any readily obvious findings like discharge, microphthalmia, slant of eyes, icterus, etc. There may be subconjunctival haemorrhage and mild lid oedema (both may be passed off as normal phenomena due to stress of delivery); both these are of no special concern.
  See if the cornea is clear.
  Look for the red reflex; white reflex could be abnormal (cataract, retinoblastoma, etc). Rocking the baby up and down may induce eye opening (do not force open the eyes for examination).
  Newborn may appear to have strabismus off and on as the coordinated conjugate movements of eye in newborn is only intermittent.
- Ear: Any abnormality in shape/low set, preauricular tags/pits, etc.
- Mouth:
  Sucking pad: Some babies will have localized thickening of mid upper lip; this is supposed to be due to intrauterine sucking by the baby.
  Look for cleft lip/palate. Slightly pressing down the lower jaw will make the baby open the mouth. Isolated cleft palate may be missed unless looked for. Submucus cleft needs palpation. There may be natal teeth; so make sure you look for it.
  Look for oral thrush.
  Protruding tongue: Could be due to hypothyroidism, Down, Wiedemann Beckwith syndrome, etc.
  Epstein pearls
- Nose: Is the nasal bridge depressed. Patency of each nostril can be tested by placing a glass slide and looking for misting or by the movement of a cotton wisp.
- Neck: Any readily noticeable abnormalities, like webbing of neck in Turner (Fig. 24.61, p 518). Palpate the thyroid (where indicated) and the clavicle (unnoticed fracture clavicle may present as a swelling due to callus formation).

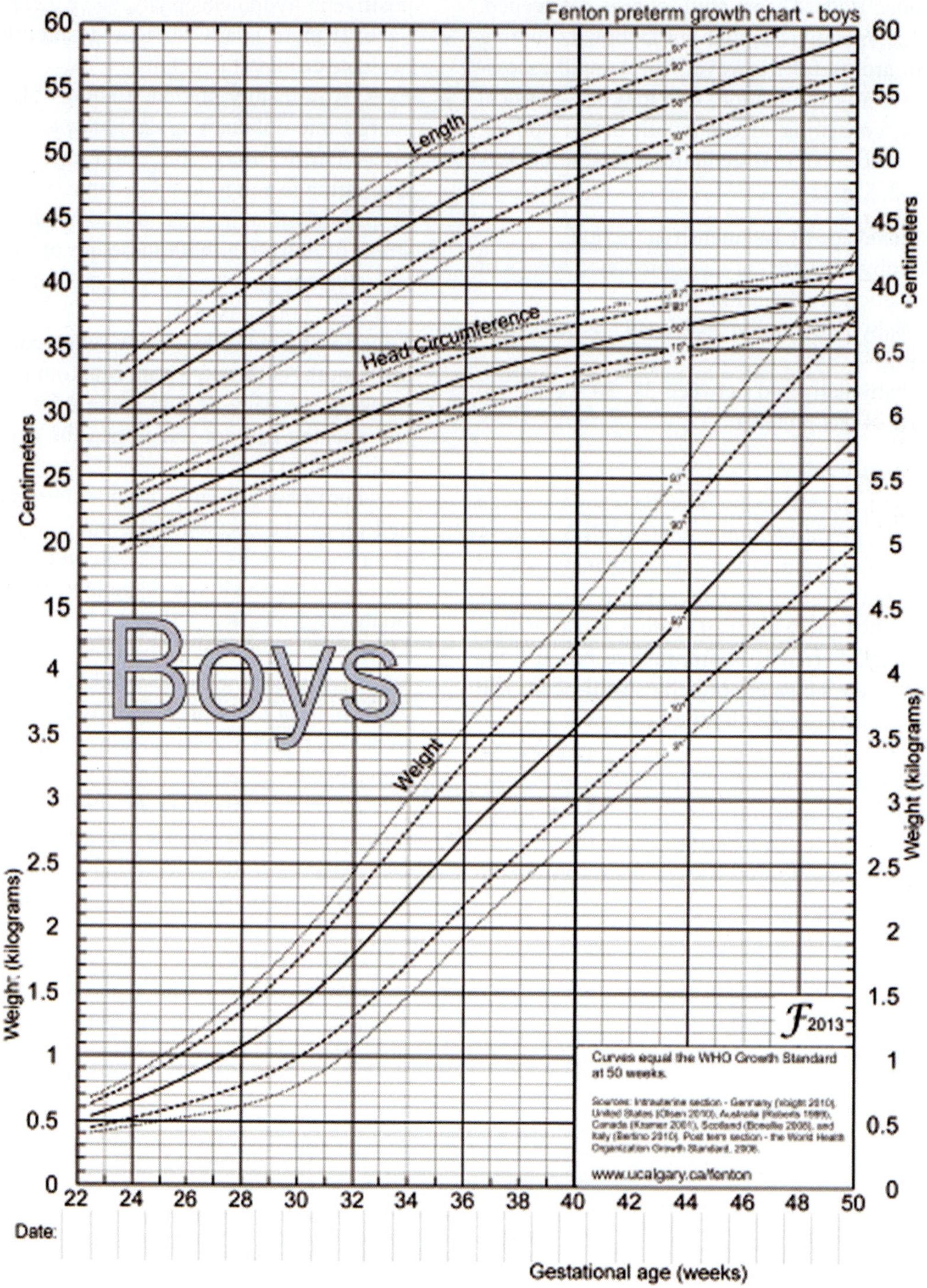

Chart 2.1 Fentons chart

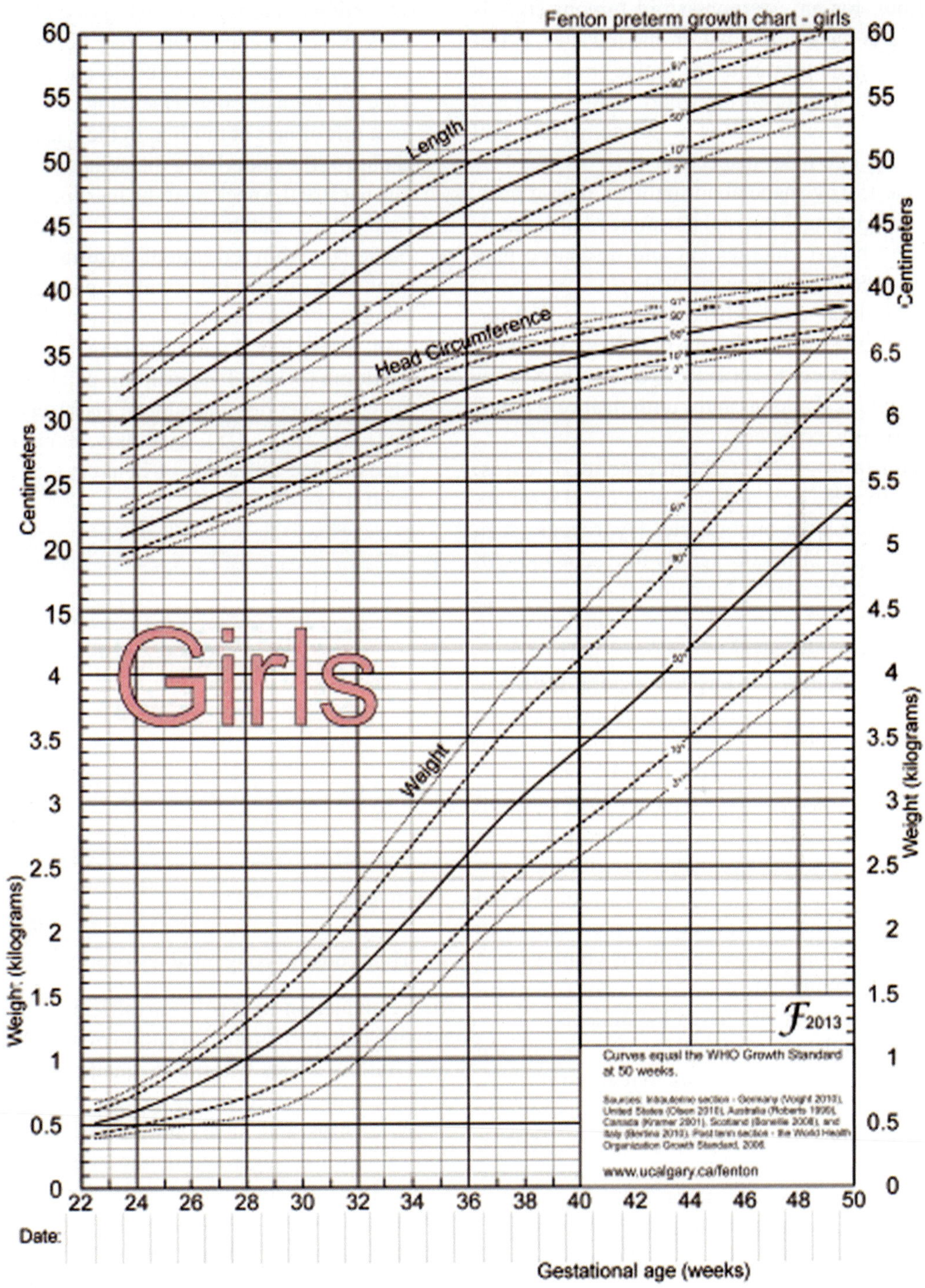

Chart 2.2 Fentons chart

Look for any sternomastoid tumour (this is due to haematoma within the muscle). Fistulous openings from the primitive branchial arch system may open anywhere from ear down to the anterior border of sternomastoid and hence one must inspect for it.

- Chest: Any shape abnormalities, nipple position/spacing. Maternal hormone induced transient breast enlargement and discharge may be seen (mastitis neonatorum).
- Umbilical cord (shriveled, foul smelling, erythema surrounding the umbilicus, bleeding, etc; if the cord is still fresh one may look for 2 umbilical arteries and 1 umbilical vein that is normally expected).
- Genitalia: Look for undescended testes, hydrocoele, hernia, poorly pigmented scrotum, exposed labia minora, etc. Hydrocoele seen soon after birth is generally transient and will get absorbed soon. Mucoid vaginal discharge on days 2–3 is normal. So is vaginal bleeding (due to withdrawal of maternal hormone effects). Phimosis is physiological at birth and as long as urinary stream is good, nothing need be done about it. The scrotum of a full-term baby has rugae all around and is more pigmented than the rest of the skin. Testes will have descended to scrotum in term baby. In case of ambiguous genitalia, describe the genitalia as is seen and mention the site of urethral opening (may get history from mother who will tell from where the urine is coming).
- Anal opening: Must be looked for (imperforate anus is often missed by students).
- Arms and legs: Erb's palsy may be missed unless the candidate has that possibility in mind. Any anomalies; e.g., oedema of the hands and feet in Turner syndrome; look at the proportions: e.g., in achondroplasia, there is rhizomelic shortening. Look at the number of fingers, palmar creases, club foot, etc. Constriction band, if seen could be amniotic constriction band. Look for club foot, if any.
- Back and spine: Look for obvious anomalies, e.g., meningomyelocoele, sinuses, sacral pits, etc. Pilonidal dimple at the top of cleft of buttock is very common and may be passed off as a normal variation. They do not communicate with spinal canal. Haemangioma, lipoma or a tuft of hair at midline in the back may be a clue to the underlying diastematomyelia. At the back of the neck near the hairline, one may find salmon patch.
- Skin: Note thin red skin of preterm/thick pale pink skin of term baby; pallor, plethora, mottling ("cutis marmorata"), jaundice, Mongolian spots (Fig. 2.7), milia (Fig. 2.6), haemangioma (p 140–141), salmon patch (reddish macules over lids and nape of neck), erythema toxicum (Fig. 2.5), cyanosis, ecchymosis (mostly due to trauma of delivery), etc. Also read p 18–19.

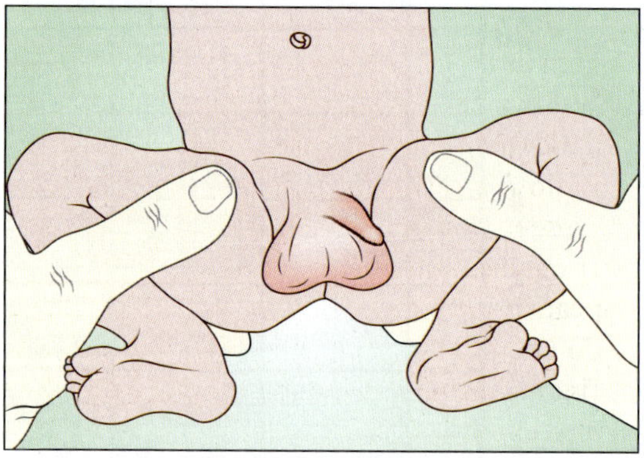

Fig.2.1 Ortolani test

- Hip: Look for congenital dislocation (Fig. 2.1).

If the abduction of hip is unrestricted, one may assume that there is no dislocation of hip. Ortolani and Barlow's tests determine whether the femoral head is dislocated or dislocatable, respectively.

With hips and knees both flexed, hold the thighs between finger and thumb: the thumb medially at the inner thigh crease, and index and middle fingers at greater trochanter. Now, pushing the greater trochanter upward away from bed, abduct the hips fully starting from the midline.

A palpable clunk will be felt as a posteriorly dislocated hip slips back into the acetabulum (if it has already been dislocated). Barlow test is to see if hip is "dislocatable." During examination, a condidate is not expected to dislocate a "dislocatable" hip and hence Barlow test is not to be done.

Examination of Systems

Neurologic Examination

It is best done beyond 24 hrs of postnatal age. Mention about the gestation, sickness, drugs, feeding, posture, behavioural state and alertness.

Higher Functions

Mental state of wakefulness, irritability, consolability, cuddlability.

Cranial Nerves

- I: Mother's milk (if history suggests the newborn turns towards breast by smell, not touch).
- II: Fixing at soft light (light from window of a dark room).
  Follow a red wool ball. Pupillary reflex is present from 28 weeks onwards.
  If ophthalmoscopy is attempted, the disc appears pale by usual paediatric standards (hence do not diagnose optic atrophy because of this finding alone). Retinal haemorrhages without any clinical effect on the baby may also be seen normally. Chorioretinitis may be seen in intrauterine infections (generally need an ophthalmologist to pick up).
- III, IV, VI: Eye movements—spontaneous and elicited by doll's eye manoeuvre; pick up the baby and gently rock backwards and forwards and from side to side observing the eye movements. Tonic deviation to one side could mean seizure.
- V: Rooting reflex (child turns with snout towards the side where the corner of mouth is touched).
- VII: Observe the child cry. Trauma of forceps delivery is the most common cause of LMN facial palsy in the newborn.
- VIII: Behavioural response to sound (startle, blinking, change in heart rate, etc). Bilirubin encephalopathy and intrauterine infection may cause deafness.
- IX, X: Position of uvula during crying. Choking during feeding.
- XI: Lift the head off the bed by holding at wrists and watch for sternomastoids.
- IX, X, XII: Suck and swallow.

Motor

- Observe spontaneous movement.
- Tone: Passive and active. Posture at rest; various angles (see p 21–24).
- Caudo-rostral progression: By 32 weeks of gestation, the lower limbs tone increases; there is flexion at hip and knee. By 36 weeks, elbow flexion appears.
- Neck (see "pull to sit" later in this chapter).
- Trunk (ventral suspension).

Reflexes

Knee, ankle, biceps, etc. Knee jerk may have crossed adductor response till about 7–8 months of postnatal age.

Ankle clonus of 5–10 beats is normal provided there is no other abnormal neurologic examination findings or asymmetry. Ankle clonus disappears rapidly and more than a few beats after 1–2 months age may be abnormal (Ref. 16). However, isolated ankle clonus without any other neurological abnormality for a few more weeks may be just a variation of normal.

Neonatal Reflexes

Several primary neonatal reflexes are described, but the most useful ones for routine clinical examination are Moro, palmar grasp and tonic neck reflex.

1. **Moro reflex**: It is elicited best by sudden extension of head in relation to the trunk (and catching the falling head).

2

The response consists of:

- Opening of hands (by 28 weeks gestation)
- Extension and abduction of upper extremities (by 32 weeks)
- Anterior flexion and adduction (embracing) of upper extremities (by 37 weeks)
- Audible cry

Moro reflex disappears by 3–4 months in most normal infants. It is a very sensitive indicator of infant's level of alertness. Depressed or absent Moro indicates generalized depression of the CNS. Bilateral exaggerated, hung up Moro is found in kernicterus. Unilateral absent Moro could mean local pathologies like fracture of clavicle, fracture of humerus, Erb's palsy, etc.

2. **Startle reflex** is different from Moro. Here, a sudden loud noise produces a Moro-like movement, but unlike Moro, elbows remain flexed (not extended as in Moro) and hands remain closed.
3. **Palmar grasp**: It is elicited by stroking the ulnar aspect of the palm taking care to see that the dorsum of the baby's hand does not touch the examination cot. At 37 weeks, the palmar grasp is strong enough to allow lifting up of the infant from bed. It appears by 28 weeks, and usually disappears by 2–3 months (when the voluntary grasp appears). Marked retention of this reflex beyond 6 months of age is characteristic of athetoid CP (and not spastic CP) because of the role of extrapyramidal system maturation in the disappearance of this reflex.
4. **Plantar grasp**: Press with thumb on the sole, in the space under the toes. The toes will plantar flex. The reflex disappears by the time the baby starts standing.
5. **Sucking and rooting reflexes**: Are present at birth if the baby is 34 weeks or more mature and persist up to 4 months when awake and up to 6 months when asleep. Rooting is elicited by touching the corner of mouth with finger and the baby turns toward it to latch on to it.
6. **Stepping reflex**: Holding baby under the axillae and leaning forward, place his sole on the table; he makes walking movements.
7. **Placing reflex**: Holding baby under the axilla, rub the dorsum of foot or leg on to the underside of edge of table. The baby lifts the leg and places it on top of the table. Placing and stepping reflexes are present at birth in term babies and disappear by 6 weeks.
8. **Pull to sit (traction response)**: Grasp the baby at his wrists and fingers and pull to sit. Flexors of neck contracts; full term baby can momentarily lift the head to the level of body.
9. **Doll's-eye response**: Hold the baby's eyelids open and briskly rotate the head first to one side and then to the other. Intact brainstem is indicated by the full conjugate deviation of the eyeballs to the opposite side. Vertical eye movements are tested by briskly flexing and extending the neck.
10. **Gallant's (trunk incurvation) reflex**: Elicited by holding the infant horizontal in prone position (ventral suspension), and running the finger down the paravertebral area on one side. The response is swinging of the pelvis towards the stimulated side. It usually disappears by 1 year of age; may occasionally persist in older children. Clinical value is in mapping a sensory level on the trunk, sensation may be absent in some spinal cord disorders below the level of lesion.
11. **Landau reflex**: When the baby is held in ventral suspension, and the head is flexed by the examiner, the hip, knee and elbow should flex. This reaction is normally present from 3 months onwards, but becomes difficult to demonstrate beyond 1 year of age. Absence of this reflex beyond 3 months of age may indicate a motor weakness.
12. **Crossed extension (adduction) response**: One leg is held in extension and the sole of the foot is rubbed. The other leg first withdraws

and then extends with fanning of the toes. The third and the final component seen only in term babies—bring the other foot towards the side that was stimulated (as though to push away the noxious stimuli).

13. **Asymmetric tonic neck reflex**: It is elicited by rotation of the head. The response is extension of the upper extremity on the side to which the face is rotated and flexion of the upper extremity on the side of the occiput; lower extremities respond similarly but less strikingly. Reflex appears by 35 weeks but is prominent 1-month post term. It disappears by 4–6 months (although tone changes may be palpable even later). Tonic neck posture is abnormal if maintained 'obligatory'; i.e., the child cannot escape from the posture imposed on him by the head turning.
14. **Symmetric tonic neck reflex**: On extending the neck, the extensor tone in arm increases and flexor tone in leg increases; i.e., on extending the neck, the upper limb extends and lower limb flexes (this is easy to remember if one can visualize a dog howling; its neck and upper extremities are extended and lower extremity flexed). This reflex is useful for a prone child to rise on its arms and ultimately on its legs. On flexing the neck, the opposite happens, i.e., the arm flexes and leg extends (this is easy to remember if one can visualize a dog drinking from a pond; its head and upper limb will be flexed and lower limb extended). In cerebral palsy, this reflex is overactive so that when the child tries to get up, he cannot, as the leg remain obligatorily flexed; the child can extend the leg only if the neck is made to flex.
15. **Parachute reaction**: This is not a neonatal reflex. It appears only by 6–9 months and persists throughout life. Hold the child in ventral suspension and suddenly lower him to the couch. The arms extend as if to protect him from falling. In cerebral palsy, it may be absent or incomplete due to abnormalities of tone.

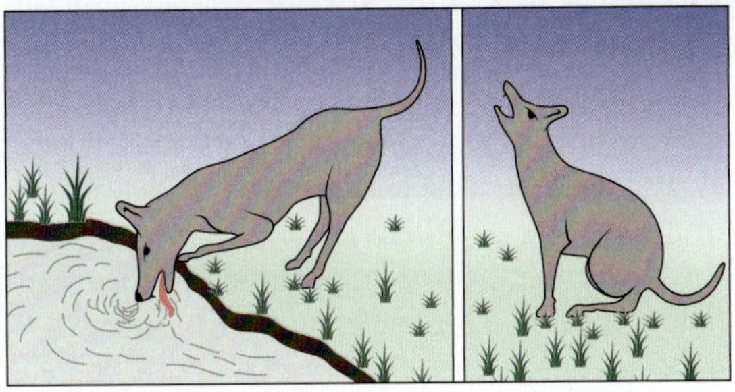

Fig.2.2 (See text on symmetric tonic neck reflex)

EXAMINATION OF SYSTEMS

System examination scheme is similar to paediatric system examination. Use the following points to decide if one has to examine the system in detail or not.

Respiratory

- Respiratory rate, retractions, nasal flaring, other accessory muscles use, breath sounds.
- Grunt indicates serious respiratory illness like hyaline membrane disease.
- Most common cause of stridor in the newborn is congenital laryngeal stridor, which clinically manifests by around 2 weeks of age, not in the immediate newborn period.

Inspection

Barrel-shaped chest indicates air trapping like meconium aspiration syndrome, but normal newborn also have a somewhat barrel chest. So do not take it as abnormal unless baby has distress. Look for any chest wall indrawing.

The physical examination methods are same as in children. Palpation, percussion and even auscultation may not be helpful in newborn to localize a pathology. Auscultation generally helps only to detect the difference in air entry.

CVS

Pulse volume, precordial pulsation, heart sounds, murmur. Attempts to evaluate JVP will fail due to short neck and so best not attempted.

Remember that TOF does not present with cyanosis in the newborn period. So, heart disease presenting with cyanosis is likely to be TGA, or if the baby is in shock, consider hypoplastic left heart syndrome. Also must consider non-cardiac causes of cyanosis (e.g., PPHN).

Inspection, palpation, percussion and auscultation must be done as per standard format.

Note: Heart murmur in newborn period is quite common, due to pulmonary flow murmurs or peripheral pulmonary murmurs. Peripheral pulmonary murmurs will disappear as the physiological fetal pulmonary hypertension regresses. Conversely, congenital heart disease may be present in the newborn without any murmur at all (e.g., transposition of great arteries). Thus, the diagnosis of congenital heart diseases must rely more on cardiomegaly, haemodynamic effects and cyanosis rather than heart murmurs.

Abdomen

Distension, organomegaly. Scaphoid abdomen is not normal in newborn; it could mean congenital diaphragmatic hernia.

Umbilical cord falls off by 7 days and the remaining wound heal by 14 days in normal babies. Persistent low grade infection is one of the causes for a granuloma remaining at umbilicus (umbilical granuloma); it may be chemically cauterized. Purulent discharge from umbilicus and periumbilical redness indicates umbilical sepsis. Exceptionally, urinary discharge (patent urachus) or fecal discharge (persistent vitello intestinal duct) may be seen. Liver is generally palpable 2–3 cm below costal margin. Liver span is usually 4.5 cm. Normally spleen is not palpable. Kidneys may be bimanually palpated with thumb over the abdomen and other fingers at loin.

The format for examination of abdomen is same as that of paediatric patients.

Some Normal Phenomenon in the Newborn

Many of the "complaints" of mothers of newborn given for clinical examination are actually normal phenomena. To help candidates realize this, the common normal phenomena are listed below.

- Normal newborns pass meconium and urine within 24 hrs of birth. Assuming that the passage of urine at birth went unnoticed, one can wait maximum 48 hrs for passage of urine.
- Regurgitation soon after feeding is a normal phenomenon and can be reduced by taking the baby on the mother's shoulder and burping after each feed. Vomiting associated with abdominal distention or bilious vomiting or bloody vomiting is pathological.
- Frequent greenish-yellow stools is normal in the first week of life and represents the transition from meconium to normal stool. Once breastfeeding is well established, the stools become golden yellow, with a frequency a few times per day, mostly soon after feeding.
- Grayish blue Mongolian spots mostly in the lumbosacral area are normal variation. They start fading by the second half of infancy and completely disappear in the first couple of years of life.
- Retention cysts called Epstein's pearls are located in the midline near the junction of soft & hard palate and they resolves by itself.
- Lacy pattern of skin (mottling, net-like Fig. 2.4) in the newborn is mostly a normal phenomenon due to vasomotor instability. Apart from this, the usual causes could be hypothermia, hypothyroidism and sepsis.
- Erythematous maculopapular rash, usually appearing by the second day of life is called erythema toxicum. It fades off without treatment within a few weeks. (Fig. 2.5)
- Milia is subaceous retention cysts, will disappear in a few days. Nothing need be done. (Fig. 2.6)

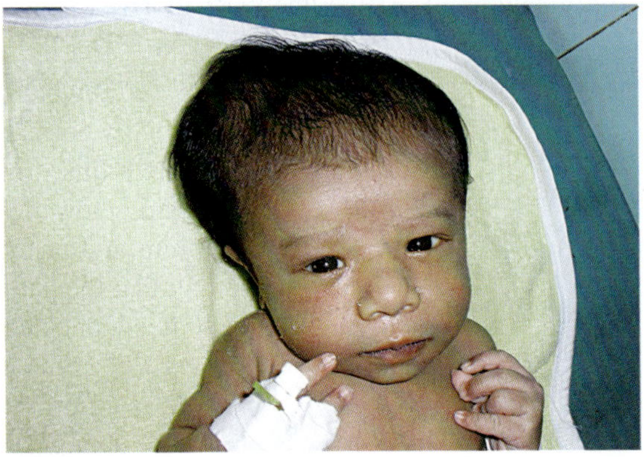

Fig.2.3 Cephal hematoma

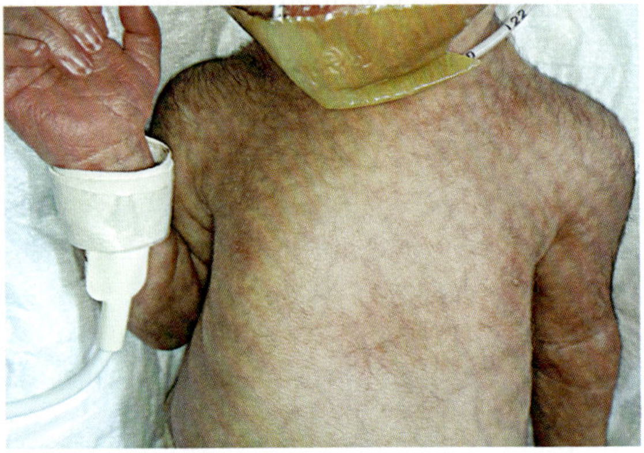

Fig.2.4 Cutis marmorata

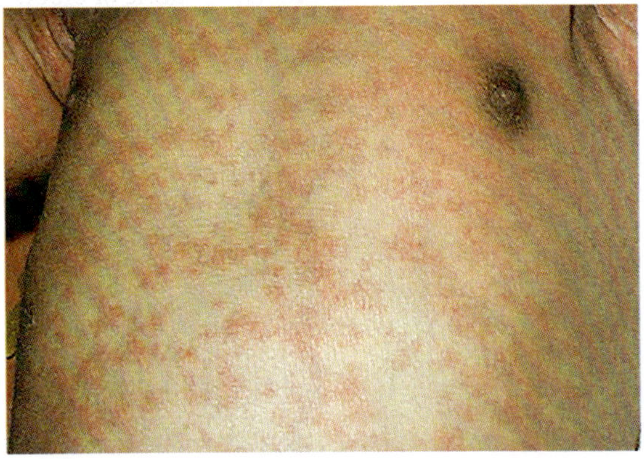

Fig.2.5 Erythema toxicum

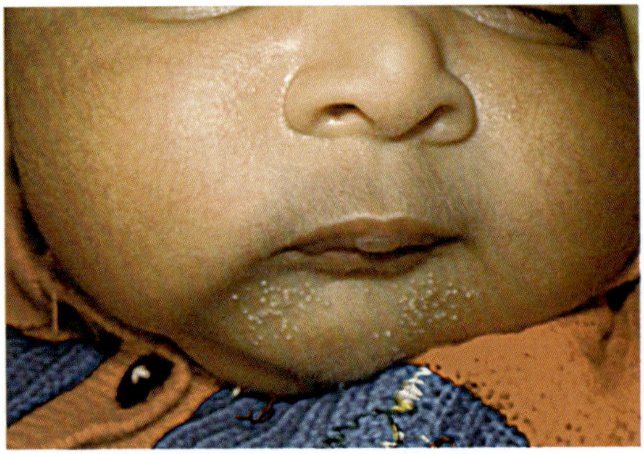

Fig.2.6 Milia

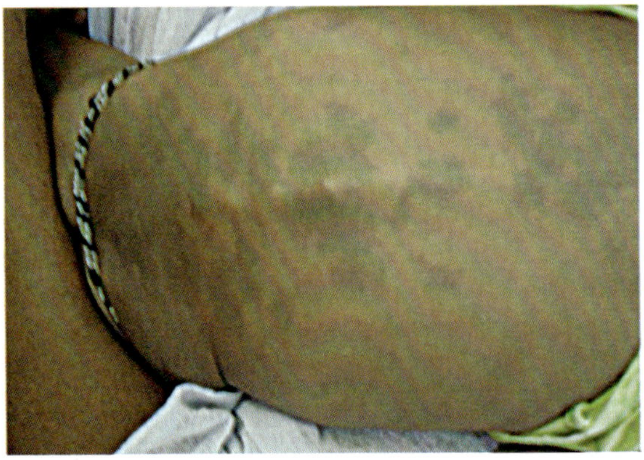

Fig.2.7 Mongolian blue spots

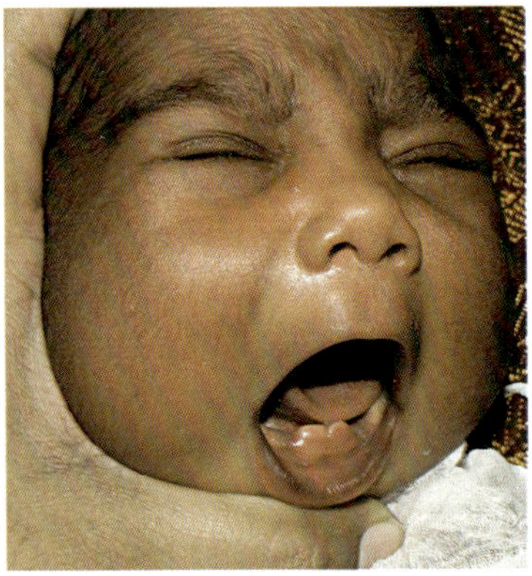

Fig.2.8 Neonatal teeth

- Whitish discharge from the vagina (Fig. 2.11) (usually 2–3 days of life), vaginal bleeding (end of first week) and breast engorgement are due to the effect of maternal hormones to which child was exposed in utero. The breast should be left alone without squeezing or massaging. The bleeding, which actually is a hormone withdrawal bleed, will settle by itself.
- Subconjunctival haemorrhage is due to the pressures during delivery. It will disappear in a few days and needs no treatment.
- Neonatal teeth is harmless. Need to be removed only if it is loose for fear of aspiration. (Fig. 2.8)
- Physiological jaundice becomes clinically detectable by 2–3 days of life, peaks in 3–5 days and disappears in about 7–10 days in a normal full-term newborn. The baby appears perfectly well. If a child has clinically detectable icterus on the first day of life, it is always pathological.
- The aetiology of physiologic jaundice is thought to be due to: (a) the increased bilirubin production due to the breakdown of fetal RBCs (fetal RBCs have a shorter life span), (b) the immaturity of hepatic conjugation mechanisms to handle the bilirubin load, (c) delayed establishment of effective feeding, which contribute to the increased entero hepatic circulation perpetuating the jaundice (see breastfeeding jaundice below), (d) defective uptake and excretion of bilirubin by the immature hepatocyte may also contribute to physiological jaundice.
- Excessive crying in a normal looking child beyond newborn period may be due to trivial problems like wet nappy, insect bite, etc. It can also be due to "***evening colic***," an unusual colic during evening hours in early infancy (>6 weeks); the cause is uncertain.

Some dangerous symptoms of newborn period.

- Newborn with respiratory distress and *scaphoid abdomen* may have a ***congenital diaphragmatic hernia***. The abdomen is scaphoid as the abdominal contents have gone into the chest, which in turn is the cause for respiratory distress.
- A child with ambiguous genitalia may be having a congenital adrenal hyperplasia (CAH).
- Baby with non-bilious vomiting in the second week of life may be having congenital hypertrophic pyloric stenosis.
- Choking during feeding may indicate aspiration of feeds as in tracheo-oesophageal fistula.
- Constant drooling in a newborn should prompt work up for oesophageal atresia. An X ray taken after passing a stiff rubber tube will show the failure of the tube to reach the stomach.

The most common newborn cases kept for examination are premature baby and jaundiced baby. The following gives essential details needed for examination in these cases.

LOW BIRTH WEIGHT BABY

- Low birth weight infants: <2500 g
- Very low birth weight infants: <1500 g
- Extreme low birth weight infants: <1000 g
- Incredibly low birth weight: <750 g

A baby can be low birth weight because it is preterm or because its intrauterine growth is retarded (IUGR). In examination setting, where graphs are not provided to know the expected weight at different gestational age, it is best to use the following mnemonic to predict whether the baby has the weight expected for its gestational age. If the weight is less than that expected for the gestational age, it is small for gestational age baby.

Table 2.1 Expected wt for gest. age

Gestational age	Expected weight for a normally growing fetus (in g)	Mnenonic
28	1000	
30	1200	1000 + 200
32	1500	1200 + 300
34	1900	1500 + 400
36	2400	1900 + 500
38 (any baby >37 weeks is full term)	3000	2400 + 600

Differentiating Preterm Baby from Term Baby by Neurologic Criteria

Preterm babies are hypotonic in general. Hence, the examination should be performed keeping that in mind.

POSTURE

Observe posture with infant not crying and in supine position. Arms and legs are extended in preterms, while full flexion of arms and legs is seen in term babies.

Term baby has universal flexion (full flexion of arms and legs); very preterm baby of 28 weeks or less will have less flexor tone, and thus both upper and lower limbs remain extended.

Table 2.2 Differentiating preterm baby from term baby by physical criteria (Fig. 2.9–2.13)

Signs	Term baby	Preterm baby
1. Sole creases	Many deep creases.	Absent deep crease or single deep crease anteriorly.
2. Male genitalia	Scrotum pigmented with multiple rugae. Testes descended into the scrotum.	Scrotum small, poorly pigmented and pinkish, few rugae. Testes may not be fully descended.
3. Female genitalia	Labia majora covers labia minora and clitoris.	Labia majora are widely separated exposing labia minora & clitoris.
4. Ear cartilage	Ear cartilages well formed; ear folds are well formed; recoils instantaneously when the ear is folded and released.	Ear cartilage is thin, ear folds are not well formed (pinna feel soft). Pressed against head, it may remain so for a few seconds, before recoiling slowly.
5. Breast nodule	5–10 mm palpable nodule.	Small, <5 mm, and in very premature, there is no palpable breast nodule at all.
6. Tone	Limbs are well flexed. Tone is good.	Limbs are lax. Hypotonia.
7. Skin	Skin is pale and thick.	Skin is very red, thin, transparent, and somewhat gelatinous. Veins may be visible over the anterior abdominal wall.
8. Hair	Scalp hair is black and silky. Laungo hair is hardly seen.	Scalp hair less back, less thick/sparse. Lanugo hair may be seen over the body.

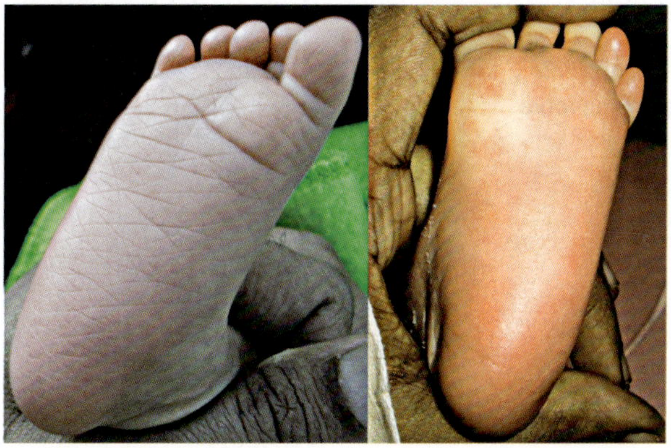

Fig.2.9 Sole of full-term and preterm baby

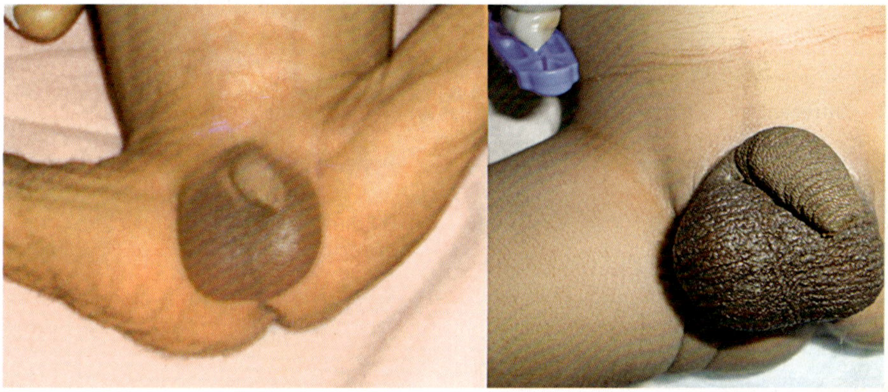

Fig.2.10 Male genitalia in preterm and full-term baby

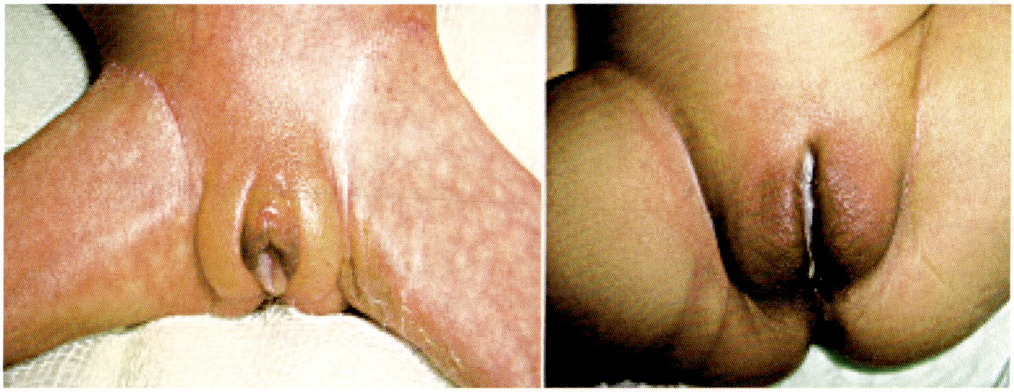

Fig.2.11 Female genitalia in preterm and full-term baby

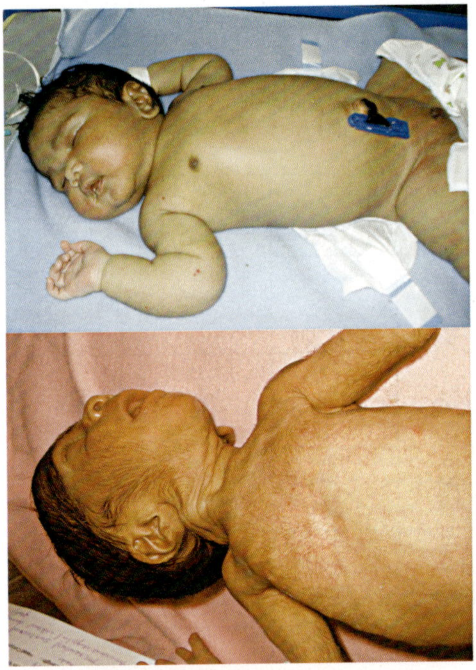

Fig.2.12 Full-term baby has more pale and opaque skin and has palpable breast tissue.

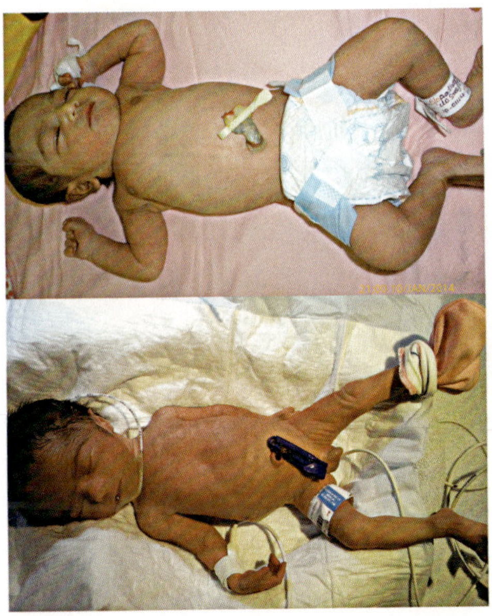

Fig.2.13 Muscle tone at rest. Full-term and preterm baby.

By around 32 weeks, baby has flexion of lower limbs but upper limbs still remain largely extended. By 36 weeks, both upper and lower limbs have less flexor tone, almost like a term baby.

SQUARE WINDOW (Fig. 2.15)

Baby's hand is flexed on the forearm between the thumb and index finger of the examiner with reasonable pressure. Measure the angle between the hypothenar eminence and the ventral aspect of the forearm. (Care is taken not to rotate the infant's wrist while doing this manoeuvre). In full-term babies, the hypothenar eminence touches the forearm and hence the angle is nearly zero. In the extreme preterm, it is less malleable, and the angle may be as much as 90°. Here, the student should not get confused. In term babies, these joints are malleable to facilitate delivery and not in preterm where the nature has not yet prepared the baby for delivery. The same is true with ankle dorsiflexion. 2

ARM RECOIL (Figs. 2.16 & 2.17)

Keep the infant in the supine position; flex the forearms for 5 sec, then fully extend it by pulling on the hands, and then release. The sign is fully positive if the arms return briskly to full flexion (i.e., in full-term babies, the arm recoils fully, which means the angle that forearm makes with the arm will be less than 90°). If the arms return to incomplete flexion or the response is sluggish, it is graded accordingly as per chart. They will remain extended without recoiling in extreme pre-terms.

POPLITEAL ANGLE (Fig. 2.18)

Keep the infant supine and the pelvis flat on the examining couch. Hold the thigh in the knee–chest position using the left index finger and thumb to support the knee. Extend the leg by gentle pressure from your right index finger behind the ankle and measure the angle. Compare the angle with

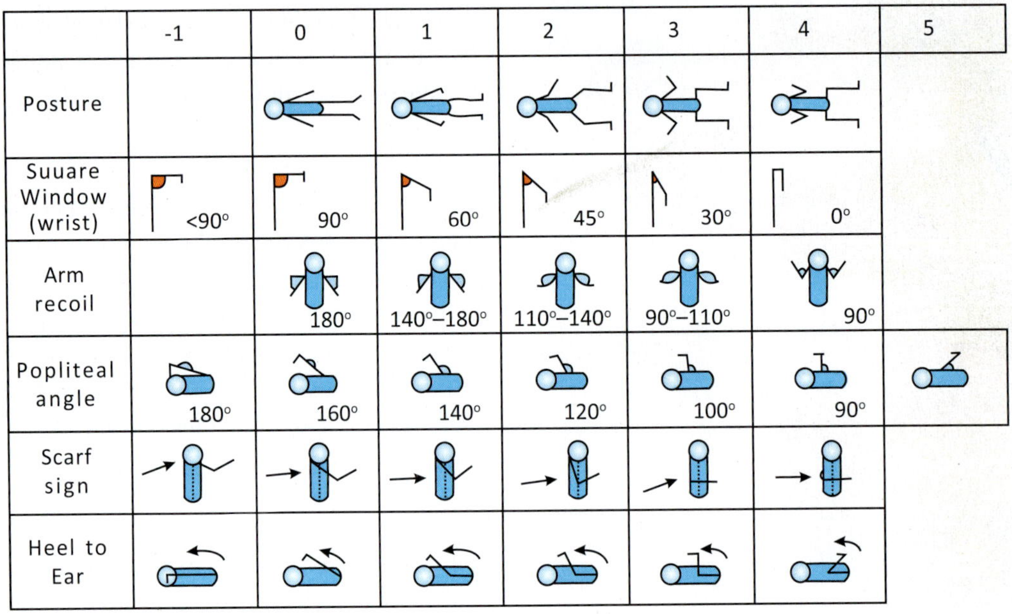

Fig.2.14 Neuromuscular maturity scoring *(Adapted from: Dubowitz L, Dubowitz V Goldberg. Clinical assessment of gestational age in the newborn infant. J Pediatr 1970;77:1).*

the standard charts. In term babies, the angle is less than 90°. In extreme preterm babies, it may be as much as 180°.

SCARF SIGN (Fig. 2.19)

With the infant in supine position, take the infant's hand and try to put it across the chest as far as possible towards the opposite shoulder. This manoeuvre will need lifting the elbow across the body. See how far the elbow goes across and grade it as per chart. Elbow will not cross the midline in term babies.

HEEL TO EAR MANOEUVRE (Fig. 2.20)

With the infant lying supine, pull the infant's foot as near to the head as it will go without forcing it. Observe the distance between the foot and the head as well as the degree of extension at the knee.

Common problems expected in preterm babies:

- Hypothermia
- Hypoglycaemia
- Hypocalcaemia
- Respiratory:
  - Apnoea of prematurity
  - Respiratory distress syndrome (HMD)

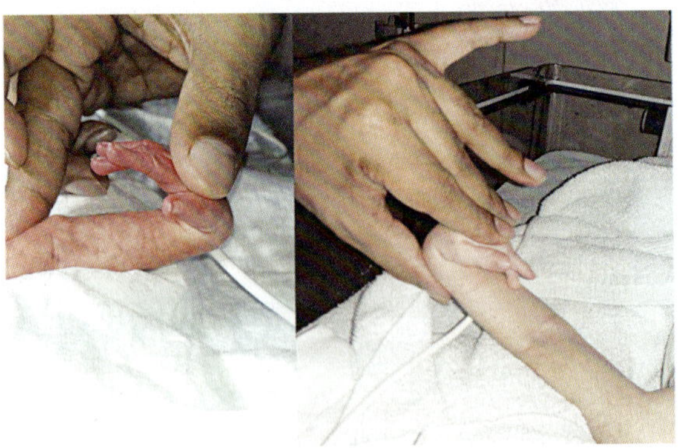

Fig.2.15 Square window in preterm and full-term baby

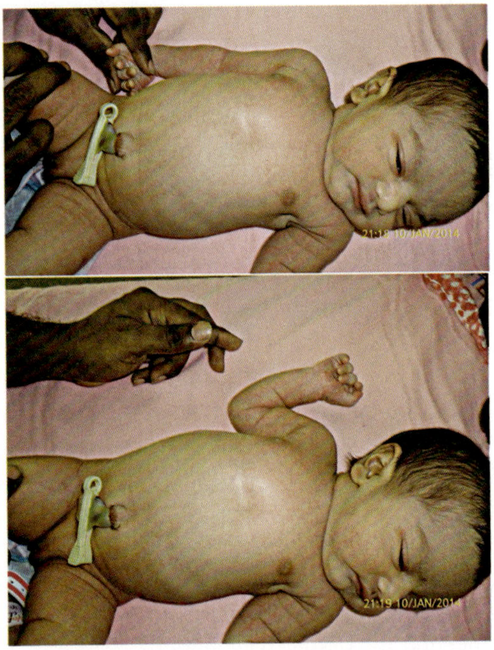

Fig.2.16 Arm recoil in full-term baby

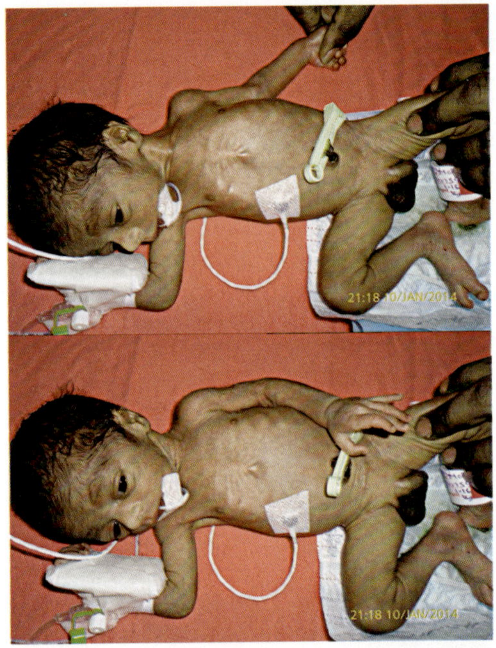

Fig.2.17 Arm recoil in preterm baby

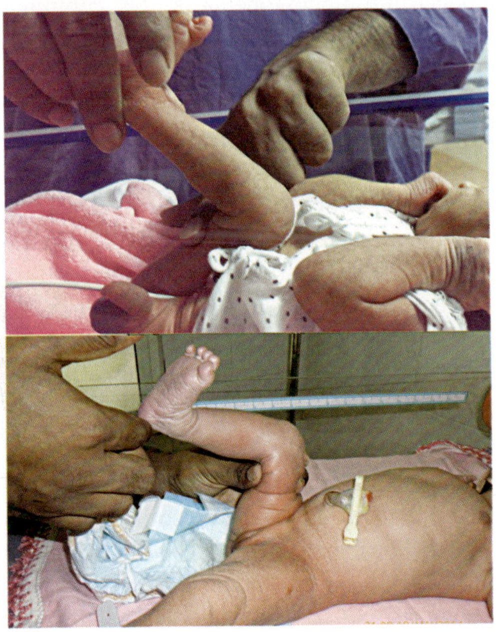

Fig.2.18 Popliteal angle in 34-week preterm and 38-week full-term babies. No more than 90° in term baby.

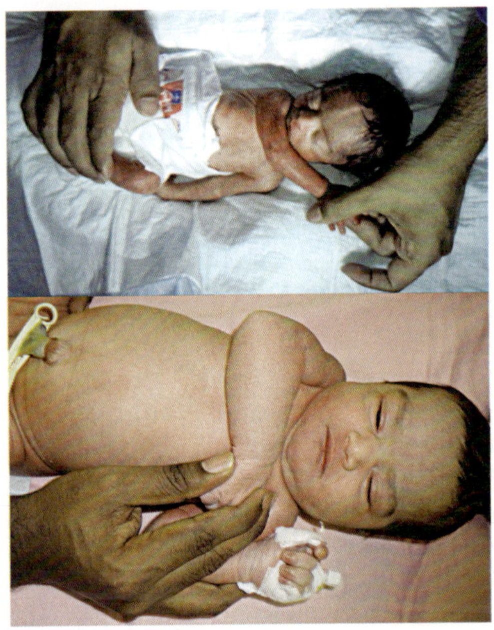

Fig.2.19 Scarf sign in preterm and full-term baby.

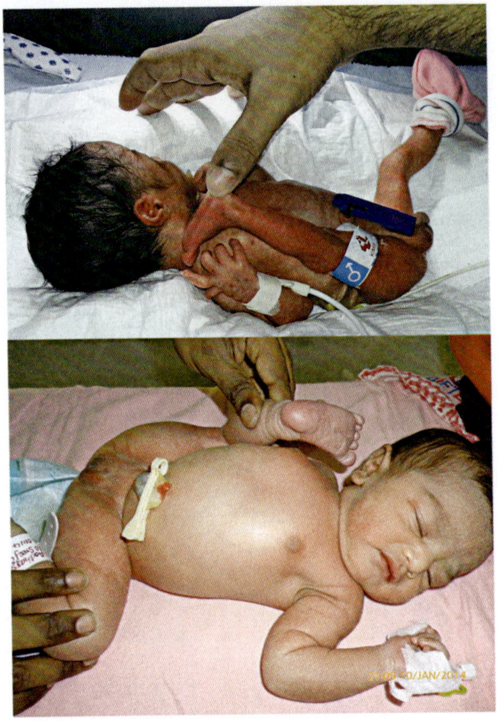

Fig.2.20 Heel to ear in preterm and full-term baby.

- GIT:
  - Feeding problems
  - Necrotising enterocolitis
  - Hyperbilirubinemia
- CNS: Intraventricular haemorrhage
- Sepsis

The difference in complications of SGA (IUGR) babies compared to a preterm babies of the same gestational age are explained as follows:

Note: SGA & IUGR are not exactly the same. SGA baby has poor growth potential (e.g., chromosomal anomaly). Normal growth potential got curtailed due to various insults in IUGR (e.g., placental insufficiency, IU infection, etc).

- Hypoglycaemia is more common in SGA; the SGA baby was stressed in utero (that is why the baby is growth restricted) and hence may have depleted glucose stores (glycogen and fat); since the brain of SGA baby is comparatively more developed compared to preterm baby, the need for glucose is more in SGA, hence hypoglycaemia is more likely in SGA.
- Hypothermia is common because of poor fat stores (fat has been used up in utero for energy); thus, there is lack of insulation and lack of fuel for heat production.
- Meconium aspiration is more common in SGA babies; this is because the stressed baby is more likely to pass meconium in utero.
- Birth asphyxia is more common in SGA babies; the baby must have been suffering from oxygen deprivation in utero as well and hence tolerate additional postnatal asphyxia very poorly.
- Polycythemia is more common in SGA, as the bone marrow responds to intrauterine hypoxia (because during hypoxia, more RBCs are needed for tissue oxygenation).
- Although hypoxia stimulates RBC production, hypoxic marrow depresses other elements and hence thrombocytopenia is very common in SGA babies (transient; normal production ensues with good postnatal oxygenation).
- Respiratory distress syndrome is less likely in SGA compared to preterm; this is because the stressed baby will have high steroid levels in the body, which protects against RDS.
- Apnoea: There is less chance. SGA baby has a relatively more mature nervous system.
- PPHN is more common in SGA babies. SGA (IUGR) babies have been suffering from chronic intrauterine hypoxia, which results in pulmonary vascular constriction.

JAUNDICED BABY

History should be directed to identify any risk factors. Jaundice may be assessed by Kramer's scale.

History

- **Time** of onset of jaundice: Clinically detectable jaundice within the first 24 hrs of life is pathological.

- **Gestational age**: Lower the gestational age, greater the risk of developing jaundice and greater the risk of bilirubin crossing the blood-brain barrier.
- **Family history**: Neonatal jaundice in previous siblings, exchange transfusion for previous siblings, history s/o haemolytic anaemia in family, liver disease, history suggestive of intrauterine infection, etc. G6PD deficiency is likely only in males (X-linked recessive).
- **Blood group incompatibility between mother and baby**: Rh incompatibility (mother Rh -ve, baby Rh +ve) or ABO incompatibility (mother O group and baby A or B blood group).
- **Natal history**: Asphyxia, traumatic delivery, oxytocin administration, delayed cord clamping and so on.
- **Drugs**: Especially important in G6PD deficient individuals.
- Total parenteral nutrition.
- **Adequacy of breast feeding**: Inadequate lactation and underfeeding predisposes to exaggeration of physiological jaundice (e.g., baby urinating less than 5–6 times a day is a good evidence of inadequate feeds).

Examination

- Icterus:
  Clinical assessment of the probable level of jaundice by **Kramer's scale**.
  - When the face alone is clinically jaundiced, the level is likely to be around 5 mg%.
  - When the chest is stained, it is around 8 mg%.
  - When abdomen is stained, it is around 12 mg%.
  - When the thighs and legs are stained, it is around 15 mg%.
  - When the sole is definitely stained yellow, the level is 20 mg% or more.
  - Clinical assessment of icterus may not be reliable if the baby is under phototherapy.
- Pallor
- Splenomegaly (Combination of pallor, jaundice and splenomegaly makes the diagnosis of haemolytic anaemia with certainty. Blood group incompatibility is the most common cause.)
- Polycythemia (SGA baby, infant of diabetic mother). Polycythemic babies look rosy red.
- Bruises, scalp swellings.
- Evidence of sepsis.
- Stigmata of IU infection (SGA, microcephaly, hepatosplenomegaly, petechiae).
- Stool/urine colour.
- Signs of kernicterus (listed below):
  - Lethargy, poor feeding, hypotonia, incomplete moro, etc, may be danger signs of impending kernicterus (stage I).
  - Seizure, opisthotonus, rigidity, etc, indicate more advanced kernicterus (stage II).
  - Survivors of kernicterus may develop choreoathetoid CP, hearing loss, dysplasia and yellow discolouration of teeth, paralysis of upgaze palsy and mental subnormality. It is said that mental retardation is not severe, but there is no way to formally assess because of the various problems this child may be having.

2

Clinical discussion on newborn is generally focused on management and hence postgraduate students are encouraged to read **Manual of Newborn Care** by same the author and publisher. This book provides plenty of photographs of newborns with various problems so that the students will find it easier to identify the same when they encounter them in clinical settings. Among the various topics, the "must read" topics for an exam going students are listed below.

- Resuscitation of newborn
- Five cleans (clean surface to place the baby, clean hands of healthcare provider, clean blade to cut the cord, clean cord tie, clean stump, which means no application to cord stump)
- Kangaroo mother care
- Cephalhaematoma
- Cutis marmorata

- Epstein pearl
- Mastitis neonatorum
- Baby friendly hospital initiative
- Counseling on breast feeding (proper position, proper latching, how to know the baby is getting adequate breast milk, management of retracted nipple and sore nipple, expressed breast milk).
- HIV and breast feeding: Current recommendations and practices.
- Common advices given to prevent hypothermia, hypoglycaemia, sepsis, etc.
- Composition, advantages of colostrum and breast milk.
- Causes of premature births, problems of preterm babies and how to prevent/manage them, difference between problems of IUGR (SGA) and preterm babies.
- Respiratory distress syndrome/Hyaline membrane disease
- Meconium aspiration syndrome
- Surfactant
- Breast feeding and jaundice
- Haemolytic disease of newborn (Rh/ABO incompatibility)
- Haemorrhagic disease of newborn
- Phototherapy
- Kernicterus
- Identification of a sick baby (please read STOPS protocol from Manual of Newborn Care by the same author).
- Warm chain: Warm chain is a set of 10 interlinked procedures carried out at birth and later, which will minimize the likelihood of hypothermia in all newborns. Warm chain is most important in low birth weight babies.
  - Warm delivery room.
  - Warm resuscitation station.
  - Immediate drying of baby after delivery.
  - Skin-skin contact between baby and the mother after drying the baby.
  - Breastfeeding as recommended in BFHI.
  - No baby bath at birth.
  - Appropriate clothing and bedding (covering the scalp is the most neglected part). Alternative is Kangaroo mother care.
  - Mother and baby are nursed together (rooming in as recommended in BFHI).
  - Warm transportation (temperature maintenance during transport is the weakest link in warm chain).
  - Training of healthcare providers.

CHAPTER 3

History and General Examination

The paediatric case sheet is an elaborate one and the student will tire the child and reach nowhere near a diagnosis if he is to follow the case sheet format faithfully. Good students will pick up the major problems quickly and direct themselves to the necessary clinical examination to have a general idea of what the child's problem is and then do a thorough and focussed systematic examination depending on the time available. Do not expect sympathy from the examiner for not completing the examination in time. It is annoying for most of the examiners to hear that a candidate could not finish the examination within the allotted time.

Personal Data

Patient's Name: This is to identify the patient. Practice addressing child by name. This gives a personal feeling and will help a lot when you start establishing medical practice of your own.

Age: Preferably in years and months after the last birthday, especially if the case is given for the assessment of development (difference of a few months will make assessment of development of infants erroneous). If a small infant, number of days—e.g., 84 days old. The age is part of diagnostic criteria of some diseases like Kawasaki disease. Thalassemia never clinically present in the first months of life. VSD presents with cardiac failure at around 4–6 weeks of life and not earlier.

Sex: Some diseases are inherited as sex-linked recessive, like haemophilia, Duchenne muscular dystrophy, etc and hence can affect only the males. Some problems are more common in females—SLE, primary pulmonary hypertension, etc are examples.

Address: This is mainly for the identity. However, some diseases have regional clustering like fluorosis, pellagra, etc. Urban areas and industrial towns may have more pollution and hence may trigger asthma.

Race/religion: These need not be routinely mentioned, except where certain heritable diseases are known to be prevalent in a community or region (e.g., thalassaemia is common in certain communities). In some non-heritable diseases also, mention of religion takes importance, e.g., Indian childhood cirrhosis is common in first-born males of Hindu families, possibly related to the custom of boiling milk in copper vessels and preferential feeding of male child.

Informant: One will have to mention whether the informant is reliable or not, which is important when the informant is not the mother or when the mother is not the primary care taker. If the informant is not a close relative, duration of stay with the child, literacy, etc, may help to deduce if history is likely to be reliable.

HISTORY

History taking is an art to be mastered by repetition so that during examination the student will feel relaxed and will be able to focus his attention on elaborating only the relevant parts of history. It is most important not to miss relevant details in history that leads to the specific diagnosis. At the same time, it is equally important not to go on elaborating irrelevant details, irritating the examiner.

Presenting Complaints

The major complaints with their duration are recorded in chronological order in the patient's (or informant's) own words. Example:
Fever: 7 days
Cough: 5 days
Difficulty in breathing: 2 days

History of the Present Illness (ODP or Onset, Duration and Progress of Symptoms)

This should be in your own words and not in parents' words. Do not blindly accept terms given by parents (like asthma, arthritis, allergy, migraine, etc). Description of ODP usually starts like "the child was apparently normal till——and then the symptoms started."

ODP is the most important part of history and will determine how you perform in the case discussion.

- Start with *Onset, Duration and Progress*. Mention ODP of each symptom, also in chronological order. Description of the symptoms must be in good detail, like their duration, character, severity, frequency, diurnal variations, postural variations, precipitating/aggravating/relieving factors, etc. Of course, the enquiry varies depending on what the symptom is.
- Other *symptoms of the involved system,* e.g., if the child has cough and fever, ask for other respiratory symptoms like breathlessness, haemoptysis, chest pain, etc. Specifically ask for associated symptoms expected (parents may not volunteer them as they may consider this insignificant) so as to make your own conclusions regarding the possible diagnosis.
- *History related to possible aetiologies*: This includes all positive and relevant negative history to rule out all the possible differential diagnosis. History of travel to areas of endemic diseases. After finishing the physical examination, the candidate can come back to elicit additional history related to differential diagnosis.
- *History of complications*: Ask for the development of complications involving the concerned illness anytime during the course of illness.
- *Course in hospital and treatment*: Should include treatment in the form of injections, IV fluids, oxygen, intensive care unit (ICU) stay, etc. Always ask if the child has been advised special diet, physiotherapy or any particular counseling by the managing team.
- *Activities of daily living*: Includes sleep, eating, dressing, toilet and ambulation (EDTA). Adult case sheets have a column on personal history to include these items. This gives an overall assessment of well-being.

It is best to conclude with a summary of the present condition of the patient.

> A sample statement: "Fever to start with was low grade, but for the last 2 days has become high grade with chills and rigor. It appears to be continuous, except for brief periods of normalization following antipyretics. Cough was dry and infrequent 5 days ago, but now is paroxysmal, productive, more frequent at night and while lying down and at times terminates with vomiting."

History of Past Illnesses

Significant illnesses in the past (particularly those requiring hospitalization) may be mentioned here. Usual ones of relevance are wheeze, seizures, travel to known endemic areas of diseases, treatment history, illness similar to the present one, tuberculosis, measles, jaundice, etc. It may be a good idea to enquire what is the established diagnosis in chronic cases; one may also try to obtain a clue from the treatment the child is on (e.g., penicillin prophylaxis in rheumatic fever, steroids in nephrotic syndrome, anti-TB treatment, digoxin in CCF, etc). After completing the examination, the student may come back to the history, now with a mental picture of the possible differential diagnosis to enquire about any illness in the past, which may have a direct bearing on the present condition. It is important to give relevant negative history; e.g., history of haematemesis in a case of suspected portal hypertension.

Antenatal, Natal and Postnatal History

Unless relevant to the case at hand, this history must be brief.

Antenatal

- How elaborate the antenatal history must be depends on the type of case at hand.
- Inquiring whether the child is born out of consanguineous marriage becomes important in heritable diseases and hence may be inquired into.
- Married since when, whether any treatment for infertility taken.
- Age of mother (age at time of pregnancy is the relevant one; e.g., advanced maternal age is associated with Down's syndrome)
- Birth order
- Past obstetric history including neonatal deaths, abortions, NICU admissions, any illness or complications during past pregnancy, etc may be inquired into.
- How did the abdomen look (to have an idea on poly/oligohydramnios). Comment if the weight gain during pregnancy was adequate, if the same is known.
- Number of antenatal hospital visits (usual minimum is three hospital visits/visits by anganwadi workers), tetanus toxoid (2 doses), illness/complications during pregnancy.
- Ask for iron-folic acid tablets, immunization, weight gain, time of appreciation of quickening. Results of investigations like HBsAg, VDRL and blood group if known in relevant cases.
- Any maternal illnesses like hypertension, diabetes mellitus, antepartum haemorrhage, hyperemesis, previous abortions, etc. Possibility of intrauterine infections must be enquired into, like fever with rash (rubella), close contact with cats (toxoplasma), genital vesicles in mother (herpes simplex), etc.
- History of hyperemesis, spotting PV, folic acid supplementation in the first trimester may be inquired into. 3
- History of UTI, maternal fever, foul smelling discharge, abdominal tenderness, etc in 3rd trimester could be risk for early onset sepsis.
- When did she start perceiving fetal movements? If a multipara, were the movements same or less compared to previous pregnancy? (may become significant in some cases, like decreased fetal movements in Werdnig-Hoffman disease or unusually brisk periodic fetal movements that is perceived in the case of fetal seizure).

The effects of common maternal illnesses could be:

- ***Hypertension***: Causes uteroplacental circulatory insufficiency and hence intrauterine growth restriction (IUGR).
- ***Diabetes***: High maternal glucose levels cross over to fetal circulation to produce hyperglycaemia, islet cell hypertrophy and hyperinsulinemia. Hyperinsulinemia results in somatic growth (large for gestational age baby). As the baby is born, the maternal supply of glucose is cut off and the prevailing high insulin levels produce hypoglycaemia. The other issues of babies of gestational diabetes are hypocalcaemia, respiratory distress syndrome, shoulder dystocia during delivery due to the large size of baby and the unusual caudal regression syndrome.

- *SLE*: Congenital heart block.
- Severe maternal malnutrition during pregnancy: Low birth weight baby. Borderline malnutrition of mother has no effect on the weight of the baby.
- Drug intake during the antenatal period or X-ray exposure?
  Examples of drug effects on fetus include: phenobarbitone (CNS depression), sodium valproate (neural tube defects), phenytoin embryopathy (resulting in dysmorphism), warfarin embryopathy, fetal alcohol syndrome, androgenic hormones (virilization of fetus), lithium (Ebstein anomaly of heart), maternal smoking (IUGR).
  Permissible X-ray exposure in the entire pregnancy is 500 millirads.
- Antenatal ultrasound scans? (In relevant cases; e.g., a hydronephrosis may have been detected antenatally). 1st trimester USG is to confirm intrauterine pregnancy. II trimester USG is anomaly scan.

Natal

- Hospital/domiciliary delivery.
- Term or preterm delivery.
- Onset of labour pains (spontaneous/induced), hospital delivery or not, normal or otherwise (CS/forceps/vacuum; reason for assisted delivery if known; could be emergency CS was done for intrauterine hypoxia).
- History of premature rupture of membranes or prolonged second stage or meconium-stained amniotic fluid. Membrane rupture-delivery interval if known.

Postnatal (Neonatal)

- Did the child breathe/cry immediately after birth (if not, details of resuscitation provided if the same is known).
- Birth weight of baby; term/preterm.
- NICU admission needed or not; any oxygen, IV medicines, umbilical catheterization, blood transfusion or phototherapy.
- When was meconium/urine passed?
- When was breastfeeding initiated and were there any problems?
- Ask for common problems like respiratory distress, jaundice, seizures, vomiting, poor feeding, cyanosis, cephalhaematoma, umbilical sepsis, etc. How was the activity, feeding and weight gain in the early neonatal period.
- Day of discharge (uneventful normal deliveries get discharged on day 3; so delayed discharges give a clue towards neonatal problems if the delay was not due to maternal issues).

> Sample statement: It was a full-term vacuum delivery at hospital and the child cried soon after birth. There is no history to suggest that the child required any resuscitation at birth. There is nothing in this history to suggest any other neonatal problems. Breastfeeding was started soon after birth. The baby passed urine and meconium within 24 hrs of birth.

Immunization History

- Mention whether immunization is adequate for the age.
- History should specifically evaluate vaccines of national schedule/additional vaccines/pulse polio.
- BCG scar is to be looked for.
- If any dose is missed, or immunization is not taken, the student must try to find out the reason for the same. The usual reasons are lack of faith, ignorance, adverse reaction to previous doses, lack of easy availability, illnesses at the time of vaccination, etc.
- If vaccination is incomplete, the student may mention (during case presentation) that the mother has been advised by the student to complete the immunization. This creates a good impression.
- Additional vaccines relevant to the diagnosis in a particular case must be inquired into (e.g., nephrotic syndrome, vaccines before splenectomy).

National Immunization Schedule

Table 3.1 National immunization schedule

Age	Vaccine
At birth, before discharge from the hospital (usually 3 days)	BCG (0.05 mL intra dermal is the recommendation up to 1 month of age, but uniformly 0.1 mL for all ages is also acceptable), OPV ("zero dose") and HBV (within 24 hrs)
1½ months or 6 weeks	Pentavac 1 (DPT, Hib, HBV), OPV 1, f IPV 1 (0.1 mL intradermal), PCV 1, Rota 1.
2½ months or 10 weeks	Pentavac 2, OPV 2, Rota 2
3½ months or 14 weeks	Pentavac 3, OPV 3, f IPV 2, PCV 2, Rota 3
9 months (completed)	MR 1, f IPV3, PCV 3, JE 1 (only in endemic areas)
1½ years or 18 months	DPT (1st booster), OPV (1st booster), MR 2, JE 2 (only in endemic areas)
5 years	DPT (2nd booster)
10 years and 16 years	One dose of Td each HPV vaccine for 9–14 yr aged girls will soon be introduced

It's easy to remember as Penta, OPV & Rota at 6, 10 & 14 weeks. f IPV & PCV at 6 & 14 weeks and 9 months. MR and JE at 9 & 18 months. At 18 months DPT & OPV booster and at 5 yr only DPT booster.

For defaulters, BCG is advised up to 1 year of age and DPT up to 7 years of age.

Additional Vaccines

1. **MMR**: Any time after 9 months of age, subcutaneous. Adolescents who have not been vaccinated can be offered this vaccine.
2. **Hib vaccine**: Primary doses are 3 (if <6 months of age) or 2 (if 6 months to 1 year of age) or 1 (if 12–18 months of age) if given as stand alone vaccine. One booster IM at or after 18 months of age. Vaccine is not required for children 5 years of age or above as the Hib disease is rare in older children. In national program it is given as a combination vaccine of DPT, Hib, Hep B (pentavac) at 6, 10 and 14 weeks. No booster for Hib in national program.
3. **Pneumococcal Conjugate vaccine** (PCV, 10, 13 or 14 valent) is now available. The schedule is 6 & 14 weeks and 9 months. **23 valent polysaccharide vaccine** is used for high-risk children above 2 years of age (asplenia, sickle cell anaemia, nephrotic syndrome, HIV infected) 0.5 mL single dose IM. Revaccination is recommended just once after 5 years only in high-risk patients.

   No further boosters are allowed. The advantage is it covers more serotypes; the disadvantage is that being a polysaccharide vaccine it is not immunogenic in those less than 2 years of age and it results in poor long-term immunologic memory.
4. **Hepatitis B**: Ideal schedule is 3 doses at 0, 1 and 6 months IM. Paediatric dose (10 μg) is enough up to 18 years of age.

   The Govt of India now recommends a birth dose of hepatitis B vaccine (HBV) in all institutionalized deliveries, followed by three doses at monthly intervals along with DPT/OPV. No further boosters are currently recommended by the Govt of India. The vaccine will be provided free of cost as part of pentavac.
5. **Hepatitis A**: 2 doses (720 units) at 0 and 6 months IM. Anytime at or after 1 yr of age. Paediatric dose is adequate up to 18 yrs of age.
6. **Varicella vaccine**: Two doses at interval of 8 weeks subcutaneously at any time after one year of age.
7. **Typhoid vaccine**: Three types of vaccines are available. Whole cell vaccine (TAB) can be given subcutaneous or IM 2 doses at 1-month interval. Vi vaccine can be given as single dose, IM, any time after 2 years of age. Capsules of oral vaccine (Ty 21a) must be swallowed with

3

out breaking it and are suitable only after 6 years of age. Typhoid Conjugate vaccine has become available, a single dose for above 6 months of age. For all other Typhoid vaccines, boosters are required after 3 years.

8. TdaP vaccine: One dose of TdaP can be given instead of Td at 10 years of age.
9. Rotavirus vaccine: Two types of vaccines are available .Monovalent (RV1- Rotarix) is given as 1ml orally at 10 and 14 weeks. The Pentavalent vaccine (RV5- Rotateq) is given as 3 doses at 6, 10, 14 weeks. for national schedule please see Table 3.1.

Development History

A detailed account is a must if the case is one with developmental delay (see p 60).

Assess the developmental age from the history of achievement of different milestones—social smile, head control, turning over, sitting, standing, walking, self-feeding and dressing, bladder and bowel control, speech, etc. Find the developmental age from the milestones of development in *various* domains. Special attention must be paid to the history suggestive of any impairment of *hearing* or *vision* (e.g., a child not turning to the side of a loud noise or not looking at the mother when spoken to). In bigger children, school performance also may be taken into account.

Note that aberrations like standing before sitting up (may be a sign of spasticity), bottom shuffling (may be due to cerebral palsy), etc, must make one cautious before committing to a normal development. Compare with siblings (any difference recalled by the mother).

Conclude by commenting if any developmental retardation is present or not and, if present, whether it is global or confined to one specific area (e.g., isolated motor delay in cerebral palsy).

Dietary History (Nutrition History)

History must evaluate the child's diet before the present illness and not the diet during the present illness. For an older child, dietary history taken by 24-hr recall method. Daily food intake before the illness is of relevance in the assessment of malnutrition.

Until what age was the child on exclusive breastfeeding? If not breastfed adequately, try to elicit the reason (examiners are likely to ask the reason).

When was the complementary feeding started, with what? Is it nutritionally adequate?

When was cow's milk/formula started? (If started, enquire about its dilution; whether using feeding bottle or spoon; if using feeding bottle, how the bottle and nipple are cleaned)

Any change in bowel habits in relation to introduction of any specific food items? (May give a clue to malabsorption. For example, celiac disease starts with the introduction of wheat.)

Enquire about the consumed food items and calculate the calorie and protein gap, if any. If the child is still being breastfed, ask how many times the child is being fed to know the approximate quantity of milk obtained by the baby. The ideal method of finding out the amount of milk obtained by the baby is to weigh the baby before and after the feed to know the weight of milk per feed, then multiply it with the number of times the child is fed. In clinical scenario, if the child comfortably sleeps 3–4 hrs after feed, passes urine many times a day and if there is let down reflex from the other breast, the milk output is possibly good enough.

The calorie requirement is roughly calculated as 100 cal/kg until 1 year of age. At 1 year, the required calories are taken as 1000 and thereafter for each additional year of age, 100 calories are added. Protein requirement is calculated as 2 g/kg till 1 year of age, the protein requirement at 1 year is about 20 g. Beyond 1 year of age, the protein requirement drops to 1.5 g/kg during toddler age. The calculated value should not go above the normal adolescent requirements (e.g., adolescent male 2400 cal and female 2000 cal). At present, calorie and protein recommended are much less. (see Table 4.10 & 4.11, p 67).

Calorie Requirement by Holliday & Segar Formula
Up to 10 kg – 100 kcal/kg
10–20 kg – 1000 + 50 kcal/kg for each kg above 10
>20 kg – 1500 + 20 kcal/kg for each kg above 20

Note: Same formula may be also used to calculate 24 hrs maintenance IV fluid requirement in children.

Calculate calorie gap and protein gap (average Indian adult diet has 300–400 kcal and 15–20 g protein gap).

Does the diet contain sources of iron, calcium, etc?

Any food allergies or intolerance?

Is the child on any food supplementation, vitamins, iron or on any special diet? (e.g., specific exclusion diets in metabolic diseases).

The nutritional values of common food stuffs are discussed in the chapter on "Growth, Development and Nutrition," p 65.

> Usually the student's impression from the nutrition history is expected. A sample statement would be: the child's diet is adequate in calories and proteins, but lacks dietary source of iron.

Family History

1. Age of parents at the time of conception of the child patient. Mention may be made on the birth order, spacing, sterilization, etc. Marital disharmony may have relevance in case of PEM, child abuse, etc.
2. Any consanguinity? If so, state the degree of consanguinity. In relevant cases, draw pedigree chart.
   - 1st degree consanguineous relationship: Dizygotic twins; siblings; parent-child. One may wonder whether such marriages are permitted in any society. True, they are not. But, unfortunately children have been born in such relations. So they are described as being born of a 1st-degree consanguineous relationship rather than 1st-degree consanguineous marriage.
   - 2nd-degree consanguineous relationship: uncle (aunt)–niece (nephew); half siblings.
   - 3rd-degree consanguineous relationship: 1st cousins.
3. Illnesses in siblings/family members: History of allergy or asthma in the family is an example. It is also important in cases of heritable diseases (e.g., jaundice and neuropsychiatric illnesses in family must strengthen the suspicion of Wilson's disease) and contagious diseases (e.g., chicken pox at home).

   Special emphasis must be given to tuberculosis in our country. Is there any elderly person in the family or neighbourhood with chronic cough and/or haemoptysis (suggestive of tuberculosis)? If so, get details. Was his sputum positive? Is he getting treatment regularly? Any adult with tuberculosis in the family who is not on treatment or completed treatment in the past 2 years can be taken as a contact who can spread the disease to the child. Any neonatal/unexplained infantile deaths? (may make one suspicious of inborn errors of metabolism).
4. Family customs/beliefs/routines: In relevant cases, inquire about any beliefs that has adverse effects on health: like obligatory prelacteal feeds before breast feeding, blowing oil into the nose (prevalent in some parts of Tamil Nadu), starvation during diarrhoea, obligatory indoor care of child (lack of sun exposure may predispose to rickets), strict vegetarianism (could cause deficiencies like B_{12}), any discrimination to the female child for schooling/nutrition (could explain the situation of only female child getting malnourished), etc.

Does the child use footwear while walking in the courtyard?

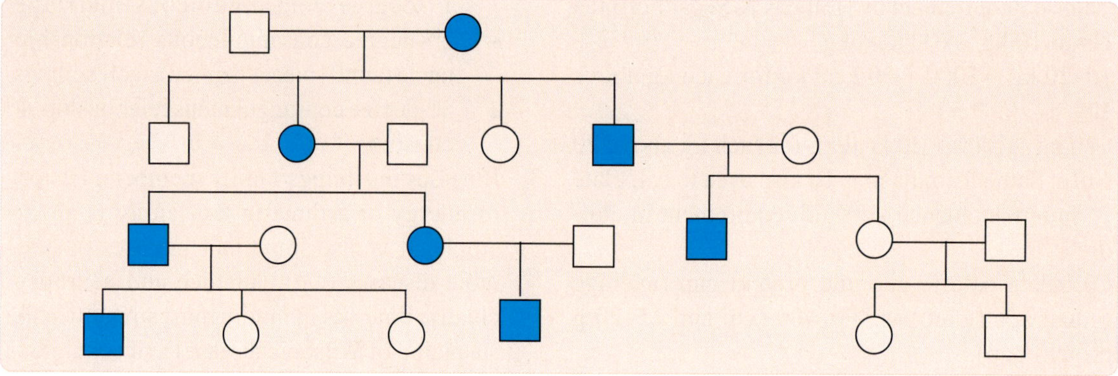

Fig.3.1 Autosomal dominant inheritance

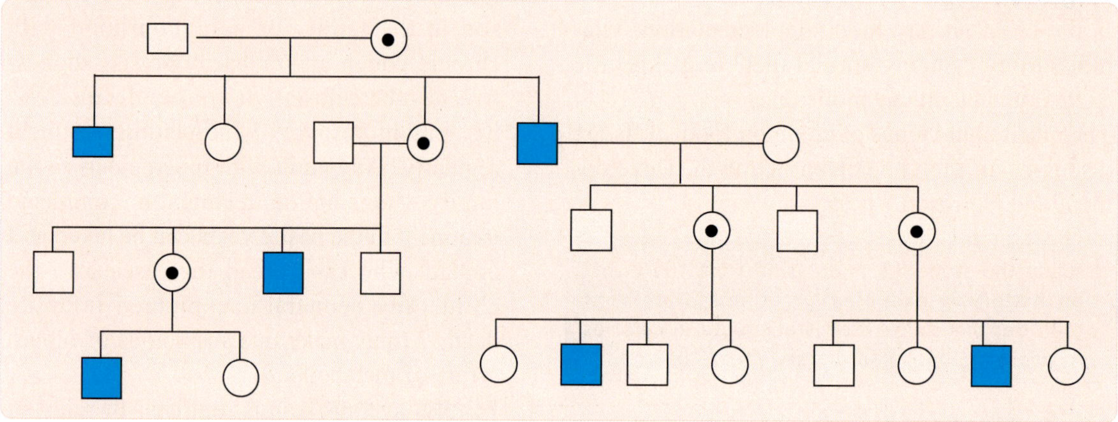

Fig.3.2 X-linked recessive inheritance

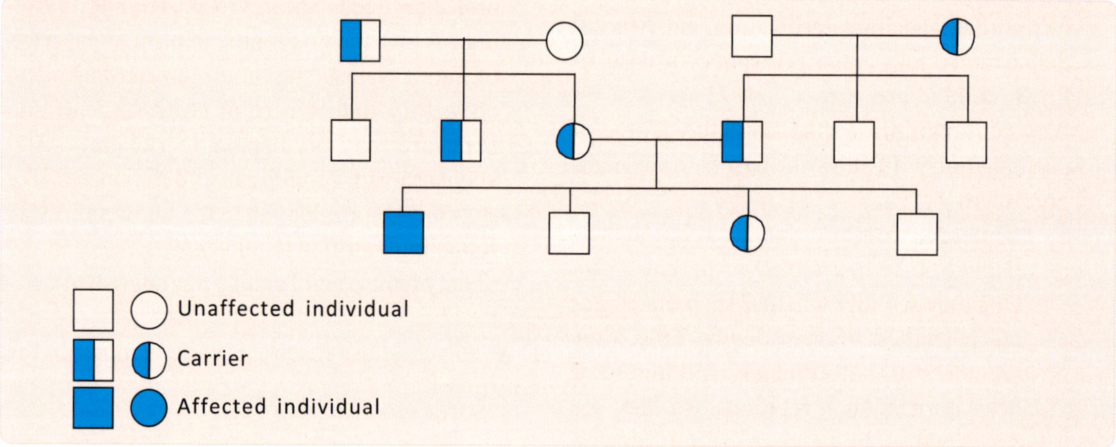

Fig.3.3 Autosomal recessive inheritance

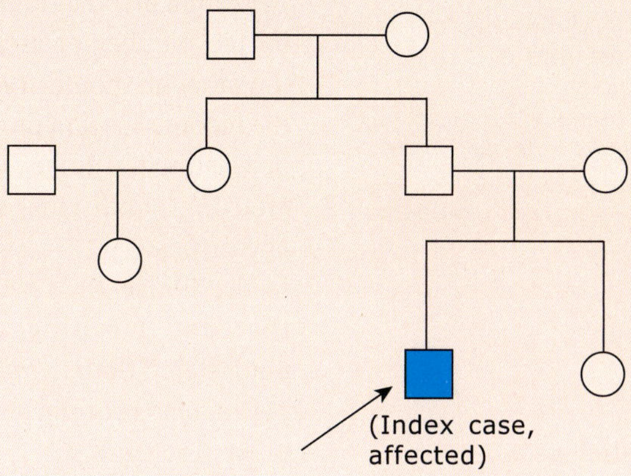

Fig.3.4a Sample drawing of pedigree chart

Symbols used in Drawing a Pedigree Chart *(Courtesy: Dr Sankar VH)*

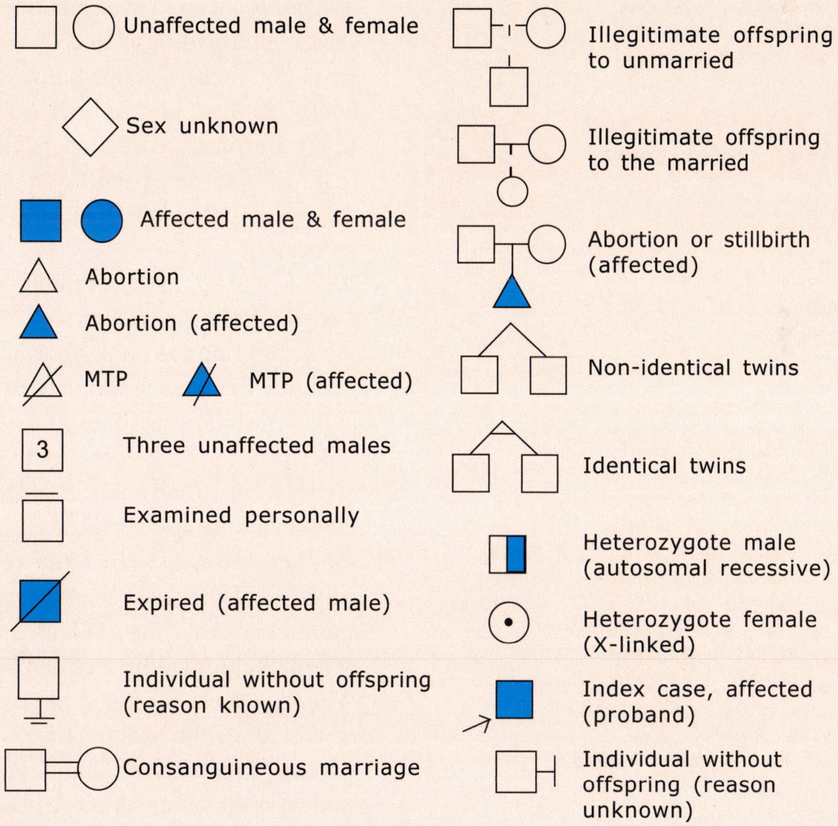

Fig.3.4b Symbols used in drawing a pedigree chart

Socioeconomic History

1. Socioeconomic status and income

Table 3.2 Modified Kuppuswamy scale of social classification *(updated – IJP, Dec 2007)*

	(A) Education	Score
1	Profession or honours	7
2	Graduate or postgraduate	6
3	Intermediate or post high school diploma	5
4	High school certificate	4
5	Middle school certificate	3
6	Primary school certificate	2
7	Illiterate	1
	(B) Occupation	**Score**
1	Profession	10
2	Semi-profession	6
3	Clerical, shop-owner, farmer	5
4	Skilled worker	4
5	Semi-skilled worker	3
6	Unskilled worker	2
7	Unemployed	1
	(C) Family income per month (Rs) (modified for 2007)	**Score**
1	>19,575	12
2	9788–19,574	10
3	7323–9787	6
4	4894–7322	4
5	2936–4893	3
6	980–2395	2
7	<979	1

Total score	Socioeconomic class
26–29	Upper (I): E.g., top business people, IAS, etc
16–25	Upper middle (II): Professionals like doctors, engineers
11–15	Lower middle (III): Trained workers like plumbers, electricians, etc
5–10	Upper lower (IV): Untrained workers, i.e., manual labourer
<5	Lower (V): No jobs (like street dwellers)

Per capita income (total family income divided by the number of members). In PEM cases, the student should try to elicit how much of the income is spent on food (bread winner may be wasting the money on alcohol, betting, etc).

2. Housing conditions, water source and sewage disposal.
   Is the house *Katcha* or *Pukka*? (*Katcha* is thatched building with mud walls and unplastered floors. *Pukka* house is the one with permanent roofing, brick walls and cement/ other flooring).
   Number of rooms in the house and members in the family? (to evaluate if there is overcrowding, which contributes to spread of communicable diseases). Two adult persons of the opposite sex, not husband and wife, obliged to sleep in the same room is considered overcrowding (*Park*,).
   Does the kitchen smoke pollute the inside of house? Is there atmospheric pollution due to heavy traffic, construction work or factories (e.g., relevant in case of asthma)?
   Any pets at home? If so, are they allowed indoors.
   What is the source of drinking water? If it is from well, is it a protected well? Are they boiling or filtering the drinking water?
   Are they having sanitary latrine? Is the child in the habit of using the sanitary latrine? Is the toilet very near the water source?
3. Social security and public health schemes: Are they aware of any social assistance schemes for the chronically ill child (e.g., cerebral palsy)? This history becomes important if the examiner wants the student to counsel the parent of chronic illnesses like hemophilia.
   Where is their nearest *Anganwadi*? Are the mother and child beneficiaries?
   These are just a few common questions. The student is encouraged to use his or her imagination to modify suitably or add more questions to suit the individual case.

It is very important that the student does not waste his time taking all these histories when it is not relevant to the case at hand.

GENERAL EXAMINATION

Uncomfortable procedures like throat examination, examination of hips of newborn etc, should be reserved for the last but when presenting the case before the examiner, the scheme of case presentation should be according to the case sheet format.

To get the cooperation of the patient: A small infant may be examined on the mother's lap, preferably while feeding at the breast. A toddler also prefers to be with the mother and may be distracted with colourful toys.

Older children may be examined while being seated near the mother or on an examination table with the mother nearby.

Note: Always remember to take the consent of the parent and the child before proceeding to examination.

1. General Comment

Is the child sick looking/tachypnoeic-dyspnoeic/ or comfortable? Give a visual impression on the build and nourishment of the child (must keep in mind the anthropometry while making the comment on nourishment).

The usual factors considered to make this general comment are level of consciousness, posture, mental (emotional) status, and attitude towards the examiner.

There is no need to score in detail, the GCS for students taking paediatric examination. This is because the scoring is best for serial monitoring and not for one time assessment. In addition, Glasgow coma scale is validated in head injury rather than medical illness. **(Refer pg 180.)**

Posture or decubitus is the position that the patient prefers to have. Examples are:

- Child lying on the same side of effusion or pleurisy (in effusion, if the patient lies on the normal side, there will be restriction of expansion of normal side as well. In pleurisy, lying on the affected side restricts movements of the affected side, thus minimizing the pain).
- Meningitis: Lies on the side, totally curled up except for the neck which is hyperextended.
- Decerebration: Upper and lower limbs totally extended, forearm pronated.
- Spastic cerebral palsy: Crossing of legs (scissoring).

The usual comments on the emotional status:

- Alert and playful: Normal child.
- Anxious: Anticipation of painful procedures or painful lesions that produces pain on movement.
- Apathetic (dull and uninterested): Kwashiorkor.
- Restless: Attention deficit hyperactive disorder; pain; generalized itching; headache (as in meningitis).

Any obvious anomalies of gait or abnormal movements?

Any peculiar odour? Examples would be halitosis (foul smelling breath) in lung abscess and bronchiectasis; acetone smell in diabetic ketoacidosis; fetor hepaticus in liver cell failure.

Peculiar body odour/odour of urine/sweat in inborn errors of metabolism is not of any good help for students facing examination. The following are standard examples:

Sweaty feet	Organic acidaemias
Burnt sugar	MSUD
Musty or mousy	PKU
Rotten fish	Tyrosinaemia
Tomcat urine	Multiple carboxylase deficiency

A sample statement in a TB meningitis child: This is a malnourished, ill-looking, drowsy child lying in curled up position except for the head, which is kept hyperextended and responds to pain with weak cry and avoidance movements.

A sample statement in a child with chorea: A well-nourished, conscious, well-oriented child with constant jerky movements of limbs, unsteady gait, and emotional lability.

contd.

A sample statement in a child with Kwashiorkor: The child is ill-looking, oedematous, apathetic and resents handling.

A sample statement in a child who is recovering from asthma or other illnesses: The child is well looking, co-operative, alert and playful.

2. Vital Signs (compare with normal values for the age)

Pulse rate, respiratory rate, blood pressure and temperature.

Pulse, BP and respiratory rate are discussed along with cardiovascular and respiratory systems.

Normal BP (mnemonic): 90 + (2 × age in year) gives the approximate systolic BP.

A sample statement of BP: BP is —— mm of Hg in the right upper limb in supine position using the appropriate cuff size.

A sample statement of pulse: Pulse is —— per minute, regular in rhythm, normal in volume and character, no radiofemoral delay and all peripheral pulses are felt equally on both sides.

A sample statement of respiratory rate: The respiratory rate is —— per minute, regular in rhythm and is abdominothoracic in type. Accessory muscles of respiration are not active.

Temperature

There is no consensus on the time for which the thermometer should be kept for recording temperature. If placed under the tongue, 1 min may be enough, but in the axilla as much as 3 min may be needed. The axilla must be dried before placing the thermometer and the bulb should be towards the apex. Normal temperature is 37 C or 98.4 F. 37 C is not an absolute cutoff but an average normal temperature. Some variation of temperature may be there normally as well, the maximum being not more than 37.7 C (100 F), usually in the evening.

The rectal temperature is more than the oral temperature, which is more than axillary temperature, each by ½ °C or 1°F. There is a diurnal variation of temperature normally (normal diurnal variation is 1°F), with > 99°F being normal in the evening. Hence, any child with fever may have a higher peak in the evening hours. Due to the same reason, mild degrees of fever are most likely to be recognized only in the evening and may present as evening rise of temperature. Tuberculosis was the classic example in yesteryears.

Rectal temperature is needed only in rare cases, like severe PEM. It is recorded by a rectal thermometer, which has a rounded bulb.

Fever is defined as rectal temperature of more than 100.4°F or 38°C. Exact recording can be made using the Digital thermometers which are available nowadays.

Patterns of Fever

There are three classical patterns of fever:

1. *Continuous fever*: In which daily fluctuations do not exceed 1°C (1.5°F). Note: According to some authorities, this value is 0.6°C (1°F).
2. *Remittent fever*: In which daily fluctuations exceed the above norms, but never touches normal. In typhoid, the rise of temperature is *as a stepladder pattern*, without touching the baseline inbetween. Obviously, it is a remittent fever, but in addition has step ladder pattern.
3. *Intermittent fever*: Is called quotidian if it occurs daily (as in juvenile rheumatoid arthritis, or JRA); tertian fever if it occurs every other day, in other words, fever on days 1 and 3 (malaria due to *Pl. falciparum*, ovale or vivax); quartan fever when it occurs every third day, in other words, fever on days 1 and 4 (quartan malaria due to *Pl. malariae*). In intermittent fevers, the elevated temperature touches baseline in between.
4. *Relapsing fever*: Recurrent episodes of abrupt onset high grade fever of 3–7 days duration; Presently this term is reserved for the fever. Pel Ebstein fever (periodic fever) is a type of fever where fever cyclically increases and then decreases over an average period of 1–2 weeks

(seen in Hodgkin's lymphoma). The afebrile phase in the febrile periods last for >24 hours.

Naturally to detect temperature patterns, one must be provided with a temperature chart. All these temperature patterns considered so important in yesteryears have no meaning in the modern era as antipyretics modify the fever pattern.

Fever with rigor and chills may be seen when the temperature is rapidly rising from its baseline normal value. Chill is a subjective sensation of cold by the patient and indicates a sudden rise of temperature from the baseline. Chills and rigors go together. This is because for the sudden rise of temperature, heat must be generated, and the body does it by peripheral vasoconstriction (hence the feeling of cold, which makes one cover oneself so that the heat is further conserved) and production of heat by muscle action (the rigor). Such a sudden rise of temperature from baseline producing chills and rigors is classical of malaria. It may also be seen in urinary infection, lobar pneumonia, etc, where sudden high fever is the rule.

Fever normalizing suddenly is called "fall *by crisis.*" (Typically seen in pneumococcal pneumonia when antibiotics are used. May be seen in other conditions also where the response to treatment is dramatically fast). Normalization of fever gradually is called "fall *by lysis*" (typical in typhoid).

With each degree F rise in temperature, pulse rate rises by 10 and respiratory rate rises by 4. Fever with relative bradycardia is classically described in typhoid fever. However, in children it is more common in meningitis (effect of intracranial tension), and viral fevers (myocardial involvement).

Hyperpyrexia: It is the elevation of core temperatures above 41°C (106°F).

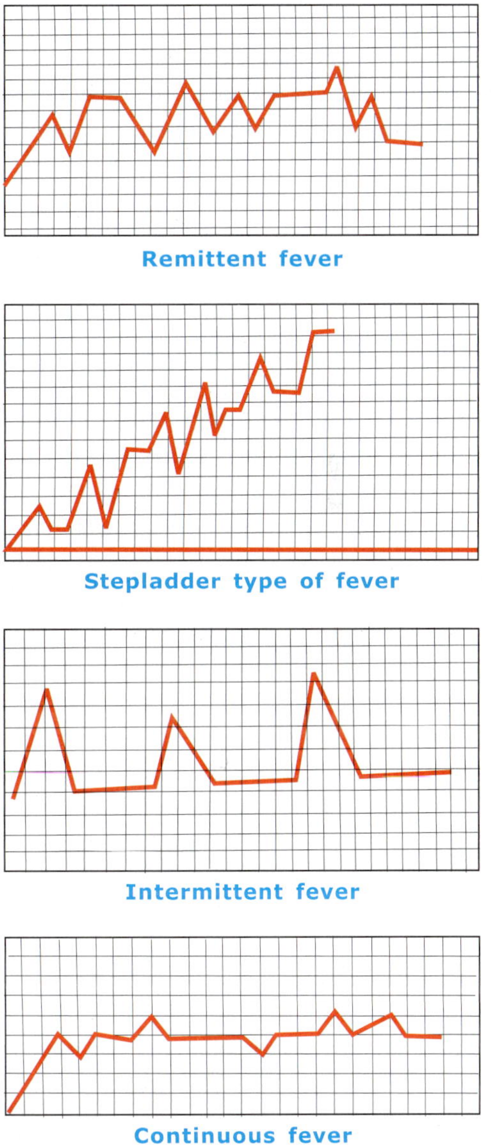

Fig.3.5 Fever patterns

It may be seen in:

- Heat stroke
- Pontine haemorrhage
- Malaria
- Septicaemia/meningitis
- "Malignant hyperthermia," that may occur in myopathy patients when halothane anaesthetic is used.

3. Anthropometry

It is discussed in Ch. 3.

4. Assessment of Development (p 60)

5. Head to Foot examination (Hand to head and head to toe) Examination

Head to foot examination is to be done in all cases, but is of prime importance in dysmorphic child, endocrinology cases and severe nutritional deficiencies. In case of musculoskeletal examination, it is advantageous to proceed hand to head and then head to toe.

Head, fontanels, hair and hairline, face, eyes, ears, oral cavity, neck, chest, skin and hair changes, abdomen back and limbs are examined for any abnormalities and noted in detail.

This topic is discussed is detail in Ch. 6. The following are a few examples.

Head: Take the head circumference: Either now or as part of anthropometry to decide whether there is micro/macrocephaly (see p 79).

Head and face examination may be done in a flow; start with back of neck (webbing, low hair line, etc), proceed upwards to back of skull (flat or prominent occiput in trisomy 21 and 18, respectively), proceed to the vertex (hair, fontanel, parietal or forehead bulging, etc), come down to forehead, eyes, ears, nose, maxillary prominence if any (e.g., haemolytic facies), mouth and down to front of neck (e.g., thyroid swelling).

Hair: Hypopigmentation, sparseness, etc. Look for pediculosis, seborrheic dermatitis, etc (see p 86).

Fontanelle: Closed/open, pulsatile/non-pulsatile, normal/depressed/bulging (see p 82).

Face: Dysmorphism, coarseness, mid-face hypoplasia (mid-face structures appear crowded compared to rest of the face), micrognathia, retrognathia, thick or thin lip, long philtrum, prominence or hypoplasia of maxilla, etc (see p 88).

Eyes: Hypertelorism, hypotelorism, upward/downward slant, microphthalmia, coloboma, synophrys, corneal clouding, cataract, nystagmus, strabismus, evidence of vitamin deficiencies, etc. Also look for pallor, icterus, conjunctival congestion, muddy conjunctiva, blue sclera, etc (see p 91).

Mouth: Oral hygiene, dentition, tongue, throat and tonsils, cleft lip/palate, inverted V-shaped upper lip, number of teeth, abnormal shape or colour of teeth, evidence of vitamin deficiencies, etc (see p 109).

Tongue: See p 109.

Ears: Anomalies, low set ears, preauricular tag, sinus, discharge ear, etc (see p 103).

Nose: Flat nasal bridge, upturned nostrils, etc (see p 91).

Neck: Short neck, webbing, low hair line, lymph nodes (see p 114).

Limbs: Over-riding of fingers and toes, arachnodactyly/brachydactyly, polysyndactyly, clinodactyly/camptodactyly, short/long limbs, broad thumbs, dystrophic nails, hypermobility of joints, dermatoglyphics, arches of foot, etc (see p 119–132). Capillary refill may be tested on finger nails. Central capillary refill may be tested over the sternum.

Chest: Pectus carinatum/excavatum, absent pectoralis major/clavicles, wide-spaced nipples, shield chest, etc (see p 117, 337).

Abdomen: Umbilical hernia, divarication of rectus muscle, distention, dilated veins, etc (see p 132, 370).

Genitalia: Hernia, hydrocoele, micropenis, undescended testes, macro-orchidism, ambiguous genitalia, precocious puberty, etc. Comment on phimosis if relevant in the case in question. SMR rating is to be done if indicated (see p 133, 498).

Spine: Dimples, hairy patches, swellings (e.g., meningomyelocoele, Pott's spine, etc), kyphosis/scoliosis/excess lordosis, etc (see p 464).

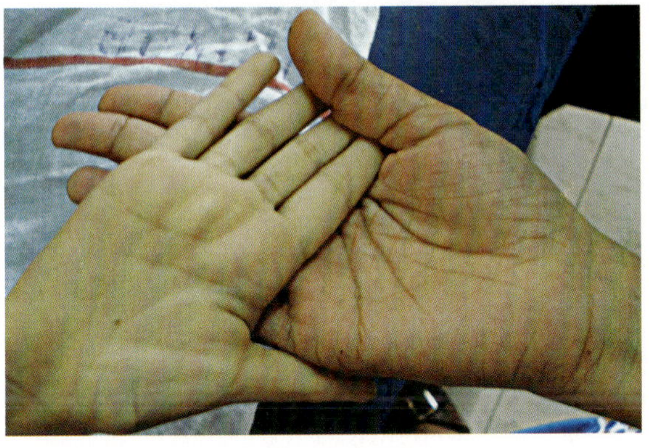

Fig.3.6 Pallor of hands: Many a time, examination of conjunctiva for pallor can be misleading (the child may have rubbed the eyes or cried recently); examining the palm of child side by side with that of the examiner gives more reliable information on pallor. Pallor of skin may be because of skin oedema (nephrotic syndrome) or vasoconstriction (circulatory shock, exposure to cold). In these situations, examination of tongue and mucous membranes help to detect true anaemia.

Skin and Nails: Changes suggestive of PEM (p 487), neurocutaneous markers. Subcutaneous emphysema, if present, may be detected by the palpating hand over the neck and chest.

Look for pyoderma, scabies, fungal infections, rash, phrynoderma, skin turgor, etc.

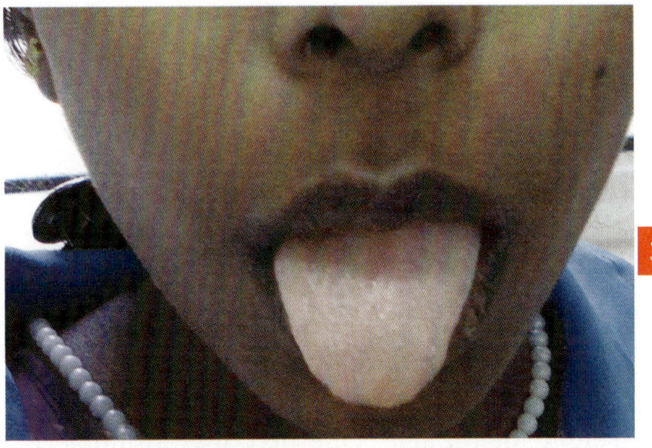

Fig.3.7 Pallor of tongue. Also note the bald tongue due to atrophic papillae.

Routinely look for **P**allor, **I**cterus, **C**yanosis, **C**lubbing, **L**ymph node enlargement, **E**dema (acronym: **PICCLE**) and neurocutaneous markers. In a case of diarrhoea, comment on any signs of dehydration. See p 114 for method of examination of lymph nodes.

To detect pallor, look at the lower palpebral conjunctiva, tongue, soft palate, nails, palms, etc. If the child has been crying, palpebral conjunctiva may not reveal pallor. Examination of palms as shown in figure may be more rewarding in that case. In severe pallor, the palmar creases also will become lighter. Icterus can be detected in good daylight, by asking the child to look down to examine the bulbar conjunctiva at upper lateral margin. Cyanosis can be looked for in fingernails, tongue, inner surface of lips, gums etc.

CHAPTER 4

Growth, Development and Nutrition

ASSESSMENT OF GROWTH

Growth is assessed by various anthropometric measurements.

Weight

Find out whether the child falls into any grade of PEM by comparing the weight with the expected weight for the age. One may use formulae or mnemonics to find out the normal, but many examination centers now provide standard growth charts for use by the candidates.

Birth – 3 kg
5 months – 6 kg
1 year – 9 kg

A full-term newborn doubles his weight by 5 months (4 months as per Nelson's Paediatrics) and triples it by 1 year.

1. Weight gain during infancy: 30 g/day for the first 3 months, 20 g/day for the next 3 months, 15 g/day for the next 3 months, and 12 g/day for the next 3 months.
   Weight of infants 3–12 months of age: (Age in months + 9) ÷ 2
   After the first year of life, children gain 2 kg per year of age (>8-year-old child gains 3 kg/year of age)
2. (Age × 2) + 8 (1–6 years); Age × 3 (> 8 years)
3. (Age × 2) + 8 (for children 1–6 years);
   $\frac{\{(\text{Age} \times 7) - 5\}}{2}$ for children 7–12 years age.

Young infant is best weighed naked except for nappy. The weight of nappy may be subtracted afterwards. If the child is not cooperative, the parent can hold the child and the combined weight recorded; afterwards, weight of the parent may be subtracted.

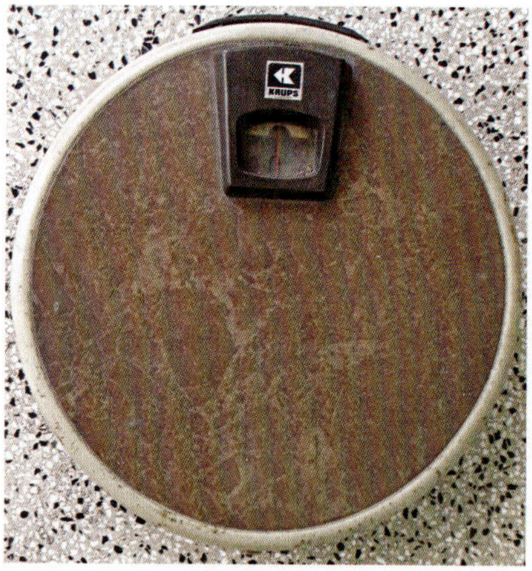

Fig.4.1 Bathroom scale: Although it is used widely, it is highly inaccurate and hence is not recommended. A beam scale must be used for recording weight. Electronic machine is another option.

Malnutrition

A child is said to be malnourished if he does not have the weight expected for his age. Conventionally it is termed PEM, though all cases of underweight are not exactly due to PEM (Protein Energy Malnutrition).

Weight Age

It is the age of a normal child who will have the

same weight as the child under evaluation. For example, if a child of 3 years has a weight of only 9 kg, his weight age is only 1 year.

Table 4.1 IAP classification of malnutrition

Grade of PEM	Percentage of ideal weight expected for the age
Normal	>80%
Grade I PEM	71–80%
Grade II PEM	61–70%
Grade III PEM	51–60%
Grade IV PEM	<50%

Post fix "K" if there is oedema indicative of kwashiorkor, e.g., grade IV K.

Table 4.2 Wellcome Trust classification of malnutrition

Percentage of ideal weight expected for the age = (Weight ÷ Ideal weight for age) x 100	Oedema present or not	Categorization of PEM
>80%	Nil	Normal
60–80%	Nil	Undernutrition
60–80%	Present	Kwashiorkor
<60%	Present	Marasmic kwashiorkor
<60%	Nil	Marasmus

Grading of Kwashiorkor

1. Peripheral oedema alone
2. Mooning of face
3. Presacral and abdominal wall oedema
4. Ascites

Grading of Marasmus

Mnemonic: ABCB

1. Loose skin folds in **A**xilla and groin
2. Loose skin folds in thigh and **B**uttocks
3. Loose skin folds in **C**hest and abdomen
4. Loss of **B**uccal pad of fat

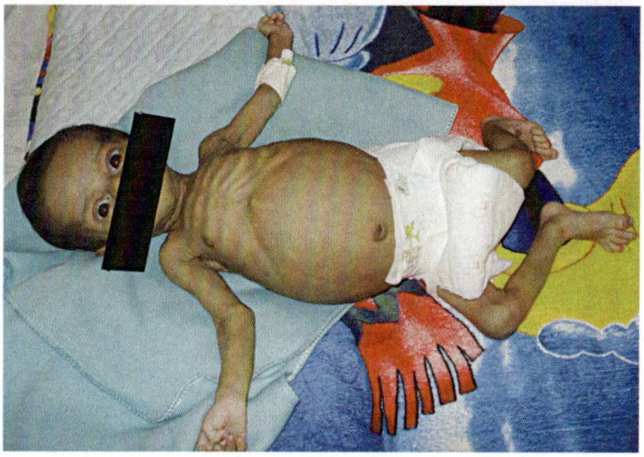

Fig.4.2A Marasmus

4

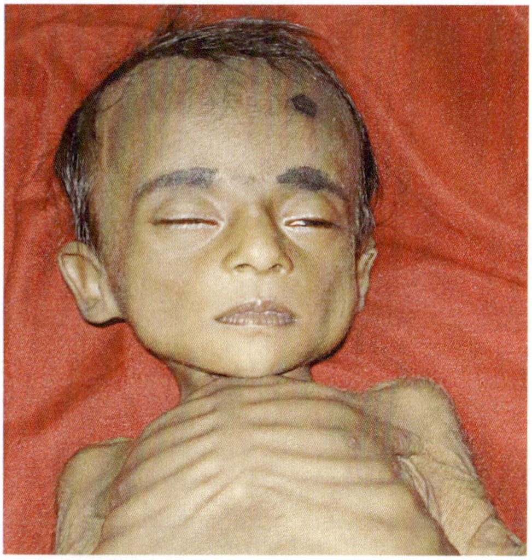

Fig.4.2B Note the loss of buccal pad of fat

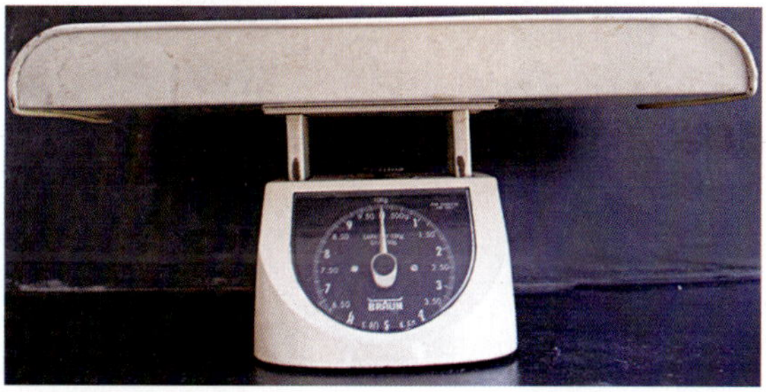

Fig.4.3 Pan type weighing scale for infants

Height

Comparison of the height with the expected height for the age will identify a child with stunting. When measured in the lying down position (in child < 2 years), it is mentioned as length. Length is measured using infantometer, and the height using stadiometer. In infantometer, the footboard can be moved to touch the foot to measure length, whereas in stadiometer the stick at the head end is moved. One can also use the wall of the room and a tape to measure the height. The child should stand against a wall with his bare feet touching each other, the heel, calf, buttock, upper back and occiput touching the wall and the child looking straight ahead. A firm scale is placed pressed to the head to mark the point indicating the height. Height may be a bit less than length due to lumbar lordosis, vertebral compression, etc, but the difference is usually less than 1 cm.

In rare situations like a quadriplegic child with contractures, the child cannot stand for height measurement and length measurement is not possible as limbs cannot be extended due to contractures. In such situations, the length of various segments of body are measured separately and added together to get the length.

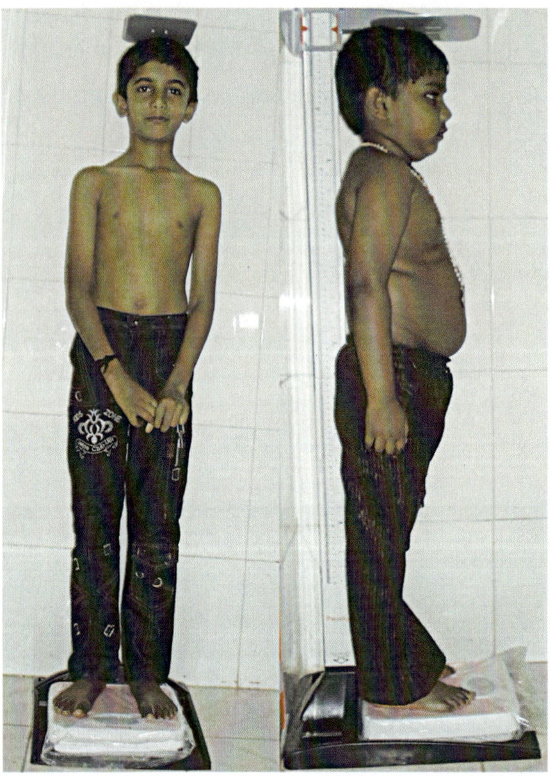

Fig.4.4 Stadiometer. Chin should be perpendicular to the scale.

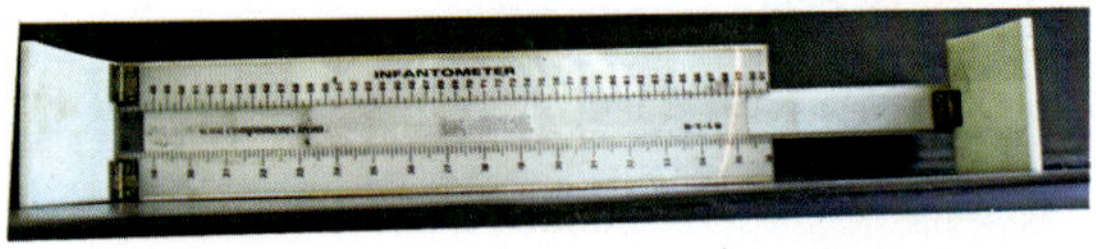

Fig.4.5 Infantometer. Before taking measurement, make sure that the legs are completely stretched and foot is perpendicular to the horizontal.

Birth – 50 cm
3 months – 60 cm
6 months – 65 cm
9 months – 70 cm
1 year – 75 cm
(Total gain in 1st year = 25 cm)

Approximate gain in length: 3.5 cm per month for the first 3 months of age, 2 cm per month for the next 3 months, 1.5 cm per month for the next 3 months 1.25 cm per month for next 3 months. At 2 years—87.5 cm (a gain of 12.5 cm in second year). Then gains around 5–6 cm per year of age. OR, use Weech formula: (Age × 6) + 77 (useful for children over 1–2 years of age)

Mnemonic: At 4 years, the height is about 100 cm, at 8 years about 125 cm and at 12 years 150 cm. Normal expected growth velocity from 2 to 10 years (before pubertal spurt) is 5–6 cm per year and any gain less than 4 cm per year is abnormal.

Stunting: A child is said to be stunted if he does not have the height expected for his age.

Height age: This is the age of a normal child who will have the same height as the child under evaluation. For example, if a child of 7 years has a height of only 100 cm, his height age is about 4–4½ years.

Table 4.3 Waterlow classification of stunting

Percentage of ideal height expected for the age = (Present height ÷ Ideal height for the age) × 100	Grade or degree of stunting
>95%	No stunting
90–95%	I
85–89%	II
<85%	III

Weight for Height

Wasting: A child is said to be wasted if he does not have the weight expected for his present height. **If growth charts are provided, mark the child's height, weight and head circumference on it and interpret in centiles or Z score**. A child with PEM need not always be wasted. For example, a child of 4 years having a weight of 10 kg and a height of 75 cm is having PEM and stunting, but is not wasted as both weight and height are reduced proportionately.

Weight for height is the objective criteria for commenting on wasting.

Weight for height = Weight of the child divided by ideal weight of a normal child of same height × 100 (to make it %).

Table 4.4 Waterlow classification of wasting

Weight for height as % of expected = (Present weight ÷ Ideal weight for the present height) × 100	Grade or degree of wasting
>110	Overweight
91–110	Normal
81–90	I
70–80	II
<70	III

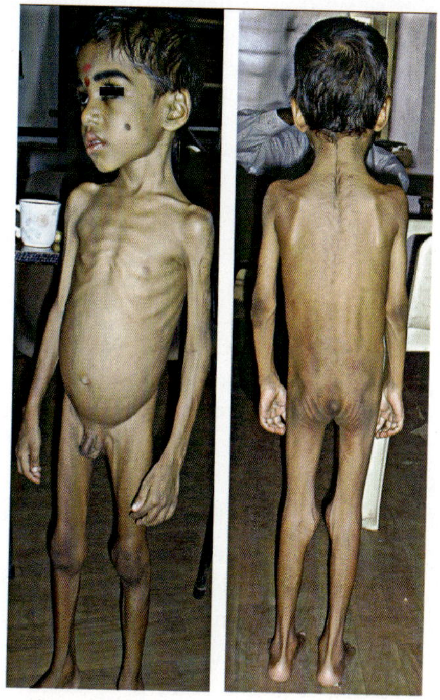

Fig.4.6 Wasting

The descriptive presentation of anthropometry must be followed by a comment on the inference as given below.

- *Normal weight, normal height and normal weight for height*: Normal nutrition.
- *Decreased weight, normal height and decreased weight for height*: Acute malnutrition.
- *Decreased weight, decreased height and normal weight for height*: Chronic malnutrition.
- *Decreased weight, decreased height and decreased weight for height*: Acute-on-chronic malnutrition (without a superadded acute event the weight should have been appropriate for height. With some acute insult the weight has further gone down acutely.)

Note: **When one simply says weight, it means weight for age. When one simply says height, it means height for age**.

Table 4.5 WHO classification of undernutrition in under-five children

	Moderate undernutrition	Severe undernutrition
Symmetrical oedema	No	Yes Oedematous malnutrition (includes kwashiorkor and marasmic kwashiorkor)
Weight for height (measure of wasting)	70–79% of expected **Wasting**	<70% of expected **Severe wasting**
Height for age (measure of stunting)	85–89% of expected **Stunting**	<85% of expected **Severe stunting**

Note: WHO now recommends Z scores: Undernutrition, stunting or wasting is moderate when Z score is <-2 standard deviation and severe when Z score is <-3 SD.

Ponderal Index

It may differentiate symmetrical and asymmetrical small-for-date babies.

PI = [Wt in grams divided by $(\text{Ht in cm})^3$] × 100. A value above 2.5 is normal. In asymmetrical (malnourished) newborns, it is less than 2. In symmetric IUGR, it is 2–2.5. PI 3 or more is over weight.

Upper Segment–Lower Segment Ratio

The upper segment–lower segment ratio may be calculated.

Lower segment = Measure from pubis to toes.

Upper segment = Height minus lower segment.

Measure from the top of pubic ramus to the toes. Top of pubic ramus is palpated and marked with the child standing and looking straight ahead. Make sure that the child does not bend forward to see the marking being made. Because as the child straightens up, the mark gets displaced from the actual site! Steel tape is advised for the measurement. Although it sounds simple, it is not easy to mark the top of pubic ramus in obese children.

Normal crown–rump length of a newborn is 35 cm, the upper segment–lower segment ratio being 1.7:1. It becomes 1:1 by 7–10 years of age. In adolescents, the upper segment–lower segment ratio is about 0.9. US/LS > normal = short lower limb. US/LS < normal = short trunk.

Upper segment remains longer than lower segment in situations where there are short limbs, like achondroplasia, rickets (because of bow legs and compression and flaring of metaphysis), and hypothyroidism (retarded growth retains infantile proportions).

Upper segment will be shorter in situations where the trunk is short, like spondylo epiphyseal dysplasias, kyphoscoliosis, mucopolysaccharidosis, etc.

Mid Parental Height

If the predicted growth curves are available, the child's height may be compared with the height curve corresponding to the mid parental height (MPH):

MPH for boys = (Father's Ht + Mother's Ht + 13 cm) divided by 2

MPH for girls = (Father's Ht + Mother's Ht – 13 cm) divided by 2

All values are taken in cm. The constant 13 is the mean difference between the heights of adult females and males.

Head Circumference

Head circumference is measured with a non-stretchable tape passing through the maximum point of occipital protuberance posteriorly and at a point just above the glabella anteriorly. However, the maximum size of head circumference is accepted instead of this conventional measurement in a child with an abnormally large or odd-shaped head.

Head circumference must be compared with that of the mother to know any familial variations. This is especially important if one finds the head circumference to be low or high in an otherwise normal child.

When the head circumference is more than expected, always measure the both parents' head circumference (if they are present at the time of examination), because benign familial megalencephaly is fairly common. If the head circumference is too small, palpate for any bony ridges along the fused sutures (may be premature craniosynostosis). Sometimes only one of the sutures may be prematurely closed, giving rise to various abnormal shapes of head (pg 83-84).

Although measurement of head circumference is in no way a threatening procedure, most children resist this measurement. If the child is trying to resist and cry, the measurement may be postponed to a later time, after finishing the essential

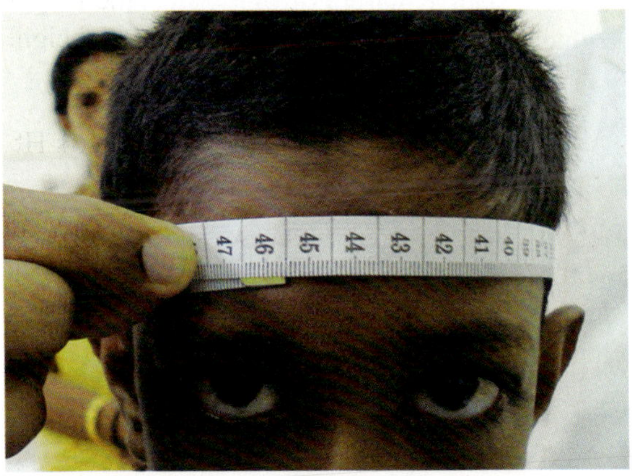

Fig.4.7 Head circumference. In case a transparent tape is available, the measurement can be easily read out from the site where the tape overlaps. However, metal tapes or fibre glass tapes, which are non stretchable are ideal though not transparent.

examinations which need a quiet and cooperative child.

Mnemonic: 2 monthly increments of (4+3+2+1+1+1)

Birth – 34 cm
2 months – 38 cm
4 months – 41 cm
6 months – 43 cm
8 months – 44 cm
10 months – 45 cm
1 year – 46 cm

Gains 2 cm in the 2nd year (48 cm) and 1 cm in the 3rd year (49 cm).

Another mnemonic is HC increases by 2 cm/month for the first 3 months, 1 cm/month for the next 3 months and 0.5 cm per month for the next 6 months. Measurement of head circumference may be inaccurate till the 3rd day of life because of moulding, etc. Hence, the baseline head circum-ference must not be measured earlier than 24 hrs of age. Also refer to the section on macrocephaly and microcephaly (p 79–80). Dine's formula for head circumference up to 1 year of age

$$= \left(\frac{\text{Length}}{2}\right) + 9.5 \pm 2.5$$

Chest Circumference

Chest circumference is measured just below the level of nipple, avoiding the breast in mid-inspiration. In a term baby, head circumference may be 2 cm more than chest circumference, and in a preterm baby the difference may be greater. They somewhat equalize by 9–12 months of age, beyond which chest circumference is normally greater than head circumference. If head circumference remains larger than chest circumference beyond 1 year of age, it may indicate malnutrition (in PEM, the brain growth is least affected); in hydrocephalus, chest circumference is relatively less because of large head. Chest circumference is usually measured up to 2–3 years of age (sometimes beyond this age in severely malnourished child).

Allowance for Prematurity

Corrected chronological age should be used for premature babies for sometime to give them the time for catch up.

Time allowance for catch-up growth:

- 18 months for head circumference
- 24 months for weight
- 40 months for height

Mid-arm Circumference (for children from 6 months to 5 years of age)

The accepted area for measurement is over the left triceps. With the arm hanging by the side, a non-stretchable tape is passed around the circumference of the arm (the tape should not be held tight enough to produce an indentation) and the measurement is noted at the midpoint of left arm, i.e., midway between acromion process and olecranon process, with arm hanging loosely by the side. Above 13.5 cm is normal, 12.5–13.5 is moderate PEM and below 12.5 is severe PEM (some consider 13.5–16 as mild malnutrition and above 16 as normal). Shakir's tape used for quick monitoring in community gives green colour if mid-arm circumference is more than 13.5 cm, yellow if between 12.5 and 13.5 cm, and red if less than 12.5.

Kanawati and McLaren's Index (1970)

Mid-arm circumference is divided by head circum-ference:

- >0.31: Normal
- 0.31–0.28: Mild PEM
- 0.28–0.25: Moderate PEM
- <0.25: Severe PEM

Skin-Fold Thickness

Skin-fold thickness need not be measured in routine clinical examination, but is required when PEM is suspected. It is measured over triceps on mid left arm hanging loosely by the side, using Harpenden's calipers. 11 mm or more is normal.

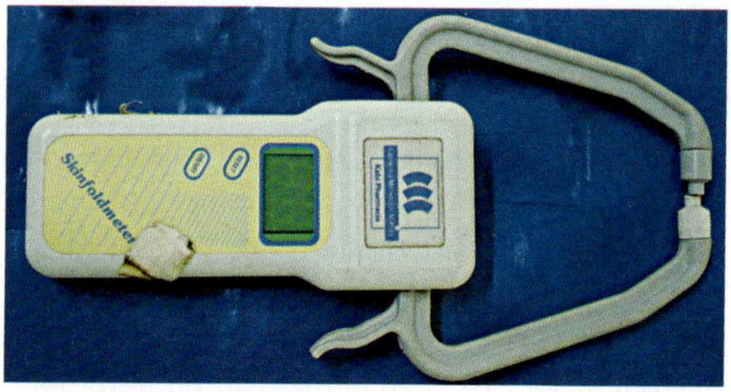

Fig.4.8 Skin-fold calipers

Arm Span

This is the distance between the middle fingers when the upper limbs are stretched across at right angle to the body. Compare it with height. Arm span may be up to 2 cm less than height in toddlers, equals height by about 7–10 years and thereafter, the arm span is slightly more than height, by about 2–3 cm in adolescents (the changes parallels the upper segment–lower segment ratio discussed above). The arm span is disproportionately more than the height in Marfan syndrome, homocystinuria, short trunk dwarfisms like spondyloepiphyseal dysplasias, etc.

Arm span > Stature (lower segment > Upper segment) is found in:

- Marfan's syndrome
- Homocystinuria
- Klinefelter's syndrome

Height > Arm span (upper segment > Lower segment) may be found in short limbed dwarfism and situations of early epiphyseal fusion like precocious puberty.

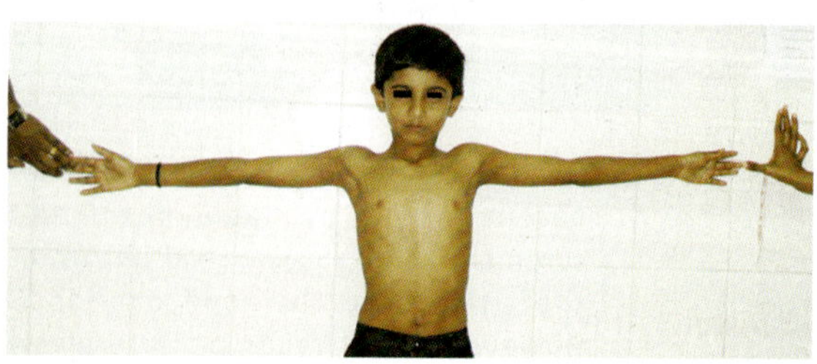

Fig.4.9 Arm span

Teeth (Primary)

(I = Incisor, M = Molar, C = Canine, P = Premolar)

Deciduous Teeth (in months) (order–**IMCM**)

Table 4.6 Primary teeth eruption and shedding

Primary teeth	Eruption	Shedding
Incisors	6–10 mo	6–9 yrs
Molars (first)	10–16 mo	10–12 yrs
Canines	16–20 mo	9–12 yrs
Molars (second)	20–30 mo	10–13 yrs
No. of primary teeth = (Age in months - 6)		

Total number of deciduous teeth is 20. The first tooth to appear is the lower central incisors.

Permanent Teeth (time of eruption in years) (order–M I P C M)

M (6)
I (7–9)
P (10–12)
C (11–12)
M_2 (13–14)
M_3 (17–22)

Table 4.7

Surface area (approx)	Wt in kg	Formula
Birth—0.2	1-5	0.05 x wt + 0.05
3 mo—0.3	6-10	0.04 x wt + 0.1
1 yr—0.45	11-20	0.03 x wt + 0.2
3 yrs—0.6	21-40	0.02 x wt + 0.4
6 yrs—0.75		
9 yrs—0.9		

Mosteller's formula for surface area = $\sqrt{\dfrac{\text{Ht (cm)} \times \text{Wt (kg)}}{3600}}$

Body Mass Index (BMI)

BMI = wt in kg divided by (height in meter)^2
Normal range for adults is between 18–25. In children, the corresponding figures may be 15–22.

Above 25 is overweight and >30 is obesity in adults; for a child, >22 may be taken as overweight; and >25 as obesity.

<15 and <13 in children indicates moderate and severe malnutrition, respectively.

BMI is traditionally used to assess body fat reserves (obesity) and not loss of body fat (PEM).

Stages of Sexual Development (SMR by Tanner)

Boys: Genital Development

- Stage 1: Preadolescent stage. The testis, scrotum and penis are of about the same size and proportion as in early childhood. *No pubic hair.*
- Stage 2: Enlargement of scrotum and testis. Skin of *scrotum reddens* and changes in texture. Little or no enlargement of penis at this stage. Scanty *lightly pigmented pubic hair*, mainly at the base of penis.
- Stage 3: *Enlargement of penis*, which occurs at first mainly in length. Further growth of testes and scrotum. Pubic hair becomes *darker and begins to curl.*
- Stage 4: Increased size of penis with growth in breadth and *enlargement of glans*. Testes and scrotum are larger; scrotal skin is darkened. Adult type of pubic hair but less in quantity, with no spread to medial surface of thighs.
- Stage 5: Genitalia is *adult in size and shape* (penile length 10 cm or more; volume of testis 20 cc or more; length of testes 4 cm or more). Pubic hair spreads to *medial thigh.*

Girls: Breast/Pubic Hair Development

- Stage 1: Preadolescent, elevation of papilla only.
- Stage 2: Breast bud stage; elevation of breast and papilla *as small mound.*

4

Enlargement of areola diameter. Scanty lightly pigmented pubic hair, mainly at labia.

- Stage 3: Further enlargement and elevation of breast and areola, with no separation contours between them. Pubic hair *becomes darker* and begins to *curl.*
- Stage 4: Projection of areola and papilla to form a *secondary mound above* the level of the breast. Adult type of pubic hair but less in quantity, no spread to medial surface of thighs.
- Stage 5: Mature stage: *Projection of nipple* only, due to recession of the aerola to the general contour of the breast. *Adult feminine triangular type* of pubic hair; spread to medial thigh is rare.

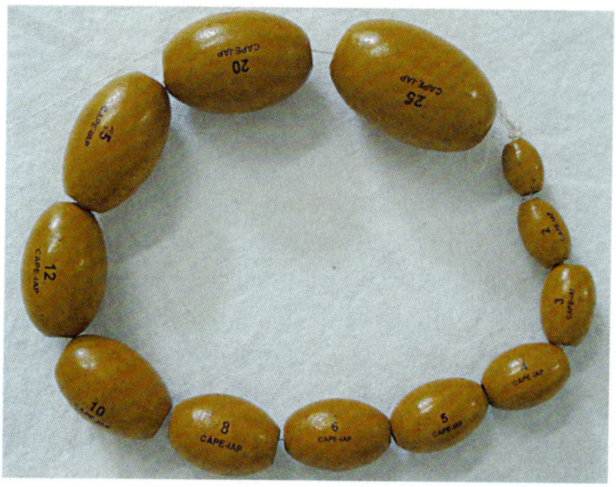

Fig.4.10 Pradder's orchidometer: There are 12 beads. Volume of each bead is marked on it (1–25 mm^3); by placing the bead side by side with the testes, one can compare the size and directly read out the volume of testes.

1½ years	I
2 years	–
3 years	+ O
4 years	□
5 years	△
6 years	◇

Fig.4.11 Copying skills

Using the Growth Charts

Age and sex specific growth charts are available nowadays that are region specific. WHO charts are used for children till the age of 5 years and the IAP charts are used thereafter till 18 years. The age must be correctly calculated from the date of birth for using the growth charts accurately. Age is plotted in completed weeks from birth until age 3 months; in completed months from 3 to 12 months; and then in completed years and months. Though a single measurement can be interpreted usefully, in practice interpreting the trends is more useful.

Plotting the weight for age

This indicator is used to assess whether a child is underweight or severely underweight, but it is not fully useful to classify a child as overweight or obese. It is important to note also that a child may be underweight either because of short length/ height (stunting) or thinness or both.

Drop a vertical line upwards from the age of the child (x- axis).

Drop a horizontal line corresponding to the weight (y- axis). (E.g. If the weight is 10.5kg plot between the lines)

Plot the intersection of these lines.

E.g. 1year old boy weighing 9 kg. Weight for age is between the 15th and the 50th centile in a centile chart or between 0 SD and -2SD in a Z score chart **(see Fig 4.11a)**

Plotting Height/ length for age

This indicator can help identify children who are stunted (short) due to prolonged undernutrition or repeated illnesses or due to systemic disorder

Weight-for-age BOYS

Birth to 2 years (percentiles)

World Health Organization

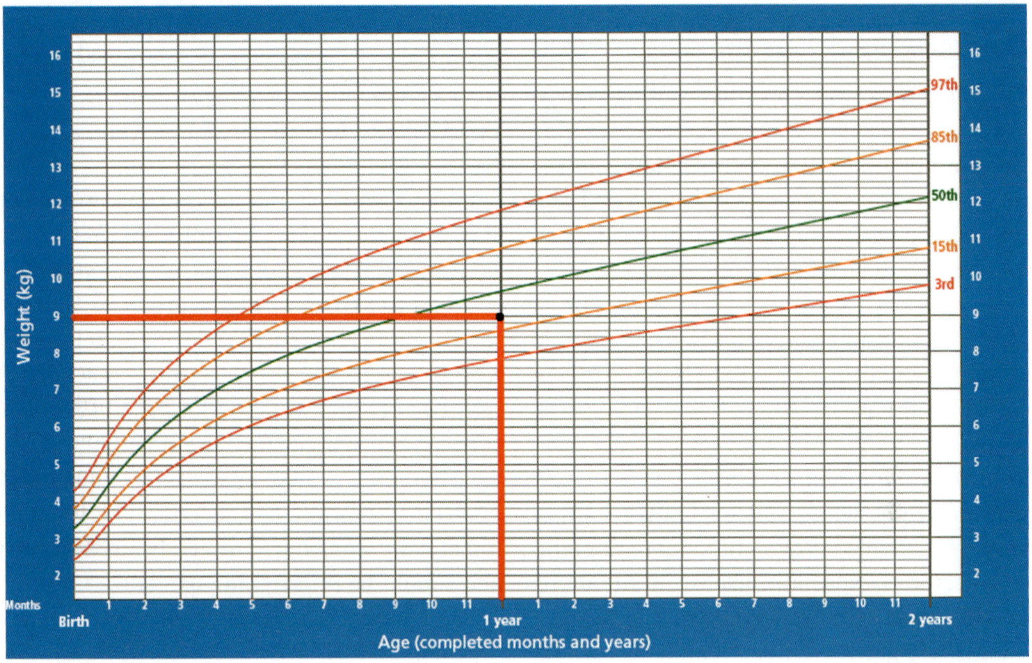

WHO Child Growth Standards

Weight-for-age BOYS

Birth to 2 years (z-scores)

World Health Organization

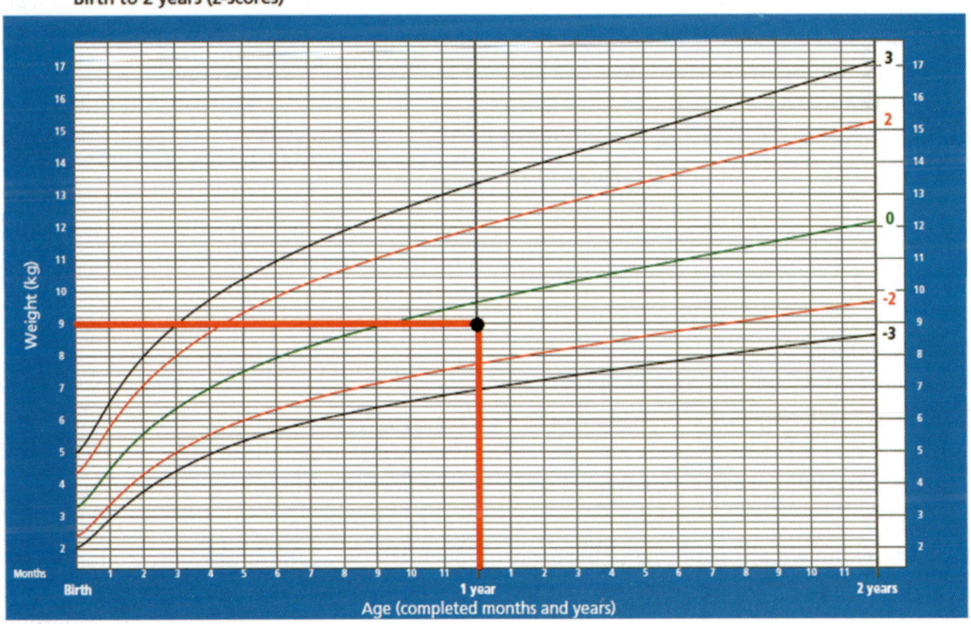

Fig.4.11a

or hormone deficiencies. Children who are tall for their age can also be identified, but tallness is rarely a problem unless it is excessive and may reflect uncommon endocrine disorders.

Drop a vertical line upwards from the age of the child.

Drop a horizontal line corresponding to the height (y-axis) (E.g. If the length is 60.5 cm, plot the point in the middle of the space between horizontal lines)

Plot the intersection of these lines.

E.g. 9-month-old baby girl with a length of 70 cm is plotted. **(see Fig. 4.11b)**

Plotting Weight for Height/ length

Weight-for-height/ length reflects body weight in proportion to attained growth in length or height. This indicator is especially useful in situations where children's ages are unknown (e.g. refugee situations). Weight-for- height/ length charts help identify children with low weight-for-height who may be wasted or severely wasted. Wasting is usually caused by a recent illness or food shortage that has caused acute and severe weight loss, although chronic undernutrition or illness can also cause this condition. These charts also help identify children with high weight-for-height/length who may be at risk of becoming overweight or obese. In these charts height/ length is given in the x -axis and weight in the y axis.

Plot length or height on a vertical line. It will be necessary to round the measurement to the nearest whole centimetre.

Plot weight as precisely as possible given the spacing of lines on the chart.

Plot the intersection of these lines.

E.g. A child of 80 cm height has a weight of 9kg. **(see Fig. 4.11c)**

In IAP charts the weight for height charts are not discretely available. To calculate the weight for height in IAP charts, drop a perpendicular from the point where the actual height of the child meets the 50th centile line for height. The point where this line meets the 50th centile line for weight is the expected weight for height obtained by dropping a horizontal line to the y-axis. So graphically on IAP charts we can only know whether the child has the actual expected weight for height or not and not quantify the variation from the median.

E.g. A 7 year old boy has a height of 125cm and he weighs 20 kg. The expected weight for height is 24 kg as shown in **Fig. 4.11d**

If a child has oedema of both feet, fluid retention increases the child's weight, masking what may be very low weight. Plot this child's weight-for-age and weight-for-length/height, but mark clearly on the growth charts (close to the plotted point) that the child has oedema. This child is automatically considered severely undernourished and should be referred for specialized care.

Plotting for BMI

BMI-for-age is an indicator that is especially useful for screening for overweight and obesity.

E.g. 10 year old child weighing 35 kg has a height of 135 cm and BMI of 19.2. as shown in **Fig. 4.11e** he is overweight.

What are percentile or z scores on charts?

The curved lines printed on the growth charts will help you interpret the plotted points that represent a child's growth status. The line labeled 50th on centile charts and 0 on z- score charts represents the median. The other curved lines are the percentile lines or z-score lines,which indicate distance from the median.

How to find the expected weight or height or BMI?

The expected height or weight (50th centile) can be obtained by dropping a line vertically from the x axis corresponding to the age of the child till it meets the 50th centile line. Drop a horizontal from that point to the y- axis.

E.g. Expected weight for a 3 ½ year old boy is 15.4 Kg **(Fig.4.11f)**

Length-for-age GIRLS

Birth to 2 years (percentiles)

World Health Organization

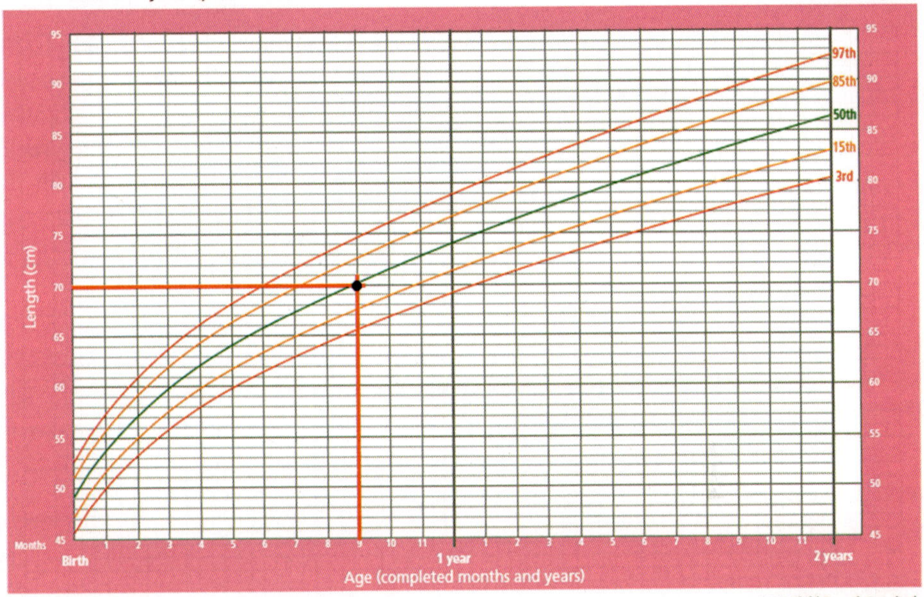

WHO Child Growth Standards

Length-for-age GIRLS

Birth to 2 years (z-scores)

World Health Organization

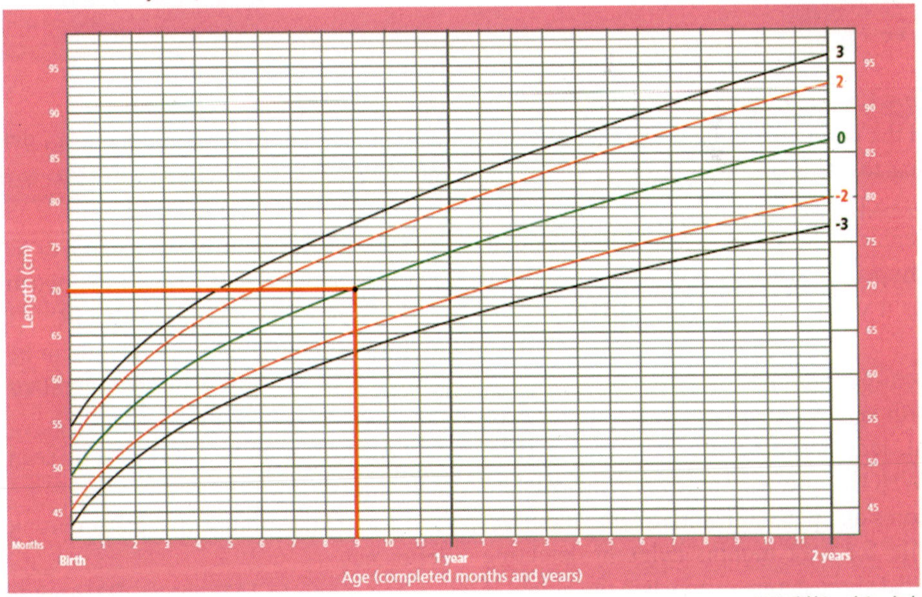

WHO Child Growth Standards

Fig.4.11b

4

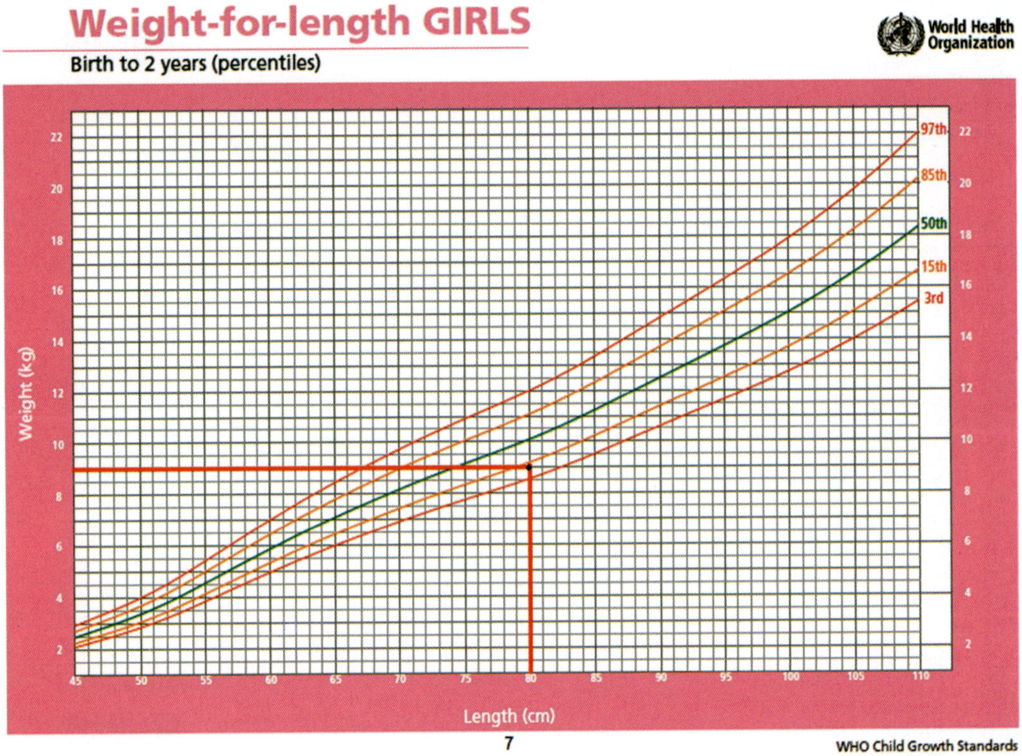

Fig.4.11c

How to find the height age, weight age?

First find the point where the horizontal line corresponding to the actual weight or height of the child intersects the 50th centile curve. Now drop a perpendicular to the x axis (age), from this point.

E.g. Expected age of a boy with a height of 105 cm is 4 years 3months. **(Fig. 4.11g)**

Growth velocity charts

The growth velocity charts are available for each of weight, length and head circumference **(Fig. 4.11h)**. (WHO has provided only the velocity tables with z scores and percentiles). Growth velocity < 25th centile for 6-12 months helps in detecting pathological short stature even when the height is normal. To comment on the growth velocity at least 3 recordings 6 months apart must be there.

How to interpret the charts?

Weight and height between the 3rd to 97th centile on IAP charts or 5th to 95th on WHO charts- child growing well and normally.

Low weight for age (<3rd centile or below -2 z score) is underweight seen in malnutrition, systemic diseases, syndromic or IUGR.

Low height for age (<3rd centile or below -2 z score) is short stature (pathological or normal variants).

Low weight for height is wasting seen in acute malnutrition.

Low BMI is thinness seen in chronic energy deficiency.

According to IAP charts, BMI adult equivalent of 23 is overweight and BMI adult equivalent of 27 is obesity.

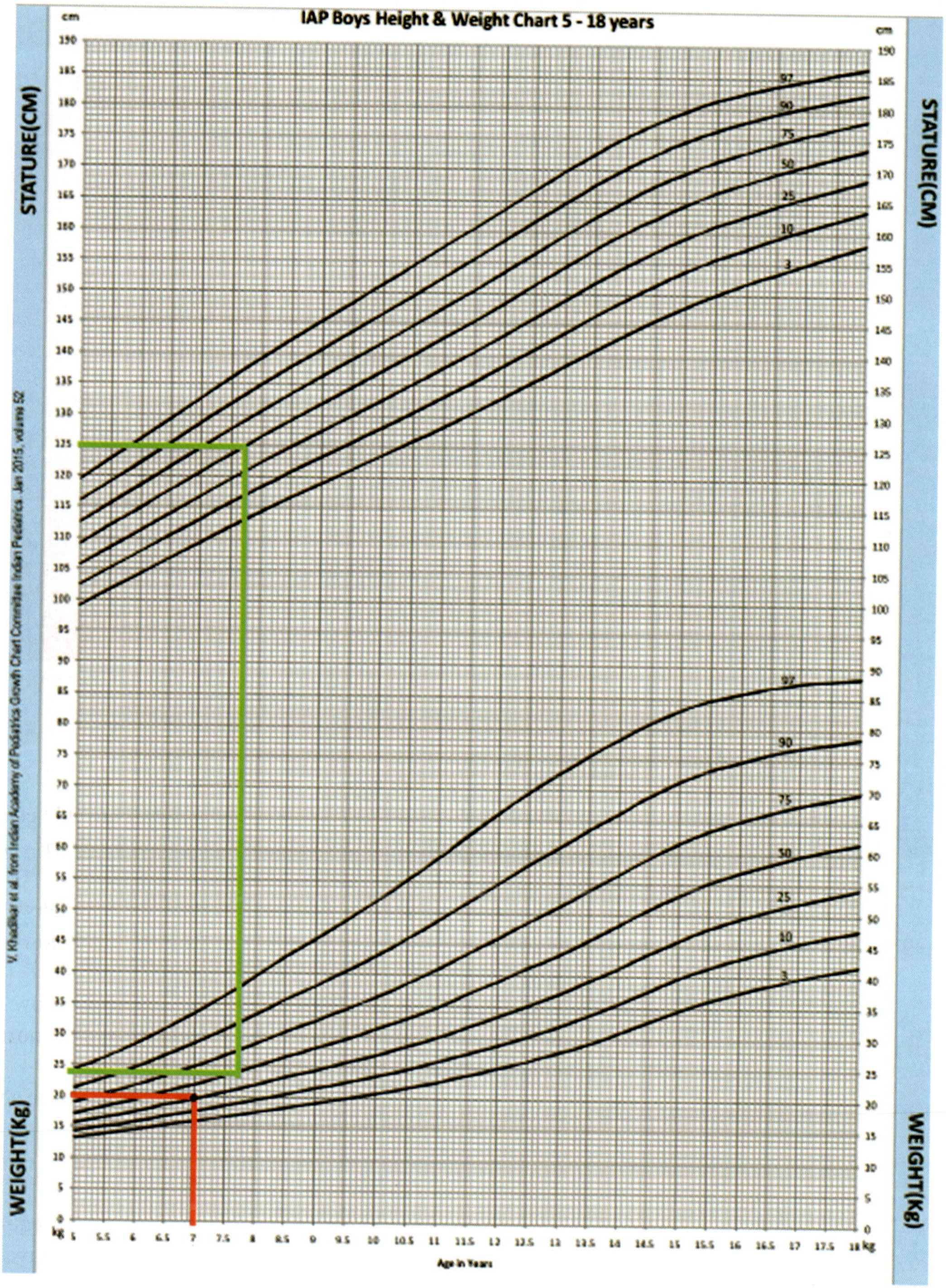
IAP Boys Height & Weight Chart 5 - 18 years
STATURE(CM)
WEIGHT(Kg)
V. Khadilkar et al. from Indian Academy of Pediatrics Growth Chart Committee Indian Pediatrics, Jan 2015, volume 52
Age in Years
97
90
75
50
25
10
3

Fig.4.11d

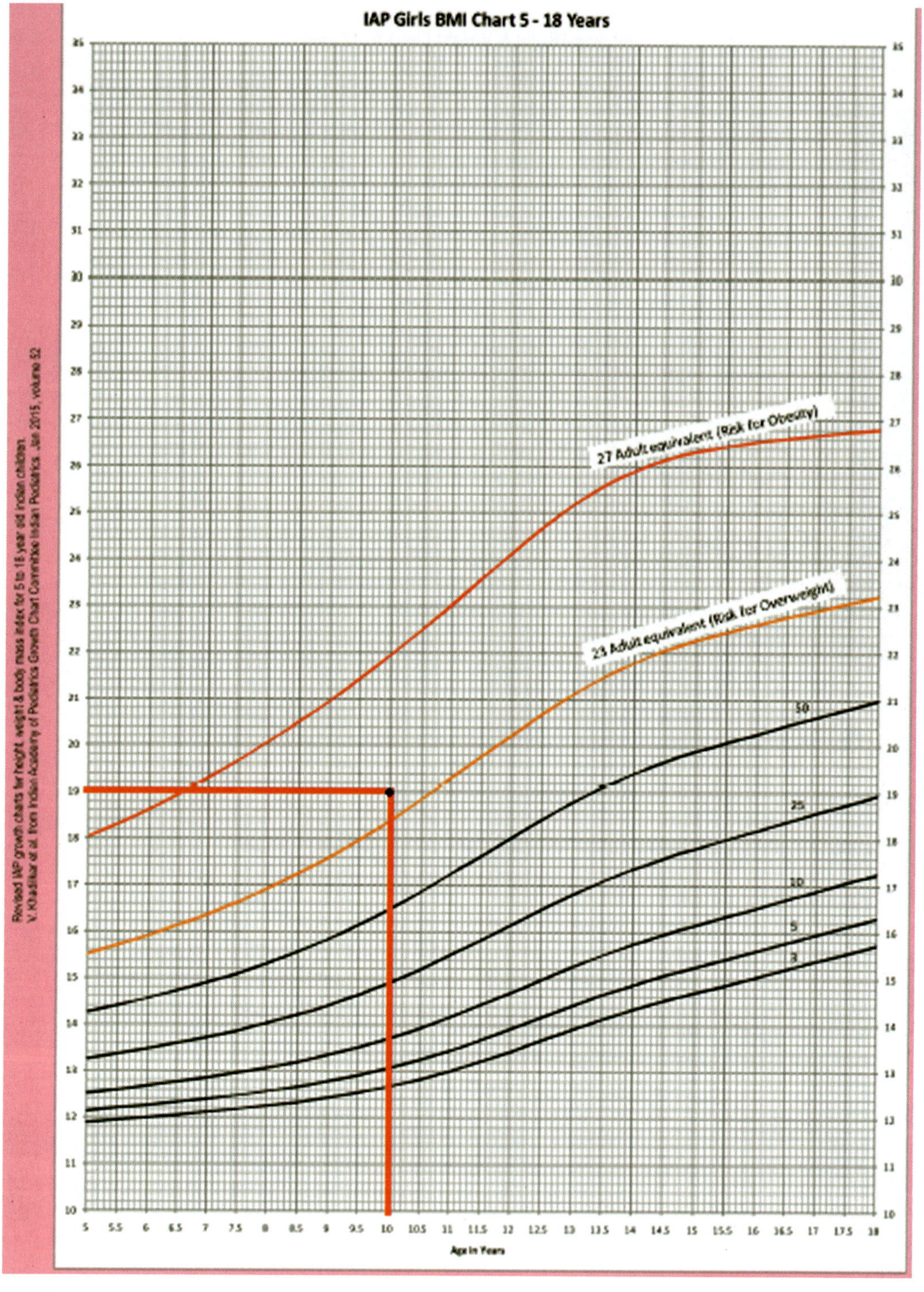
IAP Girls BMI Chart 5 - 18 Years
Revised IAP growth charts for height, weight & body mass index for 5 to 18 year old Indian children.
V. Khadilkar et al. from Indian Academy of Pediatrics Growth Chart Committee Indian Pediatrics, Jan 2015, volume 52
27 Adult equivalent (Risk for Obesity)
23 Adult equivalent (Risk for Overweight)
50
25
10
5
3
Age in Years

Fig.4.11e

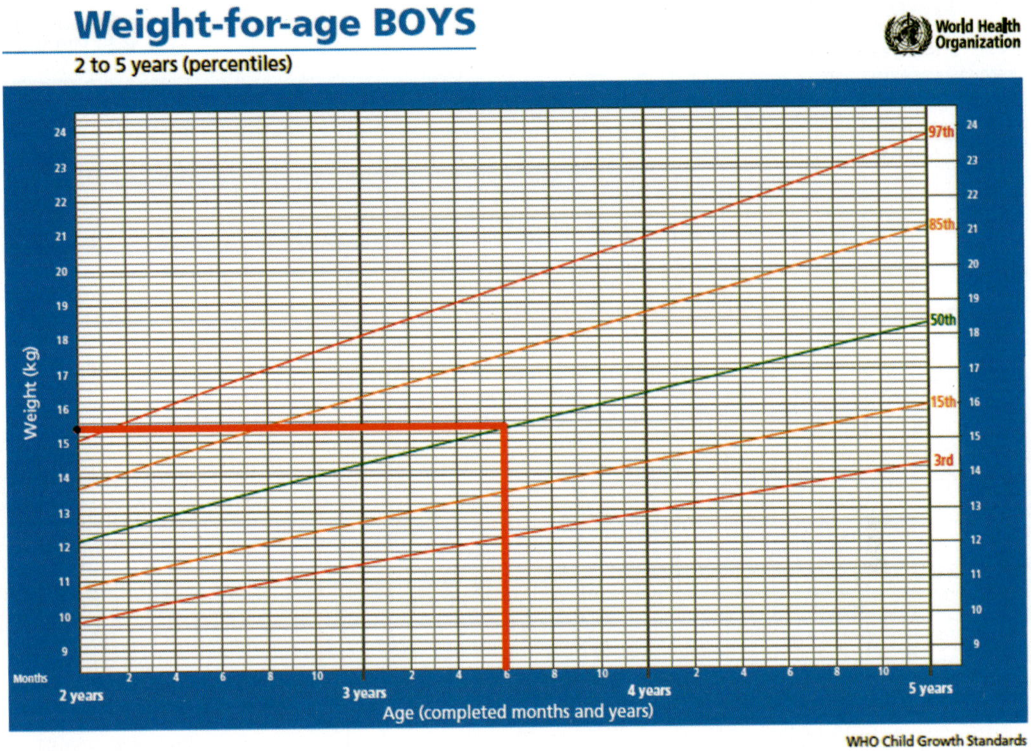

Fig.4.11f

Weight is < 3rd centile but height is normal or weight for height is < 3rd centile (weight age < height age)- a/c malnutrition.

How to go about if short stature is detected?

When short stature is detected on the growth charts, immediately calculate the Mid- Parental height (MPH= (Father's height+ Mother's height)/ 2 + 6.5 cm for boy or -6.5 cm for girl) and plot it on the graph at age 18 years with 6 cm above and below that height (target centiles). Bone age (BA) assessment using Gruelich & Pyle Atlas or Tanner Whitehouse Method, developmental age (DA) assessment and sexual maturity rating (SMR) using the tanner staging, US:LS ratio are the next data needed for interpretation. In all cases of short stature bone age is < chronological age (CA) except FSS and Precocious puberty. In addition a thorough clinical examination is needed especially to see for any dysmorphisms.

If the child's height is falling in between the target height (MPH) centiles, and the MPH is also below the 3rd centile, and the trend is parallel to the normal growth curve then it is likely to be familial short stature. Also, in case of familial short stature, bone age will be same as the chronological age.

If the MPH is normal then it may likely be, due to CDGP (if there is a history of parental delay in secondary sexual characteristics and a bone age delay not more than 2-3 years, growth velocity normal) or may be an endocrine abnormality (BA delayed by more than 2-3 years). However CDGP being a diagnosis of exclusion, these group of children need close follow up and appropriate investigations during the period of follow up.

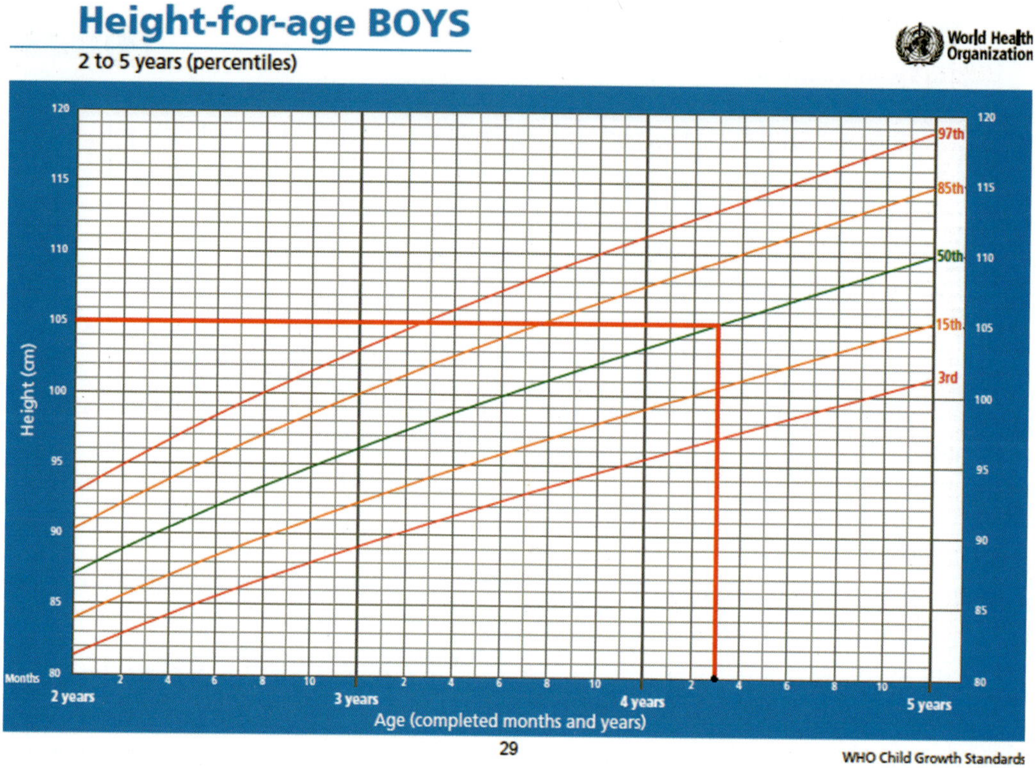

Fig.4.11g

Familial short stature	CDGP	Pathological short stature
Height <3rd centile	Height <3rd centile	Height <3rd centile
Height within MPH	Height < MPH	Height <MPH
HA<BA=CA	BA= HA<CA	BA<HA<CA

Note :

In case of pathological short stature, maximum bone age delay is seen in untreated severe hypothyroidism, then in Growth Hormone Deficiency.

CDGP:Constitutional delay in growth & puberty.

ASSESSMENT OF DEVELOPMENT

The usual tools for the assessment of development include the following:

- Rattle, bell
- Torch
- Balls
- Toys including wheeled toys (child can walk backwards and sidewise pulling on to the wheeled toy); dangling red toy
- Blocks
- Pellets (or small rounded candies, to test pincer grasp)
- Pencil and paper (to try drawing skills of child)
- Picture book of colours, shapes, animals and birds
- Bottle (to test if child can put in beads into it)

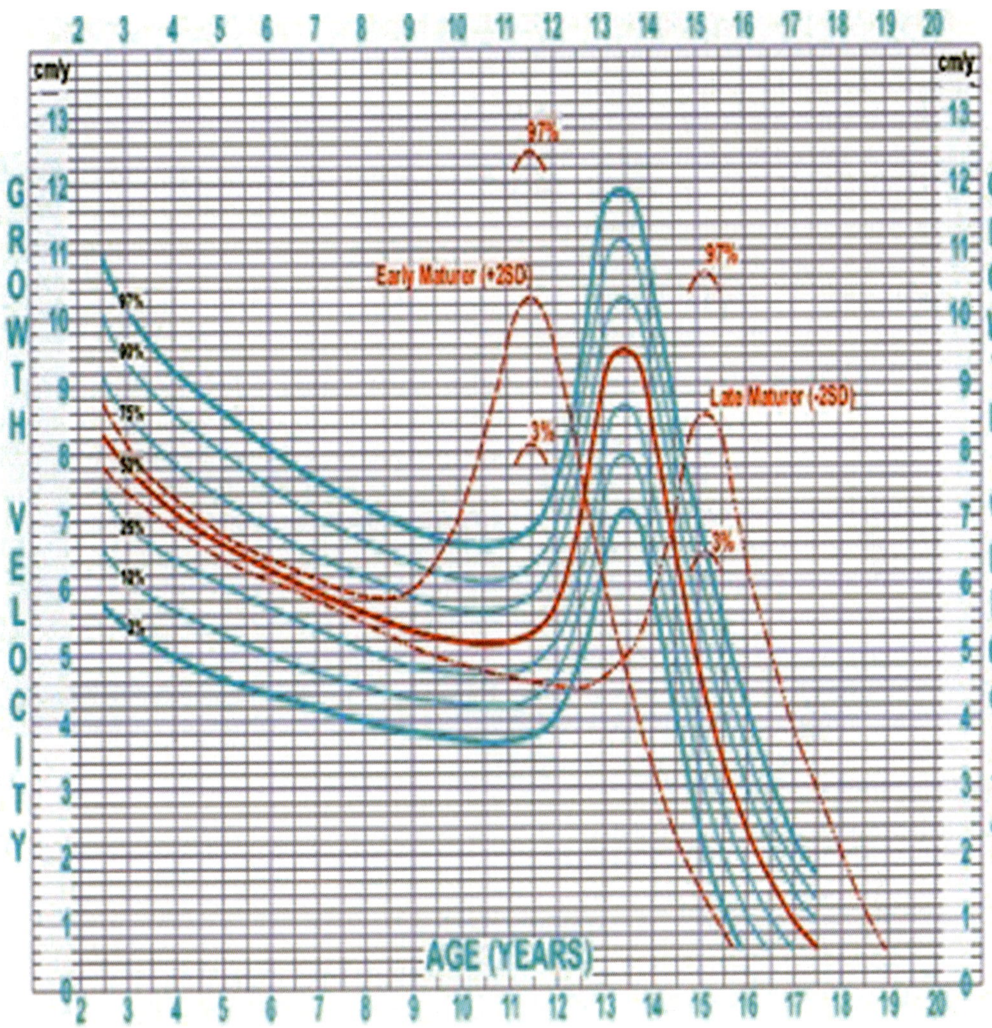

Fig.4.11h

- Form-board puzzle with removable geometric shapes (to test the child's ability to match the shapes and also to assess his fine motor skills to do so)
- Cup and spoon (to observe refinement of the child's use of these)
- A small mirror (child enjoying self image in mirror).

Each domain of development is not a watertight compartment, but are overlapping ones. For example, dressing and undressing is a fine motor skill considering the fineness of movements involved, but at the same time is a social milestone considering its implications in social development.

Addition like 1+2 may be taken as an adaptive development, as it involves adaptive development of the brain.

Fine motor (adaptive) milestones are the ones requiring skilled hand movements, hand–eye coordination, hand–mouth coordination, etc.

Variant motor development is a recognized entity. For example, some normal children may never crawl but move around by rolling, paddling or bottom shuffling. One must take extra care to meticulously look for subtle abnormalities like hypotonia, subtle cerebral palsy, etc, before committing it as a variant of normal development (because some of these variants do indicate abnormalities). For example, if a child stands up without sitting when pulled to sit, it could mean hypertonia of lower limbs and hence may be a case of CP.

Given below are selected milestones, which may be of use to the student. The best way to learn development is to observe many children of each age group. If you keep the copy of milestones in your bedroom, it helps to remember them better by sheer repetition of reading it.

Rule of thumb: A child who has attained social smile by completion of 2 months, head control by 4 months, sitting by 8 months and standing by 12 months may be taken as grossly normal. Make sure that the child sees, hears and listens. This helps in a rapid assessment of development in a case where retardation of development is not expected so that the student can spend more time on examination of relevant system.

2 Months

Gross motor: Holds the head in the plane of rest of the body when held in ventral suspension (i.e., child lifted in prone position with examiner's hand on the abdomen). In prone position in bed, the child lifts chin momentarily.

Fine motor: Eyes follow objects (e.g., diffuse light) to 180° (anything above 90° is accepted as normal).

Social smile (smile reciprocating to social contact): This is not the spontaneous smile that even a newborn may have. May stop crying when picked up to be nursed. Watches mother when spoken to, and may smile.

Language: Responds to sounds by startle or quietening to a smooth voice.

3 Months

Gross motor: In ventral suspension, lifts head above the plane of the body. Head control starts by 3 months but is fully developed only by 5 months (i.e., at 3 months, the head is held up when supported in sitting position, but bobs forwards). In prone position, the chin is lifted off the couch.

Fine motor: Grasp reflex ("passive grasp") disappears and hand is open most of the time (both are prerequisites for development of fine hand movements). Hand regard (watches movements of own hands intently: involves hand eye coordination and hence a fine motor milestone). Reaches and misses objects kept in midline.

Social: Shows interest in red dangling toy held in midline. Enjoys social contact.

Language: Babbles when spoken to. Makes sounds ahh, etc, coos, laughs, aloud.

4 Months

Gross motor: Remain on forearm support if put in prone position, lifting the upper part of the body off the bed. When pulled to sitting position, there is just an initial head lag, otherwise flexes the head beyond the plane of the body. Rolls over by 5 months (first from prone to supine position and then supine to prone, may be a month later).

Fine motor: Tries to reach objects but overshoots. Grasps objects if placed in hand and brings them to mouth. Grasp is generally with the ulnar side (ulnar grasp). Reaches for dangling red toy with both hands (bidextrous approach). Hands can come together in midline.

Social: Holds rattle when placed in hand and regards it. Laughs aloud. Excited at the sight of food.

Language: Vocalizes when spoken to. Laughs aloud.

6 Months

Gross motor: Sitting with support (back rounded). In prone position, tries to keep chest off the couch with the weight supported on hands.
Fine motor: Reach for an object with one hand (unidextrous approach). Transfers objects from hand to hand. Plays with feet, takes feet to mouth.
Social: Enjoys watching own image in mirror. Shows displeasure when toy pulled off. Stranger anxiety.
Language: Vocalizes, babbles, gaga, mama, etc (without meaning mother).

8 Months

Gross motor: Sits without support. Crawling.
Fine motor: Radial grasp starts to develop. Turns to sound above the level of ear.

9–10 Months

Gross motor: Takes a few steps with one hand held. Pulls to standing and cruises holding on to furniture by 10 months. Creeps by 10 months (remember crawling comes before creeping—as a mnemonic see the underlined letters, "a" comes first and then "e" in the alphabet! Crawl comes first).
Fine motor: Pincer grasp with ulnar support, the so-called assisted pincer grasp. Uncovers hidden toy (e.g., removes a sheet covering a toy to discover the toy).
Social: Enjoys peek-a-boo game. Waves bye bye. Stops in response to "no." Responds to name.
Language: Monosyllable sounds. Starts to understand spoken speech.

12 Months (1 year)

Gross motor: Stands without support and takes a few steps. Walks "like a bear." Starts to walk by 1 year and walks well by 15 months. At 15 months, they can walk backwards holding onto a thread to move a movable toy.
Fine motor: Unassisted pincer grasp (without ulnar support). Releases objects on request. Uses objects in hand predominantly for playing, not for mouthing. Holds blocks on each hand and bang them together.
Social: Indicates his wants, mainly by pointing. Plays peek-a-boo. Kisses the parent on request. Makes postural adjustments for dressing.
Language: Speaks two words in addition to da da, mummy.

15 Months

Gross motor: Walks well (broad based), walks backwards or sidewise pulling a toy. May crawl upstairs.
Fine motor: Tower of 2–3 cubes. Can drink from a cup with help.
Social: Starts imitating mother. Indicates needs by pointing.
Language: Adds two or three words to the vocabulary to what was there at 1 year. Uses own jargon.

18 Months

Gross motor: Runs crudely; walks upstairs with one hand held. Handedness develops by 1½ years or later but not earlier.
Fine motor: Feeds self from cup, scribbles and imitates vertical strokes. Makes a tower of 3–4 cubes. Turns pages of a book, 2–3 at a time.
Social: Mimics action of others. Dry by day. Calls mother when he wants potty. Points to three parts of body on request.
Language: Vocabulary of 10 words. Can name one part of body.

2 Years

Gross motor: Runs well. Climbs stairs one step at a time (climbs next step only after getting two feet to the previous step). Kicks ball without losing balance.
Fine motor: Turns the pages of book one at a time. Puts on shirt, pants, etc. Matches objects to pictures (e.g., a pen in hand and pen in the picture). Can build a tower of six cubes. Imitates

horizontal strokes (vertical strokes are imitated earlier, by 1½ years; imagine writing L or T, the first stroke is vertical and the next is horizontal).

Social: Points to 4 parts of body on request. Listens to stories.

Language: Starts saying 3-word simple sentences and uses pronouns. By 2½ years, refers to self as "I" and knows full name.

3 Years

Gross motor: Rides tricycle (3 wheel cycle at 3 years!). Goes upstairs one feet per step (i.e., alternating steps). Stands on one foot. Jumps.

Fine motor: Dressing and undressing with some help. Can do buttoning. Tower of nine cubes. Draws a man with three parts (three parts at three years!). Imitates a circle. Can imitate a tower of nine cubes.

Social: Dry by night. Parallel play.

Language: Knows age and sex. Counts up to 10. Vocabulary of about 250 words.

4 Years

Gross motor: Walks up and down stairs by alternating feet. Hops on one foot. Throws ball overhead.

Fine motor: Draws a man with 3–4 parts besides head. Imitates a cross.

Language: Tells a story. Knows three colours.

Social: Gives a coherent account of recent experience and events. Washes face, brushes teeth. Role play. May use toilet by self.

5 Years

Gross motor: Skips.

Fine motor (adaptive): Draws a man with head, neck and limbs. Draws triangle by imitating/copying. A child can draw a diamond at 6 years and a cylinder at 9 years.

Language: Gives descriptive comments on picture books. Additions within five (e.g., 1+2).

Social: Dresses unassisted. Domestic role play.

Drawing and Tower of Cubes

15 months: Makes a tower of two cubes.

18 months: Makes a tower of 3–4 cubes. Scribbles vertical strokes.

24 months: Makes a tower of 6 cubes. Scribbles horizontal strokes.

30 months: Makes a tower of 9 cubes (note the mnemonic relation of 3–6–9). Copies circular strokes.

36 months: Makes a tower of 10 cubes. Copies cross, circle.

48 months: Copies square. Builds gate or other forms with cubes.

60 months: Copies a triangle.

72 months: Copies diamond.

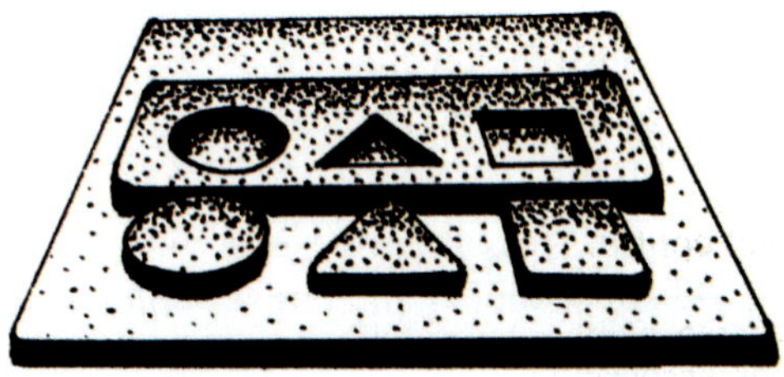

Fig.4.12 Form board

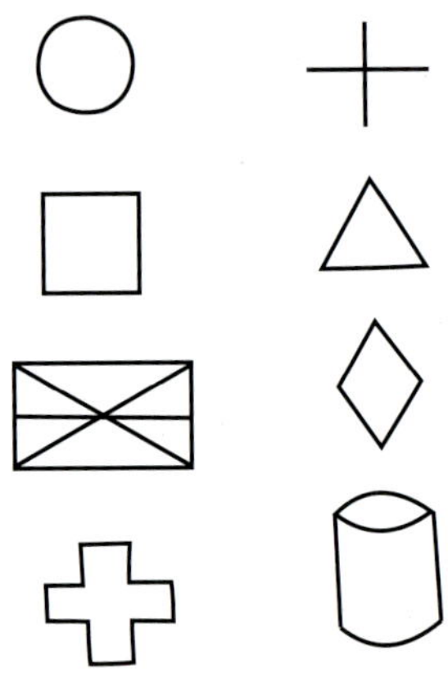

Fig.4.13 Geometric shapes

Bladder Control

1½ years: Dry by day

3 years: Dry by night (a small percentage may

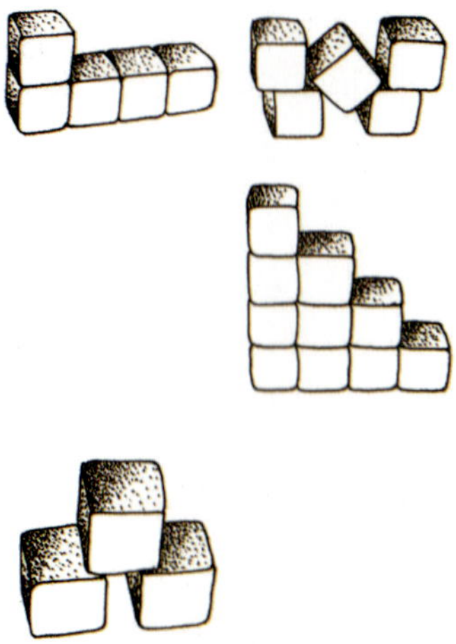

Fig.4.14 Tower & shapes using blocks *(Drawing by Dr Binoy Stephen)*

continue to bedwet without any organic pathology).

Bowel control is achieved by about 1½ years.

> Example of how to state summary of development assessment in a child with delay: Global development delay, with motor delay more pronounced. Gross motor age is 6 months, fine motor age is 4 months, social and language age around 9 months. His hearing and vision appear grossly normal.

DQ AND IQ

Child may be assigned a development quotient after clinical assessment of development in children with development delay. Developmental quotient = (Development age in any of the domains divided by chronological age) × 100. A DQ above 85 is normal

Intelligence is related to developments in various domains, but it is not the same as development. Intelligence is the ability to understand and reason out, not just performing the given tasks. One needs intelligence to understand and perform a given task, but intelligence means more than that.

The language and adaptive abilities most closely correlate with the cognitive development and future intelligence. Gross motor skills correlate least with future intelligence. Formal assessment of IQ is not feasible in children <3 years and hence DQ may be considered synonymous with IQ in young children.

Intelligence quotient (IQ) is (mental age ÷ chronological age) × 100.

- IQ 85 and above is normal.
- 70–85: Borderline MR (vulnerable to educational problems). "Mental backwardness."
- 50–70: Mild MR (educable; with special attention in classes they can attain academic skills of middle school, i.e., class 5–7).
- 35–50: Moderate MR (trainable in workshop setting under monitoring; they can take care of their own self; communication skills are reasonable to function in the society).
- 20–35: Severe MR (trainable for self-care skills).
- <20: Profound MR (needs custodian care).

Formal IQ assessments generally do not consider abilities such as perceptual, musical, practical, creative, etc and thus formally assessed IQ has got limitations in prediction of future performance of the child in society.

NUTRITION

Here, the nutritional values of commonly used foods are listed for the student to make use of in calculation of adequacy of nutrition. The values given are not exact, but a good approximation for the student to remember. Exact values are unimportant (except in research). After all, from the history, we do not get the exact amount consumed by the child.

Table 4.8 Calorie and protein content of food items

Food item	Quantity	Calorie	Protein
Cow's milk (without sugar)	Small glass (200 mL)	130	6
Cooked rice (see note below)	1 cup (150 cc)	175	4
Uppuma (contains oil, nuts, etc; so more calorie and protein)	1 cup (150 cc)	250	6
One egg/one ounce fish/meat	1 ounce, may be 8–10 small pieces	80	6
Dosa/idli/chappati/1 slice bread/ 2 small poori/2 small vadai/coffee or tea 1 glass	All are of large size unless specified otherwise	70	2
Sugar/jaggery/biscuit Fats (ghee/butter/oil)	1 tsp or 1 biscuit 1 tsp	20 40	0 (biscuit 0.5) 0
2 plantains/1 banana		100	1
Cerelac/ragi/nestum	6 teaspoons	100	2
Formula milk (for infants)	30 mL (1 ounce)	20	0.5

Food Item (100 g, uncooked)

Table 4.9 Calorie and protein content of food items

Cereals (deficient in lysine)	Calories 350; protein 7 g (rice and ragi)/11 g (wheat and maize)
Pulses (deficient in methionine thus best used in combination with a cereal, e.g., dosai)	350 calories, 20–24 g protein (soya bean 430 calories and 43 g protein)
Roots and tubers (e.g., tapioca, potato)	100 calories; protein not significant
Vegetables: Green leafy vegetables and others (brinjal, ladies finger, etc)	Negligible calories and proteins; rich in calcium, iron, B complex and beta carotene
Fruits	Protein not significant. Calories around 50 only (except jack fruit and banana), because of high water content. Gives fibre, vitamin C. Yellow ones like papaya, mango, etc, give beta carotene (vit A)
Nuts (cashew nut, coconut, ground nut, etc)	550 calories and 20–24 g protein (except coconut, which contains only insignificant amounts of protein)
Meats (fish, beef, mutton, chicken, etc)	350 calories and 20–24 g protein; calories will be less if it is "low fat fraction" or meat contains lot of water
Milk (100 mL)	Calories 67 calories; protein 3.5 g (1.1 for human milk) Some selected LBW formulae contain 80 calories

Note: Proteins and carbohydrates give 4 calories per gram (400/100 g); thus 100 g glucose will give 400 calories; however, this is not true with rice or meat; in reality, the food items contain non-digestible parts like fibre or husk, etc, and hence the actual calories obtainable is a little less, like 350 cal/100 g. This calorie is applicable to uncooked weight. For example, when rice is cooked, it increases its volume by three times. So, 1 cup cooked rice (150 mL) will contain the dry weight equivalent of 50 g rice only; so it can give at the most 200 (50 × 4) calories; giving allowance for the non-digestible parts, one has to settle for a little less, about 175 calories. In contrast, potato does not swell up to increase in volume when cooked.

Table 4.10 ICMR and bedside calculation for various ages

Age group	ICMR		Bedside calculation
	Calorie	**Protein**	
0–12 mo	110 cal/kg*	2 g/kg*	Up to 1 yr: 100 cal/kg*
1–3 yrs	1240	22	Above 1 yr: 1000 +
4–6 yrs	1690	29	(100 calories for each year of age above
7–10 yrs	1950	35	1 year; e.g.,: calories for 3-year-old
Adolescents			child is 1000+200)
Male	2450	43	
Female	2060		

*Expected weight for age.
ICMR gives ideal requirement for the age; formula for bedside calculation gives the minimum requirement for the age.

Table 4.11 Revised ICMR recommendation 2020

	Energy(kcal/day)(EAR)	Protein (g/day)
Infants 0–6 months (Adequate Intake)	530	8
Infants 6–12 months	660	10.5
Children 1–3years	1110	12.5
Children 4–6years	1360	16
Children 7–9years	1700	23
Boys 10–12years	2220	32
Girls 10–12 years	2060	33
Boys 13–15years	2860	45
Girls 13–15 years	2400	43
Boys 16–18years	3320	55
Girls 16–18 years	2500	46
Adult Male (sedentary/moderate/heavy work)	2110/2710/3470	54
Adult Female (sedentary/moderate/heavy work)	1660/2130/2720	46
Pregnancy	+350	+9.5 (2nd trimester)
		+22 (3rd trimester)
Lactation	+600 (0–6 months)	+17 (0–6 months)
	+520 (7–12 months)	+13 (7–12 months)

There is no RDA for energy, EAR (Estimated Average Requirement) for energy is equivalent to Estimated Energy Requirement.
Source: Indian Council of Medical Research (ICMR), National institute of Nutrition (NIN); 2020.

CHAPTER 5

Disorders of Growth, Development and Nutrition: Case Sheet Formats

PROTEIN ENERGY MALNUTRITION (SEVERE ACUTE MALNUTRITION)

Diagnosis: Wt. for length Z score less than – 3 SD or mid arm circumference less than 11.5 cm or bilateral nutritional pedal edema.

1. Age: Classical age of Kwashiorkor is 1–4 years (taken off breast and replaced with cereals without milk protein source).
2. Sex: In families where female is not a preferred child, there may be an ill-nourished female baby and a well-nourished male sibling.
3. Presenting complaints: Usual complaints are vomiting, loose stools (these may have precipitated SAM in borderline cases; diarrhoea is common in SAM because of villus atrophy and decreased enzymes), abdominal distension, steatorrhea (sticky bulky stools), pica, decreased activity, feeding problems, oedema, failure to gain weight, etc.
4. Onset, duration and progress (history of present illness): In all cases of SAM, inquire about/look for other deficiencies: Vit A (visual problems like poor night vision, photophobia, Bitot's spots, etc); Vit D (changes suggestive of rickets); Vit K (bleeding); Vit B_{12} (unsteady gait); Zinc (alopecia, acrodermatitis enteropathica); Copper (hypopigmentation of hair/skin).

   In case of SAM with seizure, consider hypo-glycaemia.

   SAM may not be nutritional. So ask for history suggestive of cardiac failure (suck rest cycle, effort intolerence); renal tubular acidosis, chronic renal failure and diabetes mellitus present with polyuria and polydypsia, etc.
5. Past history:
   - Measles and whooping cough precipitate acute severe malnutrition in borderline cases; vomiting and diarrhoea (precipitate malnutrition); chronic infections like tuberculosis.
   - Inquire whether child has been a beneficiary of any national nutrition programs.
   - Treatment history may be elicited, as many SAM children may have underlying illnesses contributing to failure to grow. Inquire about contact with diseases like TB.
6. Antenatal, natal, postnatal:
   - Maternal malnutrition, mother working till term, short interval between pregnancies (mother may not have recouped her nutritional status), poor weight gain during pregnancy, etc may be inquired into. Primi mothers may be less equipped with regard to proper feeding practices.
   - LBW babies and poor feeding may contribute to postnatal malnutrition.
7. Immunization: Lapses are likely; parents who are unaware of proper feeding practices are also likely to be unaware of standard immunization practices.
8. Development:
   Development delay is expected in severe malnutrition. The delay is thought to catch up as the nutritional impairment is corrected; though the current concept is that some subtle delays

do persist. The postgraduate students are advised to read about this.

9. Dietary history:
   Assess whether breastfeeding is adequate (whether the child passes urine 6–8 times, sleeps well after feeds). In case of formula/cow's milk feeds, specifically inquire about the dilution. Specifically ask about complimentary feeding. Kwashiorkor is precipitated by abrupt stoppage of milk feeds, followed by substitution with carbohydrate rich diet; hence specifically try to elicit this history. Must calculate calorie and protein gap. Also must comment on the intake of dietary items that supply micronutrients.
10. Family & social history: Social factors in SAM: poverty, ignorance, food fads, cultural beliefs, male preference in nutrition (to be suspected when only the female children in family becomes severely malnourished). Other contributors to SAM are working mother, uneducated parents, closely spaced pregnancy, etc.
11. General examination:
   a) General comment:
      - Underweight (<60% of expected when measured), skin and bone appearance with no oedema in marasmus. Oedematous, apathetic, lethargic child with poor apetite who is grossly underweight (<80% of expected although oedematous) and has skin changes in Kwashiorkor.
   b) Vital signs:
      - Pulse rate could be decreased (low basal metabolic rate) or increased (cardiac failure due to anaemia, beriberi).
      - BP is likely to be in the lower range.
      - Respiratory rate could be decreased (low basal metabolic rate) or increased due to respiratory infection or acidosis (infection and starvation).
      - Hypothermia (or in case of infections, fever) are possible. It is possible to have serious infections with the child in hypothermia in case of severe SAM.
   c) Measurements (anthropometry):
      - In addition to usual weight, height, mid arm circumference and head/chest circumference, consider skin fold thickness also (see p 50). Mid arm muscle circumference can be calculated as MAC minus (3.14 × skinfold thickness). However, there are no normal standards and hence this need not be attempted.
      - Weight for age (indicates SAM), ht for age (indicates stunting), and wt of child expected to have same ht as the index child (to assess wasting) are to be calculated.
12. **Hand to head and head to foot examination**:
   It is advantageous to follow the examination scheme for dysmorphic child, as there are likely to have many relevant findings in general survey.

   General profile appraisal
   - Standard profile appraisal with the child standing may not be feasible. If child can stand, protuberant abdomen can be made out (due to hypotonia of abdominal muscles, hypokalaemia, ileus, hepatomegaly, or rarely ascites). Handling the child, like lifting up by axilla will bring out hypotonia. Look for tremor, which is an occasional finding. Along with profile appraisal, skin examination may be done or it can be done at a later stage.
   - Skin: See p 487 for typical changes in Kwashiorkor. Dermatitis limited to sun exposed areas could be due to niacin deficiency.

5

Marasmus per se can cause decreased skin turgor and hence skin turgor is not a reliable sign to diagnose dehydration in marasmic children. Papular lesions (toad skin, also called phrynoderma), especially of elbow and knee could be related to vitamin A and essential fatty acid deficiency. Petechiae could be due to vitamin C deficiency or could indicate severe sepsis. Other possible findings in skin may be hypo/hyperpigmentation, flexural ulcers, petechiae, impetigo, oedema, loss of subcutaneous fat, hypothermia, etc. Do not miss to mention pyoderma or scabies, if any.

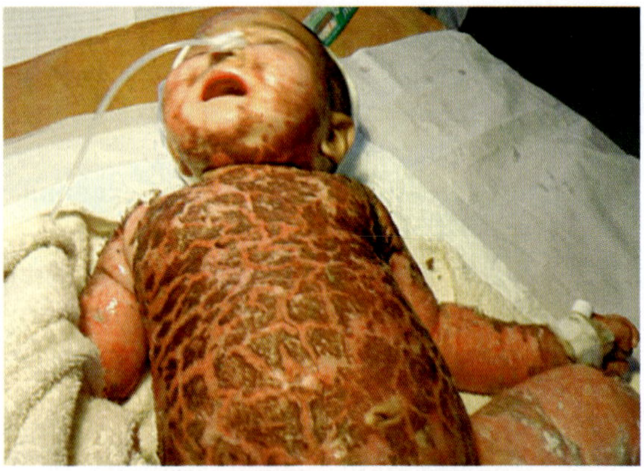

Fig.5.1 Crazy Pavement Appearance. Pg 487

- Nails (see p 123):
    - White nails (hypoalbuminemia), brittle nails (iron deficiency), spoon shaped nails (iron deficiency), transverse ridges in nails (periods of growth arrest).
- Head:
    - Alert looking or dull, apathetic. Resents handling (particularly in Kwashiorkor).
    - Microcephaly in long standing SAM.
    - Delayed closure of AF/PF in SAM, rickets.
    - Craniotabes in young infants with rickets.
    - Frontal and parietal bossing in rickets (with depressions at suture lines, it is referred to as caput quadratum). ***Note***: In severe malnutrition (Kwashiorkor, marasmus), clinical features of rickets are unlikely as growth is arrested; rickets is a disease of growing bones, not growth arrested bones.
    - Rounded face in Kwashiorkor and old man face in marasmus.
    - Loss of buccal pad of fat in marasmus.
- Hair: Easily pluckable, sparse, hypopigmented.
- Eyes:
    - Pallor, vitamin A deficiency features (dry conjunctiva, Bitot's spot).
- Ear: Chronic otitis media is quite common in SAM.
- Mouth:
    - Angular stomatitis, cheilitis, thrush, carious teeth.
    - Look for cleft palate, which could contribute to poor nutritional intake.
    - Noma in neglected cases of SAM (almost never seen in modern era).
- Tongue:
    - Magenta red (riboflavin), beefy (B_{12}), bald (niacin, iron) or gingivitis).
- Gum bleeds in vit C deficiency.
- Teeth decay due to enamel defects in vitamin D deficiency.

- May have parotid gland enlargement.
- Neck: Lymph nodes.
- Chest: Rosary (rickets), Harrison's sulcus (rickets, recurrent respiratory infections in infancy).
- Abdomen: Distention (hypotonia, organomegaly), hepatomegaly (fatty liver of Kwashiorkor).
- Anus: Dermatitis at mucocutaneous junctions in zinc deficiency; perianal excoriation (lactose intolerance); prolapsed rectum.
- Oedema limbs, sacral areas. As per WHO guidelines on SAM, oedema is to be looked for by pressing over the dorsum of foot.

13. System examination:
    - The usual systems examined are GIT, respiratory, CVS (look for cardiomegaly, cardiac failure and hemic murmurs) and CNS in that order of priority.
    - Diagnosis: See p 487.
    - Investigations: See p 488.

TREATMENT OF SEVERE SAM [SEVERE ACUTE MALNUTRITION (SAM) INCLUDES KWASHIORKOR AND MARASMUS]

1. Stabilization: Stabilizing the general condition by managing the immediate complications.
2. Rehabilitation: Restoring the weight appropriate for the age.

1. Stabilization (Mnemonic –"HIDE")

Hypoglycaemia: Blood glucose <54 mg/dL is hypoglycaemia in SAM.

For conscious child: 50 mL 10% glucose or 1 tsp of sugar in 50 mL of water to drink. Then give F75, every half hour for the first 2 hrs and then 2 hourly.

For unconscious or convulsing child: IV 10% glucose 5 mL/kg, then consider 50 mL 10% glucose or 1 tsp of sugar in 50 mL of water via nasogastric tube. Repeat blood sugar estimation.

Hypothermia (axillary temperature <35°C or rectal temperature <35.5°C): Cloth the baby including a head cap; keep the baby under warmer or in contact with the mother's body (kangaroo mother care). Start feeding. Monitor temperature 2 hourly.

Infections: Presumptive antibiotic is indicated in all hospitalized severe SAM cases (ampicillin 50 mg/kg q6 hrs and gentamicin 7.5 mg/kg once daily). All SAM babies >6 months must be given measles vaccine, with a repeat dose of MR vaccine at the routine time of 9 months.

Dehydration: Correction is similar to any child with diarrhoea and dehydration. IV fluid only if the child is in shock (Ringer lactate with 5% dextrose).

Electrolytes and micronutrients:
Electrolytes: Hypokalaemia: Potassium 3-4 mEq/kg/day orally; Hypomagnesemia: Magnesium 0.5 mEq/kg/day (inj or oral).
Micronutrients: Iron is given only after stabilization stage. Other micronutrients to be supplemented are folic acid, zinc, vitamin A, etc. Vitamin D is started once the child starts growing.

2. Rehabilitation

The various stages are feeding, monitoring catch up growth, provision of stimulating environment and follow-up. Feeding will promote growth with stimulation and follow-up (mnemonic).

Feeding

Phase 1 of feeding: Start F-75 diet as soon as possible after the initial steps of stabilization (see above). F-75: Full cream milk 30 mL + Sugar 2 tsp (10 g) + MCT oil ½ tsp + water to make it 100 mL. This provides 75 calories and 1 g protein. F-75 given at volumes to provide 100 cal/kg/day aims at recovery of normal metabolic functions and not growth (higher calories and proteins at this stage precipitate metabolic disequilibrium).

Transition phase of feeding: Replace starter F-75 with the same amount of F-100 for 48 hrs (frequent small quantity feeds). Kwashiorkor patients should remain in transition phase until the oedema starts subsiding.

Phase II of feeding: Start this phase with the return of appetite, and loss of oedema.

The options are:
F-100: Full cream milk 90 mL + sugar 1 tsp (5 g) + MCT oil ½ tsp + water to make it 100 mL. This provides 100 calories and 3 g protein.

RUTF – Ready to Use Therapeutic Food: 100 g provides 500 cal & 15 g protein. It is commercially available or can be locally prepared using available and acceptable foods.

Home available solid foods. Examples are banana, chappatti, dosa, etc.

In phase II, the amount of calorie is increased to 150– 200 kcal/kg/day and protein to 4–6 g/kg/day as per tolerance.

Catch up growth expected is >10 g/kg/day with the above feeding.

Stimulation: A stimulating environment and structured play therapy should be provided.

Follow-up: For weight gain, immunization, health education (how to avoid recurrence of SAM, care during diarrhoea and other illnesses), etc. Follow-up is best planned with the local anganwadi.

RICKETS

Age

Nutritional rickets usually presents clinically from 6 months to 2 years of life. Earlier clinical presentation is unlikely to be nutritional.

Sex

Females remain mostly indoor, more clothed, and this makes females more vulnerable. Industrial air pollution also blocks sunlight.

Race

Religious custom of purdha curtails sunlight exposure and hence more chance of rickets.

Chief Complaints

1. Deformity of limbs (noted since __)
2. Delayed motor milestones
3. Seizures (hypocalcaemic seizure rare in nutritional rickets)
4. Failure to thrive

History of Presenting Illness

Enquire the onset, duration, and progression of symptoms.

Ask for other symptoms such as repeated diarrhoea, irritability, excessive forehead sweating, history s/o seizures/tetany.

If delayed milestones is the presenting complaint mention the developmental history domain wise in the history of presenting illness itself.

History Regarding Aetiology

1. Dietary: History of milk taken per day-quality and quantity; animal products used in the diet. Milk in India is mostly unfortified and hence predominant milk feed is a risk for rickets.

   History of exposure to sunlight, clothing, use of sunscreen agents routinely.
2. Renal rickets (e.g., RTA, chronic renal failure): History of polyuria/poor urinary stream in males/recurrent UTI/failure to thrive.
3. Hepatic rickets: History of jaundice, neonatal hepatitis.
4. History of malabsorptive syndromes: Steatorrhea and abdominal distension, could point towards fat malabsorption and hence poor vit D absorption. Look for other fat-soluble vitamin

deficiencies, like vit A, vit E (ataxia), and vit K (bleeding).

5. History of drug intake: Antiepileptic drugs, outdated tetracyclines (acquired Fanconi syndrome), aluminium containing antacids.
6. History of recurrent dental abscesses: Hypophosphatasia.
7. History of bone pain/weight loss: Oncogenic rickets.

History Regarding Complications

- History of recurrent respiratory tract infections is common in rickets (recurrent respiratory infection also may be due to hypotonia interfering with drainage of respiratory secretions).
- History of fractures following trivial trauma.
- History of seizures.
- History of bony deformities (when it has not been the presenting complaint).
- **Relevant past history**
  - Antenatal, natal, postnatal:
    AN period: Whether the mother received calcium supplements; maternal malnutrition; spacing between pregnancies.
    Birth weight; was the baby born preterm; if preterm, did the child receive calcium supplementation; its dose and duration. Preterm babies may already be having osteopenia of prematurity and their rapid catch up growth requires additional calcium; hence, all the more reason to develop rickets.
  - Any NICU admission for neonatal seizures (hypocalcaemic).
- **Immunization**: As per national schedule.
- **Development**: Normally only an isolated motor delay is expected (hypotonia). If mental retardation or gross development delay or other CNS/hepatic manifestations, think of Lowe's syndrome, cystinosis, galactosemia, tyrosinemia, Wilson's disease, etc.
- **Nutrition**: History of breastfeeding, if formula fed whether fortified. Ask history of intake of calcium rich foods - milk, ragi, bony fish and phosphorus intake (nuts, milk).
- **Family history**
  - Unexplained short stature in the family (familial hypophosphatemic rickets).
  - History of renal stones in the family (could be related to renal tubular acidosis).
  - Consanguinity or similar illness in family could point towards heritable causes (non-nutritional) rickets.
  - Maternal short stature if associated with deformities, may be due to previous rickets.
- **Socio-economic status**
  Cultural practices (e.g., purdha); living in flats may be one reason for rickets (glass windows filter off sunlight of the necessary wavelength); living in areas of industrial pollution could account for less sunlight.
- **General comment**
  - Whether the child is irritable/listless and whether failure to thrive is present.
- **Vitals**
  - PR, RR
  - BP may be elevated in renal cause of rickets

Growth (Anthropometry)

Short stature is expected. Limbs may be shorter because of short limbs and bending; thus US:LS ratio may be abnormal.

Head to Foot Examination

- Head
  - Skull: Softening of skull bones allowing ping pong feel on pressing (craniotabes). It could be elicitable in normal infants near the suture lines; hence, to substantiate rickets, it must be elicitable away from suture lines.

5

Shape of skull: Frontal and parietal bossing (rarely frontal and parietal bulges with sutures in between gives the appearance of caput quadratum or hot cross bun). AF - dimension, whether PF is open (delayed closure of fontanels is expected).
- Hair- alopecia in vit D dependant rickets type 2

- Eyes:
  - Look for cataract: Lowe's, cystinosis, galactosemia
  - Icterus (hepatic cause)
  - Pallor
  - Evidence of other vitamin defeciency, e.g., Bitot spots
- Oral cavity: Dentition (Number of teeth expected = Age in months - 6).
  In rickets, there can be delayed eruption of teeth, premature fall of milk teeth or enamel hypoplasia. Enamel staining could be due to tetracyclines; out of date tetracyclines are known to cause renal tubular acidosis.
- Chest:
  - Pectus excavatum/carinatum
  - Harrison's groove
  - Rickety rosary
- Limbs:
  - Widening of wrists and ankles (p 490); for these changes to appear the child should be bearing weight on upper limbs (crawling) or lower limbs (walking)
  - Look for skeletal deformities: Genu vara (bow leg), genu valgum (knock knee), tibial bowing. Coxa vara due to alteration of femoral neck-shaft angle. Genu recurvatum is rare but can occur due to hypotonia.
  - Measure the intercondylar distance in genu valgum (>5 cm abnormal) and intermalleolar distance in genu varum (>10 cm abnormal). Both the measurements are taken with the child in supine position and both legs extended.

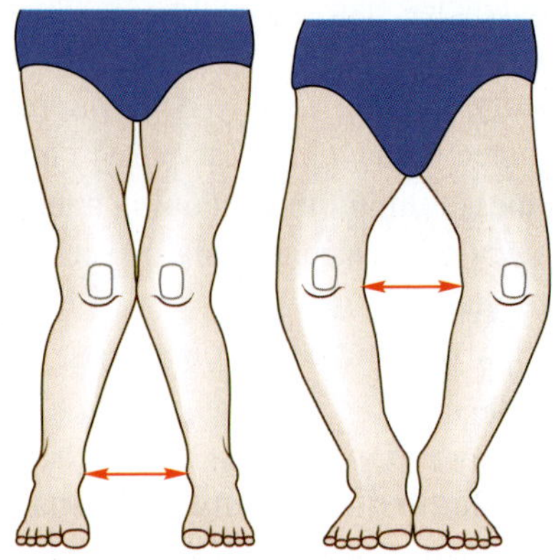

Fig.5.2 Measurements in knock knee and bow legs

- Abdomen:
  - Look for protuberant belly due to visceroptosis and hypotonia.
  - Examine the spine for deformities (kyphoscoliosis).
  - Look for other deformities (coxa vara, flat feet)/fractures.
- Abdomen:
  - Abdominal distension due to hypotonia.
  - Palpable liver/spleen (visceroptosis due to ligament laxity).
- Back: Kyphosis/scoliosis/excessive lordosis.
- Look for signs suggestive of tetany:
  - Trousseau's sign: Keep BP cuff inflated above the systolic pressure for 2–3 min carpopedal spasm like contraction is expected in hypocalcaemia.
  - Chvostek's sign: Tap at facial nerve, just anterior to ear and below the zygomatic process; twitching of ipsilateral facial muscles is expected in case of neuromuscular irritability due to hypocalcaemia.
  - Carpopedal spasm (from history).
- Systems to be examined are GIT (palpable liver, spleen), CNS (there may be a history suggestive of tetany and hence CNS examination), respiratory (recurrent respiratory infections are common with rickets).

Differential Diagnosis

The usual discussion on differential diagnosis is whether the rickets is nutritional or not.

- Renal osteodystrophy: Limbs are affected, mostly lower limbs (any rickets after infancy affects lower limbs more). Epiphyseal stippling and erosion of cortex rather than cupping and fraying in X ray.
- Alopecia and very early clinical presentation are in favour of vit D-dependant rickets type II.
- Hypophosphatemic rickets presents towards the end of infancy and lower limb is predominantly involved.
- Metaphyseal dysplasia: Usually symmetrical; usually only knee joints are affected, bilaterally; normal serum biochemistry.
- The causes of bent bones like Blount disease also may be a differential, especially by the X-ray appearance.

Investigations (p 490)

X-ray in rickets is discussed in p 567.

Double contour that may be seen in X ray is due to uncalcified subperiosteal osteoid.

Treatment

- Conventional therapy: 6 lakh units of vitamin D as a single oral or IM dose (Stross regimen) and no more vitamin D for the next 1 month. If there is no X-ray evidence of healing (no line of preparatory calcification but the aetiology appears nutritional), the dose can be repeated once more. Stross regimen is not preferred now because this mega dose is unphysiological.
- Presently lower dose is preferred. 2000 IU per day for 3 months followed by maintenance requirement daily.
- Another regimen is 60,000 units once a week for 6 weeks followed by 60,000 units monthly for a few months followed by maintenance dose daily.
- Ensure adequate sunlight exposure.
- Calcium rich food (milk, green leafy vegetables, etc).
- Vitamin D rich foods like fish, egg yolk, vit D fortified milk, etc.
- In case of non-nutritional rickets, specific therapy depends on the diagnosis.

ATTENTION DEFICIT HYPERACTIVE BEHAVIOUR

It is unlikely that a case of ADHD will be kept for examination. However, ADHD could be an association with some other disorders (like CP) and hence relevant points in history and examination are outlined here.

5

History

Try to evaluate the following by appropriate queries.

- Attention deficit: "Careless" mistakes in school work; failure to finish school work (before finishing, the attention gets diverted to something else); does not seem to listen to what is spoken to; following only part of what is instructed to do; easily distractable. The brain appears to have problem filtering off the unnecessary information; all the sensory information is appreciated with equal importance; e.g., when reading or attending class, the child appreciates sounds like birds singing, radio at a distant place, etc with equal importance. Caution: Children with ADHD can have selective and obsessive concentration if the task interests them (e.g., video games, TV shows). Consider and rule out attention seeking behaviour manifesting as ADHD. Also consider bright bored child! (bright children are bored of routine teaching schedules, which provide them nothing new or challenging).
- Hyperactivity: "On the go" always. Cannot sit in seat in class for full duration, but gets up and go around; climbs up the windows or runs around; excessive talking.
- Impulsivity: Interrupt others talk; answers before the question is completed, thus answer

gets wrong often; has difficulty to wait till his turn comes; temper tantrums.

- The symptoms must have been documented at least in two different settings (like home and school). If it is present only at home or school, consider problems at home or school rather than problem with the child.
- Ask for co-morbidities:
  - Specific learning disabilities (specifically inquire about reading, spellings, mathematics, etc).
  - Conduct disorders like aggression towards peers, animals, etc.
  - Oppositional defiant behaviour (deliberate defying, annoying, etc).
- In birth history, consider antenatal teratogens/ infections; prematurity; any CNS event is significant, hence must be sought: HIE, hypoglycaemia, seizures, CNS infections, or CNS bleed.
- Family and socioeconomic history: Family history of ADHD, learning disabilities. Marital disharmony; alcoholism; other issues in family like unrealistic expectations of parents; child abuse.
- General examination should concentrate on any dysmorphology (e.g., fragile X) and head circumference (hydrocephalus or microcephaly). Iron deficiency anaemia could cause lack of concentration (check various findings related to iron deficiency). Hyperthyroidism could cause lack of concentration (look for goitre).
- System examination must concentrate on CNS. Make sure there is no visual or auditory problems contributing to the child's problems. Test visual field and fundus (space occupying lesion).
- Iron deficiency and thyrotoxicosis can cause problems of poor attention span.

AUTISM

History

Try to evaluate the following by suitable queries.

- Poor social interaction: "Parents love the child but the child does not love back;" no eye contact while spoken to; does not smile back; "on his/her own world (loner);" pre-occupation with just one or two specific interests and plays with it all alone, without allowing friends/parents to be part of play; does not share toys.
- Repetitive and stereotyped behaviour.
- There is language delay. May go on repeating meaningless words.
- Comorbid conditions (refer to discussion on ADHD).
- Development history shows delay, more delay in language and social domains.
- Birth history: In birth history, consider antenatal teratogens/infections; any CNS event is significant, hence must be sought: HIE, hypoglycaemia, seizures, CNS infections, CNS bleed, etc.
- Most children with autism are normal on physical examination.
- Hearing impairment must be specifically looked for, because deafness could be the reason for language delay. Thyroid function is to be routinely done. Formal IQ assessment is to be considered, because mental retardation may explain all these problems. Landau Kleffner syndrome and Rett syndrome must be considered in differential.
- Postgraduate students are encouraged to refer to Manual of Pediatric Practice by the same author for discussion on management issues.

DEVELOPMENT (INTELLECTUAL) RETARDATION

- Development delay and mental retardation could be associated with syndromes and hence the scheme of examination of dysmorphic child can be used, with emphasis on development testing.
- In a case given for the assessment of development, the candidate is expected to assess

development by testing at least some parameters (all parameters cannot be tested in a given child due to the issue of non-cooperation for prolonged testing). Just the development assessment by history is not acceptable.

- Formal development testing by standard methods like Denver, Bayley or Gessell are not expected from paediatric residents. They are expected to assess development in four domains (gross motor, fine motor, social and language) plus hearing & vision.
- Age: In case of preterm babies, corrected age must be used to commit if the baby is developing normally or not (especially during infancy). Beyond 2 years of age, this correction is not acceptable as most babies are expected to have caught up with babies of same chronological age.
- Sex: The development of speech and language are generally earlier in the girl child.
- Presenting complaint: Delay in development. Sometimes, the complaint is limited to just one domain, like child is not talking.
- History of present illness: Candidate must roughly estimate, which domains are delayed. Whether the child is slowly achieving milestones or remaining static for the past few months or has lost already acquired milestones. Temporary loss of acquired milestones is possible with acute illness or severe malnutrition. Permanent loss of acquired milestones points towards a degenerative neurological/neuromuscular disorder.

  Isolated delay in scholastic performance may be due to specific learning disorder.

  History of constipation is important as hypothyroidism is a treatable cause of development delay.
- Past history: One must elicit history suggestive of head injury, CNS infections or chronic illnesses of other systems, all of which could retard the development.
- Antenatal, natal and postnatal adverse events could retard development of the child and hence must be inquired into (like IUGR, birth injuries, birth asphyxia, conception after prolonged infertility, intrauterine infection/drug/radiation exposure, etc).
- Immunization history
- Development history: This must be elicited in detail, in each domain and in addition the candidate must comment on gross adequacy of vision and hearing.
- Dietary history: Since severe malnutrition and some specific nutrient deficiencies can retard development, assess whether the diet is adequate in protein, calorie and micronutrients.
- Family history must focus on familial patterns of delay in developments (usually mild delay only); neurological disorders; mental subnormality.
- Socioeconomic history: Poor socioeconomic status, broken family, emotional deprivation, etc are detrimental to normal development.
- General examination
  - General comment
  - Vitals
  - Anthropometry: Severe SAM can be associated with developmental delay; failure to thrive may be part of dysmorphic syndromes or chromosomal anomalies.

    Short stature and development delay are the usual pointers towards hypothyroidism.

    Both large and small head may be associated with development delay.
  - Objective assessment of development: Since the case pertains to examination for development delay, objective examination of at least some of the skills of development must be attempted.
- Head to foot examination: Since mental retardation may be associated with syndromes; the hand to head and then head to foot examination is preferred. Refer to the examination scheme for dysmorphic child.
- Make sure that vision and hearing are assessed before committing development retardation.
- For infants, it is of great advantage to do the 180° flip manoeuvre as it gives more or less

accurate assessment with minimum time (see p 255).

- The retarded child is likely to have persistence of primitive reflexes beyond the usual time of its disappearance. Hence, these must be assessed (see p 233).
- Given below is the usual time of its normal persistence of primitive reflexes, beyond which time it is abnormal if present.
  - Sucking and rooting: persistence beyond 4 months of age in awake child is abnormal.
  - Palmar grasp must disappear after 3 months.
  - Placing and stepping disappears by 6 weeks.
  - Moro disappears by 3–4 months.
  - Neck righting reflex: when head is rotated to one side, the trunk rotates to be in line with the head. This reflex is active from 6 months to 2 years.
  - Asymmetric tonic neck reflex disappears by 6 months.
  - Landau reflex (see p 16).

DEVELOPMENTAL ASSESSMENT

The candidate must be thorough in developmental milestones upto 2-3 years of age. This is because most cases given for assessment is below 2 years.Introduce yourselves and spend a couple of minutes to familiarize with the child and parents, because cooperation is a must. Examine in a position comfortable for the child E.g. mother's lap.

- Developmental delay may be related to gross malnutrition, syndrome/chromosome anomalies etc. so look for syndromic features and malnutrition hence anthropometry is very important (head circumference may be taken after full examination because most children cry during measurement)
- For preterm infants use the corrected agefor the developmental evaluation upto 37 weeks (31 week old preterm examined at 8 weeks of age will have a corrected age of 2 weeks).
- Posture of the child- Floppy or less movements on one side or involuntary movement (extrapyramidal)
- Test vision and hearing before other examination as far as possible (field of vision may not be feasible in small child). Formal hearing test should be performed (avoid visual clue)- note changes of facial expression or cessation of activity in smaller children or turning to sound in older.
- Motor development- use the tools (spoon, blocks, beads, books, pencils) and do the 180° flip examination.
- Primitive reflexes- Moro if being done is to be done only after the full examination as the child may cry. While demonstrating the reflexes go on telling what you are examining and what you expect so that examiner knows that you know what to look for and how.
- Social development- assess the interaction with the examiner/ parent.

Impression: Developmental age in each domain, and additional features (E.g. Cerebral palsy, hearing defects, etc)

CHAPTER 6

Signs and Symptoms in General Examination

In this chapter, discussion on the important points encountered in the head to foot examination is attempted. Detailed evaluation of individual parts assumes significance only in specific situations like dysmorphic child, chromosomal anomaly, etc.

HEAD

Describe about the head in the following sequence-Size, Shape, Sutures, Fontanel, Swellings and Hair.

Microcephaly

By definition, microcephaly is the head circumference three standard deviations below normal **(ref. 5)**. Some authorities accept below two standard deviation as microcephaly. The point is *majority* of children with isolated microcephaly less than two standard deviations below normal do develop normally without handicaps. In contrast, *majority* of children with isolated microcephaly less than three standard deviations below normal do have developmental handicaps as they grow up.

Rule of thumb: One standard deviation is approximately 2.5% of the expected head circumference for that age and sex. For example, if the expected head circumference is 50 cm, one SD will be 1.25 cm.

Microcephaly can be primary or secondary.
Primary Microcephaly:

1. Primary asymptomatic microcephaly (familial or as a variation of normal).
2. Primary symptomatic microcephaly (familial, chromosomal, dysmorphic syndromes, etc).

6

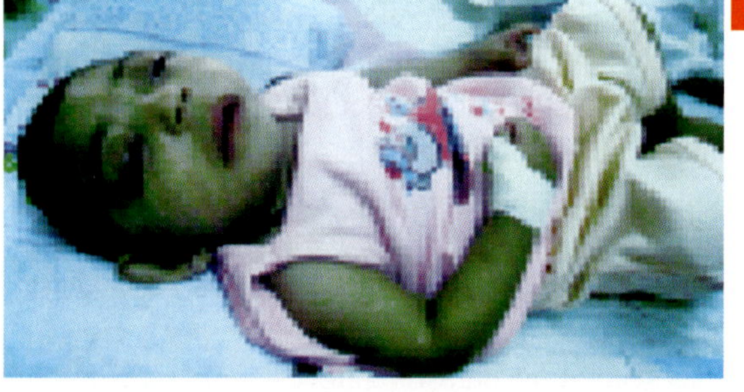

Fig.6.1 Microcephaly: Note the receding forehead, characteristic of primary microcephaly.

Secondary Microcephaly:
As a result of insults to brain development in intrauterine life or insults to developing brain postnatally.

Primary Microcephaly

In primary microcephaly, the brain is small because of genetic, chromosomal or unidentified factors or dysmorphic syndromes or as a familial characteristic. It means that the brain inherently had a very poor potential for growth.

Primary microcephaly does not always mean a gloomy prognosis. Primary microcephaly may be there in an otherwise normally developing child. This is otherwise called primary *asymptomatic* microcephaly. Primary asymptomatic microceph aly is usually familial (familial asymptomatic microcephaly). The head circumference of parents.

Also will be low and the child has normal development and is free of symptoms. Sometimes, a child with primary asymptomatic microcephaly may have no family history of microcephaly. Such children, if on follow-up develop normally and have microcephaly as an isolated characteristic, then it can be accepted as a normal variation. Here the diagnosis of familial asymptomatic microcephaly cannot be stamped for want of family history.

Primary microcephaly with abnormal development or with symptoms (like seizures) are called primary *symptomatic* microcephaly. These include genetic, chromosomal or dysmorphic syndromes and some cases of microcephaly with Mendelian inheritance. It may be inherited as autosomal recessive, dominant or very rarely X-linked character. The characteristic features of a receding forehead tapering off towards the vertex and flat occiput described in familial microcephaly are usually seen in the autosomal recessively transmitted primary symptomatic familial microcephaly.

Other causes of primary *symptomatic* microcephaly include chromosomal or dysmorphic syndromes like Down, Edward, Rubinstein-Taybi, etc.

Secondary Microcephaly

Secondary microcephaly is secondary to various insults to the brain that had normal potential for growth.

- Intrauterine infections: CMV, rubella, toxoplasma, Zika virus etc.
- Intrauterine toxins: foetal alcohol syndrome, foetal hydantoin syndrome, maternal PKU, etc.
- Perinatal and postnatal insults to the brain: meningitis, encephalitis, intracranial haemorrhage, HIE, etc.
- Craniosynostosis (skull may be odd shaped, with palpable ridging of suture lines). Failure of normal brain growth removes the force that keeps the skull bones apart so that they fuse prematurely. Primary Craniosynostosis is due to early sutural closure though the brain growth is normal, is asymmetric (only some of the sutures will be prematurely closed) and there will not be any ridging of sutures. Secondary Craniosynostosis is due to poor brain growth, is symmetric and with ridging of sutures.
- Note: Causes of Acquired microcephaly- Rett's syndrome, HIV. In Rett's syndrome the child grows normally till about 1 year after which the arrest of brain growth occurs.

Look for evidence of premature closure of fontanel, ridging of sutures, etc, as evidence of early fusion. Microcephaly with palpable ridging of sutures is craniosynostosis; microcephaly with open sutures is due to primary brain abnormality. See if the child is one of the chromosomal syndromes or dysmorphic syndromes. Look for squint, cataract, chorio-retinitis, etc.

Investigations

- CT/MRI, skull X-ray, TORCH screen, karyotype, metabolic screen.
- Neuroimaging may demonstrate structural anomalies, such as encephalomalacia, atrophy, calcification, craniosynostosis.

Macrocephaly

By definition, macrocephaly is the head circumference two standard deviations above normal. Unlike microcephaly, here two standard deviations is taken as cut off: earlier detection of macrocephaly is needed as treatment may be offered (one can do nothing about microcephaly and hence there is no hurry in picking up microcephaly!). Macrocephaly may be due to increase in:

- Soft tissue: Subgaleal bleed
- Bones (hyperostosis): Rickets, Achondroplasia (partly because of ventricular dilatation and partly because of megalencephaly) (p 545), osteopetrosis, Thalassemia major (due to bone marrow expansion)
- Brain parenchyma (Megalencephaly): Sotos

syndrome (cerebral gigantism), Alexander and Canavan disease, MPS (p 471), Fragile X syndrome (p 539).

- Ventricles (hydrocephalus): obstructive or non-obstructive. Fig 24.90
- SOL- Tumor, Abscess, Bleed.
- Familial (head circumference of father/mother also will be high).
- Neurocutaneous syndromes like tubcrous sclerosis, neurofibromatosis, etc (p 522).
- Pseudomacrocephaly: Normal sized head appears large in comparison with the dwarfed face and body, e.g., Russell-Silver syndrome (p 517).

Examine for:

- Dysmorphism
- Look for stigmata of IUI.
- Look for full fontanel.
- Separation of sutures, McEven sign or cracked pot sound (in older child with sutures closed)
- Head examination from different angles like parietal, occipital, frontal prominences.
- Describe shunt tubings if present.
- Transillumination test positive in massive hydrocephalus.
- Look for cranial bruit (vein of Galen malformation) over the temporal region, eyeballs, retroauricular region.
- Examine eyes for upgaze (severe frontal bossing can cause false restriction of upgaze palsy) and lateral rectus palsy, (sunset sign) and fundus examination (papilloedema, optic atrophy).
- spine for evidence of spina bifida, including subtle evidences like a tuft of hair (spinal dysraphism).
- Lower limb reflexes: brisk lower limb reflexes in Hydrocephalus (UMN), absent or reduced reflexes in spina bifida (LMN)
- Always measure the parents' head circumference.
- Ask for blood transfusion (haemolytic anaemia, osteopetrosis, etc).

Fontanels

There are usually 6 fontanels (1 Anterior, 1 Posterior, 2 Mastoid and 2 Sphenoid) at birth but only the anterior and posterior are palpable. Anterior fontanel is Rhomboid shaped and is usually about 2.5 x 2.5 cm, but may be as large as 4 cm, especially in A-P direction. Soon after delivery, the AF appears narrow due to overriding secondary to moulding and hence the AF apparently "increases" in size after birth. The AF is best examined with the child quiet and upright, when it is normally expected to be a bit depressed from the surface. The triangular PF is normally less than 1 cm, barely admits tip of little finger (PF is situated where the lambdoid and sagittal sutures meet). It closes by about 2 months of age. The anterior fontanel closes by 9–18 months of age. Pulsation of anterior fontanel is normal. Widened metopic suture as an extension of anterior fontanellae is most often a variation of normal. However, this could result in unusual dimensions of AF when measured in A-P direction. To avoid this, AF is best measured diagonally (not A-P and lateral) as shown in **Fig. 6.2**.

Normally, the anterior fontanel is minimally depressed compared to the adjoining bones (check in sitting or upright position). Significant depression of the anterior fontanel may be seen in dehydration. A bulging fontanel indicates increase in tension in which case the normal pulsation of the fontanel may also disappear.

A third fontanel between the anterior and the posterior fontanel is associated with Down Syndrome and Congenital Hypothyroidism.

Large Fontanel or delayed closure of anterior fontanel may be seen in:
Rickets, hydrocephalus, congenital hypothyroidism, malnutrition, osteogenesis imperfecta, achondroplasia, Down and other trisomies, etc.

6

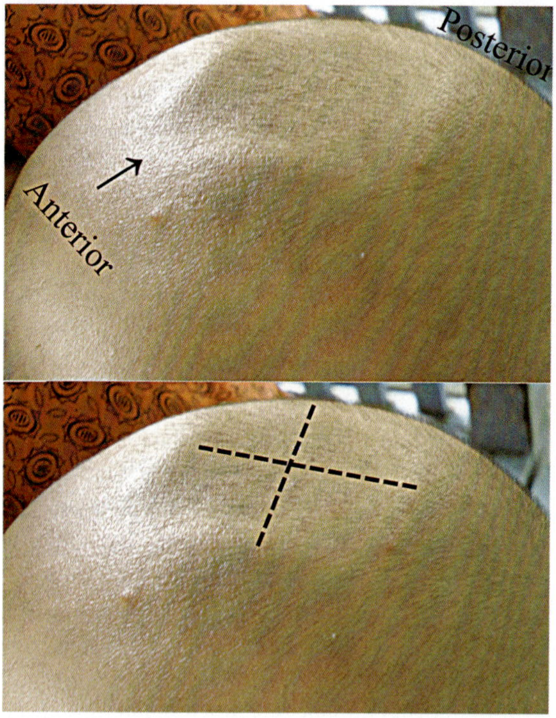

Fig.6.2 AF

Small Fontanel:

- Craniosynostosis (look for ridging of suture lines)
- Variation of normal

Sunken (depressed) Fontanel:

- Dehydration, usually when 10% weight is lost.

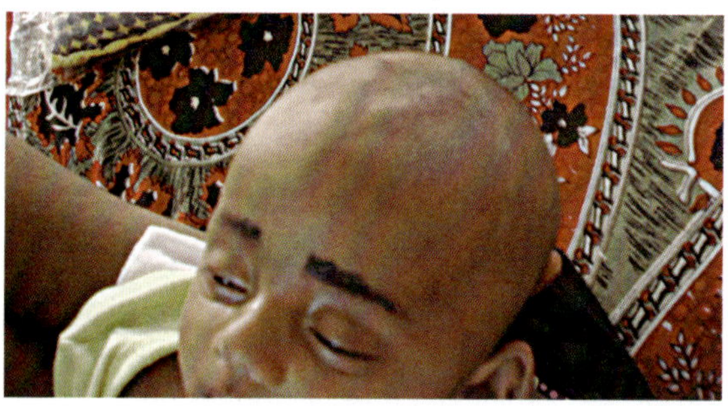

Fig.6.3 Depressed AF

Bulging Fontanel

- Raised intracranial tension: Meningitis, intracranial bleed, subdural haematoma or intracranial space occupying lesions. As the intracranial tension increases, the AF pulsations decrease and ultimately vanish. ***Note***: *Absence of pulsations of AF may be normal, but in that case it will not be bulging.*
- Hydrocephalus (AF may be bulging and non-pulsatile or pulsations may reduce from what was there previously). Scalp veins appear prominent.
- Crying child.
- Benign intracranial hypertension (nalidixic acid, tetracycline, vit A poisoning, infections like exanthem subitum).
- Rapid nutritional rehabilitation of severe malnutrition (due to disproportionate fluid retention).

Suture lines: In early infancy, the suture lines are separated and the gap is easily palpable. The suture lines are not easily palpable after 6 months of age. But in hydrocephalus, they remain palpably separated. The various suture lines of skull are the sagittal, coronal, metopic and lambdoid.

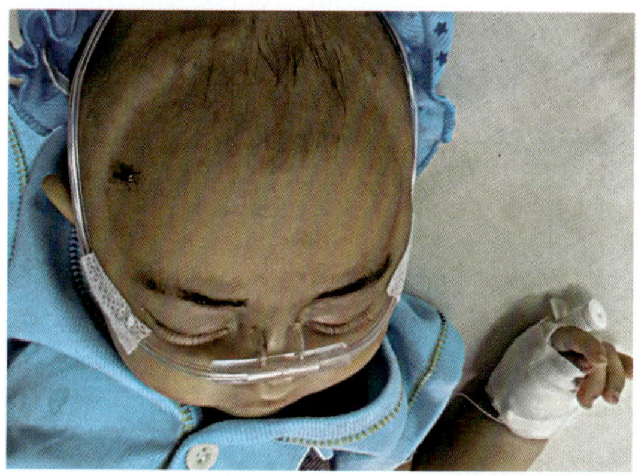

Fig.6.4 Suture over riding

Cephalic index is the head width × 100/head length. Head length is the maximal diameter through the sagittal plane using the glabella in front and the most prominent point on the occiput in the back as the landmarks. Head width is the maximal biparietal diameter.

Cephalic index	Interpretation
<76	Dolichocephaly
76–80.9	Normal
>81	Brachycephaly

Asymmetry of Shape of Head

Craniosynostosis causes shape abnormalities depending on which suture closes prematurely.

In hypotonic children, there may be flattening on one side of skull due to constant lying in the same position.

- Dolichocephaly: The antero-posterior diameter is more than the width. Here, the sagittal suture closes early. So the skull cannot grow side-wise; thus, the growth proceeds only in antero-posterior direction. This shape is sometimes called scaphocephaly.
- Brachycephaly: This is due to the premature fusion of coronal suture.
  So the head cannot grow in antero-posterior direction. Transverse diameter is more. The occiput may be flat as in brachycephaly of Down's syndrome.

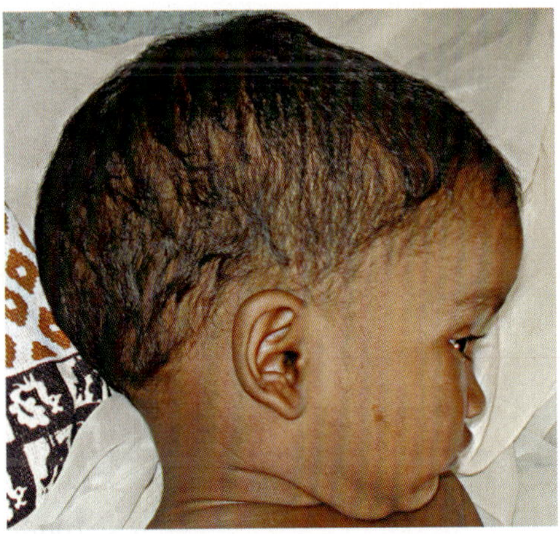

Fig.6.5 Dolichocephaly

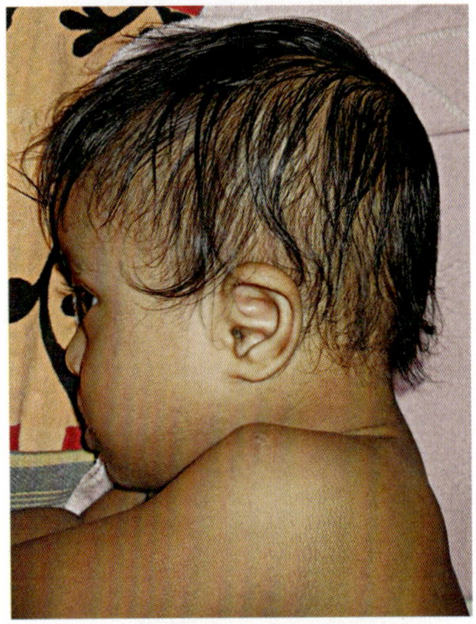

Fig.6.6 Flat occiput: Because of flat occiput, the antero-posterior diameter is less; hence brachycephaly.

- Plagiocephaly: The head shape is asymmetrical (lacks bilateral symmetry) due to premature fusion of sutures unilaterally. Examples are premature unilateral fusion of coronal or lambdoid suture or both on one side.
- A trigonocephalic skull has a triangular transverse plane (narrow anteriorly and wider posteriorly) often with ocular hypotelorism. There is a prominent mid forehead ridging due to premature fusion of metopic suture. It can be associated with midline brain defects.
- In turricephaly, the skull is high, narrow and tower (conical) shaped; the head has short anteroposterior diameter, high forehead (steep ascent of forehead) and flat occiput. It is due to premature fusion of many sutures. Other names for it are oxycephaly, acrocephaly, etc. It is found in Apert syndrome.
- Frontal and parietal "bossing:" This term is used to describe the rounded bulging of frontal and parietal bones. This may be seen in

rickets. Similar bossing may be seen in congenital haemolytic anaemia. In hydrocephalus, frontal bossing is common.

Scalp Swellings

- Dermoid
- Histiocytosis
- Osteoma
- Organized cephalhaematoma
- Secondary deposits
- Traumatic

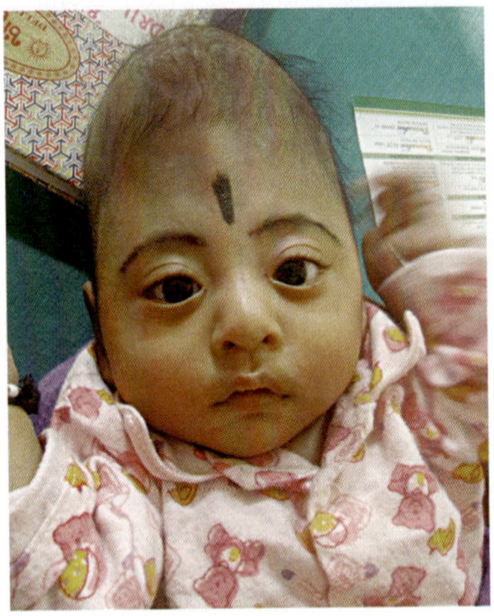

Fig.6.7 Turricephaly frontal view

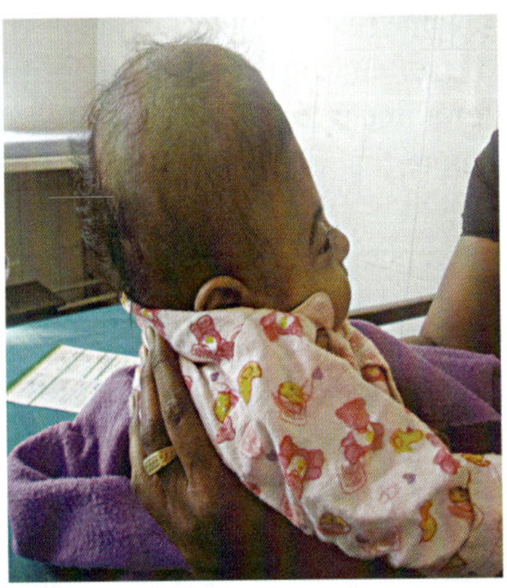

Fig.6.8 Turricephaly lateral view

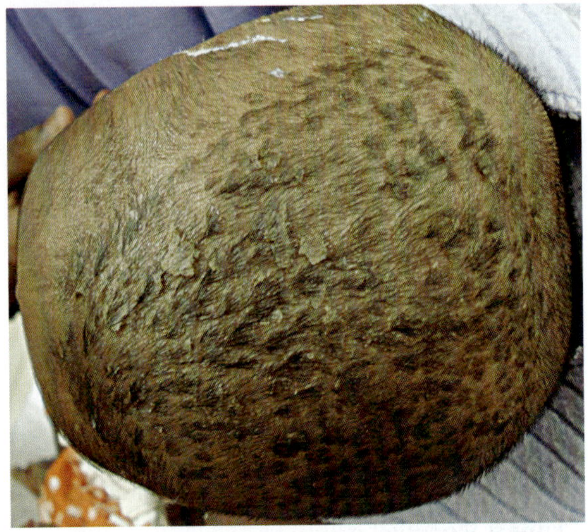

Fig.6.9 Seborrhea scalp: Note the adhesive scales.

Seborrhoeic Dermatitis of Scalp

Yellow crusted plaques in scalp (cradle cap).

Cephalhaematoma

- Subperiosteal collection of blood (due to elevation of periosteum).
- Does not cross suture lines, unlike caput succedaneum.
- Reaches maximum size by 3rd day. Almost never seen at birth.
- Usually, the parietal bone is most commonly affected.
- It may rarely be associated with skull fracture, in which case it may cross suture lines.
- Disappears by 3–6 weeks or the area may get calcified and remains mis-shapen for months, but ultimately the shape normalizes by remodelling.

Caput Succedaneum

- Diffuse, soft, baggy swelling of the scalp
- Seen at the time of birth
- Crosses suture lines
- Disappears by 1–2 days

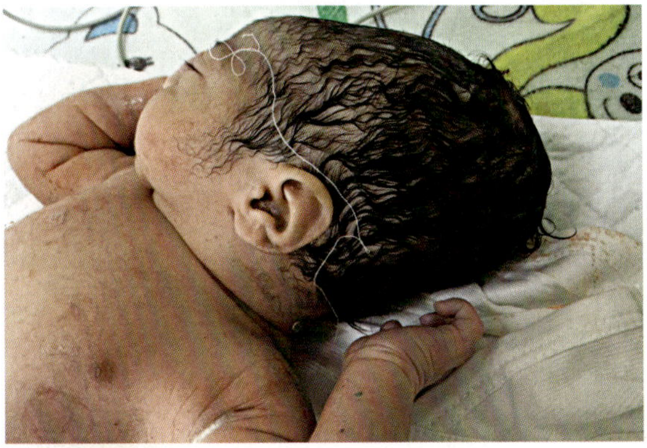

Fig.6.9a Caput Succedaneum

Cranial Bossing

It is the prominence of the central parts of parietal and frontal bones. When frontal bone alone is involved, it is called frontal bossing.

- Rounded prominences in the centre of the parietal and frontal bones may be early manifestation of rickets.
- Hydrocephalus.
- Cranial bossing may also be found in congenital syphilis, thalassaemia, cleidocranial dysostosis, Hurler's syndrome, achondroplasia, etc.

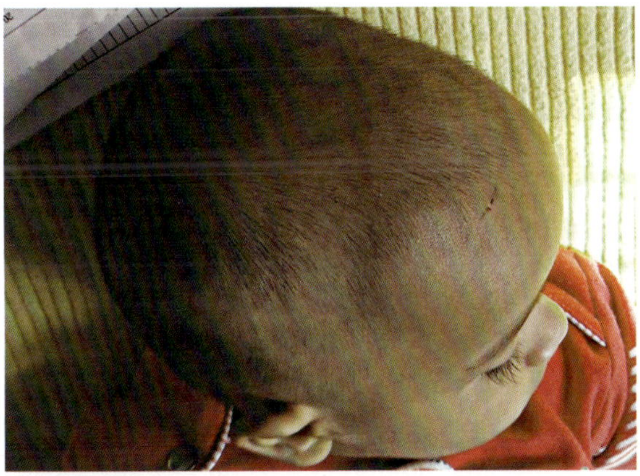

Fig.6.10 Frontal & parietal bossing in rickets

Craniotabes

It is the ability to indent under pressure and then spring back to normal contour on release of pressure like a ping pong ball. It is normal in newborn and young infants up to 3 months of age, especially near the sutures. Hence, craniotabes must be elicited away from the suture line as it may be *normally* elicitable near suture lines in small infants. In conditions of decreased bone mineralization, this may be elicitable beyond the newborn period. Craniotabes may be seen in rickets, congenital syphilis, osteogenesis imperfecta, hydrocephalus, etc.

Head Tilt (Torticollis) (Fig.6.11)

Head tilt may be due to local painful lesions causing torticollis or a compensation for visual defect.

Herniation of cerebellar tonsils may also produce head tilt. The terms 'head tilt' and 'torticollis' are used interchangeably, but they are not really synonymous as per some authors. In torticollis, the occiput is tilted to one side and the chin tilted to the opposite side. In head tilting, both the occiput and the chin are deviated to the same side.

- Sternomastoid "tumour:" It is possibly due to events in utero or during delivery that causes trauma to sternomastoid.
- Strabismus (head tilt is to compensate for it).
- Unilateral brain herniation.
- Klippel-Feil deformity.
- Dystonic reaction due to drugs.

Abnormal Head Movements

After head control is achieved, abnormal movements of head is rare. Up–down head bobbing movements may be seen in severe respiratory distress. They are described in severe aortic regurgitation, which is rare indeed. Titubation is described in p 225.

Scalp Hair

Look for the colour and texture of hair. Comment on whether the hair has a normal sheen or is dry/lusterless. White hair is seen in albinism.

6

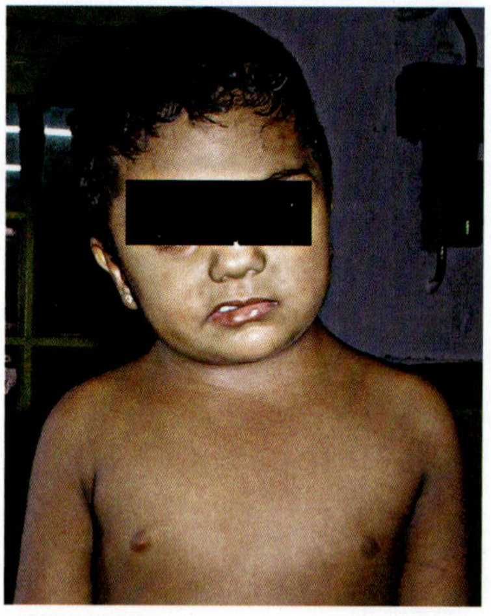

Fig.6.11 Some of the causes of torticollis are sternomastoid tumour, refractory errors and rarely posterior cranial fossa tumour. Of course, the most common cause is local pain due to trauma, sprain, lymph node, etc.

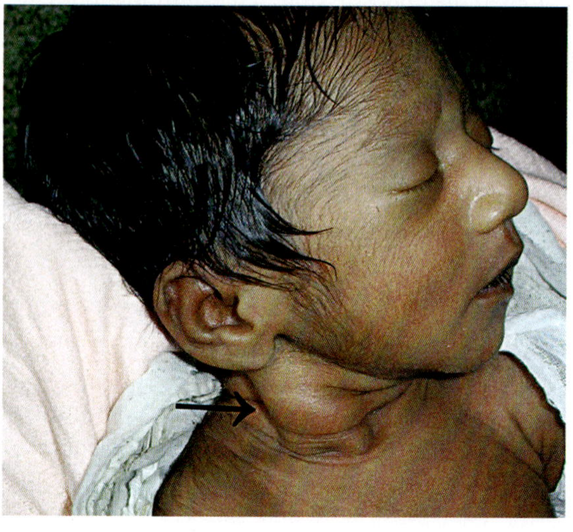

Fig.6.12 Sternomastoid tumour

Sparse to absent hair: Unhidrotic ectodermal dysplasia (p 500).

Kinky hair: Menkes kinky hair syndrome (hair shaft is twisted and brittle, called pilitorti).

Scalp Hair in Malnutrition

In severe PEM, the hair is sparse, thin, lusterless, brittle, hypopigmented, and easily pluckable. Rarely, alternatively depigmented and pigmented (flag sign) hair may be seen. Flag sign is seen in kwashiorkor where there is alternating hypopigmentation and normal pigmentation of hair, indicating periods of abnormal and normal nutrition.

Light coloured hair may also be seen in Chediak Higashi syndrome, albinism, PKU, etc.

White forelock may be seen in Waardenburg syndrome (p 501).

Hair in Microcephaly

Scalp hair pattern at least partially reflects the stretching of scalp by the growing brain. Frontal upsweep of hair ("cow lick") *may be* seen in microcephaly.

Alopecia

- Congenital ectodermal dysplasia (p 500).
- Treatment for malignancy (chemotherapy and radiation).
- Localized areas of alopecia may be seen in alopecia areata (thought to be autoimmune), over scars, fungal infection, etc. When the loss of hair is localized, also consider psychological hair pulling (trichotillomania).
- Fig. 6.14b shows localized alopecia due to friction of constantly lying in one position.

Hypertrichosis

- There may be a general increase in quantity of hair in Cushing's syndrome, deLange syndrome, etc.
- Precocious puberty due to various causes like tumours, congenital adrenal hyperplasia, etc.
- Drugs like minoxidil, dilantin and androgens can cause hypertrichosis.
- Excess hair may be a familial character without association to any diseases.

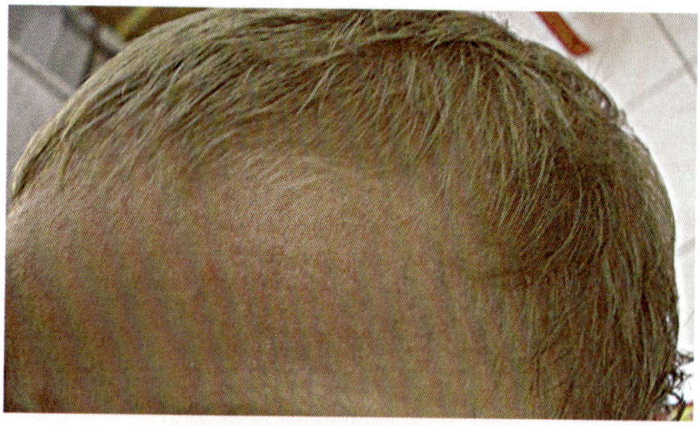

Fig.6.13 Note the hypopigmented hair. Hypopigmented sparse hair is seen in severe malnutrition. Hypopigmented hair may be seen in albinism, phenylketonuria, etc.

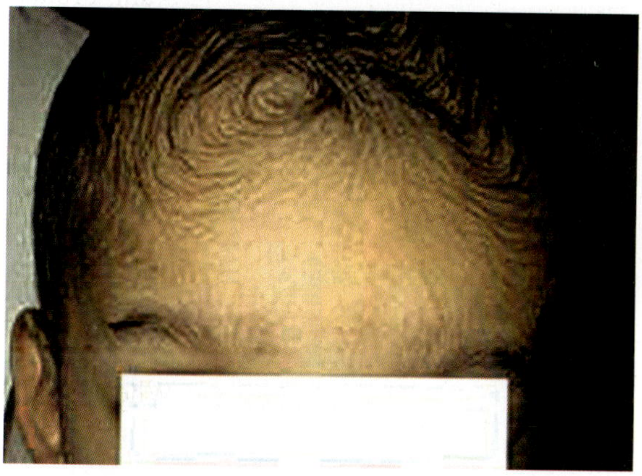

Fig.6.14a Frontal upsweep of hair

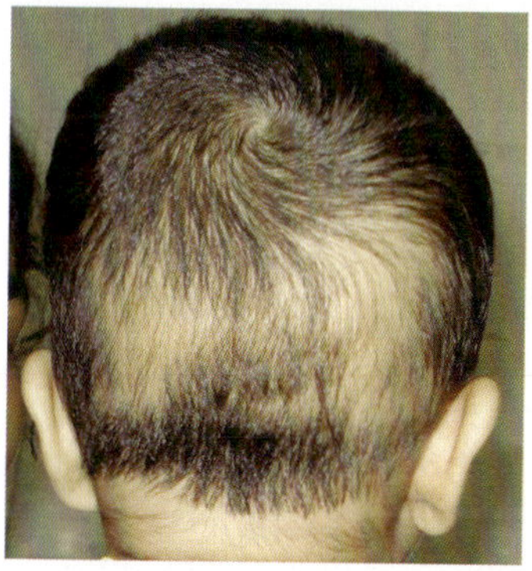

Fig.6.14b Shows localized alopecia due to friction of constantly lying in one position.

Note: *Unlike hypertrichosis, Hirsutism is the increase in the male pattern of hair growth in females.*

i

Low hairline in the back, i.e., extending below the spine of C4 (Ref. 24) may be seen in Turner's

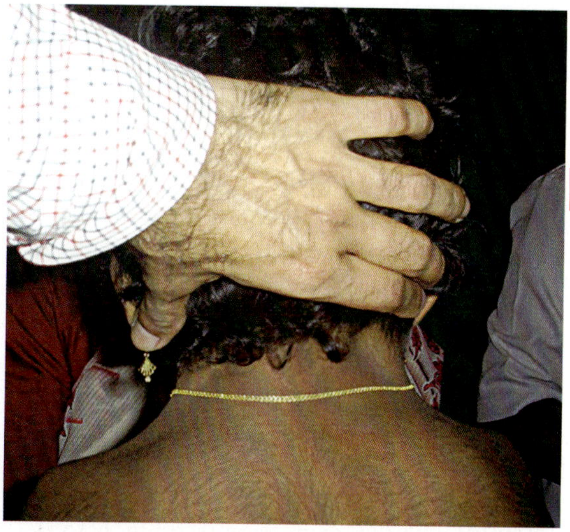

Fig.6.15a Low hairline: Low posterior hairline is usually related to short neck or webbed neck. The low posterior hairline is especially obvious at the lateral ends.

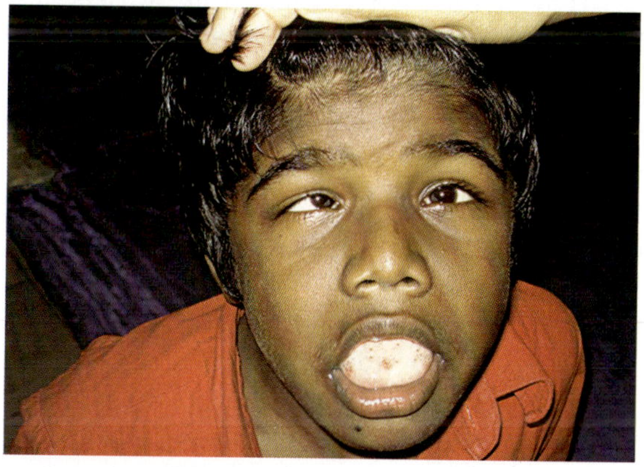

Fig.6.15b Low anterior hairline in hypothyroidism. Also note coarse facies

syndrome (p 518) and low hairline *in the front* may be seen in hypothyroidism. In hypothyroidism, the hair is coarse and sparse. A low hairline in the back, may be related to a short neck in other conditions also, like Klippel-Feil syndrome. Excess projection of hair into the cheek is seen in Treacher Collins syndrome (p 517).

Face

Myopathic Facies

The characteristic myopathic facies is long drawn, with a thin neck.

Moon Face

It is rounded face with prominent cheeks. It may be normal in the obese. It is characteristically described in Cushing's syndrome and prolonged steroid therapy.

Puffy Face

It is seen in oedema, as in nephrotic syndrome (here there is lid oedema in addition to mooning of face). Face in hypothyroidism also appears a bit puffy with dull expression (see Fig. 6.15b).

Coarse Facies

Here, unlike the face of normal babies, the face does not look "cute." There is prominent bloated cheeks and protruding tongue (Fig. 6.16, 6.17).

- Hypothyroidism (see Fig. 6.15b, 24.109)
- Mucopolysacharidosis (Hurler's) (p 499)
- Gangliosidosis
- Sotos syndrome
- Williams syndrome (Fig. 14.1, p 550)

Mask-like Facies *(face is expressionless)*

- Wilson's disease (or other diseases affecting extrapyramidal system)
- Tranquilizer overdose
- Mobius syndrome (lack of expression due to neuroparalysis). Sometimes the complaint will be "the infent does not smile."
- Infantile botulism (lack of expression due to neuroparalysis)
- Depression
- Myotonic dystrophy
- Bilateral facial nerve palsy (in GBS)

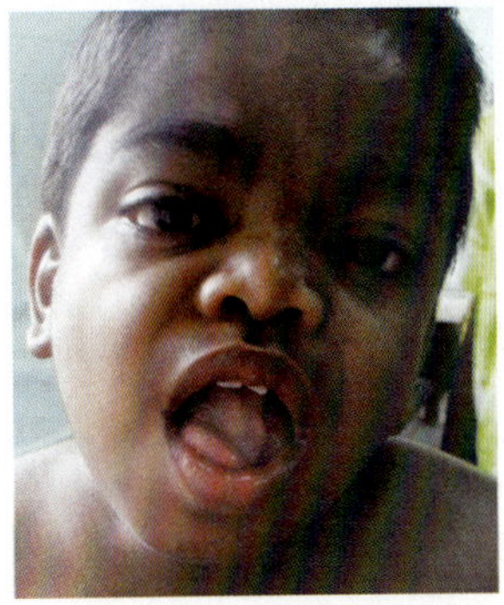

Fig.6.16 Coarse facies: Note the coarse facies of this child with MPS *(Courtesy: Dr Prameela Joji).*

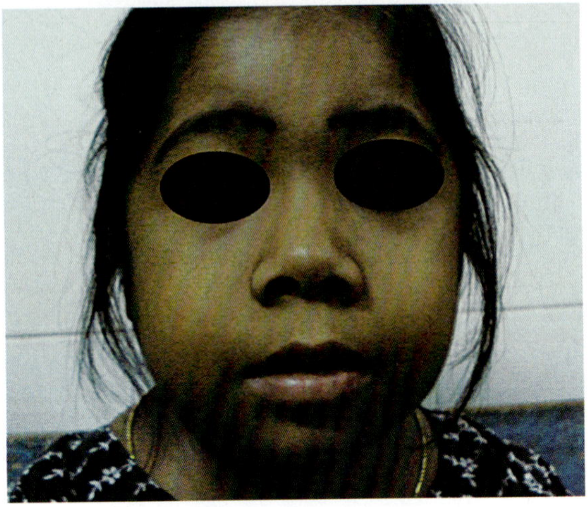

Fig.6.17 Coarse facies in hypothyroidism

Potter's Facies

- Small lower jaw (micrognathia)
- Depressed nose
- Low set ears
- Club foot & pulmonary hypoplasia are used associations.
- Face appears as though a nylon socks has been pulled through the face, flattening it in the bargain.

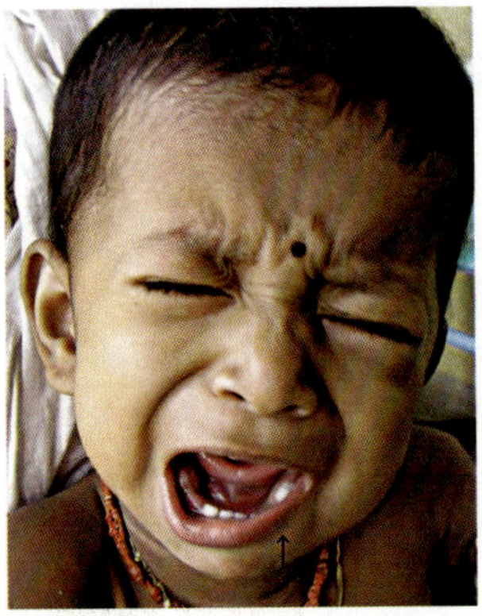

Fig.6.18 Absent DAOM: Congenitally absent depressor anguli oris muscle produces asymmetric lowering of lower lip during crying. Note the arrow. The depressor anguli oris muscle is absent on this side and hence this side does not depress during crying. Generally, it is seen in otherwise normal children. However, it may have association with congenital heart disease.

- It is the result of oligamnios in utero. Oligamnios in turn is due to decreased urine production (e.g., renal agenesis or hypoplasia, obstructed urinary tract, etc).

Haemolytic Facies

See Figs. 6.19, 6.20.

Mongoloid Facies

See p 507.

Triangular Facies (Fig. 6.22)

- Variation of normal
- Russell-Silver syndrome
- Turner's syndrome

Elfine Facies

- Upturned nose
- Broad everted lower lip
- Small mandible
- Prominent maxilla

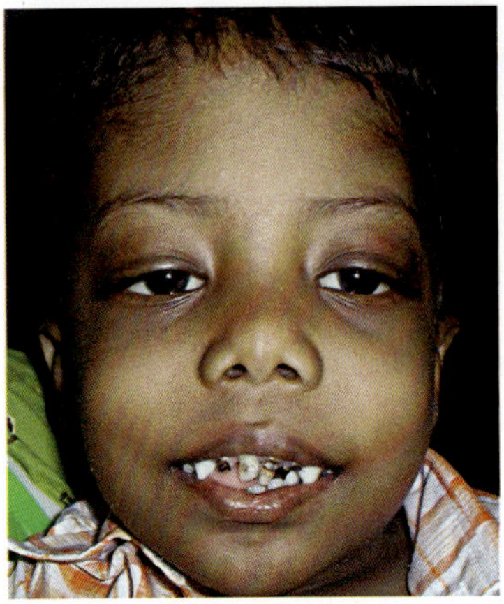

Fig.6.19 Haemolytic facies: Haemolytic facies is typically seen in beta thalassaemia. Note the frontal bossing (prominence of frontal and parietal eminences may be identifiable in lateral view), depressed bridge of nose, maxillary prominence, prominent malar eminences, and protruding malaligned teeth. In adenoid facies, the changes are confined to protruding perioral area with partially open mouth; there will be no changes over maxilla or frontal bones.

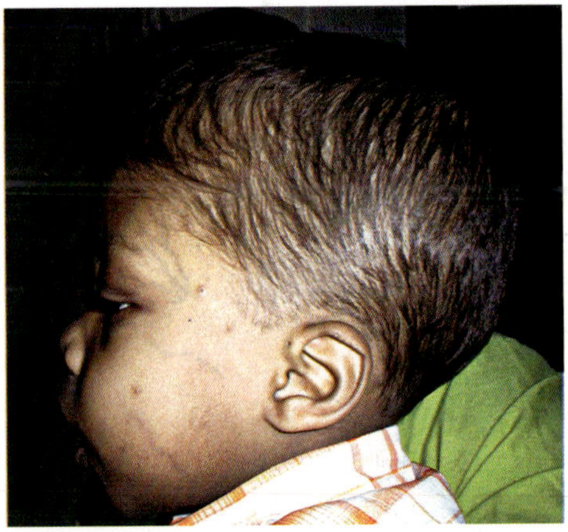

Fig.6.20 Haemolytic face (lateral). The frontal bossing is better appreciated in this lateral view; so also is dolichocephalic skull. Compare with adenoid facies (Fig. 6.21).

- Short stature
- William syndrome

NOSE

Describe about the size and shape of the nose. Small nose is seen in Trisomy 21, 18, Apert syndrome. Large nose is seen in Seckel syndrome, 13q deletion. Beaking of nose in Apert syndrome, Progeria, pyknodysostosis, Rubinstein Taybi. Rudimentary nose in holoprosencephaly.

Look also for turbinate hypertrophy, polyps in nasal cavity, foreign body, deviation of nasal septum. Always rule out choanal atresia in newborn (cyanosis reduces as the baby cries out).

Depressed Nasal Bridge

- Normal in certain races
- Down syndrome
- Congenital Hypothyroidism
- Hurler Syndrome
- Congenital syphilis (called saddle nose) (Fig. 6.24, 6.25)
- Chondrodystrophy
- Late stages of leprosy
- Part of hemolytic facies

Short columella pulls down the nasal tip and distorts the nose and gives a flat appearance to nose. **Hypoplasia of ala nasi** gives a pinched appearance and produces **beaked nose**. It is seen in infants of Diabetic mothers.(Fig. 6.69, p 108). **Broad nasal bridge** implies a palpable widening of nasal bones (Fig. 6.67, p 107). **Anteverted nose**: See Fig. 6.68, p 107.

Micrognathia

- Pierre Robin syndrome
- Treacher Collins syndrome
- Sequel of long standing juvenile rheumatoid arthritis
- Cri-du-chat syndrome
- DiGeorge syndrome
- Fetal alcohol syndrome

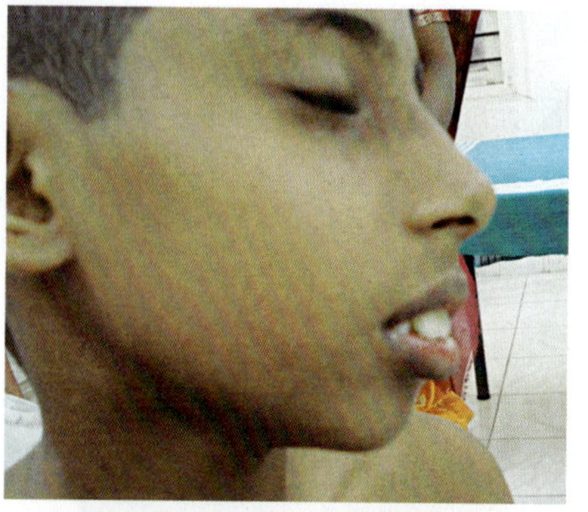

Fig.6.21 Adenoid facies

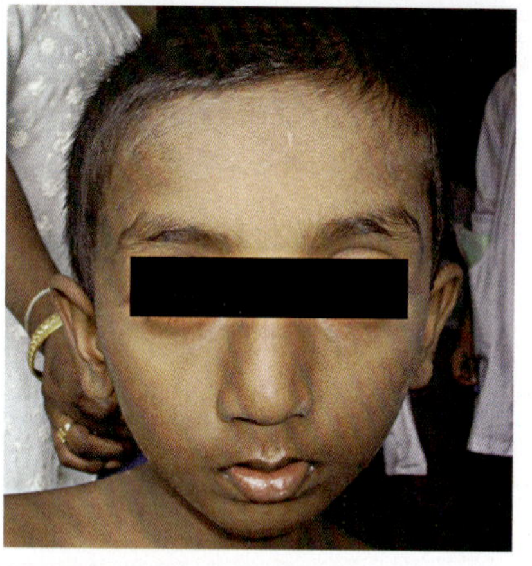

Fig.6.22 Triangular face

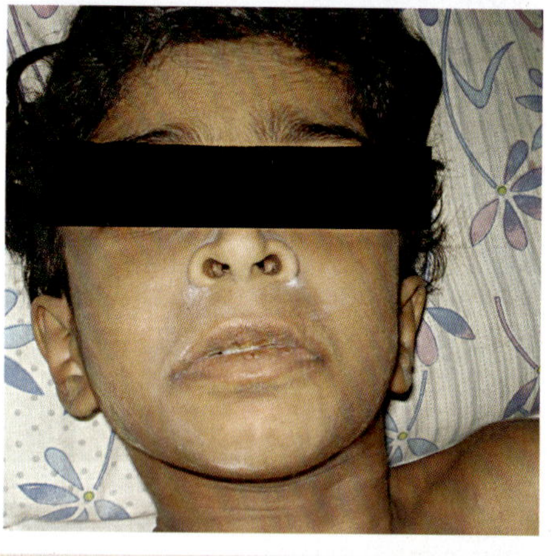

Fig.6.23 Note the fixed grin in the face (risus sardonicus)

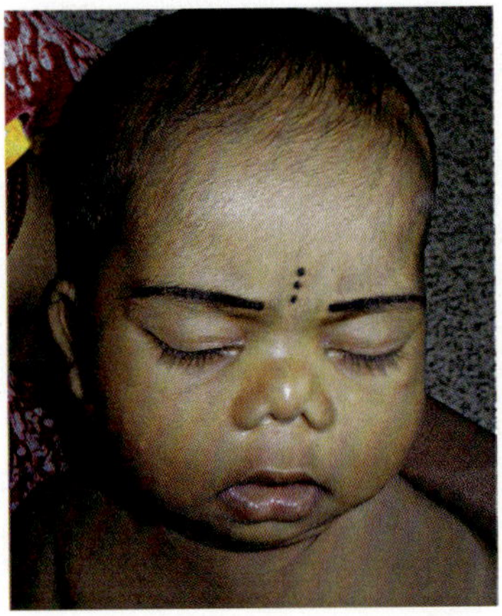

Fig.6.24 Saddle nose

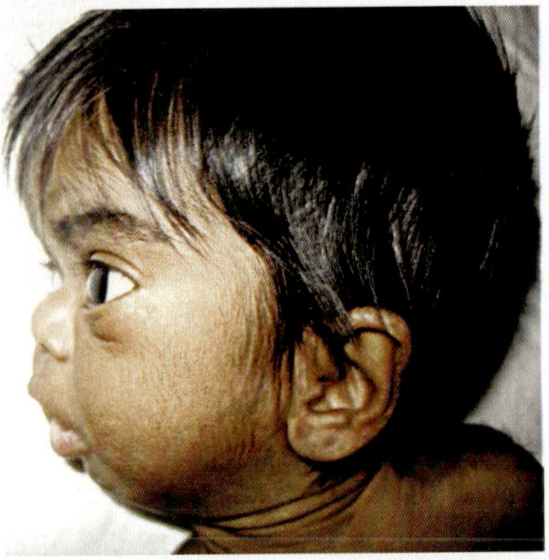

Fig.6.25 Saddle nose: In addition to saddle nose, note the low set ears.

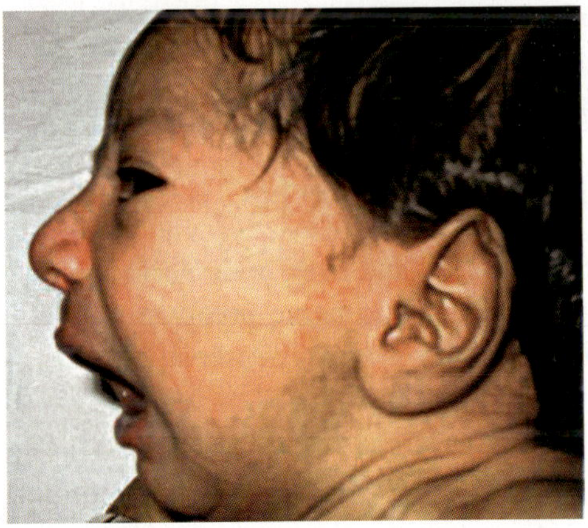

Fig.6.26 Micrognathia, and retrognathia

- Rubinstein-Taybi syndrome
- Russell-Silver syndrome

Prognathism

- Angelman syndrome
- Fragile X syndrome
- Acromegaly

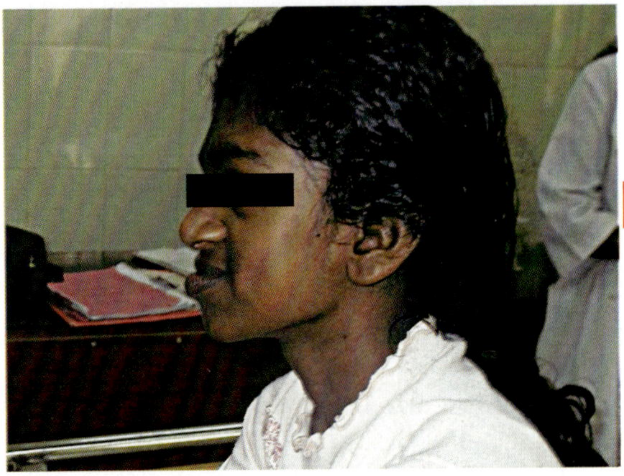

Fig.6.27 Prognathism

EYES

Eyeball Tension

To assess tension of eyeballs, palpate over the closed eyeball with the index fingers. It is raised in glaucoma. Eyes are sunken in dehydration (Fig. 6.28).

Lid Oedema

- Part of generalized oedema: Nephritis, nephrotic syndrome (p 495), cardiac failure, kwashiorkor, etc.
- Severe cough (e.g., whooping cough) or excessive crying.
- Local causes: Conjunctivitis, stye, etc.
- Allergic oedema (Fig. 8.3, p 170)
- Dermatomyositis
- Hypothyroidism
- Infectious mononucleosis (occasionally)

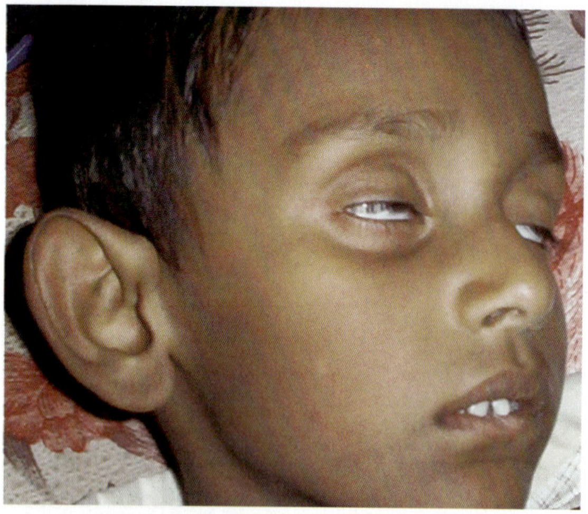

Fig.6.28 Sunken eyes (dehydration)

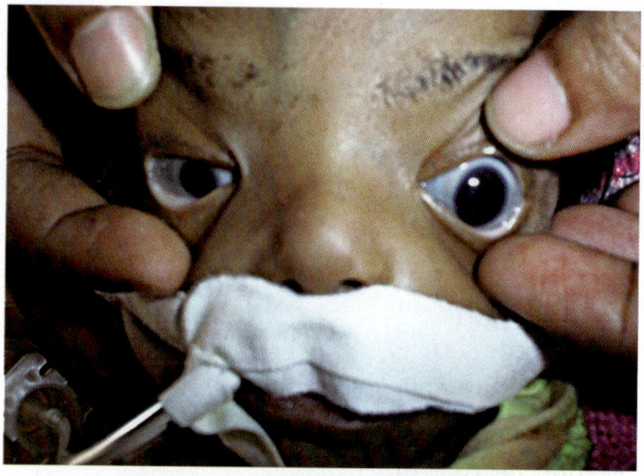

Fig.6.29 Microcornea and microphthalmos

Microphthalmos

(Reduction in size of all ocular structures, **Fig. 6.29**)

- Congenital infections—Cytomegalovirus, rubella and toxoplasmosis
- Goldenhar syndrome **(Fig. 24.44)**
- CHARGE association
- Microphthalmia associated with coloboma is usually an autosomal dominant inheritance.

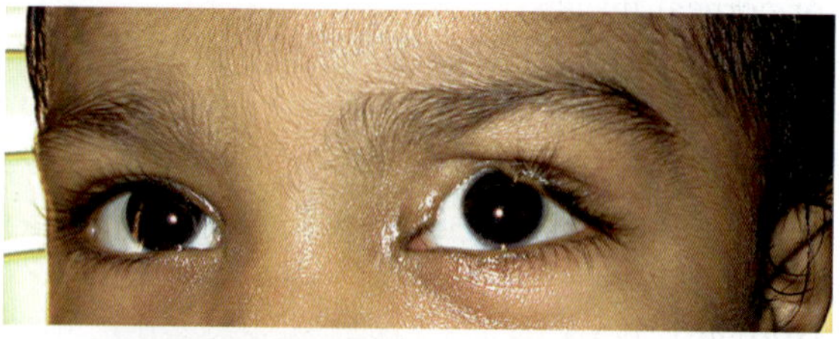

Fig.6.30 Coloboma lid

Cornea

Cornea should not be larger than in the adult. The best way is to compare with that of mother, keeping them side by side, cheek to cheek. Megalocornea may be seen in glaucoma. Cloudy cornea may be seen in mucopolysaccharidosis.

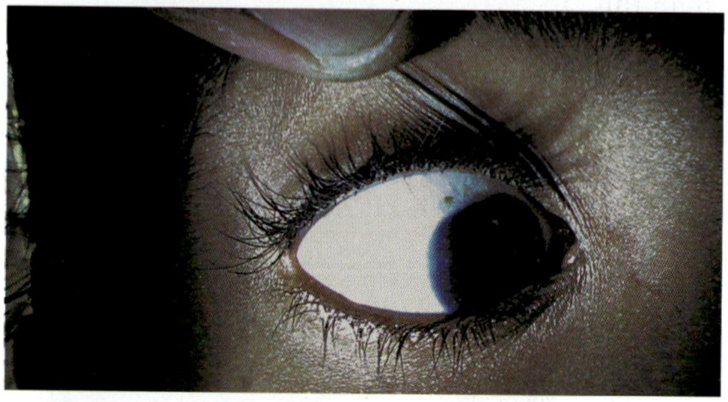

Fig.6.31 Coloboma iris

Coloboma

It is a developmental defect in some portion of the eye. Any ocular structure may be involved (eyelids, iris, lens, retina). Examples of conditions with coloboma are Goldenhar syndrome **(Fig. 24.44)**, Treacher Collins syndrome **(Fig. 24.58)**, etc.

Defect of closure of embryonic fissure of eyes results in the involvement of iris. In more severe forms, choroid and even optic nerve may be involved. With optic nerve involvement, midline defects of CNS is a likely association.

Eyelid Colobomas (Eyelid defects)

- Lower eyelid: Treacher Collins syndrome
- Upper eyelid: Goldenhar's syndrome

Coloboma by definition is a developmental defect of any portion of the eye and hence can affect other parts of eye also, the most common site of coloboma being iris. In CHARGE association, coloboma of many parts of eye may be seen.

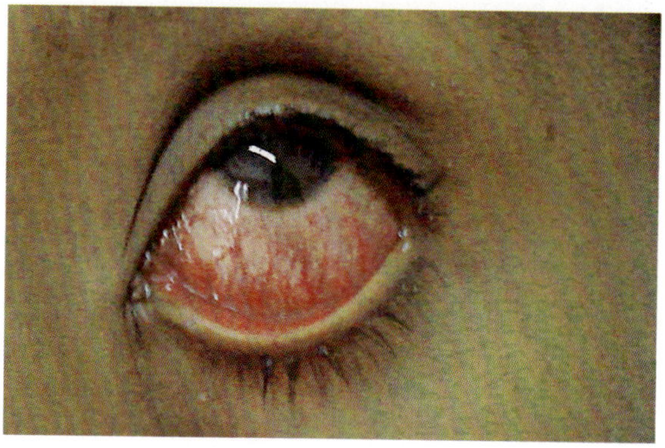

Fig.6.33 Blepharoconjunctivitis

Red Eye

Inside margin of lower lid and inferior conjunctiva are congested in early bacterial blepharoconjunctivitis **(see Fig.6.33 and Fig. 6.32A)**. The middle picture in the drawing 6.32B shows congestion all over, classical of viral conjunctivitis (e.g., adenovirus). Circumcorneal congestion (bottom pic of **Fig. 6.32C**) is typical in acute uveitis or corneal inflammation (corneal erosions or ulcers). Uveitis of rheumatoid arthritis is painless and may go unnoticed. Note the irregular pupil in a case of neglected uveitis in **Fig 6.34**.

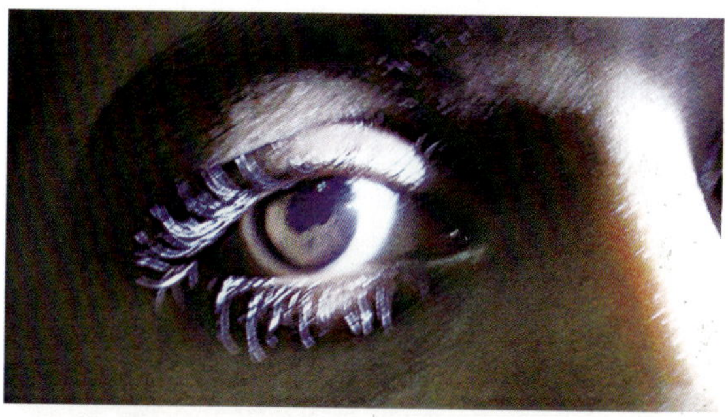

Fig.6.34 Uveitis. Note the irregular pupil.

Ptosis

Normally, only a rim of upper border of cornea will be covered by the upper eyelid when the child is looking straight ahead. If the eye lid droops more than this, there is ptosis. Note the upward movement of eyebrows in **Fig. 6.36**; the child is trying to overcome ptosis by his frontalis action.

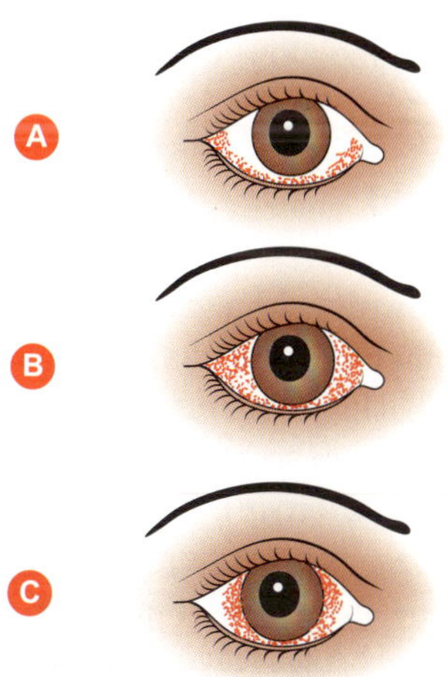

Fig.6.32 Congestion of eye

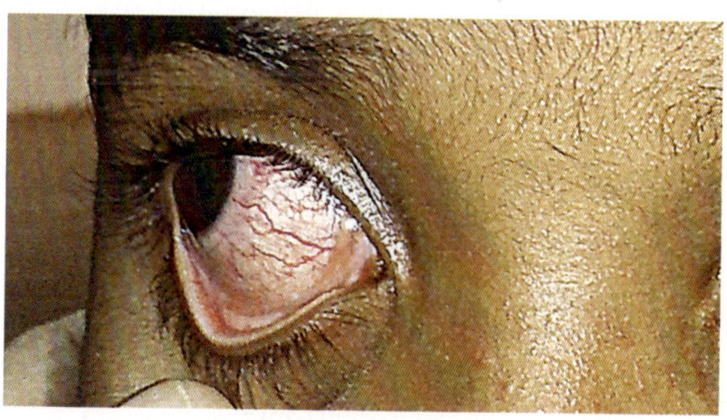

Fig.6.35 Non purulent conjunctivitis, limited to bulbar conjunctiva is seen in Kawasaki disease.

6

Causes may be:

- May be transiently seen in normal newborns.
- Congenital ptosis (may be unilateral or bilateral).
- Oculomotor palsy (in complete III nerve palsy ptosis is *complete*, there will be *mydriasis* or dilatation of pupils and paralysis of other extraocular muscles. Only IV and VI nerves will be acting so that eye is in down and out position.)
- Horner's syndrome (ptosis is *partial* and there is *miosis* and enophthalmos) **(Fig. 24.102, p 537)**.
- Myasthenia gravis (ptosis becomes worse as the day progresses) **(Fig. 6.36)**.
- Noonan's syndrome **(Fig. 24.48, p 512)**
- Myotonic dystrophy
- Local eye lesions like oedema of lids

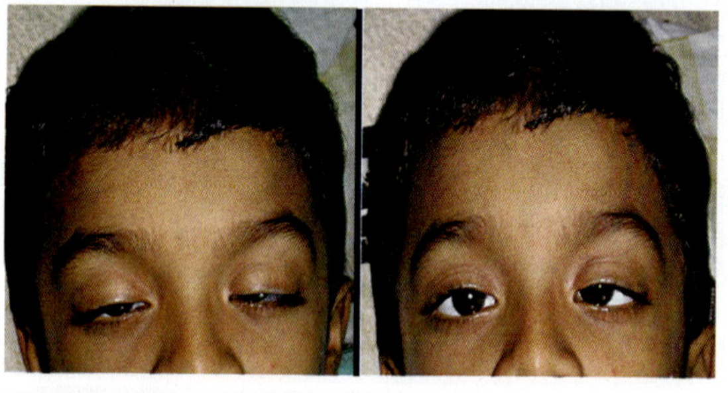

Fig.6.36 Myasthenia gravis: Note the improvement of ptosis after neostigmine (classically described drug for the test is tensilon, not neostigmine)

Proptosis

It is the forward protrusion of eye balls. Lid retraction (see below) may give an appearance of proptosis on first glance, but in lid retraction, there is no forward protrusion of eye balls.

- Malignancies: Neuroblastoma, leukaemia, retinoblastoma, etc. Chloroma of acute myeloid leukaemia and Langerhan cell histiocytosis need special mention as causes of proptosis.
- Non-malignant masses: Cavernous haemangioma, optic nerve glioma.
- Craniosynostosis: Apert's syndrome, Crouzon's syndrome, etc. Here, the proptosis is due to the small orbital cavity.
- Hyperthyroidism causes proptosis of both eyes, being classically called exophthalmos.

Enophthalmos

It is the reverse of exophthalmos (see above). Here, the eyeballs recede into the socket. The most common cause is severe dehydration **(Fig. 6.28)**. It is also seen in Horner syndrome **(see p 537)**.

Microphthalmos

Here, the eye itself is small, not just receding of normal eyeballs deep into the socket. This is commonly seen in intrauterine infections like congenital rubella **(Fig. 6.29)**.

Lid Retraction and Lid Lag

These are signs described in thyrotoxicosis. When the upper lid does not cover the upper margin of corneal limbus in a child looking straight ahead, lid retraction is said to be present. When this patient looks down, the upper lid lags behind to accompany the downward movement.

Xanthelasma

It is the swelling due to the deposition of cholesterol underneath the skin, commonly seen near the eyelids.

Epicanthic Fold

Epicanthic fold is a crescent-shaped fold of skin originating below the eye and sweeping upwards to blend with the upper lid so that the inner canthus is covered. This obscures the inner portions of both lids (so much so, it may give a false impression of hypertelorism). The epicanthic fold tends to disappear as the bridge of nose gets elevated with the growth of the child. In other words, a flat nasal bridge leaves extra skin to show up as a fold. As the bridge of the nose gets elevated, it pulls the skin up so that the epicanthic fold

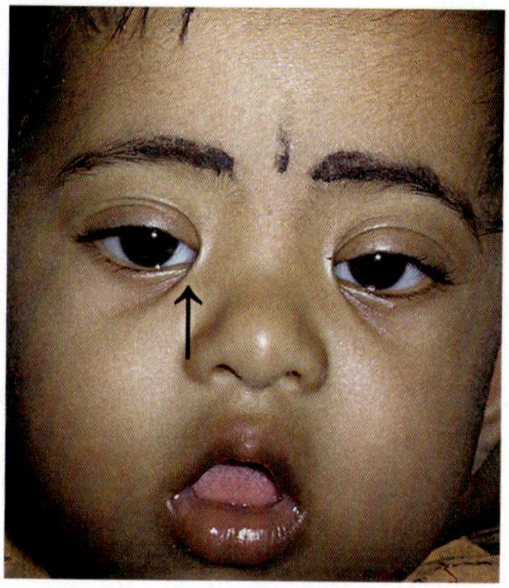

Fig.6.37 Epicanthic fold

disappears. Another reason for epicanthic fold may be syndromes with loose skin; the extra skin shows up as the fold. Unilateral epicanthic fold may occasionally be seen in torticollis, as the head position allows free skin to form a fold. Epicanthic fold is classic in Down syndrome. It can be seen in certain races (e.g., Chinese), but then it is not so prominent as to cover the inner portions of both lids.

- Seen in some normal newborns, disappears by 1–3 months as the bridge of nose grows up.
- Down syndrome.
- Other conditions like Noonan syndrome, Turner syndrome, Cornelia de Lange syndrome, Smith-Lemli-Opitz syndrome, Ehlers-Danlos syndrome, Cri-du-chat syndrome, William's syndrome, Fetal alcohol syndrome, Fetal hydantoin syndrome, etc.

Pseudostrabismus: Prominent epicanthic fold can hide nasal sclera, so that when the child looks sidewise, an apparent strabismus may be seen.

Mongoloid Slant

The slant is upwards, slanting up from medial to lateral side (Fig. 6.38). The outer canthi lie above the lines joining the inner canthi.

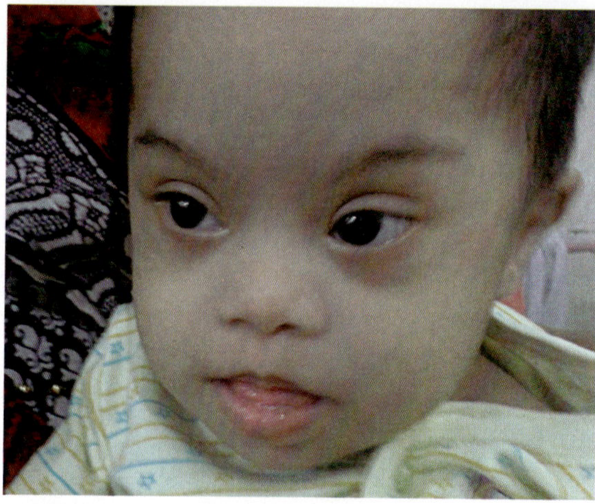

Fig.6.38 Upslant (mongoloid slant)

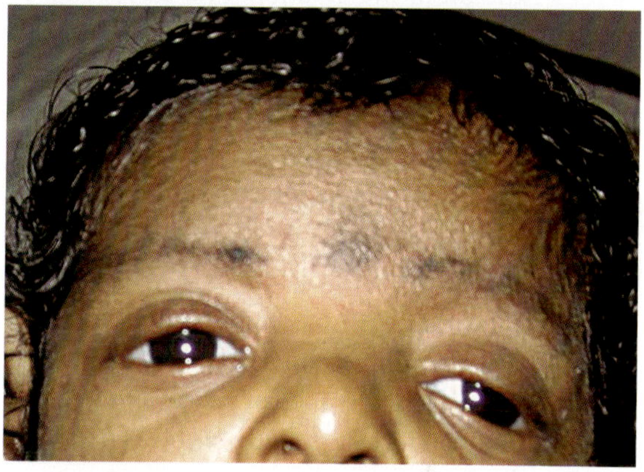

Fig.6.39 Downslant (antimongoloid slant)

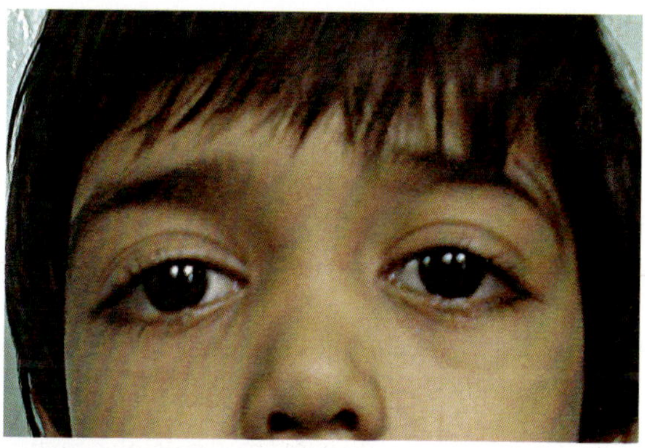

Fig.6.40 Downslanting eyes

- Racial
- Down syndrome
- Prader-Willi syndrome (some cases)

Antimongoloid Slant

It is the downward slanting of eyes (Fig. 6.39). The outer canthi lie below the lines joining the inner canthi (Fig. 6.39, 6.40).

- Treacher Collins syndrome
- Noonan syndrome
- Turner syndrome
- Apert syndrome
- Trisomy 18 (Edward syndrome)

Note: Down slant of eyes in Treacher Collins syndrome is the result of undergrowth of maxilla (with a little bit of imagination, one can see how the eyes slant down because of failure of maxilla to grow laterally). A similar visualization of undergrowth of midline part of anterior frontal brain or that part of skull can tell you why the lateral part of eyes slant up in Down syndrome (Ref. 6).

Hypertelorism

If the distance between the medial canthi of two eyes is more than the width of each eye, suspect hypertelorism, which is part of many syndromes (Noonan, Turner, Apert, Crouzon, Williams, Zellweger to mention a few) and may also be a normal variation.

In the Fig. 6.42, width of an eye is marked out for easy identification of hypertelorism.

Standard definition: The orbital spacing may be determined by measuring the distance between the centres of both pupils in forward gaze (interpupillary distance). This value can be plotted in the nomograms for interpupillary distance and **hypertelorism** (more than three standard deviation above the mean) and **hypotelorism** can be ascertained. This definition is used only for research purposes.

Telecanthus: This is depicted by the displacement of inner canthi laterally although the globes are normally situated. The main difference from hypertelorism is that there is reduction or absence of visible sclera medial to the iris along with lateral displacement of lacrimal puncta.

In hypertelorism, the interpupillary distance, inter inner canthal distance and inter outer canthal distance are all increased. In hypotelorism, all these distances are reduced. In telecanthus, the inner canthi are laterally displaced so that the inter inner canthal distance is increased but the interpupillary distance and inter outer canthal distances are normal, thus the eyes are only falsely appearing widely spaced (actually only the inner canthi are widely separated, not the eyes). Note that in telecanthus, only the distance between midline and the inner canthus is increased.

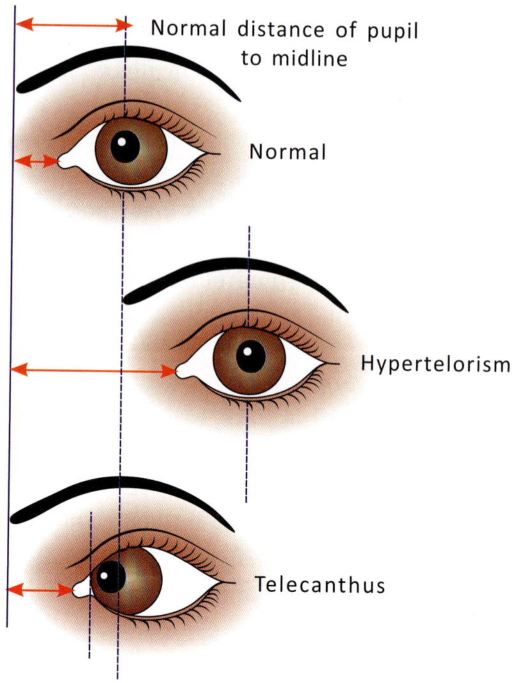

Fig.6.41 Telecanthus

Hypertelorism may be due to hypertrophy of lesser wing of sphenoid.

The inner and outer canthal distances are measured to look for ocular hypertelorism. The

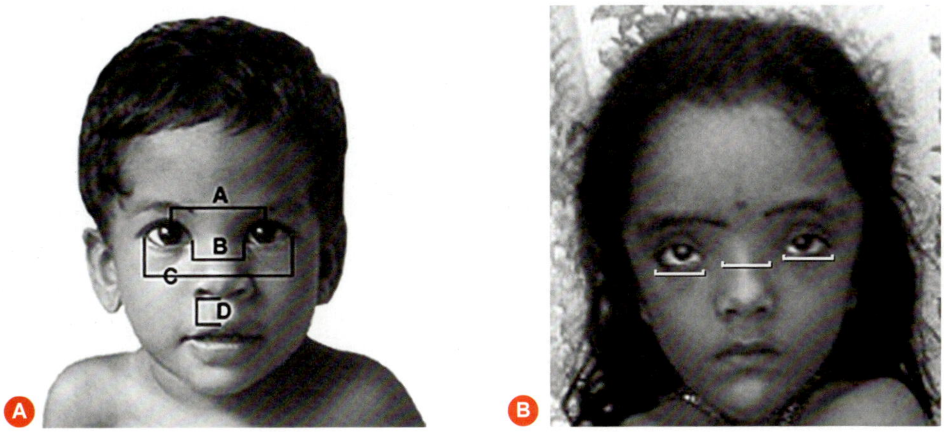

Fig.6.42 A = Inter pupillary distance; B & C = Inner and outer canthal distance; D = Philtrum

6

measurements can be done objectively if one places a transparent sheet with markings on it for measurement (see the Figs. 6.60 & 6.70).

1. The frontal view of the face from the outer edge of one ear to the other can be separated into 5 vertical sagittal planes each approximately the width of an eye in the horizontal plane.
2. The intercanthal distance should be about one eye width (half on each side of the midline). In hypertelorism, the distance between two inner canthi is more than one eye width.
3. The normal distance from the outer canthus of the eye to the edge of the ear should be 1 eye width.

The patient has hypertelorism when the ratio of the intercanthal distance (in cm) divided by interpupillary distance (in cm) is > 0.6. Other calculations are also described. For example:

Hypertelorism = Distance between the inner canthi divided by the distance between outer canthi > 0.38 (canthal index).

Flat nasal bridge will cause hypertelorism see Fig 6.44, imagine this way: Had the nasal bridge been raised, it would have drawn tissues up so that the eyes would have come closer.

Hypotelorism = Distance between the inner canthi divided by the distance between outer canthi < 0.32.

Hypertelorism may be found in:

- May be normal in certain individuals and certain races.
- Down syndrome.
- It can be part of many dysmorphic syndromes like Apert, Crouzon, Rubinstein-Taybi, Turner, Noonan, etc (Fig.6.47).

Synophrys: Eyebrows meeting each other in mid line. It may occasionally be seen in normal people. It is seen in Cornelia de Lange syndrome (Fig. 24.35).

Eyelashes: The eyelashes are unusually long in certain normal children and are no longer considered a pointer towards diseases like tuberculosis (Fig. 6.48). Sparse eyebrows are seen in hypothyroidism.

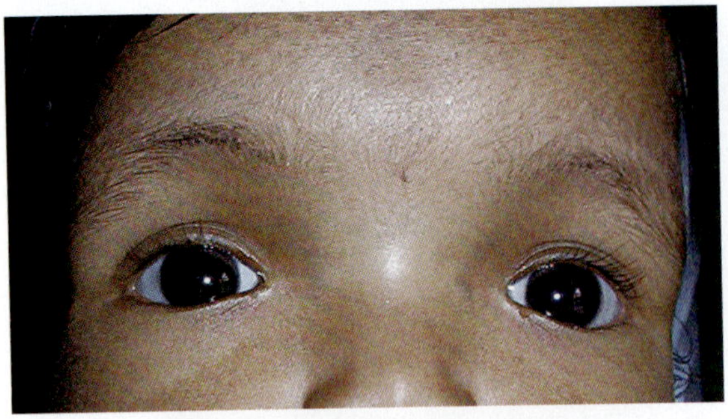

Fig.6.43 Hypertelorism

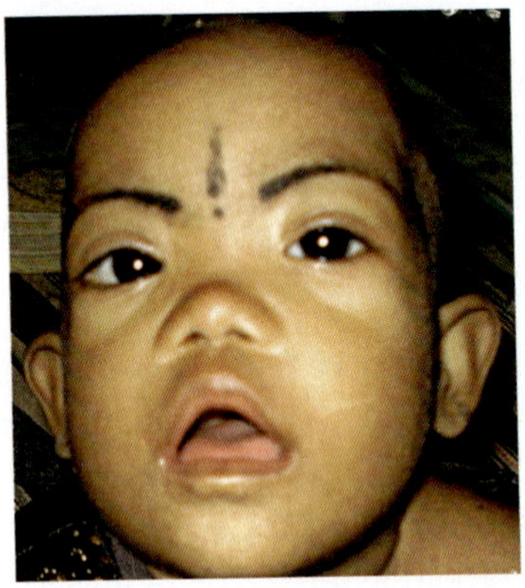

Fig.6.44 Down syndrome with hypertelorism

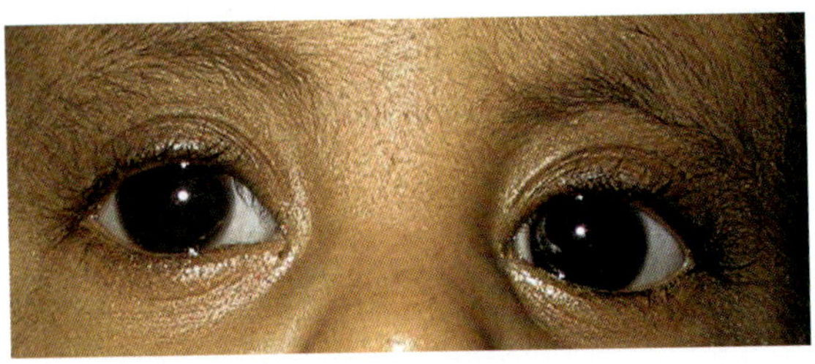

Fig.6.45 Hypotelorism

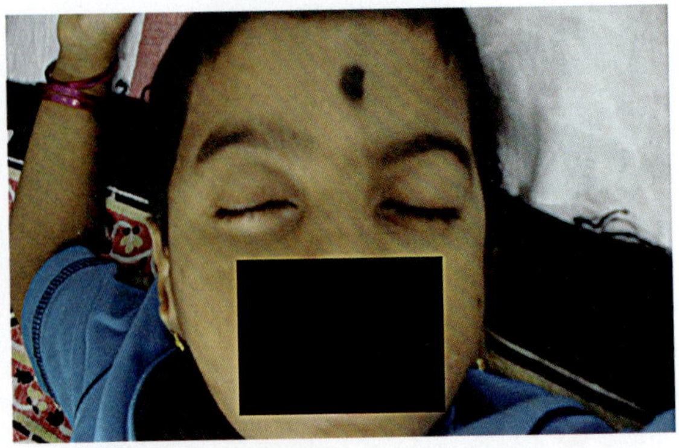

Fig.6.46 Hypotelorism. Note the inter-inner canthal distance is less than one eye width.

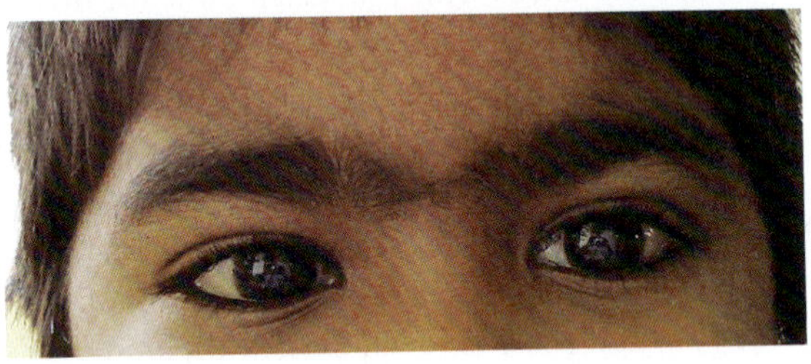

Fig.6.47 Synophrys

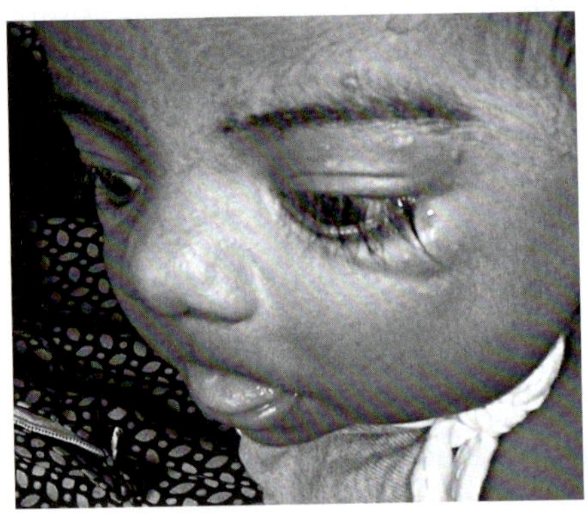

Fig.6.48 Long eyelashes

Photophobia

- Local: Corneal ulcer, iridocyclitis, phlyctenular conjunctivitis, etc.
- Meningitis.
- Vitamin A deficiency (due to its effect on cornea).

Squint and **nystagmus** are discussed under Neurology, p 197–199.

Conjunctiva

Xerosis of conjunctiva: Xerosis means dryness. Xerosis of bulbar conjunctiva is clinically detected by wrinkled appearance when viewed tangentially. Bitot's spot is a gray, rough, dry area on the temporal side of conjunctiva **(Fig. 6.50, p 99)**. Xerosis of cornea is seen as wrinkling of cornea. Keratomalacia is the cloudiness of weakened cornea, which if left alone may perforate. Phlyctenular conjunctivitis may occur on temporal or nasal side **(Fig. 24.84b, p 527)**. Telengiectasia of bulbar conjunctiva is seen in ataxia telengiectasia (p 523).

Oedema and watery discharge together with redness or follicles in the palpebral conjunctiva of upper lids characterize trachoma. Membranous conjunctivitis was characteristic of diphtheria in yesteryears. Petechiae in palpebral conjunctiva may be seen in ITP.

Subconjunctival haemorrhage may be seen in trauma, violent cough (whooping cough) or bleeding disorder (Fig.6.49).

Pupils

Discussed in the neurology section, p 200.

Heterochromia Iris

It is the asymmetry in the colour of the iris. It may be seen in *congenital* Horner syndrome (the eye with Horner is lighter in colour) or secondary to inflammation of the eye or as a sporadic occurrence. See Waardenburg syndrome, p 501.

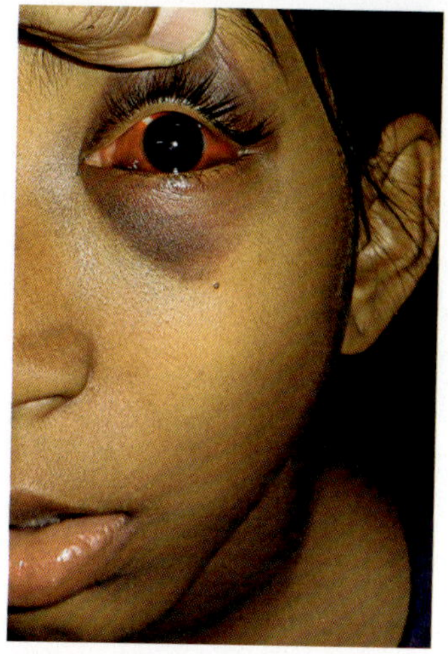

Fig.6.49 Subconjunctival haemorrhage

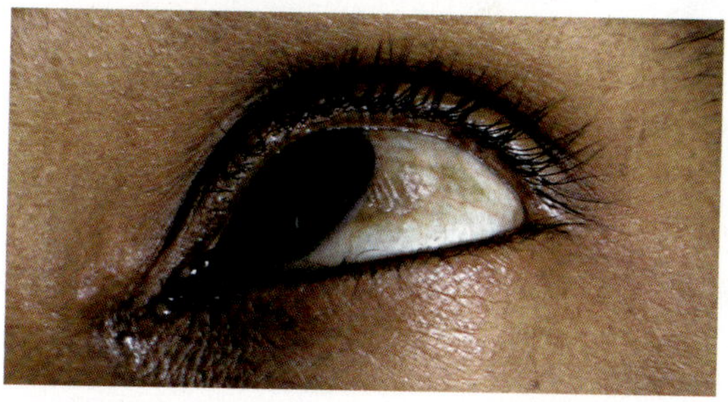

Fig.6.50 Bitot spot

In *Chediak-Higashi syndrome*, there is hypopigmentation of eyes, skin and hair; recurrent bacterial infections and a mild bleeding diathesis.

Aniridia

- Absent irises, usually bilateral
- Photophobia
- Impaired visual acuity
- Association with Wilms' tumour. Children with aniridia should be checked for chromosome 11 deletion as this carries increased risk of Wilms' tumour. Aniridia may be familial and may also be associated with hemihypertrophy.

6

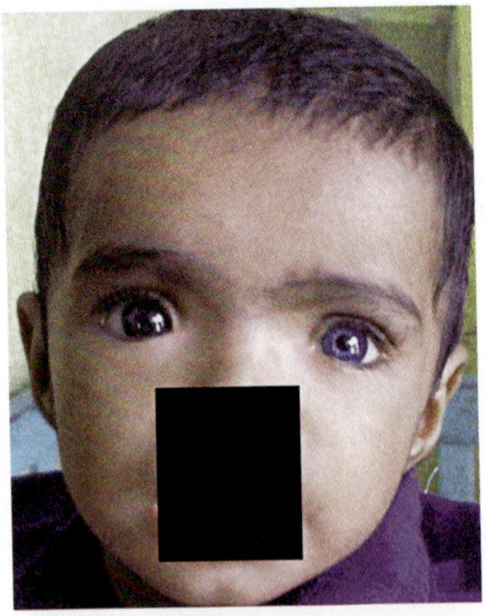

Fig.6.51a Heterochromia of Iris

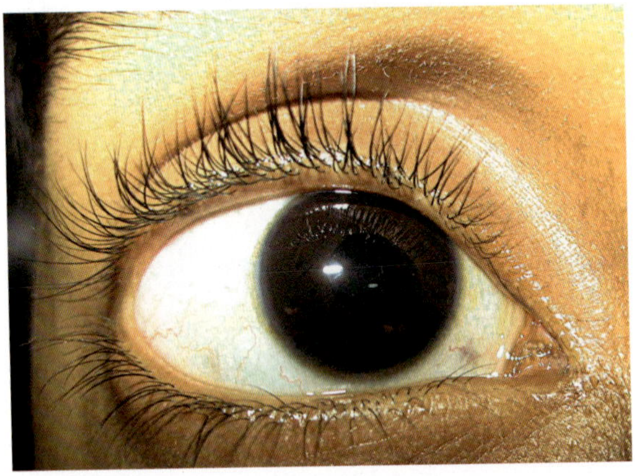

Fig.6.51b Lisch nodule (see page 522)
Courtesy: Dr Sheela Nampoothiri.

Blue Sclera

- Normal newborn or small infants
- Osteogenesis imperfecta
- Ehlers-Danlos syndrome

White Eye Reflex (Cat's eye reflex)

Normally when light is shone through the pupil, a red flare is seen. Here, it is absent and the pupil may appear white. The white reflex arises from the lens, uveal tract or retina.

Most common is cataract.

- Lens: Cataract.
- Retina: Retinoblastoma and retinopathy of prematurity (Fig. 6.52).

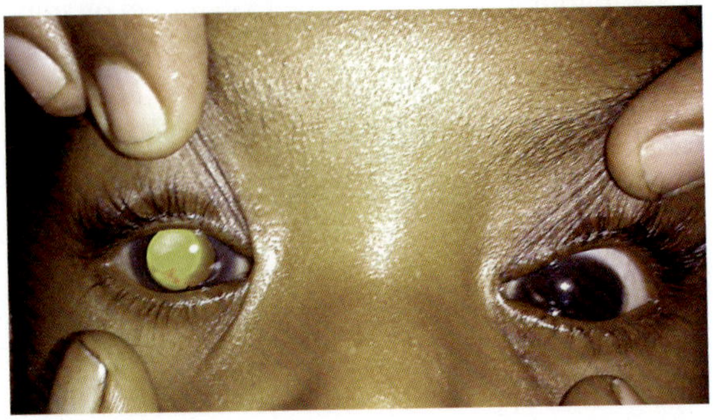

Fig.6.52 White eye reflex due to retinoblastoma

Cataract

Pupil on examination shows white appearance due to cataract (hence called white eye reflex or leukocoria). Other causes of white eye reflex are rare in paediatric practice (but may be seen in ophthalmic practice). If using ophthalmoscope, use +10 lens of ophthalmoscope to visualize the lens (to see cataract).

- Idiopathic: There is no abnormality other than cataract. May run in families. Congenital cataract may be transmitted as autosomal dominant, recessive or X-linked trait. The term 'congenital cataract' is used if it is present at birth or becomes obvious soon after birth.
- Intrauterine infections: Most common is rubella, but can occur in other intrauterine infections as well. It can occur in congenital varicella.
- Metabolic causes: Galactosaemia ("oil drop cataract"), hypoparathyroidism, Wilson disease ("sunflower cataract"), Lowe's syndrome (p 546), diabetes mellitus, etc.
- Chromosomal anomalies and dysmorphic syndromes: Trisomy 13, 18, 21; Turner's, Zellweger's, incontinentia pigmenti.

- Miscellaneous: Trauma, radiation, drugs (e.g., posterior lenticular cataract with long-term steroids) (Fig.6.53).

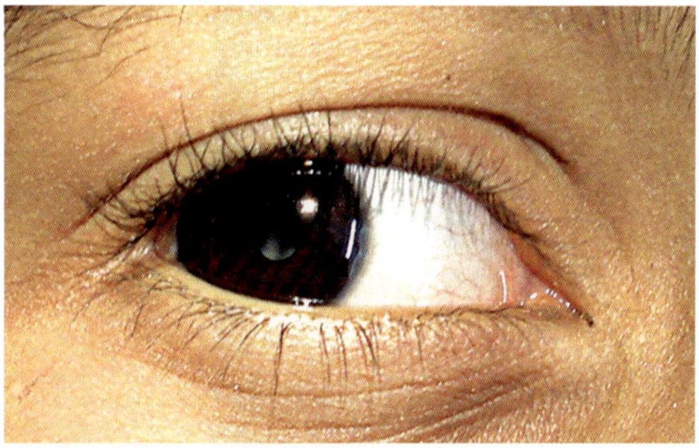

Fig.6.53 Cataract

Ectopia Lentis

Dislocation of lens is seen in Marfan syndrome (upward) and homocystinuria (downward) (Fig.6.54).

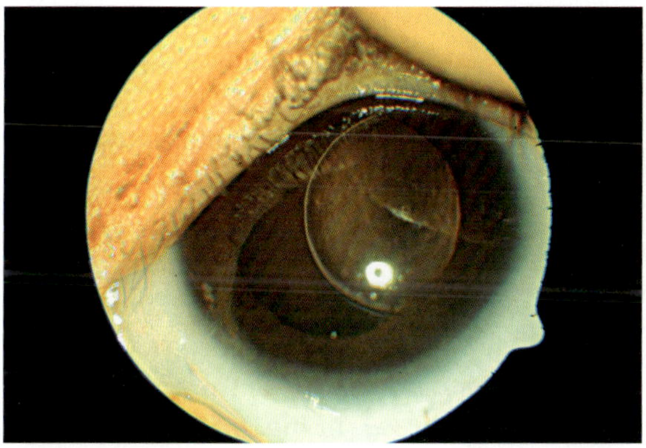

Fig.6.54 Subluxation of lens (magnified view). *Courtesy: Dr Sheela Nampoothiri.*

Buphthalmos (Congential Glaucoma)

- Hazy or cloudy cornea due to corneal oedema
- Enlarged orbital globe (bulging eyeball)
- Blepharospasm (eyelid squeezing)
- Photophobia
- Epiphora (tearing)
- Decreased visual acuity and blindness, if untreated
- Associations: Sturge-Weber syndrome; neurofibromatosis; congenital rubella syndrome (Fig.6.55).

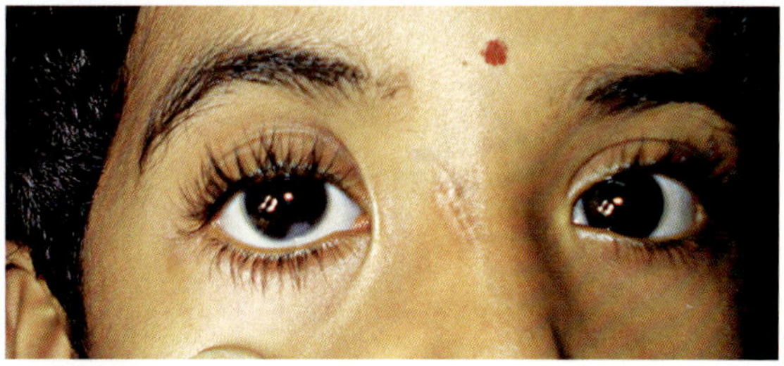

Fig.6.55 Localized corneal opacity

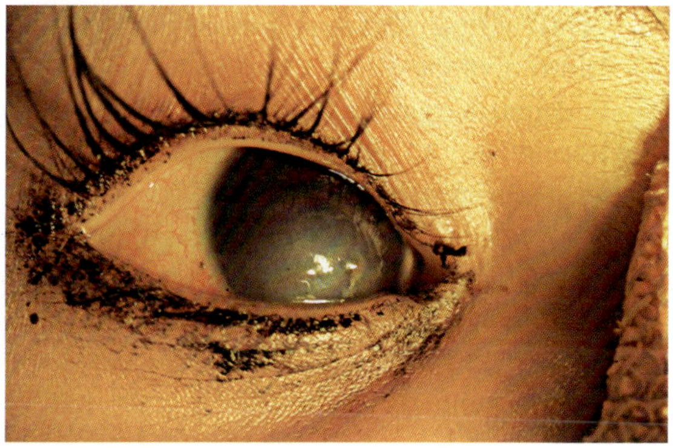

Fig.6.56 Corneal opacity

Optic Atrophy

- Pale, clearly delineated optic discs in primary optic atrophy; yellow/grey discs with blurred margins if atrophy is secondary to papilloedema (see p 191).
- Paucity and attenuation of retinal vessels crossing the optic discs. Normally, >10 vessels are expected; in optic atrophy it is less than 7.
- Enlargement of optic cup.
- Consensual reaction of pupil to light is preserved if the other eye is normal, but no direct light reaction.
- Decreased visual acuity.

6

Optic atrophy may be seen in:

- DIDMOAD (diabetes insipidus + diabetes mellitus + optic atrophy+ deafness)
- Intracranial tumours, due to long-standing increased intracranial tension
- Neurodegenerative syndromes (white matter degeneration)
- Post-inflammatory like optic neuritis
- Leber optic atrophy (male:female ratio = 6:1), where there is bilateral involvement in early adolescence

Papilloedema

Fundus changes are:

- Optic cup gets filled up.
- Hyperaemic discs; dilatation and tortuosity of veins; normal venous pulsations disappear.
- Blurring of the disc margins (usually starts at temporal margins; disc margins are not clearly traceable).
- In severe cases, "macular star" due to macular oedema (in severe hypertension).
- Normal visual acuity (in papillitis, the fundus appearance is similar but there is diminished visual acuity).
- Normal pupillary reflexes (see Fig. 9.5, p200).

Papilloedema is expected in:

- Intracranial space occupying lesions (tumour, abscess, tuberculoma, haematoma).
- Hydrocephalus.
- Foster-Kennedy syndrome: Optic atrophy due to frontal lobe tumour pressing on optic nerve and contralateral papilloedema secondary to raised intracranial pressure.
- Benign intracranial hypertension.

Retinitis Pigmentosa

- Early stages: Clumps of pigment in peripheral retina; so, examine the fundus after dilatation. Pigment deposition in peripheral part of retina giving classical 'bone corpuscle' pattern.
- Earliest clinical manifestation is night blindness. As it progresses, there may be only a tunnel vision.

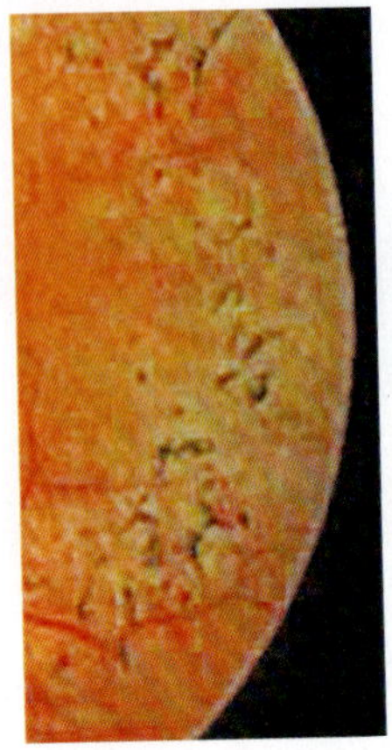

Fig.6.57 Peripheral retina showing retinitis pigmentosa

Associations

- Congenital infections.
- Refsum syndrome: Neuropathy, ataxia, deafness, ichthyosis (autosomal recessive inheritance).
- Laurence-Moon-Biedl syndrome.
- Abetalipoproteinaemia: Acanthocytes, ataxia and lipoprotein abnormalities.

KF Ring

This is seen in the periphery of the cornea, as a golden yellow, orangish red, greenish or brownish ring. There is *no space between the ring and the limbus of cornea*. In Fig. 6.58 (A,B), the arrow shows the ring, which extends into the cornea for variable length over most of the circumference of cornea (in the picture note that there is no space between the ring and the edge of cornea). That there is no space between the ring and the edge of cornea differentiates KF ring from corneal arcus (which is a lipid deposition) because cornal arcus does not extend to the limbus so that there is a *thin* rim of cornea between the arcus ring and the limbus. In addition, the corneal arcus is whitish in colour (Fig.6.58D). Please note that whatever be the colour, a ring outside cornea cannot be KF ring. A ring outside the cornea is shown in the picture (Fig. 6.58C); it is epithelial pigmentation at limbus, which is a variation of normal. At times, it is related to xerosis of conjunctiva or allergy in which case it goes off when the primary condition goes off. There is a brown ring all around the cornea in Fig. 6.58E, but there is a thin rim of clear area demarcating it from cornea.

So this is not KF ring. Fig. 6.58F shows arcus of old age.

Slit lamp examination will show the pigment in KF ring as a coalescence of fine particles (under magnification), and by changing the illumination angle, a play of colours (colours of KF ring mentioned above) may be seen.

KF ring in the initial stages is seen only in the upper and lower corneal margins. After 3–4 years of penicillamine therapy, the ring starts to regress.

KF ring was initially described by Kayser in 1902 and its relation to Wilson disease was established by Fleischer in 1912. KF ring is not specific for Wilson disease, and may rarely be seen in chronic active hepatitis, primary biliary cirrhosis, etc.

Strabismus

It is the non-parallelism of visual axes. Small infants often have a convergent squint because of poor development of coordination and also because of the fact that the medial rectus is stronger than the other muscles at this age. Refractory error can also produce a convergent squint. Since the accommodation and convergence are closely related movements, over action of the medial rectus for accommodation in refractory errors will produce a convergent squint.

Squint can be concomitant or paralytic. In concomitant squint, there is a constant angle of deviation of the eyes in all fields of vision. In paralytic squint, this is not constant and the deviation increases in the direction of movement normally produced by the paretic muscle. More discussion on it can be found under the section of nervous system (p 197) (see Fig. 24.92, 24.93, p 533).

Setting Sun Sign

Eyes are rolled downward, iris is covered by lower eyelids and the upper sclera is visible. This is due to the involvement of the centre of upward gaze in pretectal region (Fig. 24.90).

- Newborns: Setting sun sign may be seen transiently in normal newborn
- Hydrocephalus
- Kernicterus

6

EARS

Low Set Ear

Method

An imaginary line drawn joining medial and lateral canthi is extended towards the ear. Normally, $1/3^{rd}$ of the ear comes above this line. When less than 20% (10% as per some books) comes above this line, it is a low set ear. However, this old definition is not favoured now. The currently favoured definition is that the superior attachment of pinna to the side of head must be at or above the line joining the two inner canthi in normal children. If it is below this line, it is considered low set ear. This eliminates the apparent low set ear due to poorly developed helix (like in some cases of Down syndrome) and posteriorly rotated ears. If examined with the child's head extended, the ears may appear falsely low set. So examine from the front with the child's head held erect and eyes facing directly forwards. Keeping a transparent film with rulings in front of face helps in objectively assessing whether the ear is low set or not (Fig. 6.60). Small low set ears may be seen in Down syndrome. Large prominent ears may be seen in Marfan, Fragile X syndrome, etc. Deformed pinna is seen in Treacher Collins, Goldenhar syndrome, Down syndrome, etc. Low set ears may be seen in Apert's, Carpenter's,

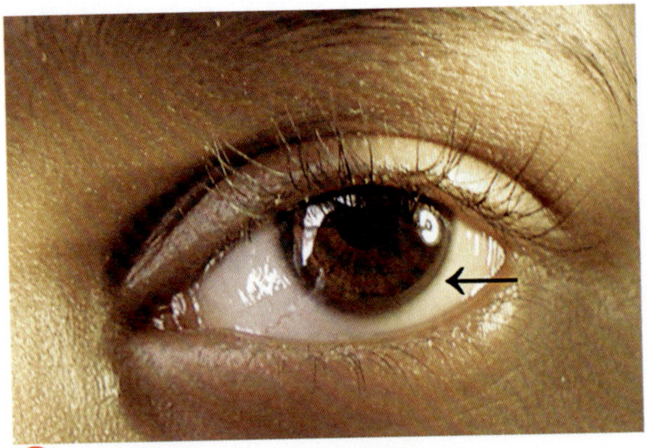

A KF ring

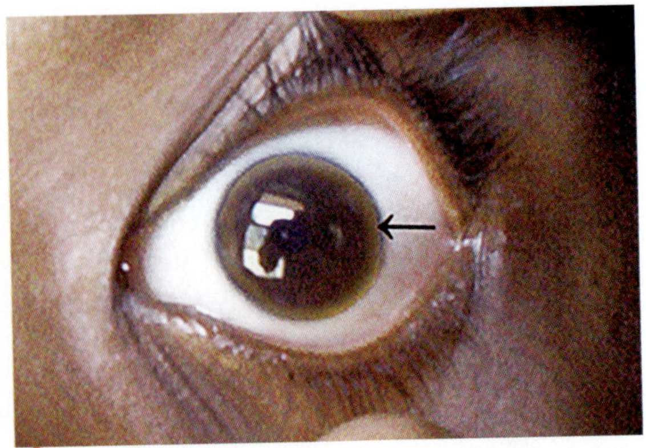

B KF ring

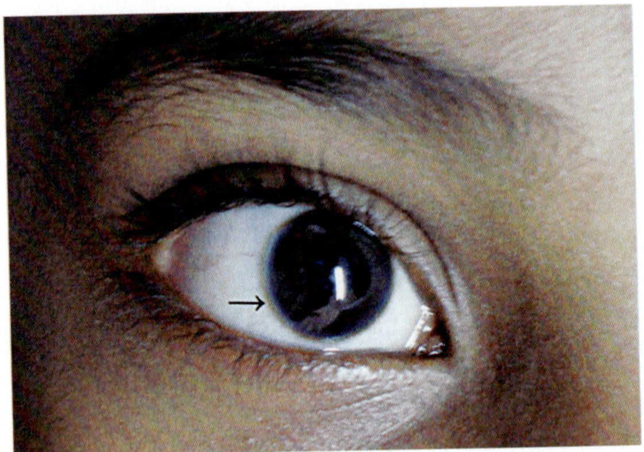

C Ring outside cornea, so not KF ring. See p 103

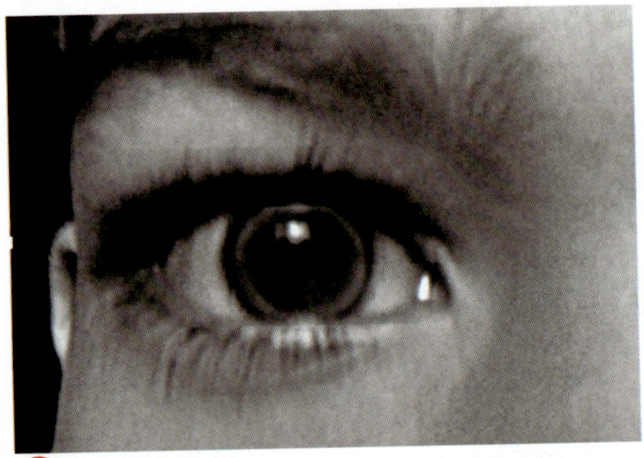

D Corneal arcus

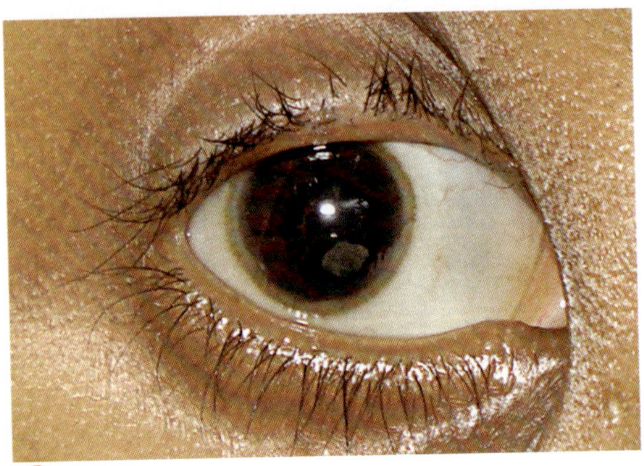

E See text p 103

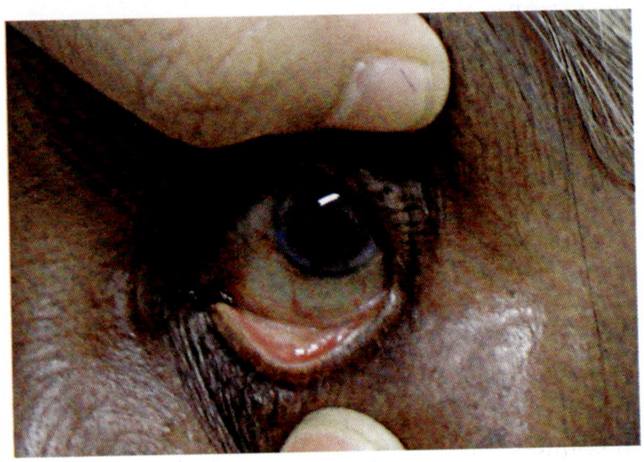

F Arcus of old age

Fig.6.58 KF ring and closely mimicking conditions

DiGeorge, Noonan's, Potter's, trisomy 13, trisomy 18, Turner's and many other dysmorphic syndromes (see low set ear in **Fig. 6.44**).

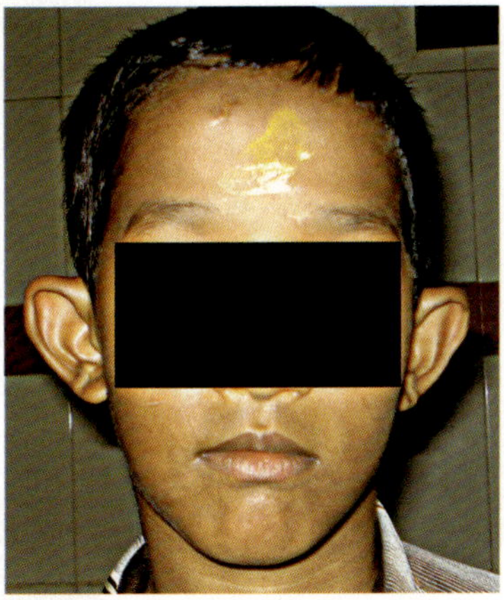

Fig.6.59 Prominent ear

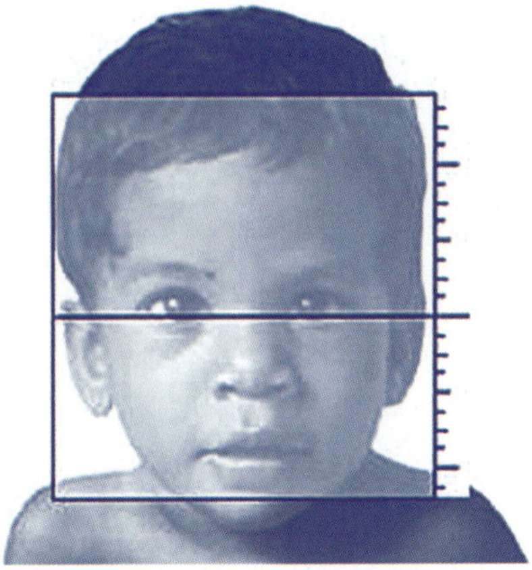

Fig.6.60 Ruled transparent sheet for face measurements

Protuberant ear: The normal ear makes angle of no more than 10° with the scalp and this should help identify a protuberant ear (Fig. 6.59).

For clinical purposes, ear that appears to "stand out" may be considered protuberant ear. The long axis of the pinna usually makes a slant of not more than approximately 15° with the vertical axis of the head. An angle of more than 20° is **posterior rotation of pinna**.

Bat ear: Protruding ears with poorly formed folds of helix (Fig. 6.61). Horizontal crease in ear lobe is described in Beckwith–Wiedemann syndrome.

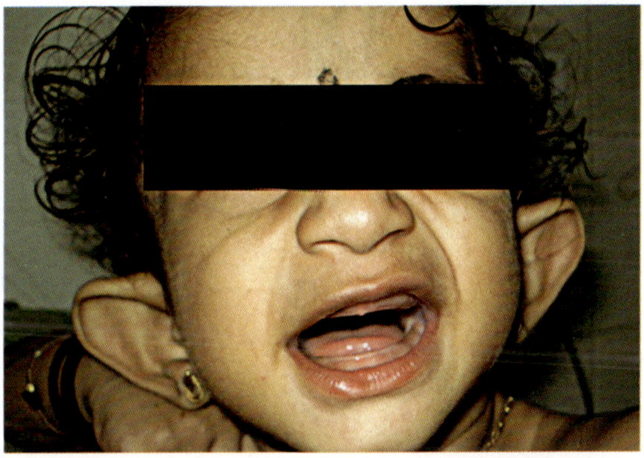

Fig.6.61 Bat ear: Note the poorly formed folds of helix and prominent protruding ears.

Preauricular Tags

Preauricular tags usually contain a bit of cartilage and hence feel firm (Fig. 6.65). It is benign condition, but hearing assessment may be considered. Preauricular pits are generally benign; it may run in families. Enquiry regarding any discharge from the pit and hearing assessment are warranted. Unilateral large ear may be positional, like in torticollis (Ref. 6).

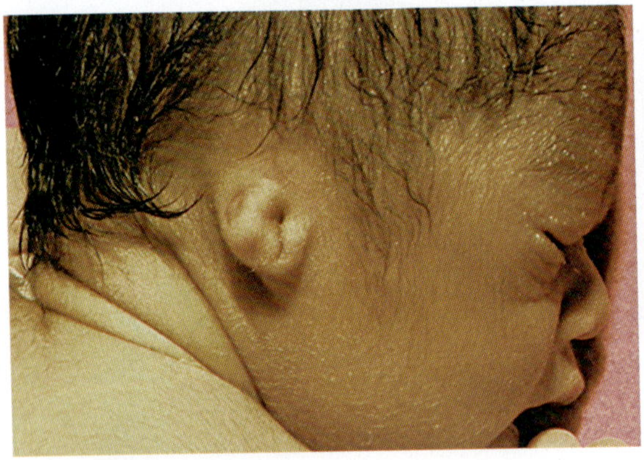

Fig.6.62 Microtia: Most children with microtia will have hearing loss, mostly ipsilateral.

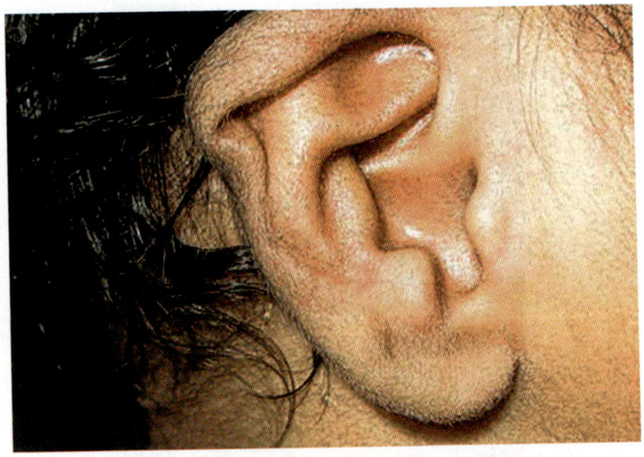

Fig.6.64 Crumpled pinna

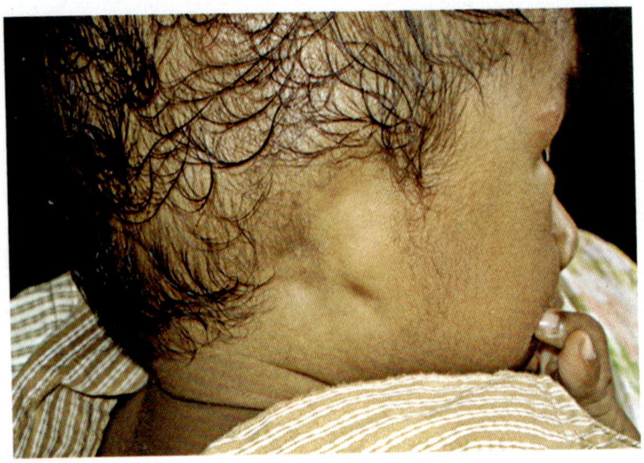

Fig.6.63 Anotia

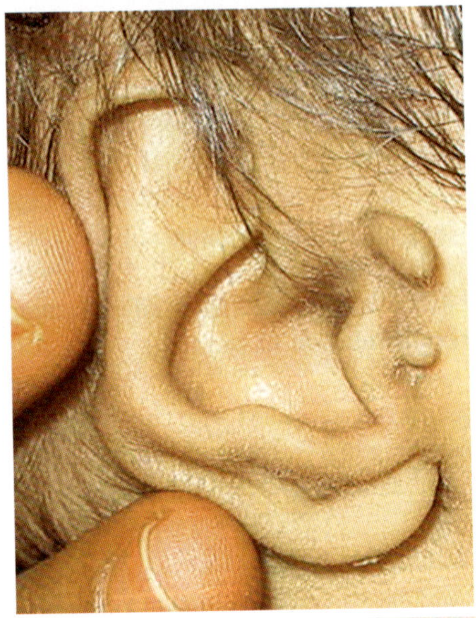

Fig.6.65 Preauricular tag

Tragus sign: Pressing over the tragus causes pain, indicative of otitis externa. See parts of ear marked in Fig. 6.66.

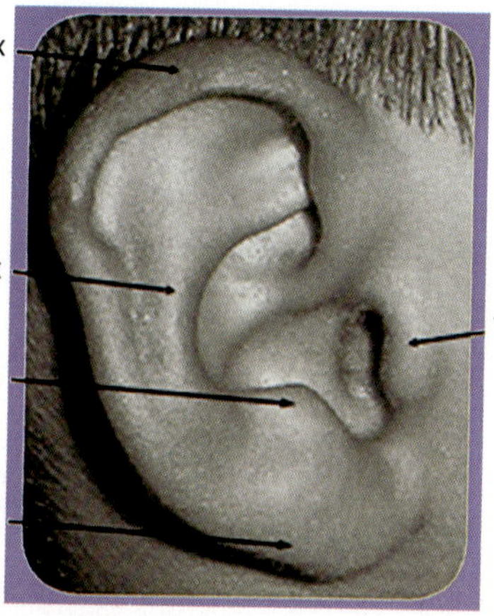

Fig.6.66 Ear parts

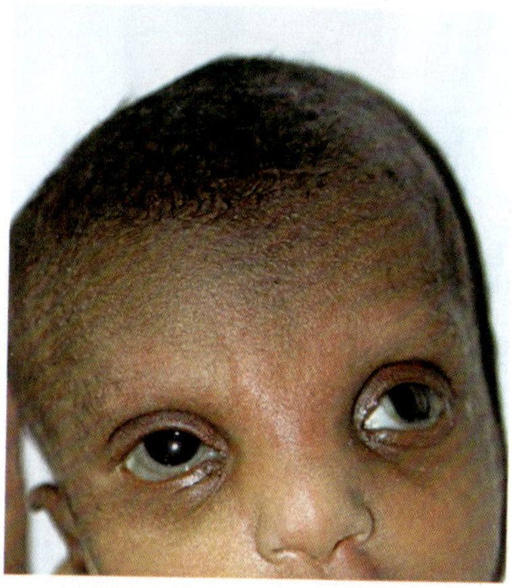

Fig.6.67 Broad nasal root: May be seen in craniofrontonasal dysplasia, GM_1 gangliosidosis, etc. Squared nasal root may be seen in DiGeorge syndrome *(Courtesy: Dr Sheela Nampoothiri).*

Acute otitis media: Tympanic membrane will be inflamed and bulging forward. There is loss of light reflex. Relief of pain is brought about by perforation. There will be conductive hearing loss.

DEAFNESS

Deafness can be conduction deafness or sensorineural deafness. Refer to section on neurology (p 206).

- Sequel of neonatal kernicterus
- Intrauterine infections like rubella
- Deafness is part of many syndromes
- Recurrent otitis media
- Otitis media with sterile effusion (OME) causes temporary conduction deafness for a few weeks to months
- Hypothyroid syndromes (e.g., Pendred syndrome)
- Drugs like aminoglycosides
- Conduction deafness is due to mechanical block, most common being wax
- Traumatic damage to tympanic membrane

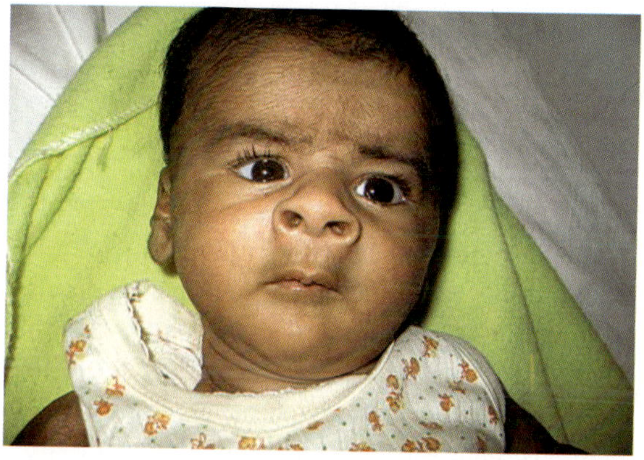

Fig.6.68 Anteverted nose: Seen in many syndromes; e.g., acrodysostosis. When the dorsum of nose is very short, the nasal tip is pulled upwards and this results in anteverted nares *(Courtesy: Dr Sheela Nampoothiri).*

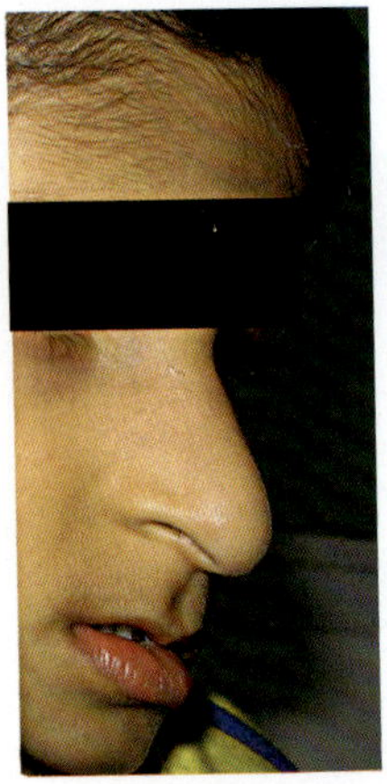

Fig.6.69 Beaked nose: The term 'beaked nose' or 'hooked nose' is used to describe an unusually pointed prominent nose; the term is also used to describe nose with poorly developed ala nasi so that the nasal septum is seen prominently. This type of nose is described in many syndromes; e.g., Seckel syndrome, some trisomies, Alagille syndrome, etc *(Courtesy: Dr Sheela Nampoothiri).*

MOUTH

Normally, the dimensions of mouth is such that the outer edge of the lips fall on a perpendicular dropped from the centre of either pupil with the eyes looking straight ahead. When the edge of the lips fall well outside these perpendiculars, the patient has macrostomia; when the edge of the lips fall well within these same perpendiculars, the patient has microstomia.

Large mouth: Goldenhar syndrome, Williams syndrome, etc. Blister or callus at the centre of upper lip in the first few weeks of life is the remnant of vigorous intrauterine sucking and is of no consequence. Red patch below or above the lip may be found in habitual lip-lickers.

Mandibular hypoplasia: Pierre Robin syndrome (see p 513).

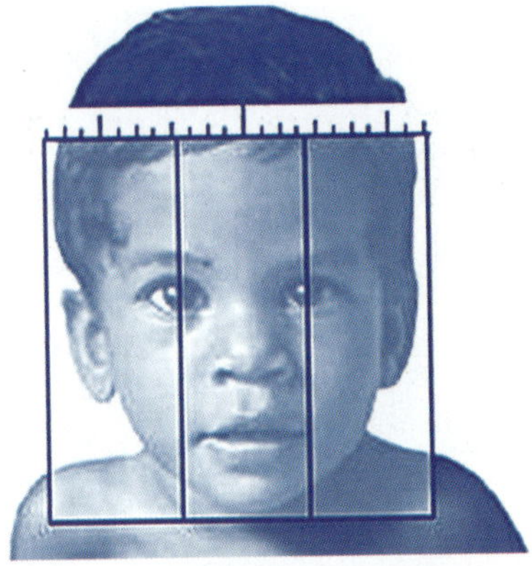

Fig.6.70 Ruled transparent sheet for mouth measurements

Angular stomatitis is found in:

- Riboflavin deficiency [cracked corners of mouth may be seen in monilial (Candida) infection also; see Fig. 17.1, p 390].
- Rhagades (in congenital syphilis)

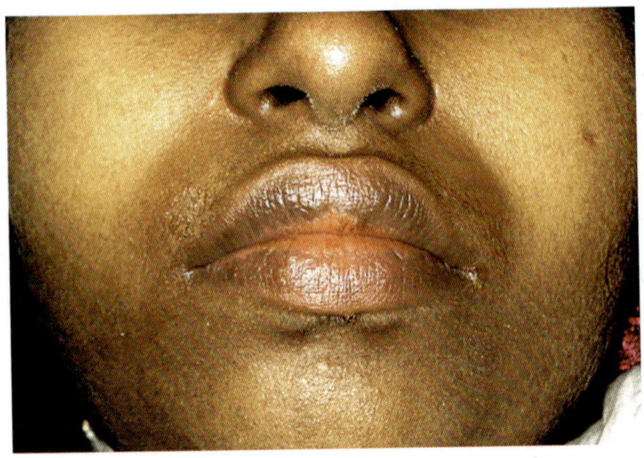

Fig.6.71 Circum oral pigmentation in Fanconi anaemia

Philtrum (See Fig. 6.42D)

Nose and philtrum occupy the cental zone of face. Hence, a change in the length of one is accompanied by a compensatory change in the length of the other. A long nose results in **short philtrum** and short nose leads to **long philtrum**.

- Long philtrum (Fig. 6.72): Williams syndrome, Cornelia de Lange (Fig. 24.35)
- Short philtrum: Cohen syndrome

- Smooth philtrum ("flat and featureless"): Foetal alcohol syndrome
  Multiple frenulum are seen in Ellis-van Creveld syndrome (see Fig.24.43, p 509)

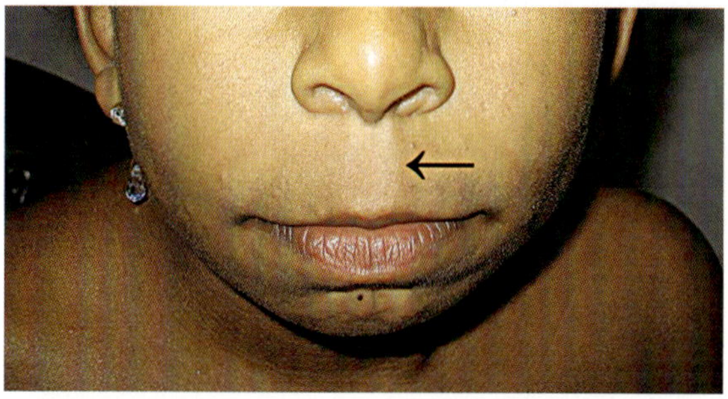

Fig.6.72 Long philtrum. Also note the thin upper lip. Long philtrum may be seen in fetal valproate syndrome *(Courtesy: Dr Sheela Nampoothiri)*.

Palate

- Normal palate is smoothly curved in all directions. Palate is high arched if the roof of palate is not seen when the examiner's eyes are at level with the upper incisor teeth and the patient keeping the mouth wide open **(ref. 23)**.
- Prominent palatal ridges (Fig. 6.76) may be due to poor tongue thrusting of the baby, which in turn could be due to neurological deficits resulting in poor sucking. These ridges make the palate look very narrow.
- Cleft palate may be seen as an isolated anomaly or in trisomy 13, trisomy 18, Pierre Robin syndrome, Beckwith-Wiedemann syndrome, fetal hydantoin syndrome, etc (Fig. 24.51, p 506).
- Look for isolated cleft palate, especially if there is a nasal twang of voice. Submucous cleft will have to be palpated for.
- Bifid uvula may be seen in Apert's syndrome, DiGeorge syndrome, Treacher Collins syndrome, etc. Bifid uvula is usually a variation of normal only. However, in the presence of bifid uvula, one must palpate for submucous cleft palate, which is a common accompaniment (Fig. 6.74).
- Painful ulcer of hard palate may be due to herpes zoster, if there is evidence for the same in the nerve distribution. Petechiae in the same location is painless (petechiae is painless, whereas ulcer is painful). Herpangina produces painful ulcers in oropharynx, soft palate and uvula.
- Exanthematous fevers may show rash in mucous membranes (enanthem) before the appearance of skin rashes (exanthem) (Fig. 6.74).

Drooling

- Normal during teething
- Stomatitis

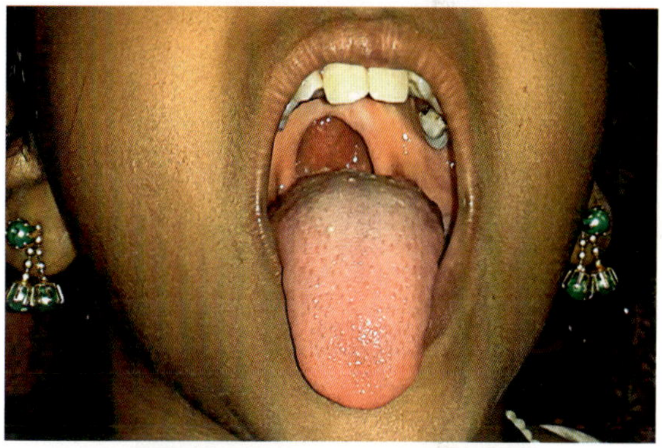

Fig.6.73 Cleft palate limited to soft palate

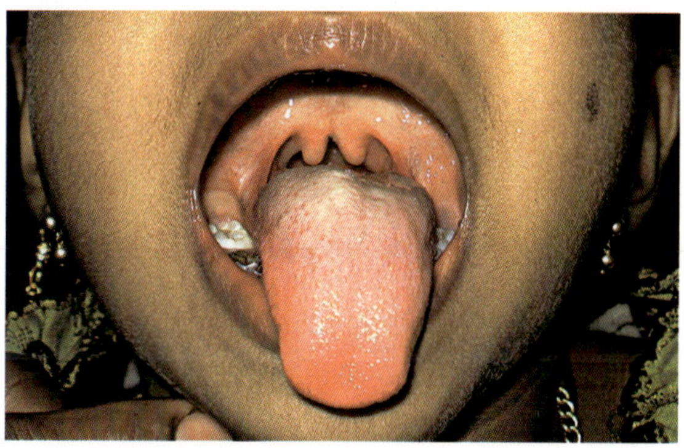

Fig.6.74 Bifid uvula

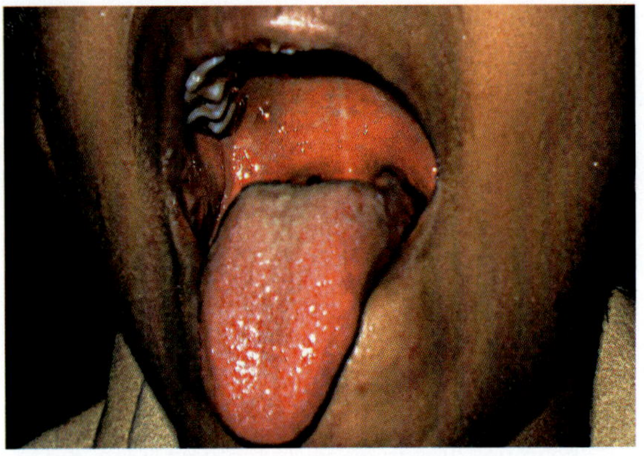

Fig.6.75 Enanthem. See exanthem of measles on p 547.

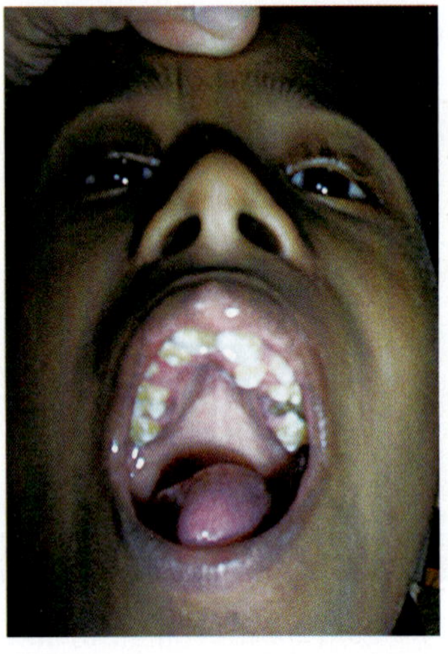

Fig.6.76 Note the high arched palate and prominent palatal ridges on the lateral sides, which make the palate very narrow.

- Acute epiglottitis/diphtheria/tonsillitis/herpangina, etc.
- Pseudobulbar palsy (e.g., cerebral palsy)

Dry Mouth

- Dehydration
- Mouth breathing
- Antihistamines, atropine-like drugs, etc

Oral Thrush

- Antibiotics
- Steroids
- AIDS
- Hypoparathyroidism
- Note: Recently ingested milk may give a thrush-like appearance to the tongue

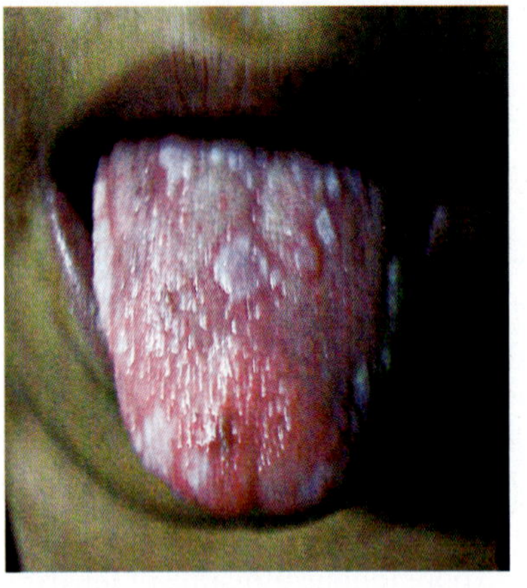

Fig.6.77 Oral thrush

Lips and oral cavity are discussed in Ch. 11 (p 390–393).

Trismus

- Tetanus
- Infantile Gaucher's disease
- Part of dystonia (e.g., metoclopramide poisoning)
- Temporomandibular joint arthritis (seen in juvenile rheumatoid arthritis)
- Encephalitis (rarely)

Cry

- Shrill cry ("high pitched cry") in CNS insults like meningitis.
  Intermittent inconsolable cry followed by sleep of exhaustion during relief is seen in infants with intussusception.
- Cat-like mewing cry in cri du chat syndrome (this cry progressively become less characteristic as the child grows).
- Weak cry in neuromuscular disorders (like Werdnig-Hoffman syndrome).
- Crying on handling is due to painful conditions like arthritis, fractures, etc. Babies with CNS insults like meningitis also resent handling.
- Hoarse cry may be due to hypothyroidism or local causes like laryngitis.

Salivary Glands

Parotid duct opens in buccal mucosa, opposite second upper molar (check for redness of exuding pus). Bimanual palpation if indicated, may be done with a gloved finger inside the mouth and the other hand over the parotid gland externally. The duct of submandibular salivary gland opens on the underside of the tongue just lateral to the frenulum. Bimanual palpation may be needed to differentiate the enlargement of submandibular salivary gland from submandibular lymph node.

TEETH

Delayed Dentition

The normal pattern of eruption of teeth is discussed in the chapter on growth and development (p 51). No teeth beyond 13 months of age may be considered as delayed dentition.

The causes may be:

- Constitutional delay
- Hypothyroidism
- Hypopituitarism
- Rickets
- PEM

During examination, count the number of teeth. See if they are permanent or milk teeth. The permanent teeth are more yellowish and have serrated cutting edges. When both permanent and milk teeth are present, the colour helps a lot to differentiate.

Mottling and discolouration of teeth is due to poor enamel formation. Such children are more prone for caries formation (see Fig. 6.79).

Discoloured Teeth

- Poor oral hygiene
- Tetracycline therapy (brownish)
- Enamel hypoplasia (brownish)
- Kernicterus (brownish)
- Porphyria (reddish)
- Iron therapy (blackish)
- Chalk white patches or dull unglazed tooth, pitting, etc, may be seen in endemic fluorosis.

Gum Hyperplasia

- Poor oral hygiene
- Dilantin therapy
- Acute monocytic leukaemia
- Scurvy
- Epulis
- Delayed dentition
- When teeth get destroyed as in nursing caries, the gum may appear relatively large compared to the tooth

Blue line along the ridge of gum may be seen in lead poisoning.

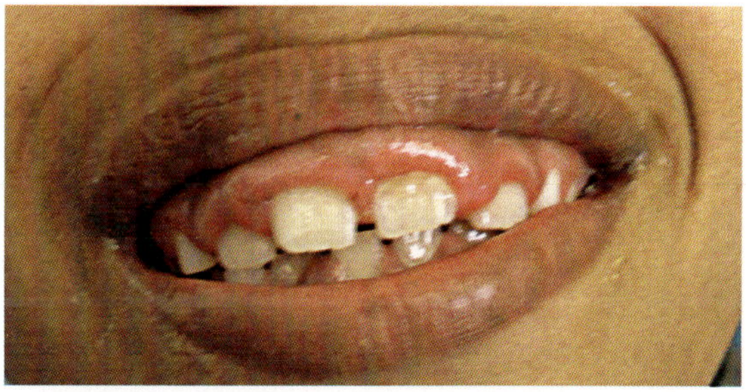

Fig.6.78 Gum hypertrophy

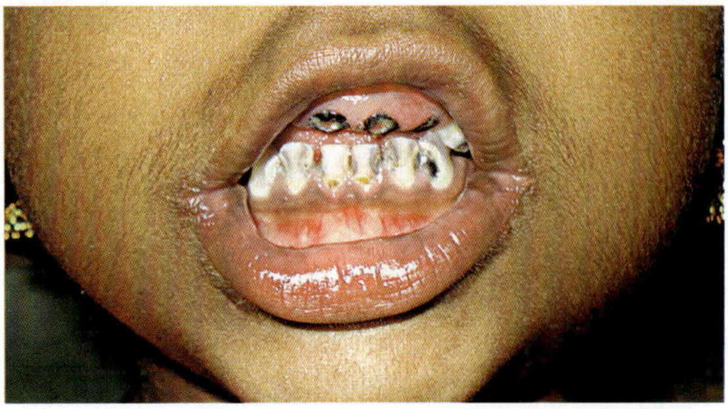

Fig.6.79 Nursing caries: Sleeping with milk feeds is strongly associated with this type of caries.

Swollen spongy bleeding gums may be seen in scurvy.

Neonatal teeth may be seen as a normal variation and in Ellis-van Creveld syndrome.

Tongue

Also see p 391.

Macroglossia

- Congenital hypothyroidism.
- Down syndrome (rarely fissured tongue, otherwise called "scrotal tongue"). In Down syndrome, tongue is relatively large compared to oral cavity.
- Beckwith-Wiedemann syndrome (Fig. 24.33).
- Local causes: Cystic hygroma, haemangioma, lymphangioma, etc.
- Glycogenosis type II, Hurler's syndrome.
- Tongue protrusion without macroglossia occurs in mental retardation.

Small tongue may be seen in spastic paralysis (UMN or pseudobulbar palsy) or flaccid paralysis (LMN or bulbar palsy).

Coating of Tongue

- Poor oral hygiene
- Typhoid fever
- Uraemia

Ulcer of the frenulum of tongue may be seen in severe cough, like whooping cough (due to mechanical injury).

Ranula is a retention cyst on the underside of tongue.

Smooth bald tongue without papillae may be seen in B_{12} deficiency.

Geographical tongue shows reddish areas of desquamation.

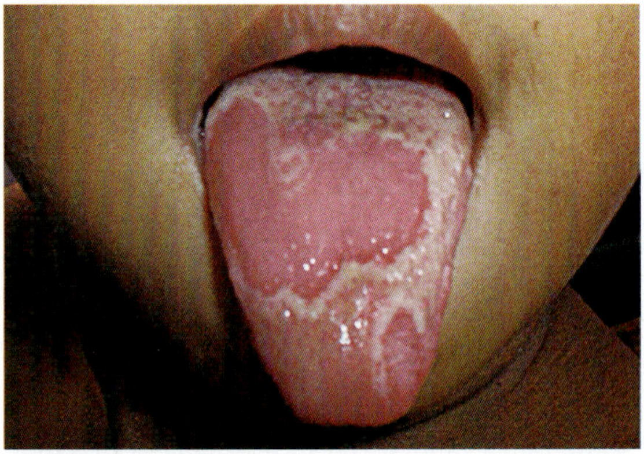

Fig.6.80 Geographic tongue

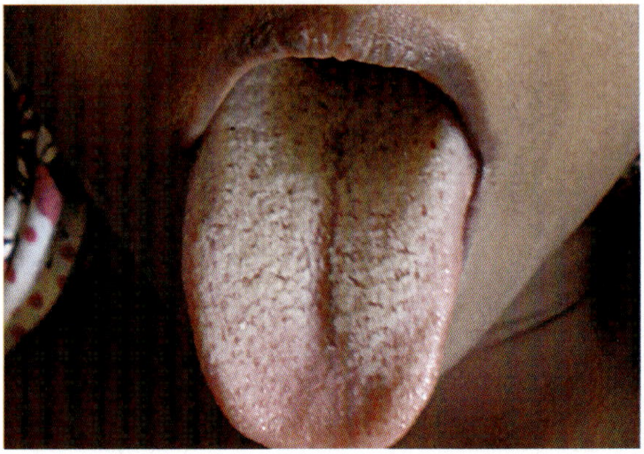

Fig.6.81 Coated tongue

NECK

Short Neck

- Turner's syndrome (Fig. 24.60)
- Noonan's syndrome (Fig. 24.48)

- Morquio syndrome (Fig. 24.18)
- Down's syndrome (pp 507)
- Klippel-Feil deformity
- Sprengel's deformity
- Platybasia
- Hypothyroidism
- Hurler's syndrome

Ratio of neck length (distance between the external occipital protuberance and the C7 spine) and height (Bird's index) is normally < 1:12.8; if it is more than 13.6, it suggests short neck (Ref. 2). This value is given as 13.6 (Ref. 24) or 12.7 as per other sources.
Neck length = 10 + (0.035 × Height) *(Ref: PV Mahajan PV, Bharucha BA. Indian Pediatrics 1994)*

Average neck length (NL) is 11.2 cm at 3 years and 15.5 cm at 12 years.

(NL/Ht) × 100 provides a mean value of 12.7, which can be used in all children across the age groups. As there are no standards, the students can follow their teacher's advice on normal standard.

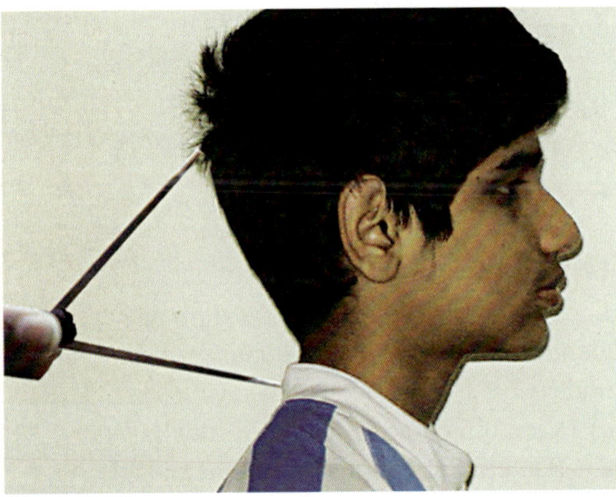

Fig.6.82 Neck length measurement

Neck length is actually the distance from the point where the neck meets the shoulder and the inferior margin of occipital bone. However, it is only subjective and there is no objective way to measure as the landmarks are very vague. Hence, for objectivity, the neck length is measured from external occipital protuberance to the spinous process of C7.

Neck length can be measured by an apparatus similar to the divider in the instrument box of school students; the measurement is made between two fixed bony points (inion and spinous process of C7) with the head held in neutral position.

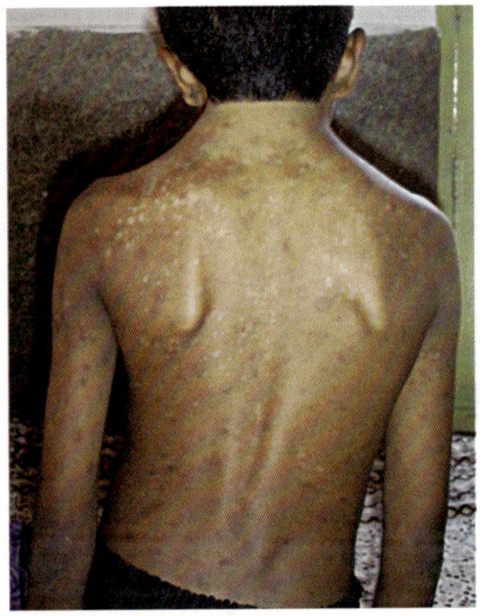

Fig.6.83 Short neck

Goitre

- Puberty goitre
- Hashimoto's thyroiditis
- Iodine deficiency
- Congenital enzyme deficiencies of thyroxine biosynthesis
- Graves disease

Thyroid gland is best appreciated when the child extends the neck or when the child swallows (thyroid gland moves with swallowing). Traditional recommendation is to palpate from the back, but most children do not like to be approached from the back. So many paediatricians prefer to examine from the front, by placing both thumbs over

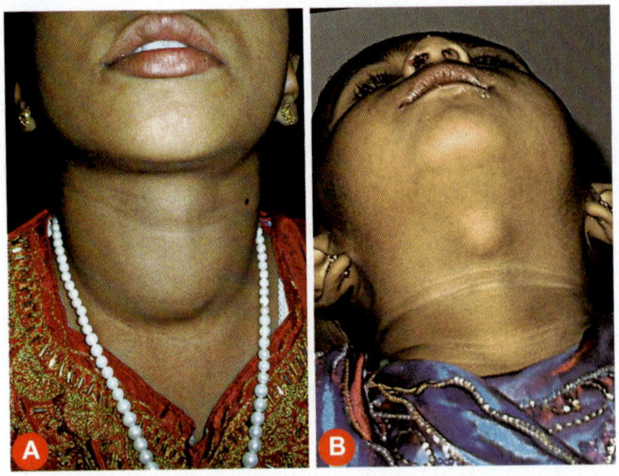

Fig.6.84 (a) Goitre, (b) Thyroglossal cyst

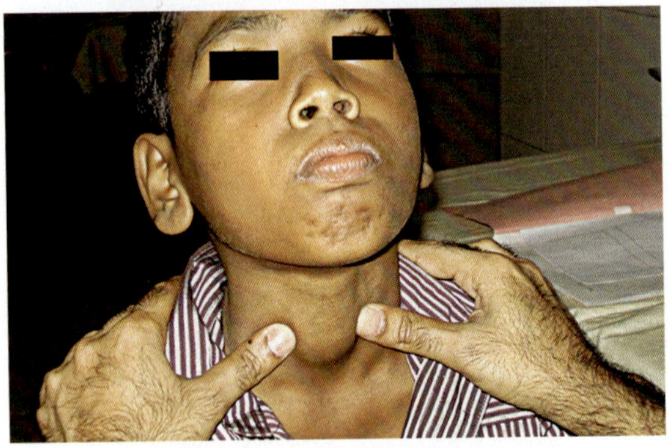

Fig.6.85 Palpation of thyroid from the front

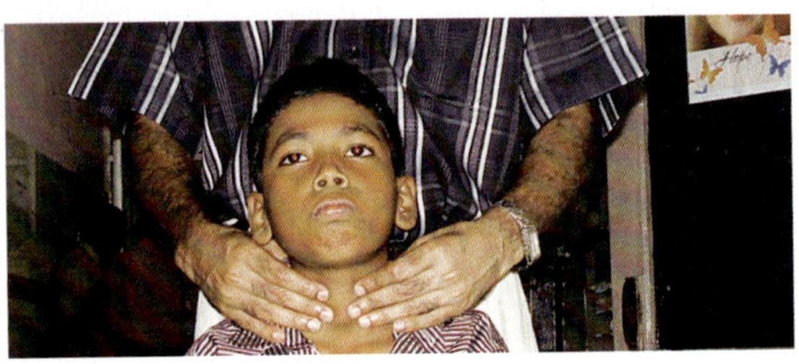

Fig.6.86 Palpation of thyroid from behind

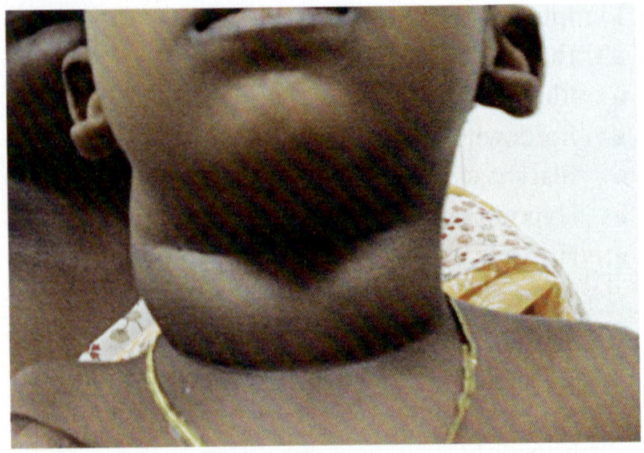

Fig.6.87 Bull neck, classically described in diphtheria

the thyroid and feeling its size, borders and nodularity as the child swallows. Palpating from the back, one can use second and third fingers placed over the thyroid to palpate it. Normal thyroid gland is soft and hence difficult to delineate the borders. The gland is firm in autoimmune thyroiditis and rather hard in carcinoma (unlikely in a child). Thyroglossal cyst when present is found in the midline somewhere between the thyroid gland and the chin; it characteristically moves with protruding tongue.

Webbing of Neck

- Turner's syndrome (Figs. 24.60, 24.61)
- Noonan's syndrome

Lymphadenopathy

Localized: Any infection in the drainage area.

Generalized (>2 non-contiguous groups of lymph nodes):

- Viral infections: IMN, HIV, rubella, etc
- Bacterial infections: E.g., tuberculosis
- Malignancy: Lymphoma, leukaemia
- Connective tissue disorders: SLE, JRA
- Drugs: Phenytoin

Lymph node may be described by its site, size, number, consistency, fluctuation, tenderness, mobility (fixity to skin or deep structures), matting and whether there is any sinus formation. Significant enlargement of lymph nodes is taken as >1 cm in cervical and >1.5 cm in inguinal regions (some authorities put it as >1.5 cm for cervical nodes as well). Regarding axillary nodes also there is no consensus, except that 0.5 cm or less is definitely not significant and >1 cm is significant. 0.5–1 cm is a grey zone, the significance attributed depending on the clinical scenario.

Facing the child, with fingers of both hands feel the occipital group of glands at the back of the head along the hairline. Now take the hands forwards to feel the postauricular glands with fingers; simultaneously both the thumbs can come forward to feel the preauricular glands. Now move the hands downwards to feel the posterior cervical glands, go still down to feel supraclavicular glands (rare to be enlarged). Then move the hand up along the anterior border of sternomastoid feeling the anterior cervical glands, still up to feel the jugulodigastric glands, then move forwards to feel the submandibular and submental glands. Unlike in adults, it is not advisable to palpate the cervical glands approaching from the back, because most children resent this and become un-cooperative.

The preauricular, postauricular and suboccipital glands belong to the horizontal group of cervical glands. The vertical groups of glands are felt along the anterior and posterior margins of the sternomastoid muscle and most of them belong to the superficial groups of cervical lymph nodes. Deep cervical nodes are hard to palpate unless considerably enlarged, as they are deep in the anterior border of sternomastoid. Jugulodigastric nodes belong to the deep cervical group whose enlargement is associated with tonsillitis.

Axillary glands of different groups are to be palpated; behind the pectoralis (anterior or pectoral), posterior wall of axilla (subscapular), upper medial arm bordering axilla (brachial or lateral) and deep into the apex of axilla and lateral chest wall.

For epitrochlear glands, palpate just above the medial condyle of humerus. Epitrochlear glands, after locating, is palpated in a cephalocaudal direction to avoid mistaking palpable ulnar nerve for epitrochlear gland. These glands are enlarged in IMN, NHL, HIV, Secondary Syphilis.

Inguinal glands are palpable horizontally along the inguinal ligament and vertically along the direction of femoral vessels and femoral triangle. Inguinal glands are palpable so frequently in normal people that enlargement more than 1.5 cm alone is considered significant, but no standard guidelines exist in this regard.

Popliteal gland, if enlarged, may be palpable in popliteal fossa.

Lymph nodes of abdomen: External iliac nodes may be palpable in the iliac fossa above the inguinal ligament, only if they are considerably enlarged. Mesenteric and retroperitoneal glands (para-aortic glands) are palpable only if hugely enlarged (e.g., lymphoma); in that case, one cannot make out whether it is a gland, so proceed to describe it as an abdominal mass rather than committing that it is lymph node. If the mass is mobile only at right angles to the line of attachment of mesentery, it may be assumed to be mesenteric gland.

Large mediastinal node mass cannot be palpated, but may be indirectly suspected by dullness to percussion (e.g., lymphoma, T cell leukaemia).

Meticulous examination of all these lymph node regions is not indicated routinely, but may be undertaken in relevant cases like malignancy.

Warm tender glands indicate infection. Soft fluctuant glands indicate suppuration. Matted glands indicate chronic inflammation (e.g., tuberculosis- due to periadenitis). Discrete hard nodes (particularly a large hard node) indicate malignancy. Cystic hygroma is usually located on one side in the posterior triangle of the neck and it trans-illuminates.

Description of lymph nodes: The nodes are examined by a combination of inspection and palpation. Percussion for lymph nodes is used only for mediastinal glands causing mediastinal widening.

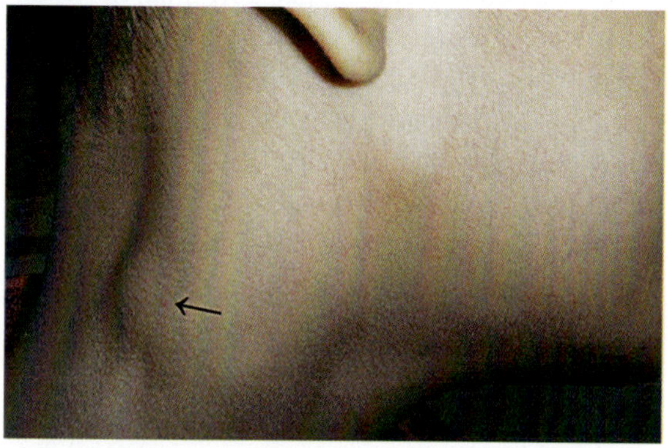

Fig.6.88 Lymph node (posterior cervical)

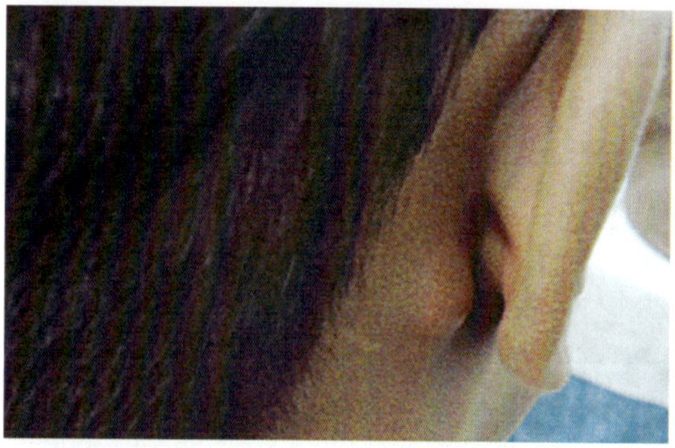

Fig.6.89 Postauricular lymph node

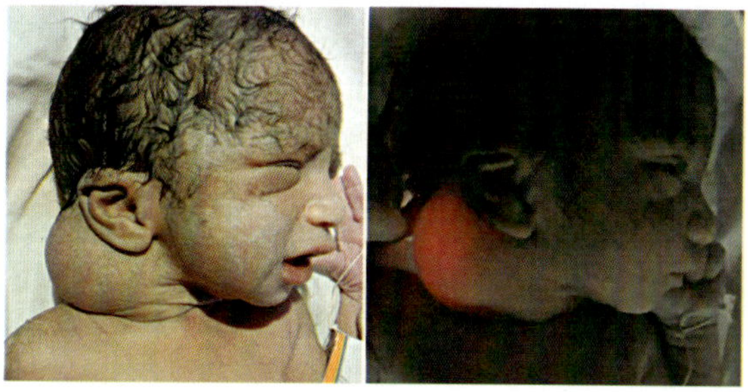

Fig.6.90 Cystic chygroma

- Site
- Size
- Number
- Consistency
- Tenderness
- Features of periadenitis: Will cause either fixity to adjacent structures or sticking together of adjacent glands (matting)
- Skin over the gland (fixity to the gland, sinus/ulcer, etc)
- Comment on any obvious focus of infection in the drainage area of the enlarged gland

Neck Stiffness

- Meningitis (stiffness on flexing the neck but not on lateral movement). When there is doubt whether it is voluntary resistance, bring the child to the edge of the table so that the head hangs loosely down. Now flex the neck and the voluntary resistance to flexion will no longer be there. It is because the head hanging below the edge of the table is uncomfortable for the child and hence he cooperates with flexion movement. Testing for neck stiffness with the child sitting with the knees extended is more sensitive than testing for it in supine position. This is because in the former position, neural elements of the whole length of spinal canal stretch fully.
- Subarachnoid haemorrhage.
- Meningism: Upper lobe pneumonia, tonsillitis, etc.
- Herniation of brain (as in space occupying lesions).
- Due to neck retraction: Tetanus (actually it is painfully retracted neck), dystonia of various causes like phenothiazine toxicity. Here, lateral movement of the neck is also restricted.
- Local causes: Retropharyngeal abscess, painful cervical adenitis, local trauma, etc. Here, lateral movement of neck is also painful.

Opisthotonus (Fig. 6.91)

- Kernicterus
- Tetanus
- Meningitis
- Infantile Gaucher's disease
- Part of dystonia (e.g., metoclopramide poisoning)
- Part of decerebration
- Local causes: Retropharyngeal abscess (usually only neck retraction)

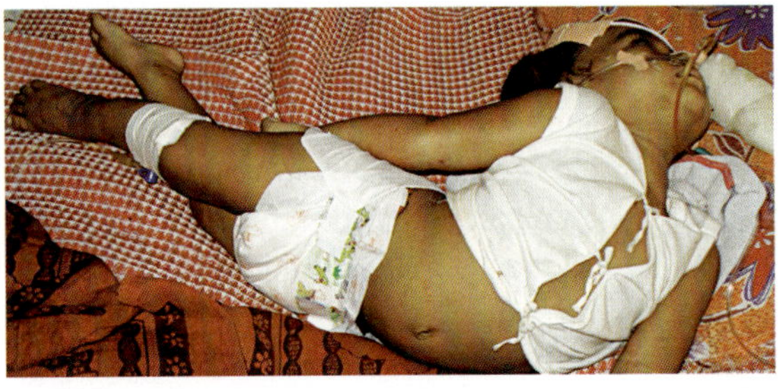

Fig.6.91 Opisthotonus

Typical Postures

- Epiglottitis: Sitting up, leaning forward, prefers not to lie down.
- Peritonitis: Lies quietly, does not move much.
- Meningitis: Lies on one side with thighs flexed on abdomen or opisthotonus posture.
- Lordotic posture: Exaggerated lumbar lordosis. Seen in muscle diseases (due to proximal weakness) and bilateral hip problems.

Refer to the section on neurology for discussion on postures in various neurological diseases.

CHEST

Relevant general examination findings in the chest are discussed under the respiratory and cardiovascular systems (see p354–369).

Some readily visible abnormalities are listed below:

- Absence of clavicle: Cleidocranial dysostosis (Figs. 24.24).
- Presternal oedema may be found in mumps.
- Widely spread nipples may be seen in Turner's (space between the nipples >25% of chest circumference) (Fig. 6.92).
- Shield-shaped chest with widely spaced nipples in Turner's.
- Narrow thoracic cage may be seen in Ellis-van Creveld syndrome, Jeune syndrome, etc (Fig. 6.93).
- Absence of pectoralis muscle is seen in Poland's syndrome. Palpate the anterior axillary fold (Fig. 24.27, p 503).

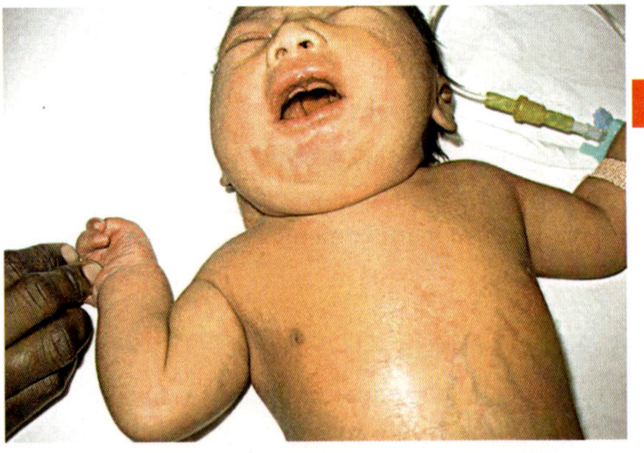

Fig.6.92 Note the wide spaced nipples and the webbing of neck *(Courtesy: Dr Sheela Nampoothiri).*

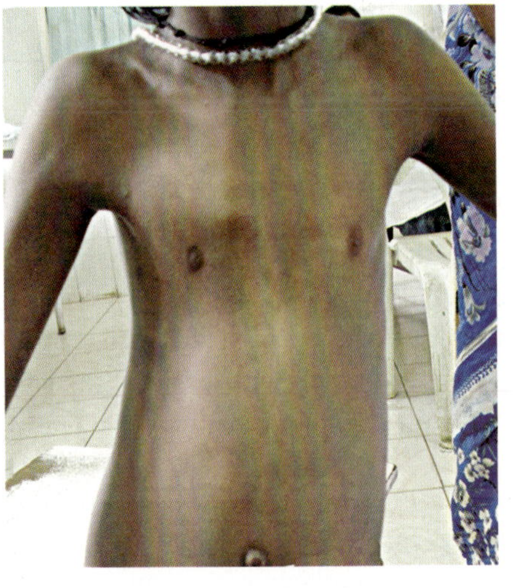

Fig.6.93 Narrow chest

6

- High position of scapula with lower angle turned toward the spine is seen in Sprengel's deformity.
- Pectus excavatum/carinatum (Figs. 15.10a,b & 15.11). Pectus carinatum may be a normal variation or may be seen in rickets.

  Pectus excavatum may be seen in rickets, Marfan syndrome and upper airway obstruction in early life (e.g., severe congenital laryngeal stridor).
- Rosary or costochondral beading (see p 490).
- Harrison sulcus (see Fig. 15.12, p 360).

Sprengel's Deformity

- Elevated scapula (normal scapula is usually between T2 and T7 levels).
- Limitation in movement in ipsilateral arm may be there.

Gynaecomastia

This is the enlargement of breast in males.

- Transient during puberty (usually disappears within 6–24 months).
- In obesity as a part of generalized fat deposition, there will be breast enlargement as well.
- In newborns, it is normal due to maternal hormones.
- Cirrhosis liver
- Drugs like digitalis
- Oestrogen-secreting tumours
- Klinefelter syndrome

SPINE

Normally, there is a concave C curve in the cervical region, convex curve in the thorax, another concave C curve in the lumbar region (lumbar lordosis). The loss of normal curvature in the cervical region may indicate juvenile rheumatoid arthritis or rarely tuberculosis. The loss of normal lumbar lordosis may indicate ankylosing spondylitis.

Scoliosis: This is the lateral curvature of spine. It is described as scoliosis with convexity to left or right. A short neck or elevated shoulder along with scoliosis may indicate the possibility of hemivertebrae. Scoliosis may be primary or secondary. Primary scoliosis is associated with rib hump. Secondary scoliosis may be due to leg length discrepancy or neuromuscular diseases (like residual palsy of poliomyelitis).

Positional scoliosis or non-fixed scoliosis: Ask the child to lean forward and try to touch his feet without bending the knees. Scoliosis that disappears with this procedure is non-fixed scoliosis. In a smaller child, lifting him up by the axilla will correct non-fixed scoliosis.

A bunch of hair in the midline in the back must raise a suspicion of spinal dysraphism. Sacrococcygeal dimple is seen in many normal children. It cannot have connection with the spinal canal as the spinal canal ends high in the lumbar vertebral region and does not extend to sacrococcygeal region. Pilonidal sinus is higher in position.

Gibbus: A prominent angle at the apex of kyphosis. It usually indicates underlying collapse of vertebra, the most common cause being TB spine (Pott's spine) in children.

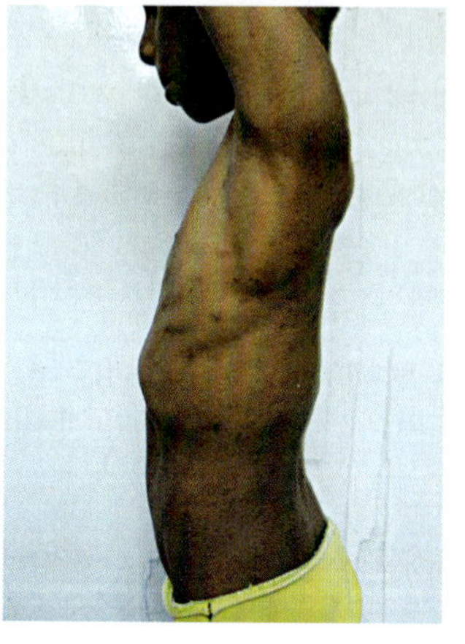

Fig.6.94 Gibbus

UPPER LIMBS

- Cubitus valgus: Forearm distal to elbow is directed away from body.

- Cubitus varus: Forearm distal to elbow is directed towards the body.

Fingers

Clinodactyly: This is the shortening of the middle phalanx of the little finger, which is more pronounced in the radial aspect so as to make the little finger curve inwards (towards the middle finger). It may be seen in a few normal children and also in Down's syndrome. There is no special term for outward deviation of fingers and so the term 'clinodactyly' can be used for this also. Of course, clinodactyly can affect other fingers also, but no specific significance has been ascribed to them (Fig. 6.95a & Fig. 6.98).

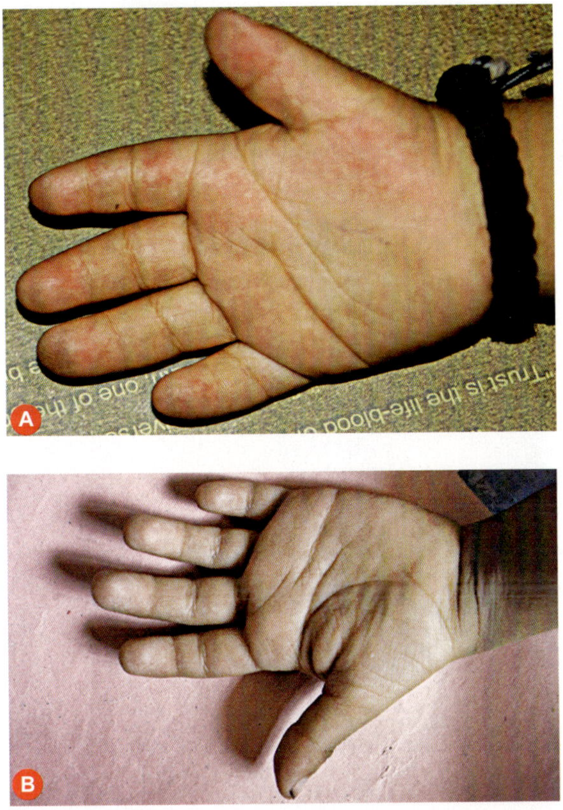

Fig.6.95 (A) Brachydactyly: Note the short palm, hypoplastic middle phalanx of the little finger and brachydactyly. Brachydactyly may be seen in Down syndorme, achondroplasia, Prader-Willi syndrome, etc (B) Note the absent middle phalanx of little finger.

Camptodactyly: This is a flexion deformity of the fifth finger (restricted extension). It is seen in a few normal people and is thought to be a heritable defect. It may be seen as part of some syndromes like Down.

Hypoplasia of the 4th metacarpal is seen in pseudohypoparthyroidism. Thus, here the ring finger will be shorter than the index finger (the reverse is true in normal children) (Fig. 24.28, p 504).

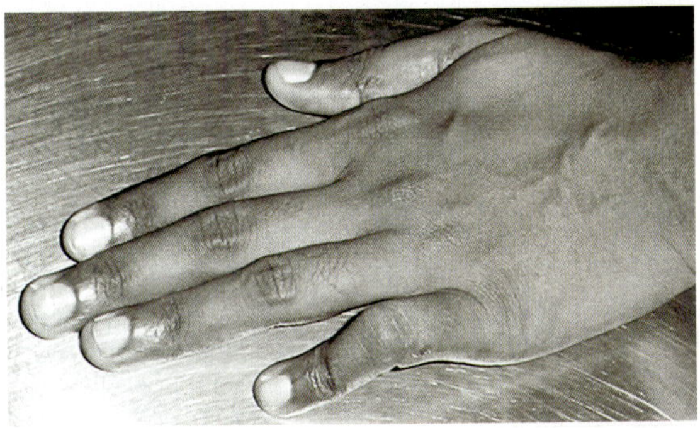

Fig.6.96 Camptodactyly

Broad thumb: Rubinstein-Taybi syndrome
Bifid thumb: This may be associated with some chromosomal anomalies. Bifid thumb (Fig. 6.97), or rudimentary thumb may be seen in many syndromes. Refer to Holt-Oram, Fanconi, etc. The picture here shows rudimentary thumb and clinodactyly (Fig. 6.98).

Arachnodactyly: Unduly long fingers. May be found in Marfan syndrome (p 511), homocystinuria, hypogonadism and in certain normal individuals.

Thumb sign: In Marfan syndrome, when the thumb is brought across the palm, it protrudes past ulnar border of palm. This sign is absent in homocystinuria, which mimics Marfan's in many ways (p 511).

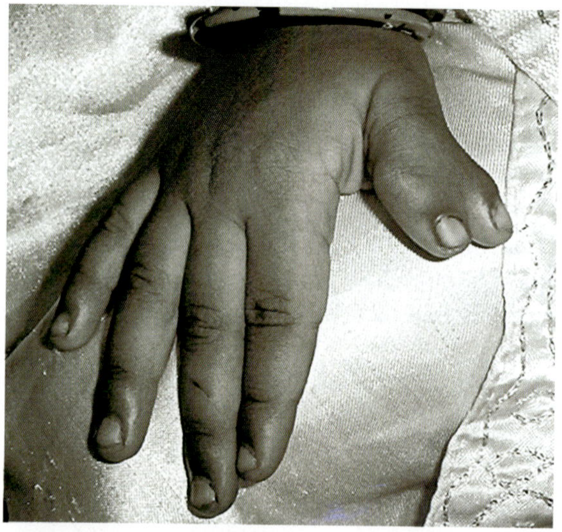

Fig.6.97 Bifid thumb

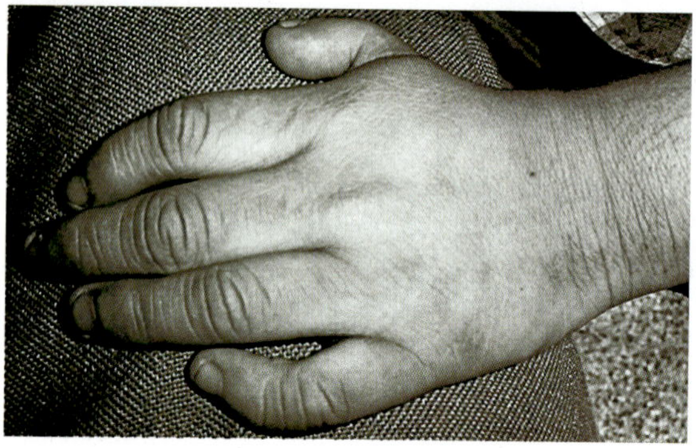

Fig.6.98 Rudimentary thumb and clinodactyly of the little finger

Wrist sign: The child can encircle his wrist by grasping it with the thumb and 5th finger (thumb and the 5th finger will overlap in this grip) (see p 511).

Trident sign: In achondroplasia, there is marked divergence between 3rd and 4th fingers so that the thumb, first two fingers and the last two fingers stand out as separate groups to give a trident appearance.

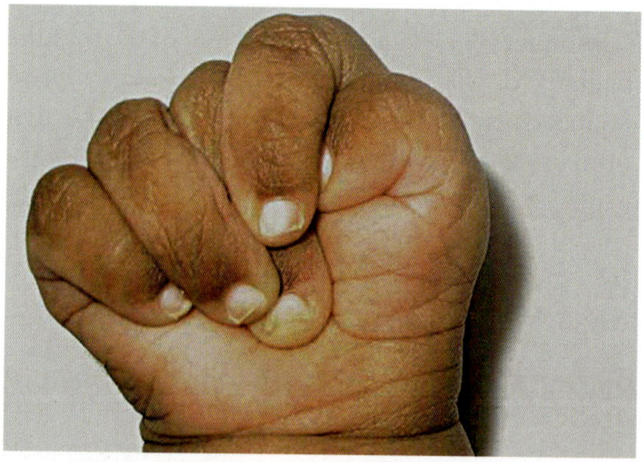

Fig.6.99 Overriding fingers: It is commonly seen in trisomy 18 (Edward syndrome).

Polydactyly

- Mostly it is congenital with no apparent reason or it may be occasionally familial.
- Ellis-van Creveld syndrome.
- Laurence-Moon-Biedl syndrome.

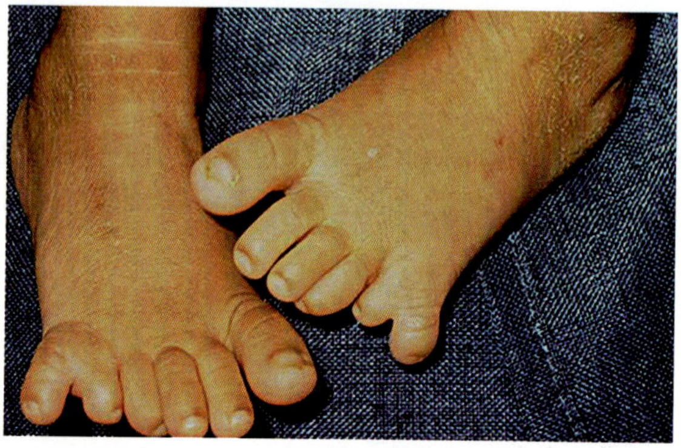

Fig.6.100 Post axial polydactyly: The concept of pre- and post axial polydactyly is easy to understand. Those associated with thumb or big toe are preaxial; those associated with little fingers are post axial *(Courtesy: Dr Sheela Nampoothiri)*.

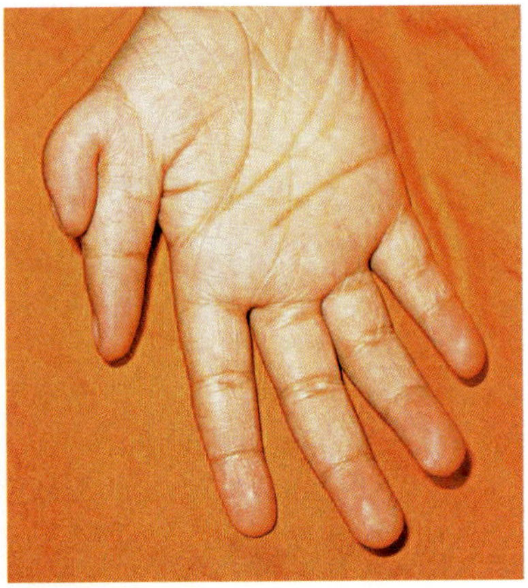

Fig.6.101 Preaxial polydactyly

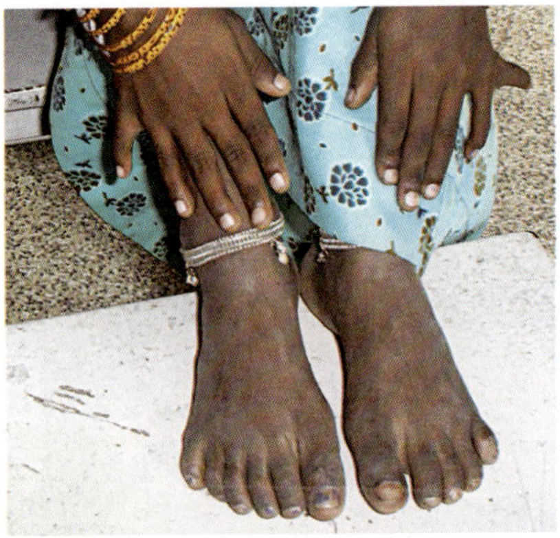

Fig.6.102 Polydactyly of four limbs: Polydactyly of all the four limbs may be seen in Ellis-van Creveld syndrome.

Syndactyly

- Apert syndrome (Fig. 24.104)
- Trisomy 13
- Smith-Lemli-Opitz syndrome

Syndactyly is most common between 2nd and 3rd digits. When the degree of fusion is less than 1/3rd the length of the digit, it may be considered as a normal variation. More lengthy fusions may be considered a minor malformation.

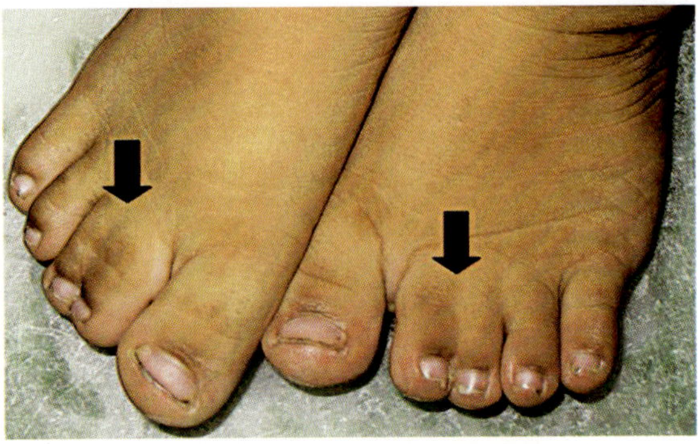

Fig.6.103 Complete syndactyly *(Courtesy: Dr Sheela Nampoothiri).*

6

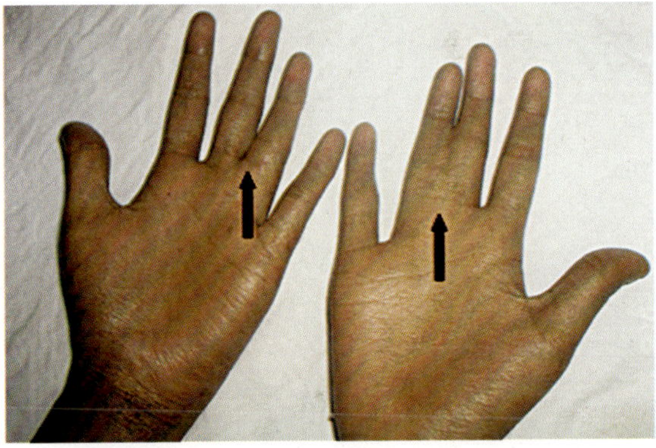

Fig.6.104 Partial syndactyly of fingers

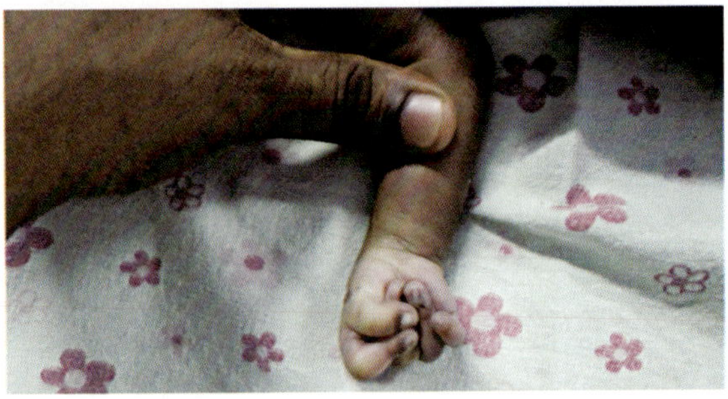

Fig.6.105 Overriding fingers in Edward syndrome

Absent Digits

- Mostly, it is congenital with no apparent associations.

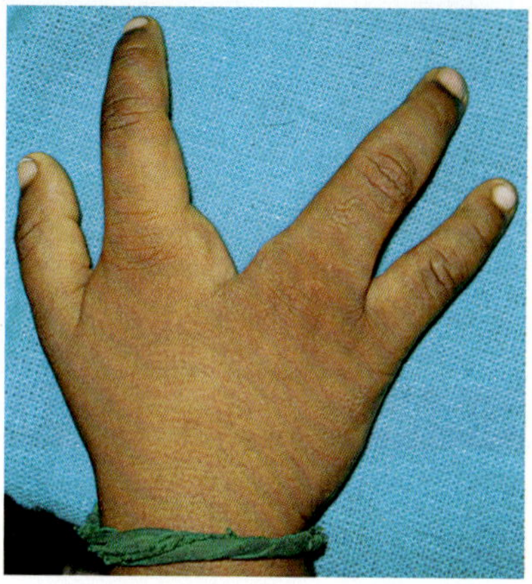

Fig.6.106 Lobster hand. Ectrodactyly or split hand. Ectrodactyly, ectodermal dysplasia and cleft lip/palate constitute EEC syndrome.

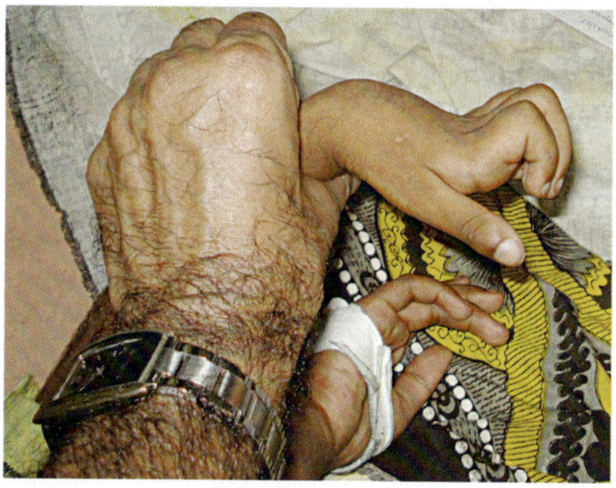

Fig.6.107 Claw hand

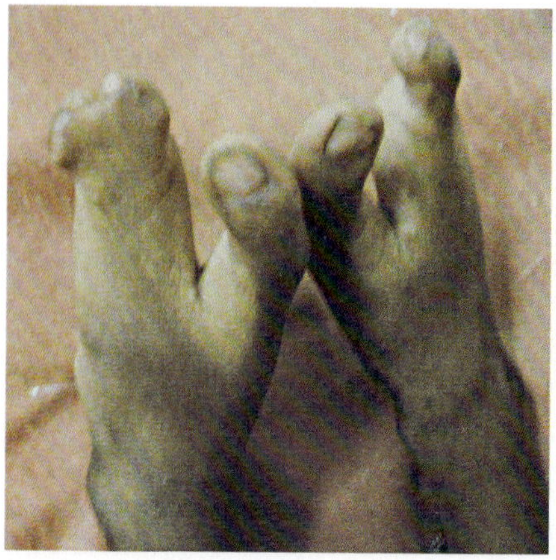

Fig.6.108 Lobster leg

Absent Thumb

- May be seen in Fanconi's anaemia, Holt-Oram syndrome, etc (Fig. 24.49).
- Diamond-Blackfan syndrome.

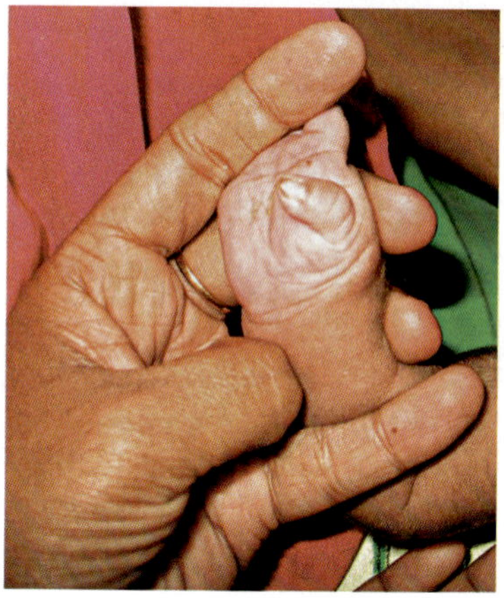

Fig.6.109 Proximally placed thumb

Triphalangeal Thumb

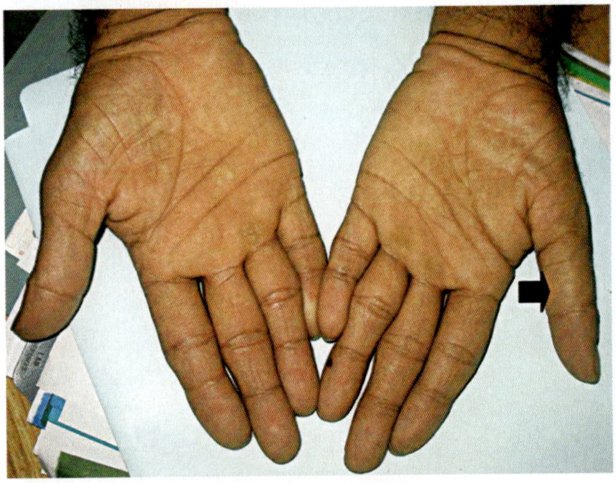

Fig.6.110 Triphalangeal thumb

Osler's nodes: Transient (lasting for a few days), small, pea-sized, tender nodules in the pulp of fingers and toes, thenar/hypothenar eminences, etc. It is classically described in infective endocarditis, but may be seen in various vasculitis syndromes. Hence, the origin of Osler's nodes is now thought to be vasculitis rather than embolic phenomena (p 304).

Janeway lesions: Painless erythematous patches over palms or soles.

Congenital absence of clavicles: The child can approximate two shoulders in front of the chest (Fig. 24.24a).

Phocomelia: Congenital absence of limb. It was the notorious complication of use of thalidomide in the first trimester of pregnancy (Fig. 6.111).

Holt-Oram syndrome: The thumb is hypoplastic or absent or triphalangeal or may be in the same plane as the other fingers or may have gross

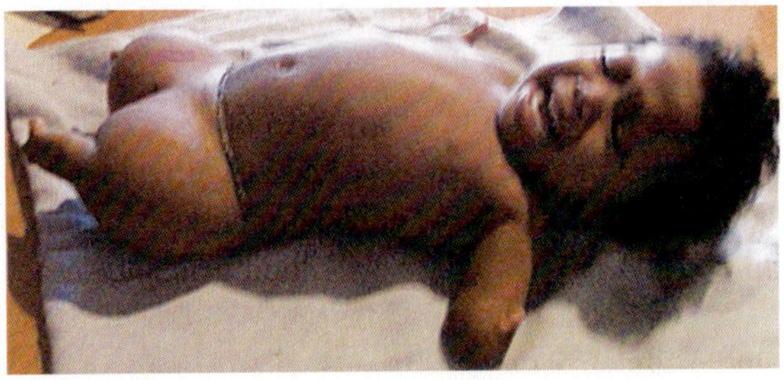

Fig.6.111 Phocomelia

anomalies of upper limb. There may be radioulnar synostosis causing restriction in supination-pronation movement.

Nail

- Koilonychia: Soft, thin, brittle, flattened or concave (spoon-shaped) nail, seen in iron deficiency. Please note that this change may not be seen uniformly in all nails. In Fig. 6.112, the third toe shows definite koilonychia. Koilonychia may also be seen rarely as an inherited family character. A drop of water cannot stay over a nail, but if there is koilonychia the water remains in the nail. Flattening of nail without concavity is sometimes referred to as platynychia (Fig. 6.112).
- Half and half nail: White proximal and red or brown distal half in same nail, may be seen in chronic renal failure (Fig. 6.122).
- White nail: Anaemia, hypoalbuminaemia (cirrhosis, nephrotic syndrome, etc), and so on.
- Red nail: Always suspect polycythaemia (as in cyanotic congenital heart disease).
- Blue lunule of nail may be seen in Wilson disease (rare) (Fig. 6.113).
- Nail fold telangiectasia is seen in dermatomyositis, systemic sclerosis, SLE, etc.
- Nail-patella syndrome: Rudimentary patellae and abnormal nails, like small nails or split nails.

- Hypoplastic nails: Ellis-van Creveld syndrome, ectodermal dysplasia, etc.
- Brittle nails: In nutritional deficiency, especially iron.
- Transverse ridges in nails: This may represent growth arrests during episodes of acute severe malnutrition. Equivalent of this may be seen in bones as transverse growth arrest lines in X ray of growing ends of long bones.
- Transverse linear depressions of the nail may be seen in long-standing diseases, marking periods of arrested growth.
- Hyperconvex nail: Seen in Turner and Noonan syndrome. It is not clubbing as nail bed is not altered (Fig. 6.121).
- Black nail: Addison's disease. Blue–black pigmentation of nails may be seen with use of certain drugs (especially antimalignancy drugs).
- Punctate white spots are not of significance; may be anonymous in origin or may indicate trivial trauma.
- Splinter haemorrhages: Linear streaks of haemorrhages under the nails (Fig. 6.114). This is classically described in infective endocarditis. However, the most common cause is trauma!
- Subungual fibroma: Warty swelling from lateral edge of nail base. Seen in tuberous sclerosis.

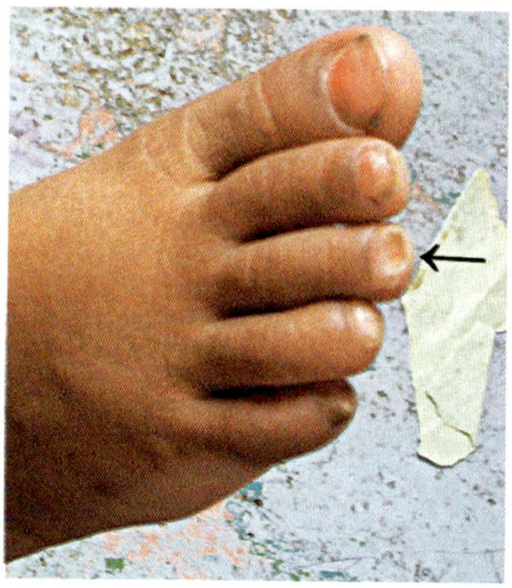

Fig.6.112 Koilonychia

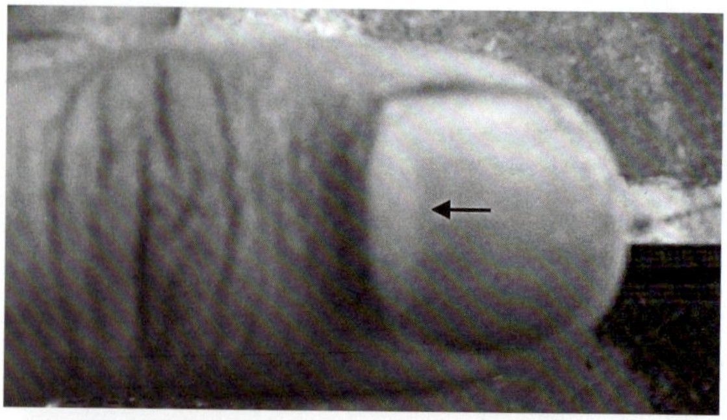

Fig.6.113 Lunule

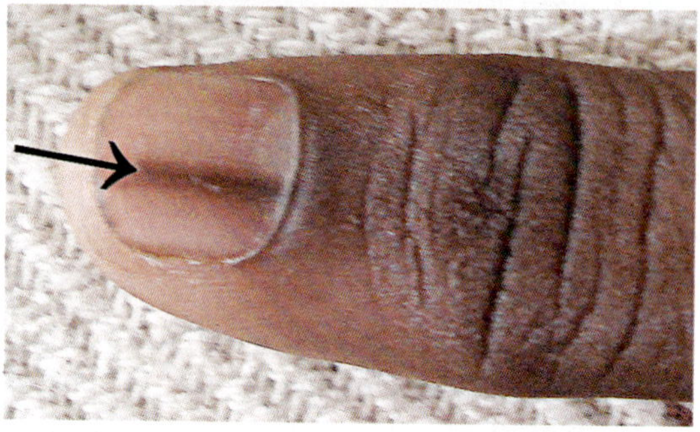

Fig.6.114 Splinter haemorrhage

- Capillary pulsations: Exert slight pressure at the distal end of nail so that only half of nail is blanched. Now observe for pulsations at the junction of blanched and unblanched areas. It is seen in severe aortic regurgitation.
- Nail represents the underlying phalanx; thus in case of bifid nail, the underlying phalanx may be bifid and in case of hypoplastic nail one must consider X ray to rule out missing phalanx bone.

Clubbing

Clubbing is probably caused by hyperactivity and the opening of anastomotic channels in the nail bed, because of anoxia or other unknown stimuli.

The normal angle between the nail and nail bed (skin–nail junction on the dorsal surface of terminal phalanx) is lost in clubbing. In Fig. 6.115, a normal and a clubbed thumb are placed side by side for comparison.

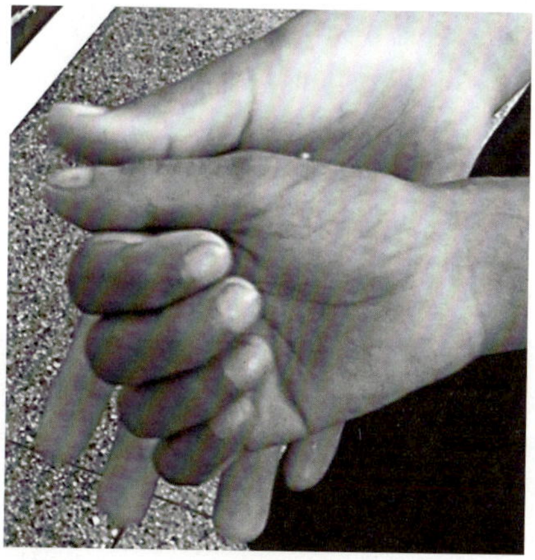

Fig.6.115 Clubbing (comparison with normal)

In normal nails when both thumb nails are placed in opposition, there is a large lozenge-shaped (diamond shaped) gap, whereas in clubbing there is reduction or disappearnce of this gap—Schamroth's window test (Figs. 6.116, 6.117).

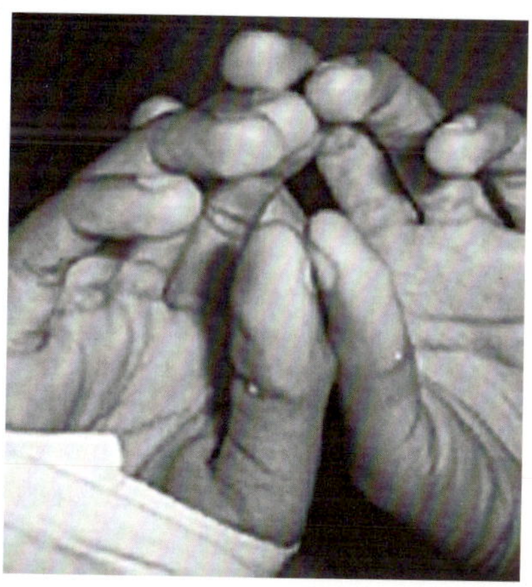

Fig.6.116 Schamroth window test (clubbing)

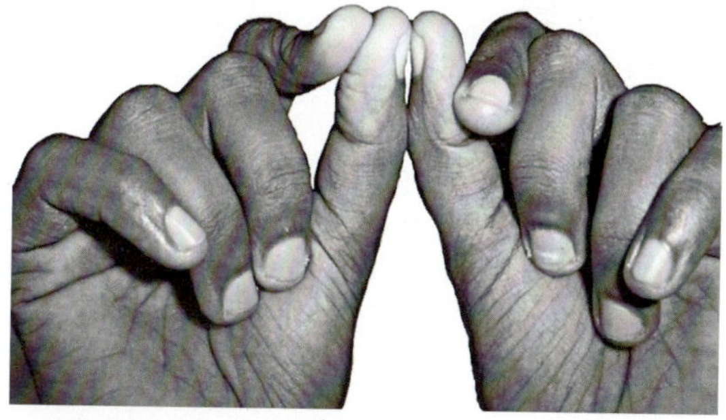

Fig.6.117 Schamroth window test (normal)

In true clubbing, the vertical height at the base of the nail is more than the vertical height of the distal interphalangeal joints. Measurement of a normal finger is shown in Fig. 6.118.

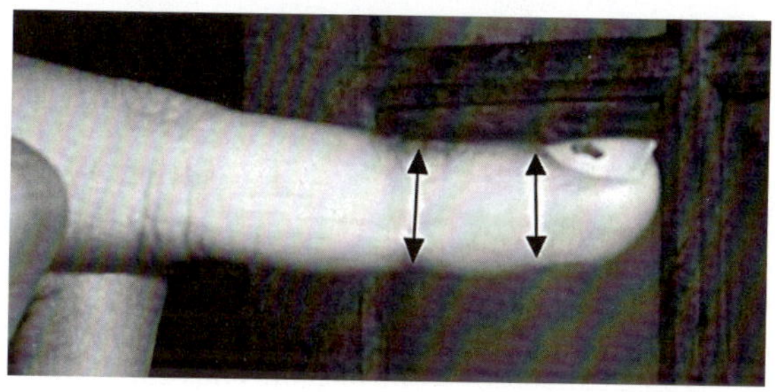

Fig.6.118 Finger measurement for clubbing

Causes

- Cardiac: Cyanotic heart disease (e.g., TOF), infective endocarditis, Eisenmenger syndrome. Clubbing may develop in 2–3 weeks in infective endocarditis. In TOF, it may take about 6 months for clubbing to get noticeable.
- Pulmonary: Bronchiectasis, lung abscess, empyema. Clubbing may develop in 2–3 weeks in lung abscess and empyema. In case of bronchiectasis, it generally takes a year or so.
- GIT: Inflammatory bowel disease (e.g., ulcerative colitis), cirrhosis.
- Hereditary clubbing: Rare. It may be familial, so look for clubbing in family members. Hereditary clubbing is usually not present at birth but appears later, sometimes only in adolescence.

- Unidigital clubbing is usually due to local insults to the digit.

Grading of Clubbing

1. Softening or sponginess of nail bed (one will be able to elicit increased fluctuation) (Fig. 6.119). On inspection, there will be glossiness and occasionally a cyanotic tinge at nail bed.

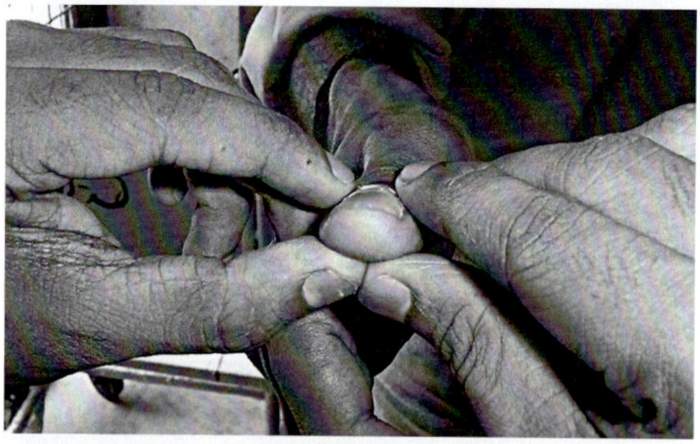

Fig.6.119 Examination for fluctuation

2. Obliteration of the angle of the nail bed (normal angle between the nail and nail bed is about 165°; called Lovibond angle). The obliteration is detected clinically by Schamroth's sign. When two fingers are held together with nails face to face, a diamond-shaped window is expected, which is obliterated in clubbing (Fig. 6.119).
3. Swelling of subcutaneous tissues over the base of nail along with increase in curvature of the nail in its long axis: parrot beak appearance. (Fig. 6.120). When fingertips are also enlarged, it takes "drumstick" appearance.
4. Swelling of the fingers in all dimensions associated with hypertrophic pulmonary osteoarthropathy causing pain and swelling of the hand, wrist, etc, thickening of periosteum of radius, ulna, tibia and fibula and subperiosteal new bone formation.

   Grade 4 is typically seen in bronchogenic carcinoma in adults; never seen in children.

Note: Curth modified profile angle is the angle between the back surface of the middle phalanx and that of the terminal phalanx. In clubbing this angle decreases from 160° to <145°.

DPD (distal phalangeal diameter) to IPD (interphalangeal diameter) of the middle finger of normal children is <1 and in clubbing it is >1.1.(Rice and Rowl interphalangeal depth ratio (Fig. 6.118)

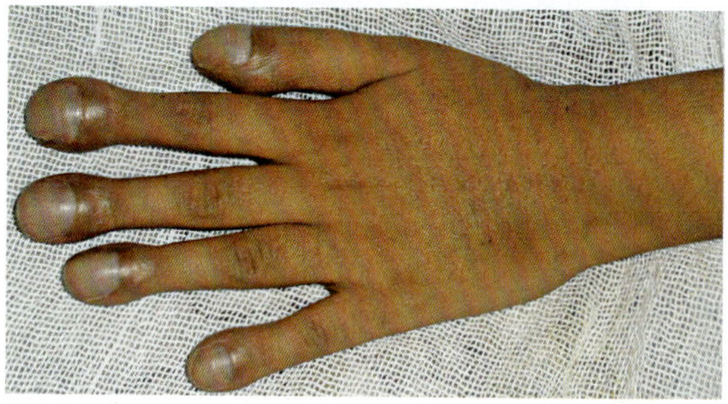

Fig.6.120 Clubbing (parrot beak) and cyanosis

Pseudoclubbing may be seen in hyperparathyroidism. Excessive bone resorption may result in disappearance of the terminal phalanges with telescoping of soft tissues and a drumstick appearance of the fingers resembling clubbing. However, the increased curvature of the nails is not present.

Hyperconvex nail is found in certain conditions, like Noonan syndrome. Here, the finger may simulate clubbing but there are no changes in nail bed.

Cyanosis: Bluish discolouration of the nails, lips and tongue due to increased amount of reduced haemoglobin (>5 g%) in capillary blood. In carbon monoxide poisoning, cherry red lips (*not* cyanosis) are found. Also refer to the section on cardiology.

- Cardiac: Congenital cyanotic heart disease (e.g., TOF); Eisenmenger syndrome.

- Pulmonary: Severe pneumonia, especially interstitial pneumonia; ARDS.
- Abnormal haemoglobin (methaemoglobin) may also produce cyanosis, presenting as cyanosis in asymptomatic child. Certain poisonings (e.g., dapsone) are known to produce methaemoglobinaemia and hence cyanosis.

Note: If the mucous membranes or nails appear very polycythaemic, it may be a subtle cyanosis, so look again.It is difficult to make out cyanosis in the presence of anaemia. Absolute quantity of reduced haemoglobin determines the visibility of cyanosis rather than the relative quantity. Pulse oximetry measurement should be done on all 4 limbs.

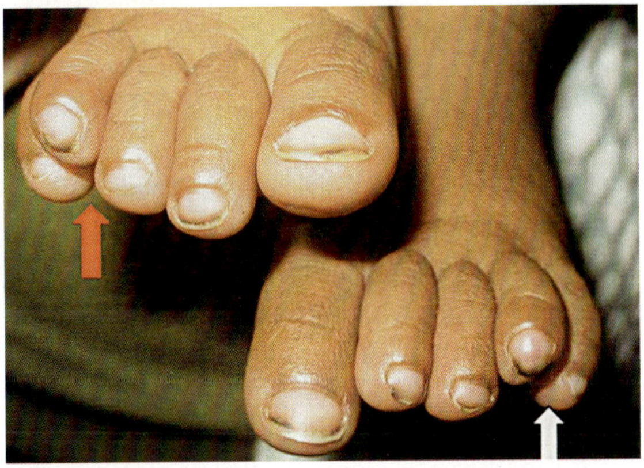

Fig.6.121 Hyperconvex nails

Differential Cyanosis

Upper limb pink, Lower limbs cyanosed.
Seen in Preductal CoA with PDA, PDA Eisenmenger, Complete TGA with PDA.

Reverse Differential Cyanosis

Upper limb cyanosed, Lower limbs pink.
Seen in TGA with PDA with increased PVR.
Hyperoxia test is done to differentiate cardiac causes for cyanosis from other causes. After taking a baseline ABG in a cyanosed infant, administer 100% Oxygen via hood or ET tube for 10-15 minutes. Then repeat the ABG and seen for increase in PaO2 values. If PaO2 values have not changed much and is <150mmHg cyanosis is due to cardiac cause. If >150 mmHg it is due to pulmonary cause. If > 200 mmHg but SpO2 reading is still low it is due to methaemoglobinemia or other abnormal haemoglobin disorders.

Half and half nails ("Lindsay's nails"): The proximal portion of nail is dull white and the distal portion is red or brown, with a sharp line of demarcation between the two halves. Note that lunula is not seen as is normally expected. This type of nail is commonly seen in renal failure patients on long-term dialysis.

6

Palmar erythema: This is more obvious over the thenar and hypothenar area.

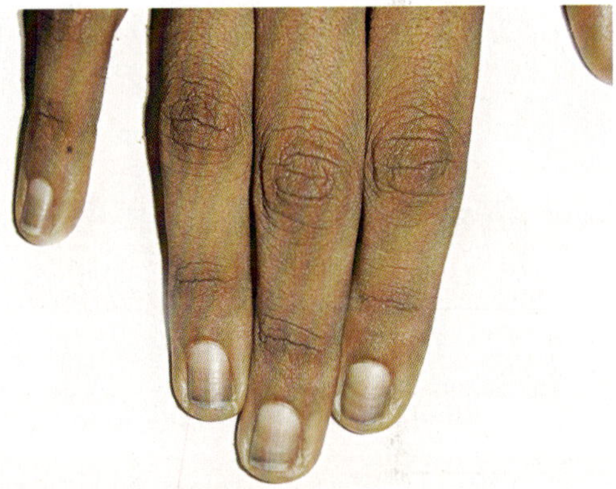

Fig.6.122 Half & half nail

Dermatoglyphics

Before the advent of cytogenetics, analysis of human hand and foot prints were given undue importance in the description of chromosomal anomalies. Now its importance is not there although it may be discussed in examinations when cases like Down syndrome are given.

Dermatoglyphics strictly refers to the configurations formed by dermal ridges, not by flexion creases. However, here we will discuss both. Ridges and palmar creases remain unchanged for life except for their size. Epidermal ridges of palm are unique to each individual and are not identical even in identical twins (that is why thumb print is taken instead of signature in the illiterate).

Finger patterns: The pattern at the distal phalanges of fingers can be arches, loops or whorls or double loops. Triradius is the junction of three sets of converging epidermal ridges (Fig. 6.125). Ulnar loop means that the ridges enter and leave from ulnar side (i.e., opening towards the ulnar side). If opening towards the radial side, a radial loop is formed. Loops have one triradius, whereas whorls have two (Fig. 6.123). The normal pattern is ulnar loop in little finger and radial loop in index finger. In Down syndrome, there may be ulnar loop in all fingers. More whorls than normal may be seen in congenital rubella syndrome. Increase in number of arches may be seen in trisomy 18.

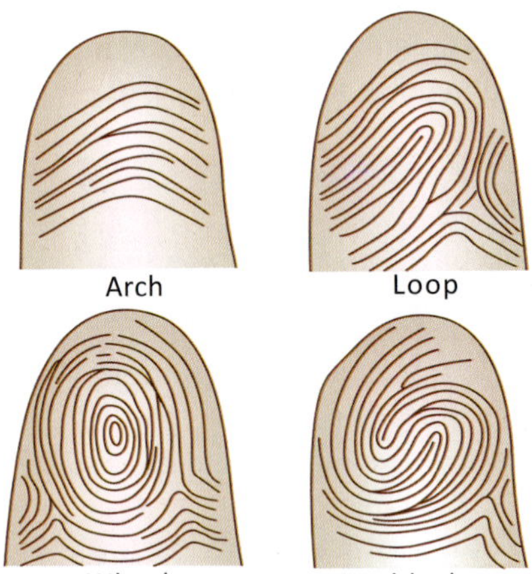

Fig.6.123

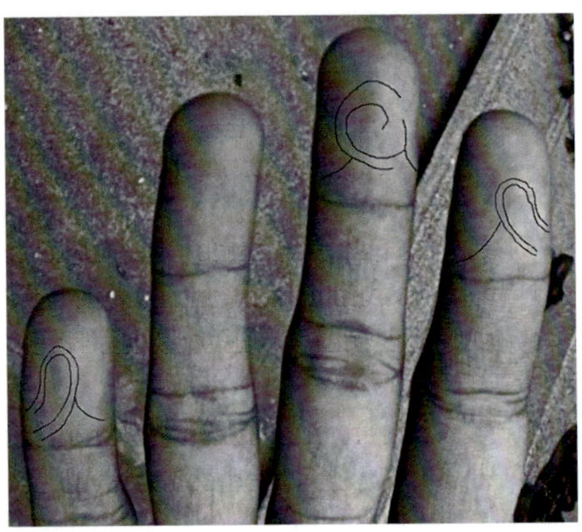

Fig.6.124 Finger loop

Ridge count: The total number of ridges from the core of the pattern up to the triradius gives the number of ridges for that finger. The average value for ridge count in males is said to be 145 and female 127 (total count from all the ten fingers).

Ridge count can be done after taking a fingerprint in a paper. The ridge count is low in Klinefelter syndrome and high in Turner, congenital rubella, etc (since they have more whorls).

Pattern in palm: Tri radii are found normally beneath each finger and in the axial line of palm. The distal tri radii are named a, b, c and d from index to little finger, respectively. The axial tri radius is called t (Fig. 6.126). Normally, t is found proximally near the wrist, but in syndromes like Down's, "t" may be displaced distally in the palm so that atd angle will be wider. Normal atd angle is about 40–45°, but in Down's syndrome it may be 75 or more (Figs. 6.126 & 6.127). More than one tri radius may be present and there may be displacement of its location towards ulnar or radial side.

Palmar crease: Normally, two deep transverse palmar creases are expected, each stopping short of reaching the other end of palm. In Down syndrome instead of two palmar creases, there is only one transverse palmar crease, extending across the entire palm (Simian crease) (Fig. 6.128a). When there are two transverse creases, but the proximal one extends across the whole of the palm, then it is called Sydney line, which may be seen in some cases of Down syndrome. It is also described in congenital rubella.

We shall try to analyze why there are two horizontal flexion creases in the palm. The creases just represent the plane of folding (flexion). Make a fist and observe the plane of metacarpophalangeal

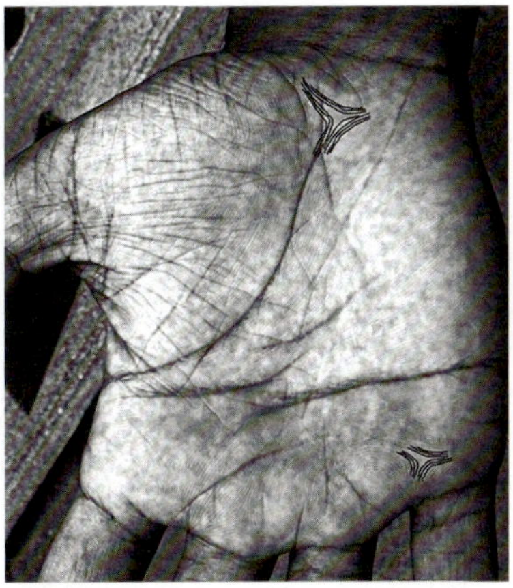

Fig.6.125

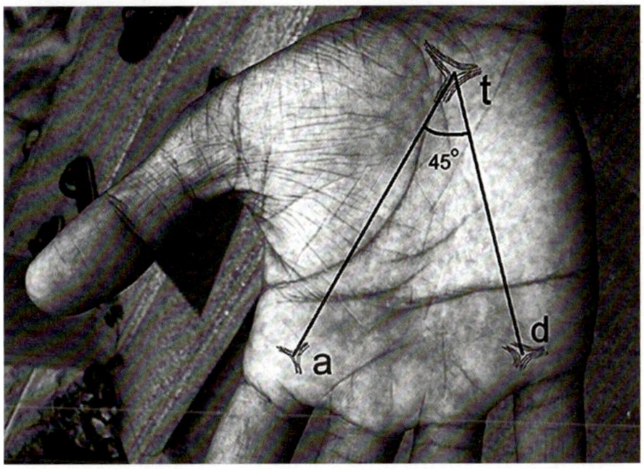

Fig.6.126 atd angle (normal)

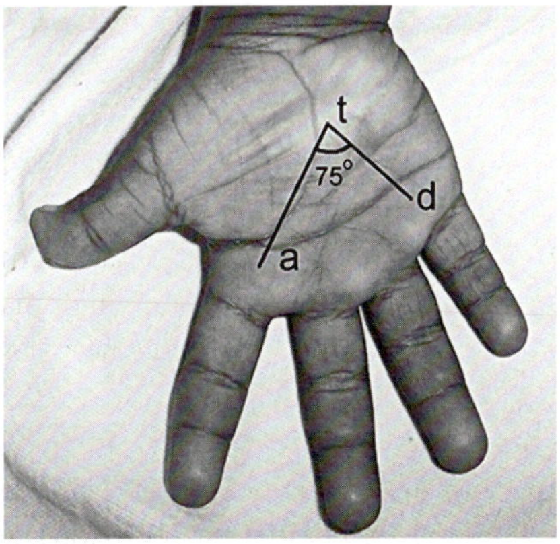

Fig.6.127 atd angle (Down syndrome)

joints. The line joining these joints take a slanting plane up to the middle finger. Then it straightens off to join the m-p joint of index finger. Thus, when we close our hands, the little finger to middle finger closes in one slanting plane to give the slanting distal palmar crease. Since the index finger closes in a different plane, it produces the proximal (middle) palmar crease. And the closing of the thumb produces the palmar crease in relation to the thumb. Closure of thumb and index finger augments the middle palmar crease. It is easy to understand if the student observes his own palm while trying the above described movements.

Now assume that all the metacarpals are in the same plane and there is no sloping plane in these joints (this is the case in Down syndrome).

Then the closure of the fingers need produce only one crease. In addition, when the palms are short as in Down syndrome, the two horizontal creases, if at all present, come too close together to produce almost a single crease.

Single palmar crease may be seen in Down syndrome and some other chromosomal anomalies. In some cases of Down syndrome, distal slanting crease is there but the proximal mid-palmar crease extends the whole breadth of the palm (sometimes referred to as Sydney crease). Unilateral single palmar crease may be seen in about 5% and bilateral single palmar crease may be seen in about 1% of normal population (Ref. 6).

A deep sole crease between first and second toe is seen in Down's syndrome (Kennedy crease) (Fig. 6.128b).

Dermatoglyphics in Certain Disorders

- **Down syndrome**: Simian crease, single flexion crease on the fifth finger, excess ulnar loops, increased radial loops in 4th and 5th finger, increased atd angle, etc.
- **Turner syndrome**: Increased whorls on fingers. Increased atd angle.
- **Klinefelter's syndrome**: Loops on digits have low ridge counts. Excess arches on fingers.

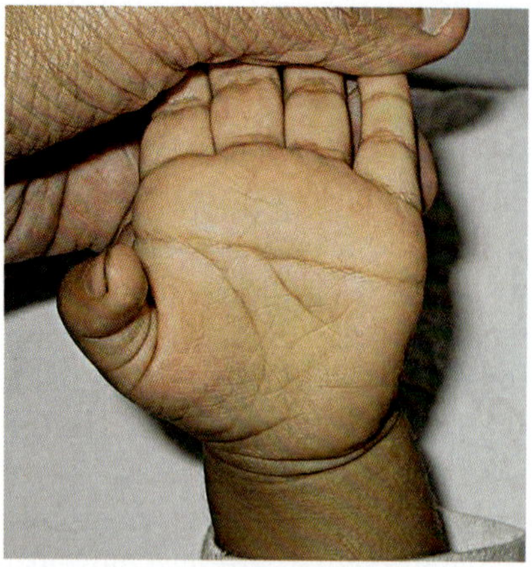

Fig.6.128a Simian crease

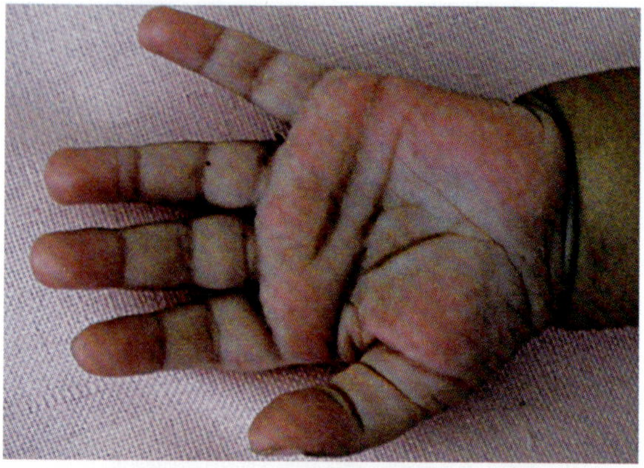

Fig.6.129 Palmar erythema

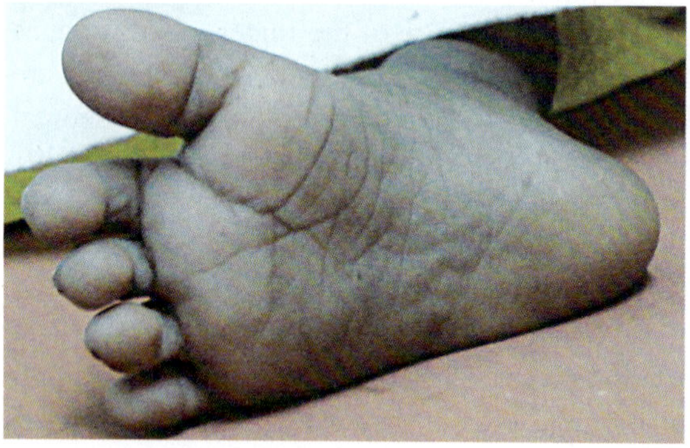

Fig.6.128b Kennedy crease

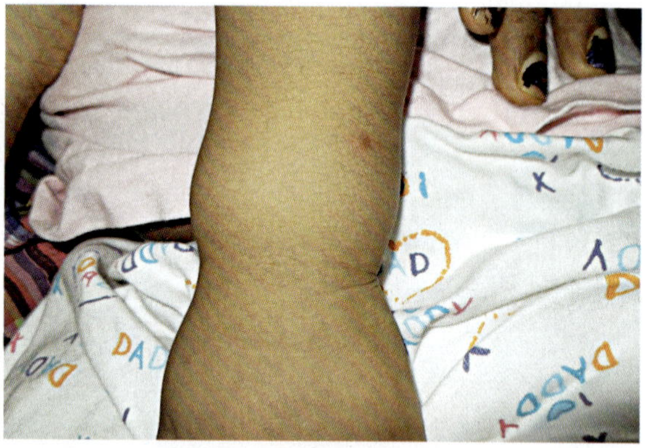

Fig.6.130 Widening of wrist in rickets

LOWER LIMBS

Varus denotes angulation towards midline of the body and valgus means angulation away from midline of the body. Talipes equinovarus is familiar to all students and so it is easy to remember that varus means angulation medially.

- Coxa valga: Angulated away from midline at hip joint. The opposite is coxa vara.
- Genu valgus: Let the child stand erect with both the medial condyles of knee touching each other. If the distance between the two medial malleoli is more than 5 cm, there is genu valgus (knock knee) (Fig. 6.131). Most often

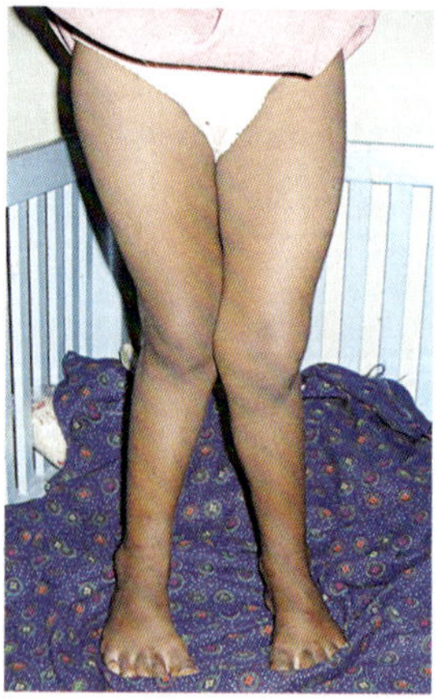

Fig.6.131 Knock knee

it is congenital, but may be seen in rickets as well.

- Genu varus: Let the child stand erect with both the medial malleoli touching.

  If the distance between the two medial condyles at knee is more than 5 cm, there is genu varus (bow leg) (Fig 6.132). Up to 5 cm is accepted as physiological. However, usually less than 10 cm is not treated by orthopaedic measures. It is found in rickets, achondro-plasia, Blount disease, etc. Lateral bowing of tibia is said to be common with rickets and anterior bowing is classical in syphilis (sabre tibia). However, anterior bowing may be seen in rickets as well.
- Both genu varus and genu valgus are physiological in children of 1½ to 2 years of age.

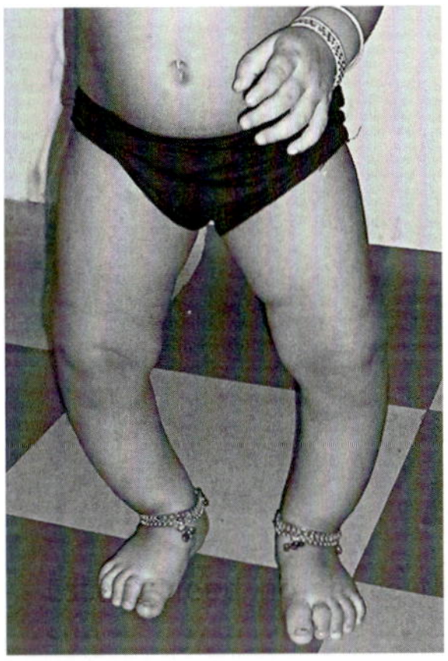

Fig.6.132 Bow legs

- Genu recurvatum: Hyperextension of the knee joint, usually associated with conditions of hypotonia. It may be congenital, secondary to hypotonic conditions, poliomyelitis, etc.
- Pes planus (flat foot): The medial border of the foot touches the floor due to inadequate longitudinal arch of foot. It is physiological in 1½ to 2 years age group. The arch forms only when walking is well established.
- Pes cavus (claw foot): Accentuated foot arches (Fig. 6.133). May be familial. It may also be seen in Friedreich's ataxia, peroneal muscular atrophy, poliomyelitis, etc.

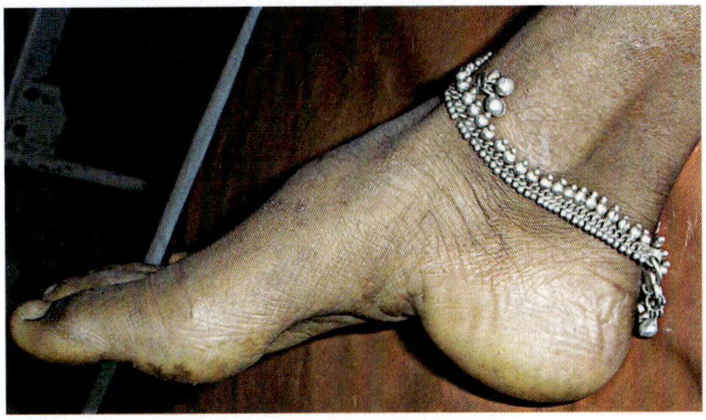

Fig.6.133 Pes cavus

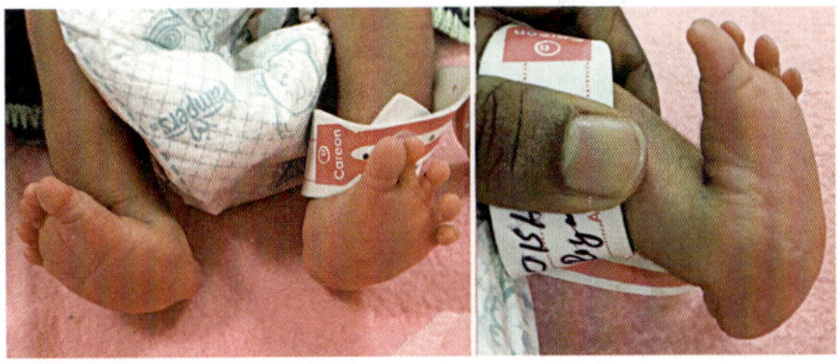

Fig.6.134 Rocker bottom foot

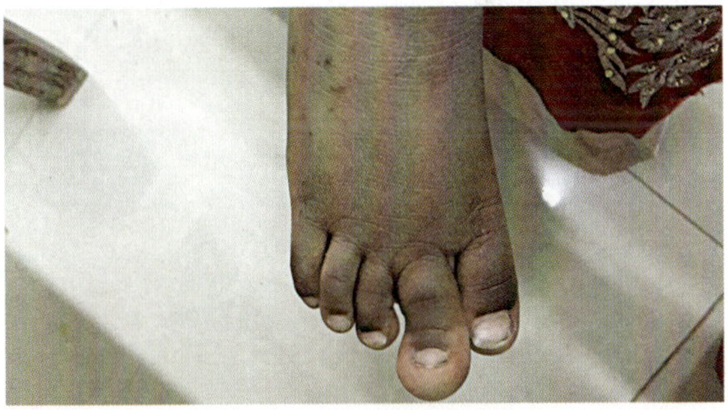

Fig.6.134a Localised Gigantism

- Talipes equinovarus (clube foot): The foot is adducted downwards and inwards with medial concavity. It is usually congenital, but may follow neurological disease (e.g., Friedreich's

ataxia). Equinus means plantar flexion. Varus means inversion and medial turning of foot.
- Hallux valgus: Lateral deviation of big toe, usually acquired because of tight pointed shoes. Dorsiflexed hallux may be seen in Edward syndrome. Flexion contracture of interphalangeal joint result in hammer toe.
- Homan's sign: Quick dorsiflexion of foot (while knee is extended) produces pain in the calf in case of deep vein thrombosis.

ABDOMEN

Abdominal Mass

- Hepatomegaly
- Splenomegaly
- Kidney mass like hydronephrosis
- Faecal mass
- Worm mass
- Intussusception
- Malignancies like neuroblastoma, lymphoma, etc

Umbilical Hernia

This is due to imperfect closure of umbilical ring (Fig. 6.135). It may be associated with diastasis recti. It protrudes during crying or straining. Most close spontaneously and surgery is only indicated for large defects persisting beyond 4 years of age.

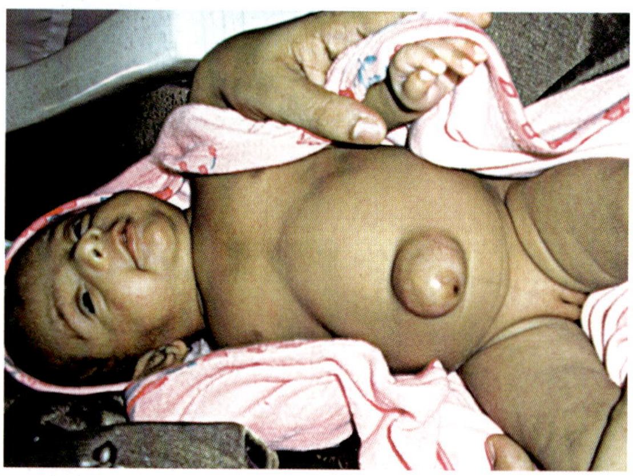

Fig.6.135 Umbilical hernia

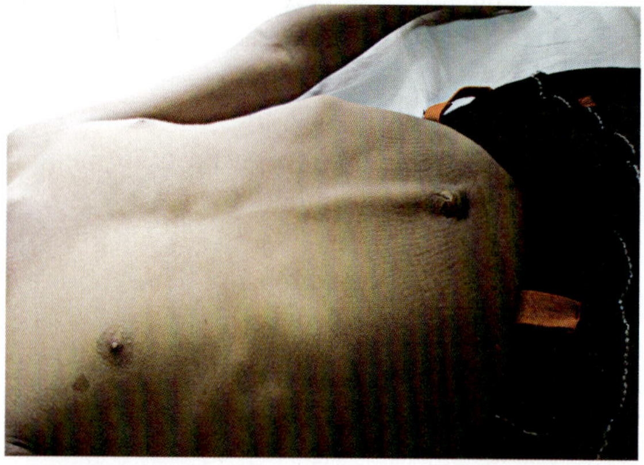

Fig.6.136 Hernia of linea alba

In contrast, paraumbilical hernias do not close spontaneously.

GENITALIA

Micropenis

Normal stretched length of penis in infants is about 4 cm. Micropenis is said to be there if the stretched length is <1.5 cm.

- Hypogonadotrophic hypogonadism
- Hypopituitarism
- Klinefelter
- Noonan syndrome
- Kallmann
- Prader-Willi syndrome
- Obesity (apparent micropenis as the penis gets submerged in fat)

Micro-orchidism

Measurement of volume of testes is done subjectively by comparing with the sizes of beads of orchidometer (see p 52).

- Hypopituitarism
- Hypothalamic disorders
- Laurence-Moon-Biedl
- Rudimentary testes syndrome (possible vascular accidents during fetal life)
- In conditions associated with micropenis

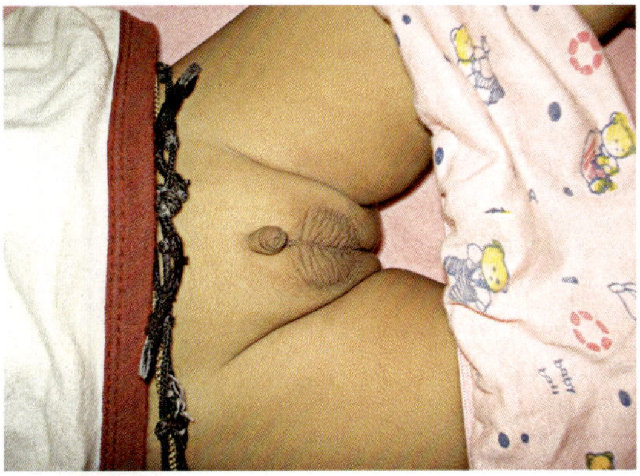

Fig.6.137 Micropenis

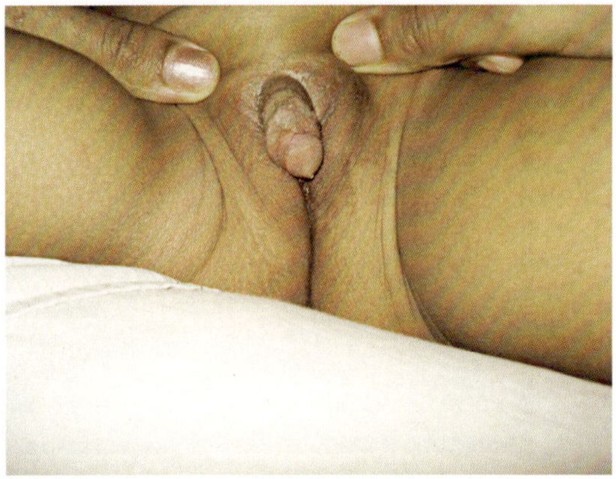

Fig.6.138 Ambiguous genitalia showing clitoral hypertrophy

Macro-orchidism (>30 mL)

- Fragile X syndrome (p 539)
- Neurogenic or idiopathic sexual precocity
- Precocity induced by hypothyroidism
- Testicular tumours (unilateral)

Ambiguous Genitalia

Genitalia, which cannot be pronounced as male or female by external appearance (see p 542).

Nappy rash and ***cutaneous candidiasis*** may look alike. Skin folds are not spared in candidiasis, but are spared in contact dermatitis (nappy rash); this is because inside the skin fold the contact with the irritant is not there for the dermatitis to develop.

ANUS

Anal atresia

Orifice counting is to be done at the time of birth itself. If an anal atresia is missed, and the baby is fed signs of distal bowel obstruction develop shortly. Always remember to see for the anal opening when mother gives a history of non-passage of meconium. It may be associated with other malformations.

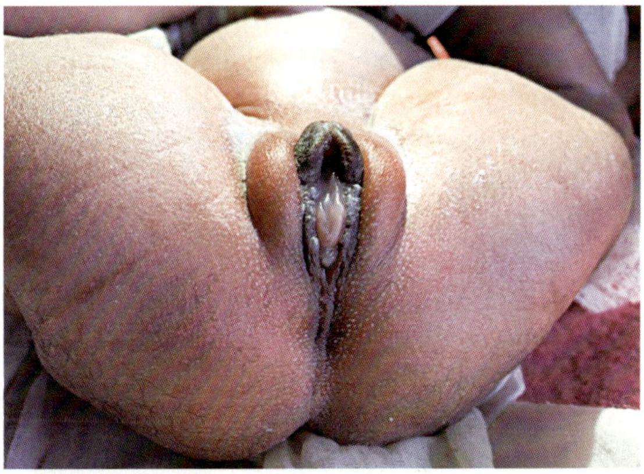

Fig.6.139 Anal atresia. Usually gets noticed in the newborn because of failure to pass meconium

Patulous Anus (see Fig. 24.87)

SKIN

Descriptive Terms for Skin Lesions

The primary skin lesions are:

- Macules: Flat, non-palpable lesions flush with the surface of the skin.
- Papules: Palpable elevated lesions that are small in size (<5 mm). Larger ones are called nodules and still larger ones are called tumours. Plaques are confluent papules. (Fig.6.140)

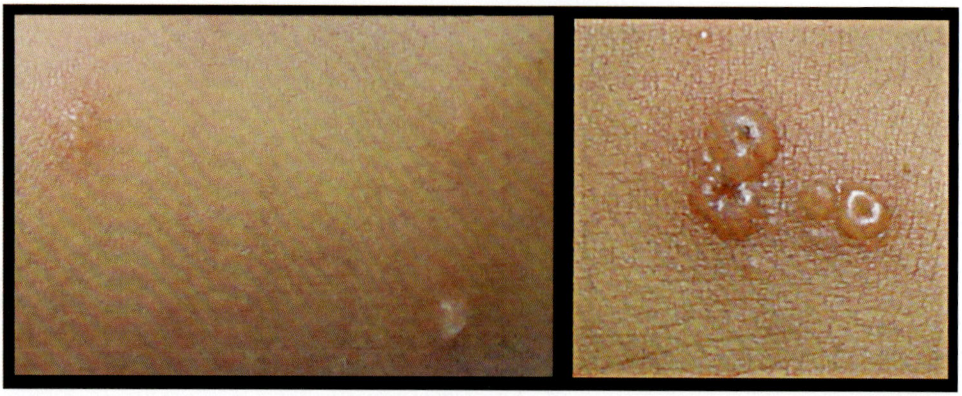

Fig.6.140 Chicken pox: Shows the vesicles containing cloudy fluid and the umbilicated vesicles.

- Vesicles: Elevated small fluid-filled blisters (<0.5 cm). Small lesions are called vesicles, and larger ones are called bullae or blebs.
- Pustules: These are superficial vesicles that contain pus. Deeper lesions with pus are called abscesses.
- Wheals: Slightly elevated lesions of the skin with the central portions of the lesion paler than the periphery (Fig.6.141).
- Petechiae: Pin head sized macules of blood. (<2mm)
- Purpura: Large petchiae, which do not blanch on pressure.(2-5mm)
- Ecchymosis: Large extravasation of blood in skin (bruise). (>1cm)

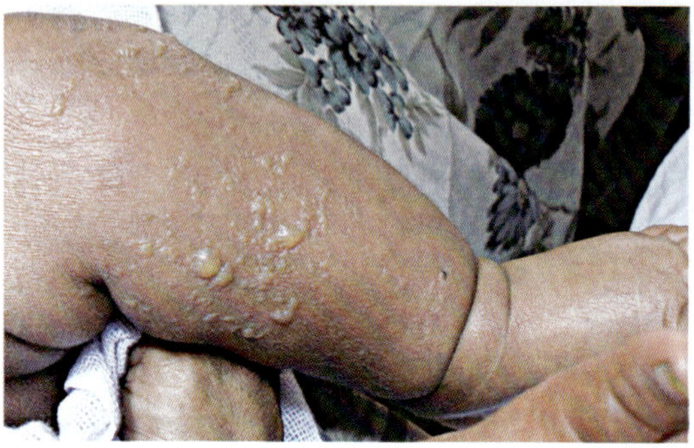

Fig.6.141 Blebs

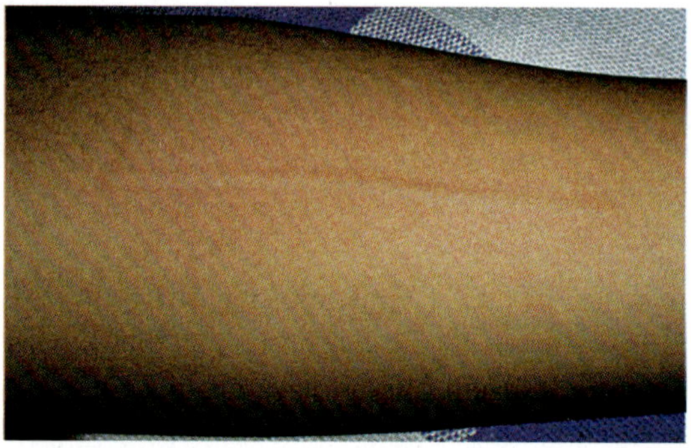

Fig.6.142 Dermographism: Stroking the skin will result in wheal; this phenomenon is called dermographism, which is a physical urticaria.

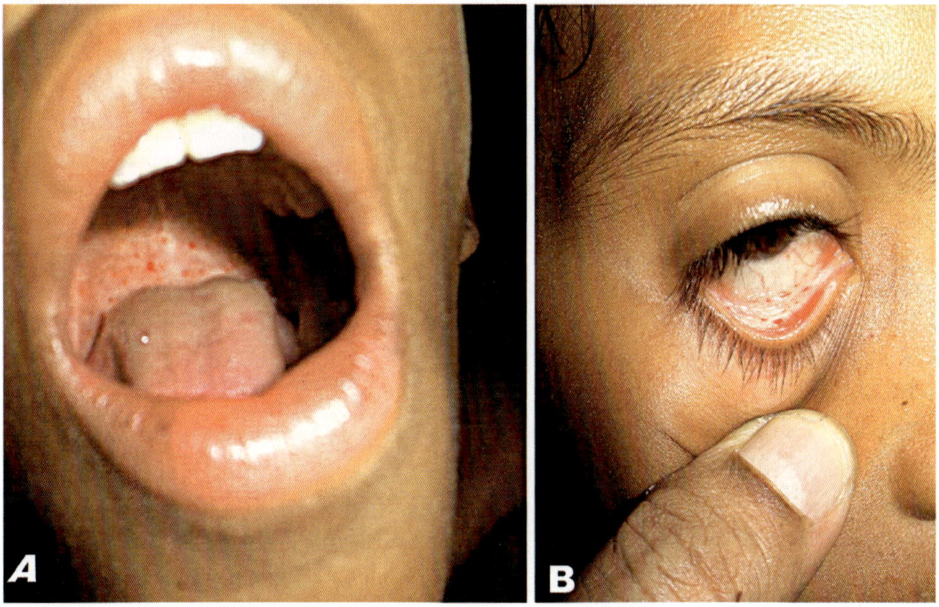

Fig. 6.142 a A) Palatal Petechiae. B) Sub Conjunctival Petechiae.

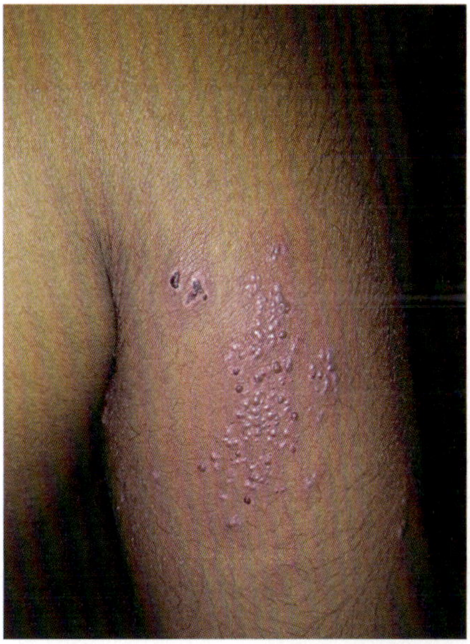

Fig.6.143 Herpes zoster: Note that the rash stops at midline and is distributed along the ophthalmic division of trigeminal nerve on the right side.

Secondary lesions are:
- Lichenification
- Crust formation
- Desquamation
- Pigmentation
- Ulceration
- Scar formation
- Atrophy

Grouped vesicles along a dermatomal distribution suggests herpes zoster (Fig. 6.143). A rough, coarse skin is commonly seen in various allergies and hypothyroidism.

Excess elasticity of the skin demonstrated over the elbow, forearm and interscapular areas is seen in variants of Ehlers-Danlos syndrome (p 502).

Generalized Hypopigmentation

- Albinism
- Chediak-Higashi syndrome
- Phenylketonuria.

Localized Hypopigmentation

- Hansen's disease
- Waardenburg syndrome (p 501)
- Hypomelanosis of Ito (p 519)
- Tinea versicolor
- Pityriasis alba
- Vitiligo (localized areas of *absent* pigmentation)
- Post-inflammatory hypopigmentation

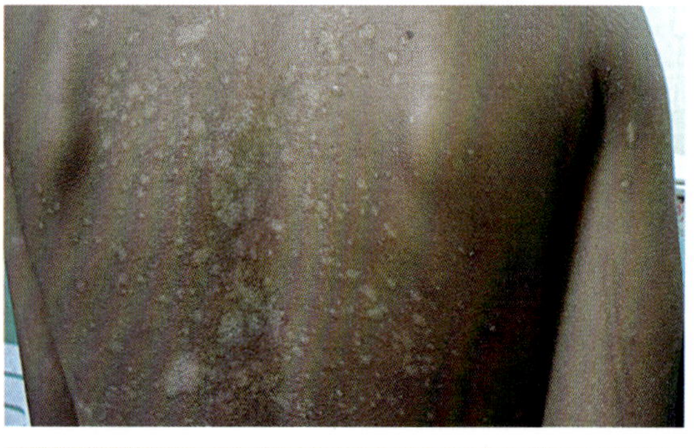

Fig.6.144 Tinea versicolor

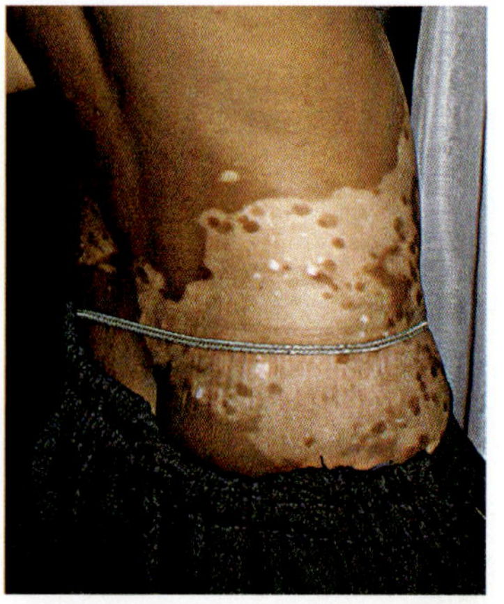

Fig.6.145 Vitiligo

Generalized Hyperpigmentation

- Addison's disease
- Congenital adrenal hyperplasia
- Haemochromatosis
- Kala azar

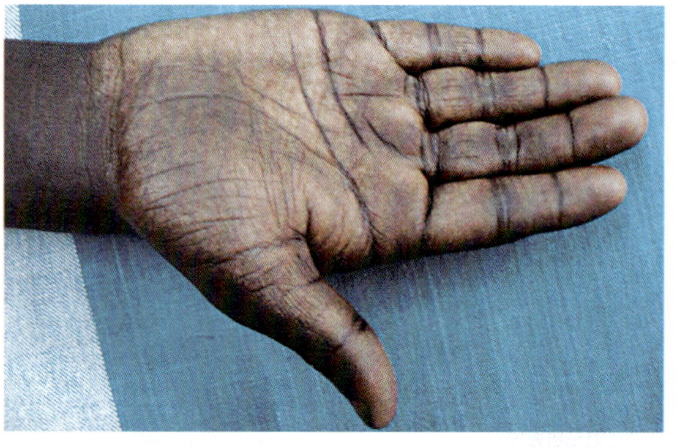

Fig.6.146 Hyperpigmentation in CAH may even involve the palms

Localized Hyperpigmentation

- Post-inflammatory hyperpigmentation
- *Acanthosis nigricans* in the obese could be a pointer towards "metabolic syndrome" or CHAOS (coronary artery disease, hypertension, atherosclerosis, obesity & stroke).
- Fixed drug eruption
- Photodermatitis (pellagra, porphyria, SLE, etc)

- Hyperpigmentation of oral cavity is seen in Addison disease and Peutz-Jeghers syndrome.

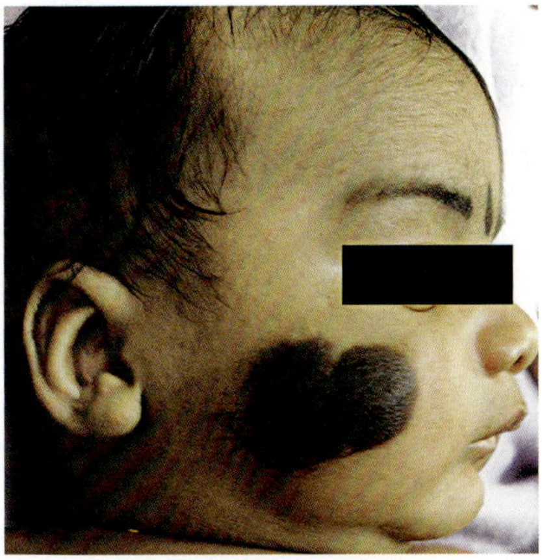

Fig.6.147 Hairy naevus

Cafe-au-lait Spots

These are coffee coloured areas in the skin. they are considered significant if:

1. Prepubertal: >5 mm in size and >6 in number.
2. Post-pubertal: >15 mm in size and >6 in number.
3. Isolated cafe-au-lait spot >15 cm in size.
4. Any cafe-au-lait spot in the centre of the body.
5. Cafe-au-lait spot associated with neurofibromatosis.

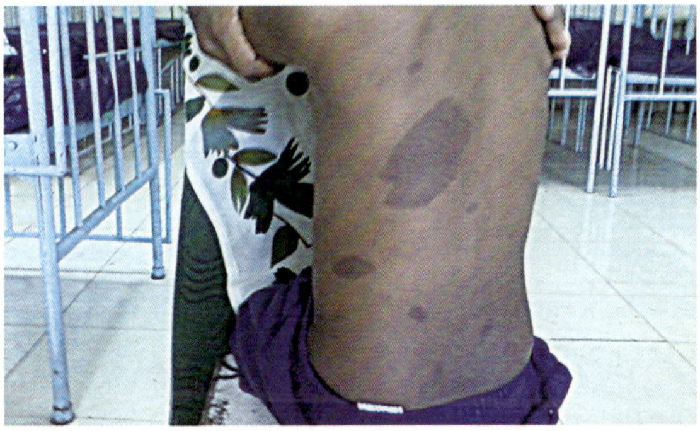

Fig.6.148 Cafe au lait spot

Causes

- Neurofibromatosis ("coast of California")
- McCune Albright syndrome (here cafe-au-lait spots have irregular or ragged margins) ("coast of Maine")
- Multiple lentigenes
- Ataxia telangiectasia
- Tuberous sclerosis
- Gaucher's disease
- Chediak-Higashi syndrome
- Fanconi's anaemia

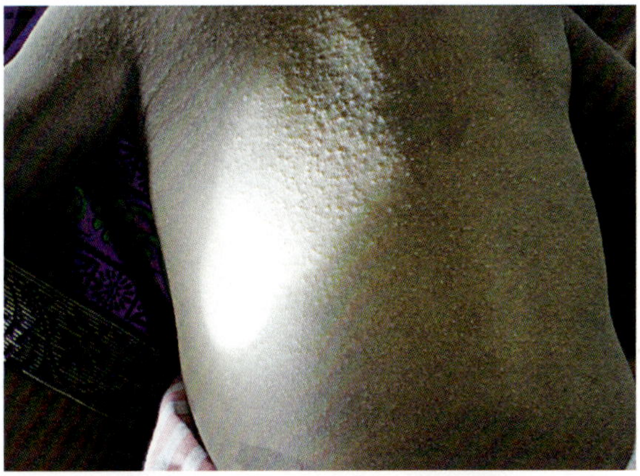

Fig.6.149 Finely papular rashes are best made out by tangential light

Pruritus

- Urticaria
- Atopy
- Scabies
- Chickenpox
- Prickly heat
- Pediculosis
- Ring worm (Tinea)
- Obstructive jaundice

6

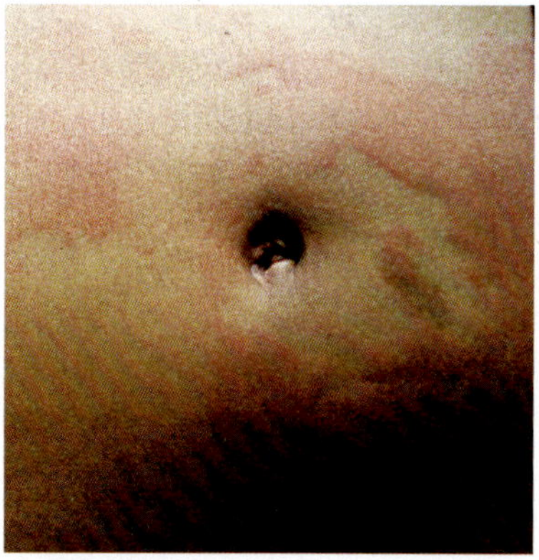

Fig.6.150 Urticaria

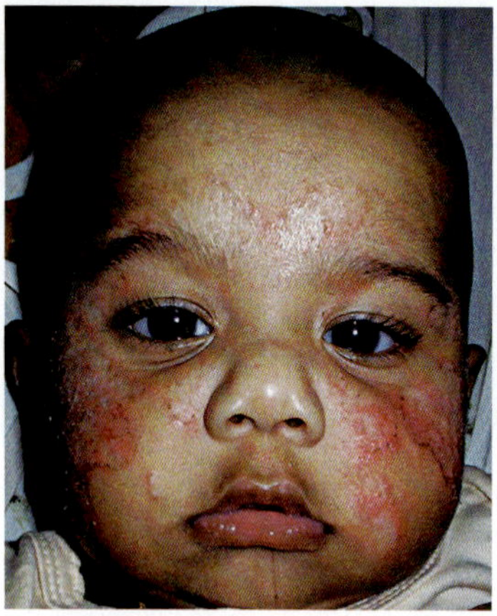

Fig.6.151 Atopic dermatitis: This is the typical area of involvement in early infancy.

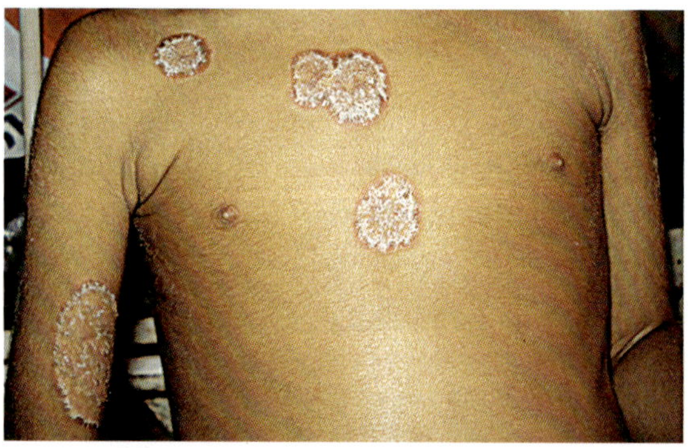

Fig.6.152 Tinea corporis

Photosensitivity

- Pellagra
- Porphyria
- Drugs
- Hartnup disease
- Xeroderma pigmentosa

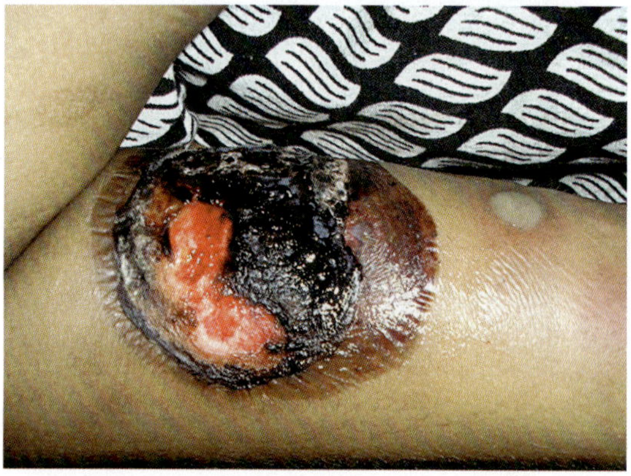

Fig.6.153 Eschar: Eschar is the black dry dead necrotic tissue that is cast off from the surface of skin. Classically described in cutaneous anthrax, the commoner causes are burns, gangrene, etc (also see Fig. 6.155).

Peeling of Skin

This is common following many viral infections, and a few bacterial infections, the examples being scarlet fever, staphylococcal scalded skin syndrome (Fig. 6.154) etc. Peeling also occurs following Kawasaki disease, see p 516.

Erythema Nodosum (p 543)

- Drugs (sulpha, phenytoin, penicillin, barbiturates, etc)
- Streptococcal infections
- Tuberculosis
- Inflammatory bowel disease

Erythema Toxicum

- Benign and self-limited lesion of term *newborns* (Fig. 2.5).

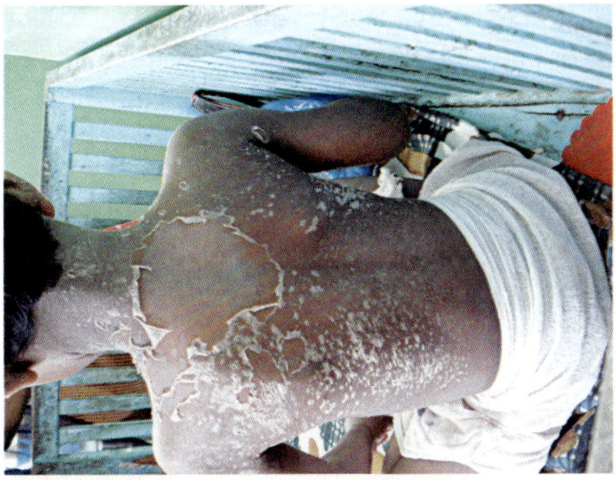

Fig.6.154 Peeling in big patches in SSSS. In viral infections, peeling is usually punctate.

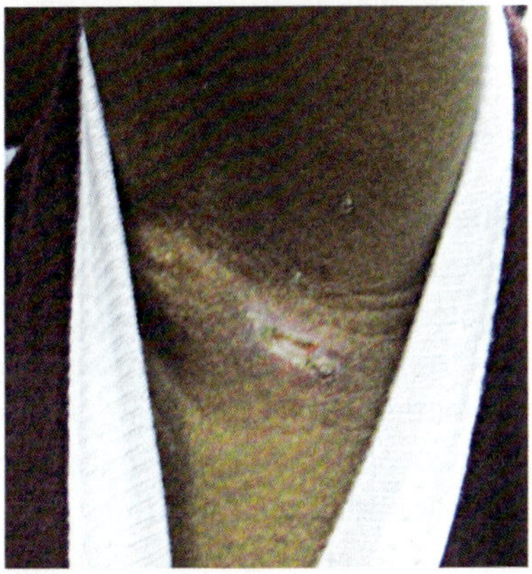

Fig.6.155 Eschar need not have the black tissue.

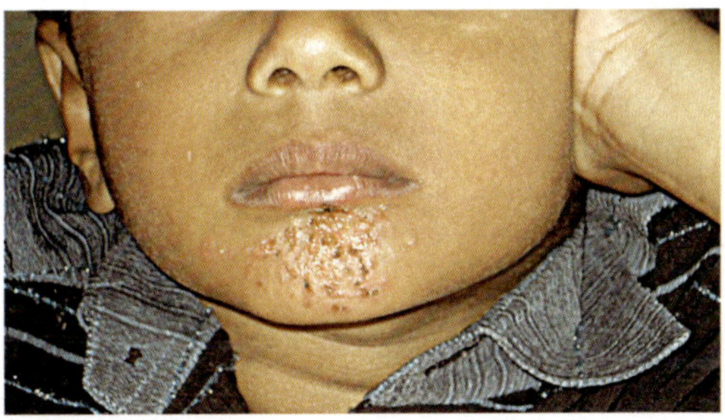

Fig.6.156 Impetigo

- Appears on 2nd or 3rd day of life.
- Numerous 1–2 mm papules and pustules with erythema in an otherwise well newborn.
- Aetiology is unknown.
- Biopsy shows eosinophils.

Molluscum Contagiosum

- Light brown multiple, raised, umbilicated lesions, may be in clusters.
- Viral in aetiology and spread by direct contact.
- Resolve spontaneously after 6–9 months.
- Treatment: Curettage, chemical cauterization or cryotherapy if not resolving spontaneously.

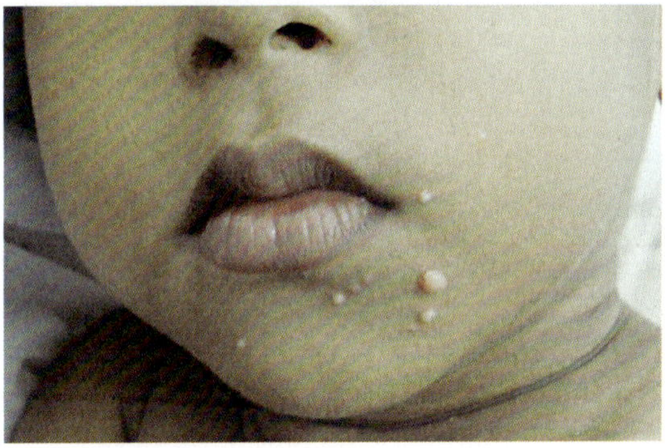

Fig.6.157 Molluscum contagiosum

Neurofibroma

See p 522.

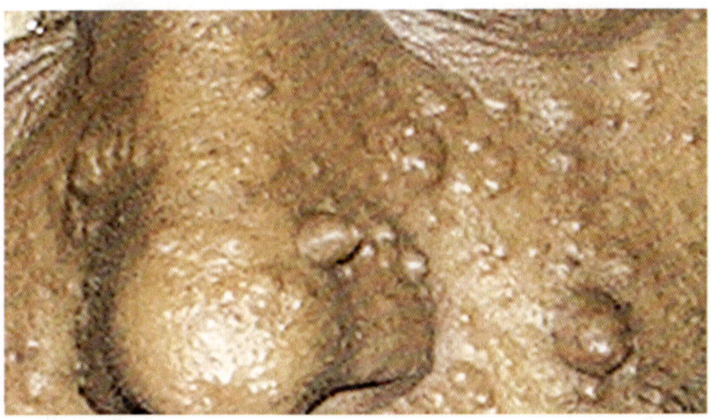

Fig.6.158 Neurofibroma

Mongolian Blue Spot

- Grey–blue pigmented macules over the lumbosacral region. May be found in other areas like buttocks, posterior thighs, back, etc.
- Benign and fades over months to years.
- More frequent in pigmented skin race, Down syndrome and GM_1 gangliosidosis.

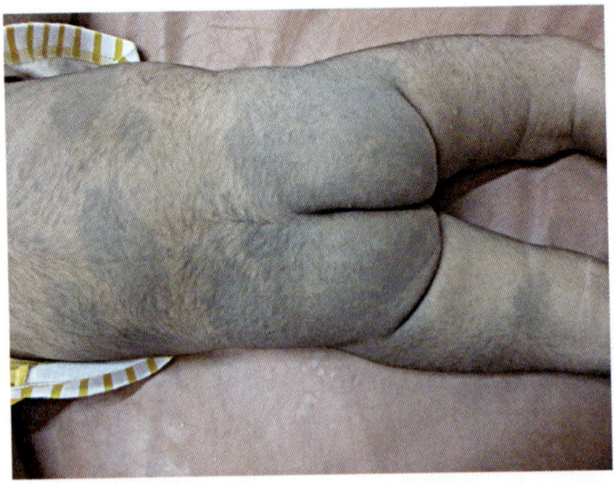

Fig.6.159 Mongolian blue spot

Haemangiomas

- Salmon patch: Pale pink macule, at nape of neck, eyelid, face, etc present *at* birth.

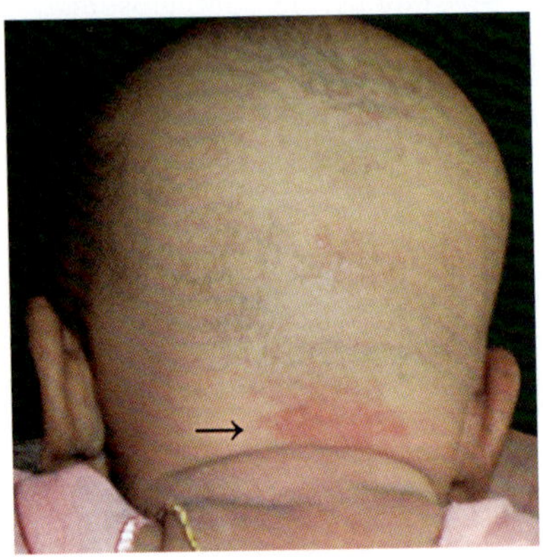

Fig.6.160 Salmon patch

- **Port wine stain**: Present *at* birth, may fade with age, but does not disappear (note that strawberry haemangioma regresses with age). It may be associated with Sturge-Weber syndrome or Klippel-Trenaunay syndrome. Skin lesions may be masked by the skilled use of cosmetics.

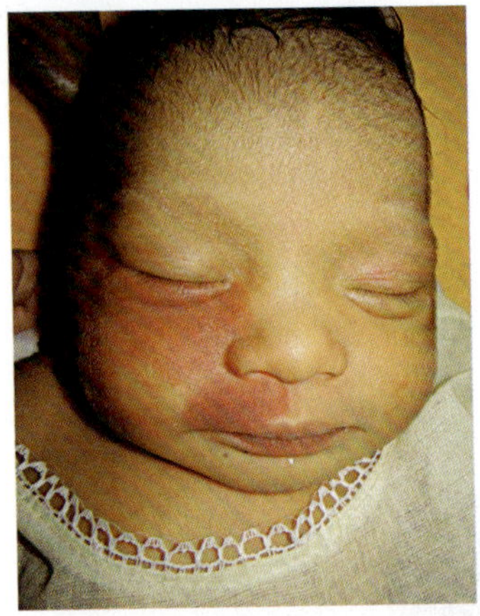

Fig.6.161 Port wine stain

- **Strawberry naevus**: The surface looks and feels like a strawberry. They are raised, well-demarcated, bright red, compressible lesions. Appears soon *after* birth, increases in size for a few months before stabilizing. As the child grows, it involutes. Bleeding due to trauma is the most common complication.
- **Cavernous haemangioma**: Located deeper and hence seen as bluish–red masses with *indistinct* borders. Very large ones may produce high-output cardiac failure. 90% cases disappear by 9 years.
- **Kasabach-Merritt syndrome**: Large, usually deep seated, cavernous haemangioma associated with platelet sequestration, thrombocytopenia and haemorrhage.

Note: The skin manifestations in relation to various diseases are discussed along with the corresponding diseases in the section on short cases (Ch.24).

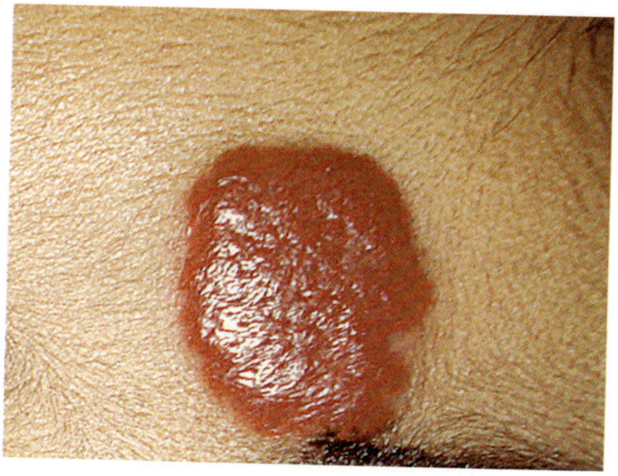

Fig.6.162 Strawberry haemangioma

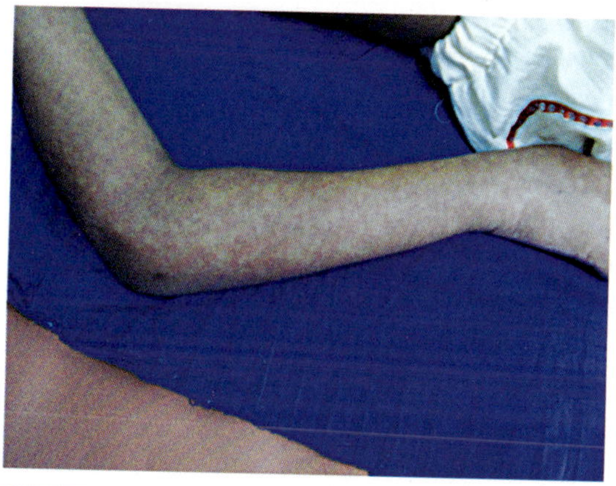

Fig.6.163 Rash of convalescent period of dengue. Note areas of clearing within the diffuse erythematous.

Hypothermia

- Exposure to cold
- Severe PEM
- Shock
- Hypothyroidism

Spider Naevus

The main vessel is an arteriole. Look for spider naevi in upper part of the body, neck, hands, etc. One must look for it in chronic liver disease (see Fig. 6.164A).

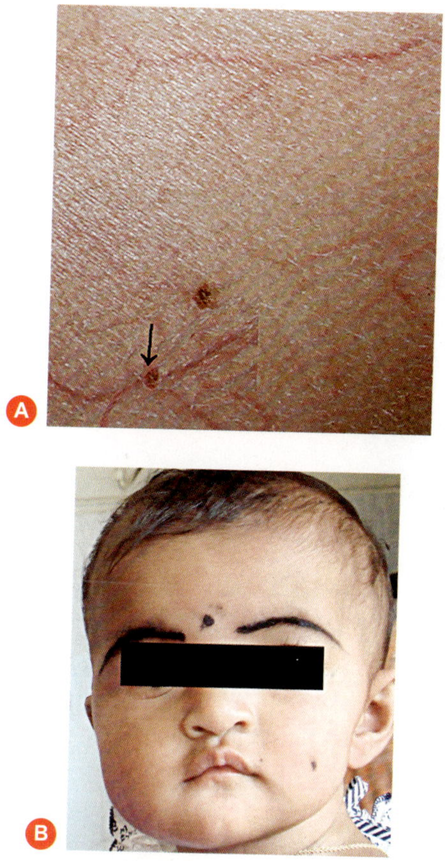

Fig.6.164 (A) Spider angioma, (B) Hemihypertrophy.

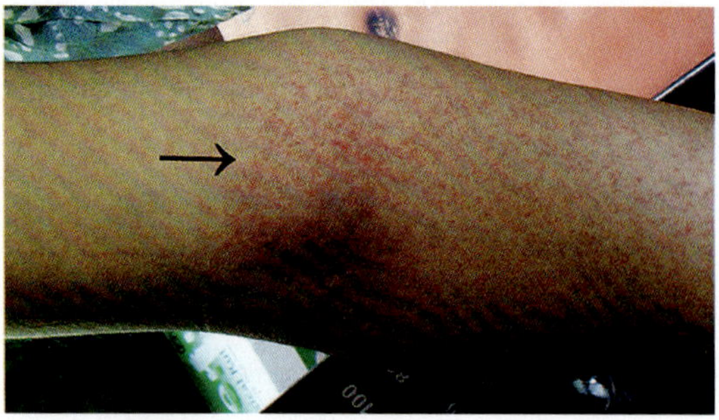

Fig.6.165 Tourniquet test

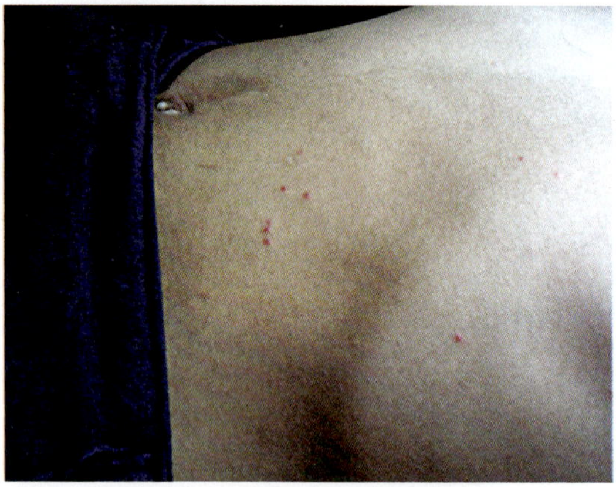

Fig.6.166 Rose spots: Rose spots over the abdomen and chest are described in typhoid fever.

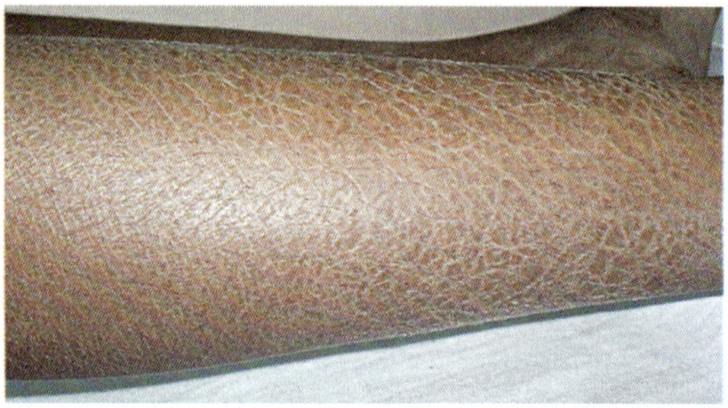

Fig.6.167 Icthyosis

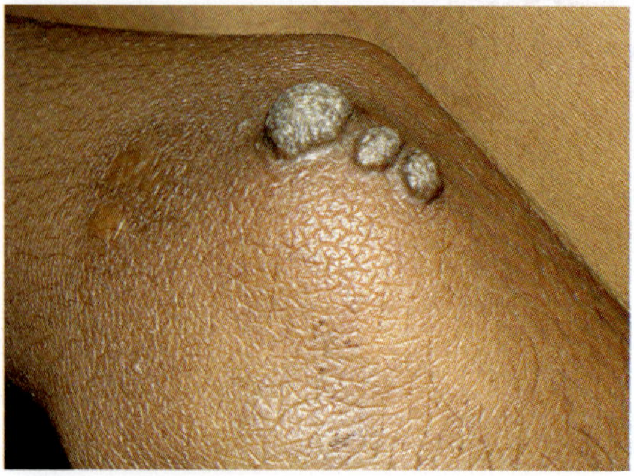

Fig.6.168 Wart

Telangiectasia

- Variation of normal
- Ataxia telangiectasia
- Osler-Rendu-Weber syndrome (hereditary haemorrhagic telangiectasia)
- Spider naevus
- Prolonged topical steroid therapy
- Collagen vascular diseases (e.g., SLE)

Hemihypertrophy

- Idiopathic
- Wilms' tumour
- Russell-Silver syndrome
- Beckwith-Wiedemann syndrome
- Klippel-Trenaunay-Weber syndrome

Hess capillary resistance test (Tourniquet test): Keep the pressure of the BP apparatus midway between the systolic and diastolic pressure for 5 min. Development of >10 petechiae over an area of 1 inch^2 on the flexor surface of forearm is +ve test. Some authorities quote >20 petechiae as positive test. This test is very popular in the screening of suspected dengue fever cases.

***Note*: It is highly recommended that all students, especially the postgraduate students see all the clinical photographs given in Ch. 24.**

CHAPTER 7

Dysmorphic Child: Case Sheet Formats

I. DYSMORPHIC CHILD

In this chapter, an approach to the clinical examination of a dysmorphic child is presented.

1. Presenting complaints:
2. History of the present illness:
3. History of past illnesses:
4. Antenatal, natal & postnatal history:
   Get birth measurements from history/charts (if available). Many chromosomal anomalies and intrauterine (IU) infections are born small for date and have lower potential for postnatal growth. IUGR is common in dysmorphic child. Birth length < 3rd centile point towards primordial dwarfism.
5. Immunization history: Many dysmorphic children are under immunized and hence must be probed into the history.
6. Development history: Development retardation is almost universal and hence a detailed development history is a must.
7. Dietary history: Take a good diet history. Poor nutrition could be an additional contributing factor to poor growth potential of a dysmorphic child.
8. Family and socioeconomic history:

II.GENERAL EXAMINATION

1. General Comment:

- Any obvious dysmorphism (details can be examined in hand to head to foot examination)

2. Vital Signs (compare with normal values for the age):
   - Pulse rate, respiratory rate, blood pressure and temperature
3. Assessment of Growth (measurements or anthropometry):
   - Height, US:LS ratio (refer to discussion under short stature p 50 & 449)
   - Head circumference
   - Weight: Obesity is part of some syndromes like Pradder Willi
   - Height chart of the particular child may be requested to know the height velocity. Percentile charts to know which centile the child's height comes to.
   - Arm span
   - Mid parental height
   - Skin fold thickness (only in relevant cases). If you want to comment on muscle mass you need mid arm circumference and skin fold thickness.
4. Assessment of Development:
   Intellectual impairment is a feature of most syndromes and hence a good development history supplemented by objective assessment is a must.

   For example, in addition to getting a reliable history, the student may test if the child can perform specified tasks (e.g., pick up a pellet from floor).

5. Hand to Head to Foot Examination:
   In the examination of dysmorphic child and skeletal system examination, it is advantageous to start with a profile appraisal followed by hand to head and head to foot examination sequence. This will help not to miss important general examination findings.

Overall Profile Appraisal

Have an overall look at the child. Familiar syndromes will be suspected by the very appearance, like Down, Marfan, etc. Short/tall stature, short limbs, etc also will be suspected by the overall appearance. Any gross limb defects, contractures, etc can be noticed on this gross inspection.

The candidate must show the child what he is expected to do and then ask them to do the same.

- View from front: Examine with the child standing with arms by the side and palms facing forward.
  - Look for asymmetry between the sides (Russel Silver). Hemihypertrophy in Beckwith Wiedemann syndrome. Localized hypertrophy in Klippel Trenauney Weber, neurofibromatosis, congenital hemihypertrophy, etc.
  - Look for cubitus valgus (over 15° in Turner).
  - How far the fingers of UL will reach. Normally, it reaches distal thigh. If fingers reach only above the mid-thigh, the limb is short. If the trunk is short the fingers may reach up to the knee.
  - Palm up: Look for numerous findings possible (clinodactyly, simian crease, etc, to mention a few; see p 105–106) (119-120).
  - Palm down: Make a fist to detect short 4th metacarpal (pseudohypoparathyroidism). Trident deformity of achondroplasia is best displayed with hands down position. Proximally placed thumb is due to short first metacarpal (Cornelia de Lange syndrome). Hypoplastic nails of Ellis-van Creveld and hyperconvex nails of Turner, Noonan are examined for in this position.
  - Joints: Look for joint laxity or stiff joints (restricted joint mobility or increased joint mobility). Look for joint laxity and tests for Marfan, if indicated (see p 469, 511). Must look for joint laxity in short child also, as this may be associated in certain short syndromes like osteogenesis imperfecta and Ehlers Danlos syndrome.
  - Tip of thumb on shoulder test (demonstrate how to do it). If the thumb overshoots, there is proximal segment shortening (rhizomelic); example is achondroplasia.
  - Shoulder approximation test for cleidocranial dysostosis.
- View from the side: Look for
  - Prominent forehead (achondroplasia, rickets, hydrocephalus, haemolytic anaemia)
  - Flat occiput
  - Proptosis (craniosynostosis)
  - Micrognathia
  - Prognathism
  - Lordosis
  - Kyphosis
- View from the back:
  - Neck: Standing at the back, look at the back of neck for short neck, webbing, low hairline, etc.
  - Spine: Have the child bend forwards to touch the toes, to detect scoliosis (true scoliosis will persist even after bending down, whereas the positional scoliosis disappears).
- Skin:
  - Pigmentation (Fanconi)
  - Cafe-au-lait spots (neurofibromatosis I)
  - Hypopigmented areas (tuberous sclerosis, vitiligo)
  - Freckling in xeroderma pigmentosa, LEOPARD syndrome

- Blue black macules in Peutz-Jeghers syndrome
- Whorls of pigmentation in incontinentia pigmenti
- Vascular malformations (Sturge Weber, Klippel Trenauney Weber)
- Telengiectasia (ataxia telengiectasia, Osler Rendu)
- Butter fly rash in malar area (telengiectasia and erythema in Bloom, Cockayne)
- Icthyosis in CHILD syndrome
- Sparse hair or alopecia in CHILD, Cockayne

■ Gait (characteristic gaits are found in muscle weakness, UMN weakness, painful limb, etc; p 168)

Hand to Head and Head to Toe Examination

■ Dysmorphic child will have definite leads to the diagnosis connected with 3 Hs: Hand, Head or Heart. Each anatomical structure in hand and head has to be examined to see if there is any deviation from the normal expected anatomy. Then a detailed CVS examination is to be done. Not just syndrome, all chronic disorders will cause deceleration of height velocity.

■ Nails: Clubbing in cystic fibrosis; hyperconvex nails in Turner; bluish in cyanotic congenital heart disease; leukonychia in chronic liver disease.

■ Palms: Palmar erythema in chronic liver disease, changes of Down syndrome if the case is Down.

■ Clinodactyly of fifth finger in Down, Russel Silver, and Seckel.

■ Short fingers or arachinodactyly.

■ Simian crease in Down.

■ Trident hand in achondroplasia.

■ Short 4th metacarpal in pseudohypoparathyroidism, occasionally Turner.

■ Polydactyly in Lawrence Moon Biedl. Syndactyly in Apert.

■ Wrist: Widened wrists (suggestive of rickets); changes suggestive of rheumatoid arthritis (like deviation of wrist).

■ Pulse: Radiofemoral delay (coarctation may be seen in Turner); bradycardia (in hypothyroidism).

■ BP: Hypertension in chronic renal failure, Cushing, etc.

■ Head: Skull shape abnormalities.

■ Dysmorphism (look at head, hand and heart whenever dysmorphism is suspected). Syndromes are Down, Turner, Noonan, Russel Silver, fetal alcohol syndrome (mid facial hypoplasia in FAS), etc.

■ Triangular facies in Russel Silver (small face with micrognathia, making the normal skull appear big apparently: the whole thing makes it look triangular face); frontal/parietal bossing in rickets.

■ Mid-line defects may be seen in hypopituitarism. Anosmia in Kallman syndrome.

■ Eyes: Look for hypertelorism, epicanthic folds, etc.

■ Partial ptosis (Noonan)

■ Pallor (in chronic renal disease; thalassemia), Jaundice (chronic liver disease),

■ Blue sclera in osteogenesis imperfecta.

■ Photophobia in cystinosis (due to cysteine crystal deposition in cornea).

■ Cloudy cornea in IU infections and mucopolysaccharidosis; cataract in congenital rubella.

■ Visual field defects (craniopharyngioma).

■ Fundus: Chorioretinitis in IU infections.

■ Mouth: Delayed dentition in hypothyroidism; oligodontia with conical teeth in ectodermal dysplasia (p 500).

■ Ears: Low set in Turner, Noonan, Seckel, etc posteriorly rotated ear is usually seen in Noonan syndrome.

■ Ask if the child is using hearing aid (in congenital rubella syndrome, Treacher Collin, Waardenburg, etc).

7

- Neck: Low posterior hairline (Klippel Feil, Turner, Noonan); short neck (Klippel Feil, Noonan). Goitre may be seen in hypothyroidism.
- Chest: Pectus excavatum (Noonan, Turner); wide spaced nipple (Turner); shield shape chest (Turner); rachitic rosary (rickets). Auscultate chest (e.g., bronchiectasis in cystic fibrosis) and heart (congenital heart disease).
- Abdomen: Distension could be because of weak muscles due to malnutrition, celiac disease, ascites or organomegaly (e.g., chronic haemolytic anaemias). Striae over abdominal wall may be seen in Cushings.
- Look for organomegaly.
- Cafe au lait spots (in neurofibromatosis, Fanconi, Russel Silver).
- Back: Scoliosis (Klipper Feil).
- Genitalia:
  Tanner staging: Advanced Tanner stage in precocious puberty. Delayed Tanner stage (in relation to the present age of the child) may be seen in growth hormone deficiency, hypothyroidism, chronic illnesses, and constitutional delay (late bloomers, meaning pubertal changes get delayed; so much so the fusion of epiphysis also get delayed; so child has more time to achieve height and so ultimate height achieved will be normal).
- Measure penile length. Micro penis in hypopituitarism. Measure testes length or better compare with orchidometer.
- Tanner stage is advanced in precocious puberty; retarded in hypothyroidism and all chronic illnesses.
- Lower limb: Bowing (rickets, metaphyseal dysplasia); Oedema of dorsum of feet may be seen in newborns with Turner (not in the grown up Turner and hence unlikely to find it in a short stature child).
- Erythema nodosum (in IBD).
- Delayed relaxation of ankle jerk in hypothyroidism.
- Flat foot in Marfan.
- Polydactyly in Ellis van Creveld.
- Wide gap between first and second toes with deep plantar crease (Kennedy crease) between them are seen in Down.
- Hallux valgus, hammer toe, etc.

DOWN SYNDROME

The history depends on the presenting complaints for which the child got hospitalized.

Past History

- Past history of surgeries (may have had surgeries for duodenal atresia, Hirschsprung disease, etc; adenoidectomy/tonsillectomy for obstructive sleep apnoea; cardiac surgery).
- Recurrent respiratory infections (invariably present in L-R shunt CHDs).
- Obstructive sleep apnoea (snoring, restless sleep, day time somnolence).
- Behavioural problems:
  - Hyperactivity, poor attention span, impulsivity, temper tantrums (ADHD).
  - Autistic behaviours (obsessed with routines, on his own world, self play, no reciprocation to parental love).
  - Any other deviant behaviours.
- History suggestive of diabetes mellitus in older Down child (excessive eating and drinking; night time urination).

Antenatal/Natal/Birth History

Age of mother at conception. Down is associated with advanced maternal age.

Inquire birth parameters. May have been small at birth.

Development: Global delay is expected. Social domain may be better than other domains.

Dietary History

Take a good diet history. This will enlighten whether the growth retardation is contributed by dietary deficiency in addition to inherent poor growth potential.

Family and Socioeconomic History

Impact on parents, siblings, finance. Whether aware of or already member of social support groups.

General Examination

Record vital as in any other case.

Anthropometry

Mention that Down syndrome specific growth charts are ideal for comparisons comparison As this is usually not provided in exams, you may use the common charts.

Weight

They generally remain underweight during infancy, but after toddler age, most are overweight.

- Obese (consider co-existing hypothyroidism; or over eating)
- Thin (poor intake)

Also measure height (short stature), mid arm circumference, head circumference.
You may mention that mid parental height was not calculated as this may not have relevance in Down child.

Development Assessment

This step may be attempted, but is not a must (because it is not always possible to get the child's cooperation). Here, the candidate tries to make the child perform the development milestones that the child has achieved.

Hand to Head and Head to Foot Examination

In any dysmorphic child, hand to head and head to toe examination is the preferred scheme of examination.

Hand: Hand is short; fingers are also short (brachydactyly). Single palmar crease (*simian crease*) or there may be two palmar creases, but the proximal palmar crease extends to the full width of palm (sydney crease); other dermatoglyphics like atd angle, etc are not looked for during routine clinical examination. Dysplastic middle phalanx of the 5th finger causing short middle phalanx of 5th finger, and *clinodactyly* (curved finger). Hypotonia and hypermobility of joints of limbs

Head: Flat occiput (flat occiput and flat facial profile are best appreciated by viewing from the side); large anterior fontanel and delayed closure of fontanel. Soft sparse scalp hair. Head circumference is less than average.

7

Face

- Nose: Flat nasal bridge.
- Ear: Ear is usually low set, though not necessarily so. Ear may be small, the upper helix may be over folded and more horizontal than rounded. Hearing impairment is common (conductive, due to otitis media; short Eustachian tube predisposes to recurrent otitis). Check hearing. Inquire whether the child is using hearing aid. Try to visualize tympanic membrane for any perforation (be sure to use otoscope).
- Eyes: Upward slant of palpebral fissures (called mongoloid slant, see p 95); epicanthic folds on the medial canthus (p 95); speckled iris (*Brush-field spots,* see p 509); Look for squint, nystagmus, cataract; inquire whether the child is using spectacles. Look for pallor (iron deficiency anaemia, leukaemia).
- Mouth: Protruding tongue (short hard palate and small oral cavity, hence the decreased number of teeth, irregular placement of teeth, carious teeth. Large tonsils may be associated with OSA, so comment on tonsils normal sized tongue remain protruded); furrowed tongue ("scrotal" tongue).

Neck: Thyroid, swelling, if any.
Neck pain, torticollis could be due to atlanto axial instability. Look for weakness of limbs, loss of bladder control and increased deep tendon reflexes. Look for low posterior hair line of neck.

Chest: Look for pectus carinatum, excavatum. Harrison sulcus may be present due to repeated respiratory infections (L-R shunt lesions are common in Down).

Full CVS examination has to be done in Down syndrome (50% have congenital heart disease). May have scars of surgeries of heart.

Endocardial cushion defect (atrioventricular septal defect) and VSD are the most common heart lesions. They are more prone for *early development of pulmonary arterial hypertension* due to abnormalities of alveoli-capillary network and hence the candidate must clinically look for evidence of PAH. Tetralogy of Fallot is a rare lesion (about 8%).

Abdomen: Look for scars of surgeries done in newborn period (duodenal atresia, Hirschsprung, etc). Hepatomegaly/splenomegaly (cardiac failure, leukaemia).

Genitalia: Consider Tanner staging in grown up children.

Lower limbs: Increased space between the 1st and 2nd toes (sandal gap) and a furrow on the sole in the space between the same fingers (Kennedy crease). Hypotonia, hyperextensibility of joints.

Back: Have the child bend forwards to touch the toes to detect scoliosis. Scoliosis is probable in children with hypotonia.

Skin

- Cutis marmorata
- Palmo plantar hyperkeratosis; generalized dry skin (as a feature of Down, or because of hypothyroidism).

Management

Since there is no definitive treatment, the management consists of counseling and management of associated deficits:

- Cardiology evaluation (congenital heart disease). Infective endocarditis prophylaxis must be advised.
- Periodic ophthalmic evaluation (cataract and refractory errors).
- ENT evaluation (obstructive sleep apnoea; otitis media; hearing evaluation).
- Dental hygiene (to prevent endocarditis).
- Thyroid function study (every 6 months till 3 years and then yearly till 12 years).
- Counseling on restriction of contact sports (atlanto-axial subluxation).
- Education as guided by IQ and competence.
- Karyotyping (see Fig. 26.11, 26.12, p 589).
- Prenatal diagnosis, (see p 509).
- The students are advised to read "Manual of Pediatric Practice" by the same author to equip themselves to answer the investigation and management related questions during examination.
- Important areas to be read are:
  Non dysjunction and translocation.
  Chances of recurrence if parents are normal, mother is carrier or father is carrier.
  Intrauterine diagnosis
- Complications
- How to follow-up Down child
- Counseling

TURNER SYNDROME

General Considerations

Consider Turner in any short *female* child, even if there are no other manifestations (can present with short stature as the only manifestation). On the other hand, if there are morphological features of Turner, but the child is male, then the diagnosis is Noonan, not Turner.

In adolescence, delayed puberty, amenorrhea, (and by investigation, elevated FSH levels) are the clues to diagnose Turner.

X-linked recessive conditions do not manifest in females. However, if a Turner child inherits any of these disease genes (e.g., haemophila, Duchenne), it may manifest although the child is female. This is because the only available X chromosome carries the disease gene.

In newborn period, there may be lymphedema of hands and feet; hence ask for the same in history.

Antenatal/Natal/Birth History

Inquire birth parameters. May have normal length at birth. Short stature manifests after 2 years.

Development

Development retardation is not expected in Turner.

Dietary History

Take a good diet history. This will enlighten whether the growth retardation is contributed by dietary deficiency in addition to inherent poor growth potential.

Anthropometry

Measurements (short stature is universal; Turner specific growth charts if available is ideal).

Weight

- Obese (consider co-existing hypothyroidism).
- Thin (elicit history regarding IBD; also bear in mind the possibility of various malignancies like gonadoblastoma, colonic carcinoma, etc).

Mid parental height will not predict the adult height of Turner.

In any syndromic child, the best scheme of examination is the one used for dysmorphic child.

Overall Appraisal

The candidate must show the child what he is expected to do and then ask them to do the same.

- View from front: Examine with the child standing with arms by the side and palms facing forward.
  - Look for cubitus valgus (over 15° in Turner).
  - How far the fingers of UL will reach. In normal child, it reaches distal thigh.
  - Palm up: Short mid phalanx of little finger. Madelung deformity (congenital subluxation of head of ulna, with resultant radial deviation of hand).
  - Palm down: Make a fist to look for short 3rd, 4th or 5th metacarpals. Hyperconvex nails.
  - Joints: Juvenile arthritis may co-exist in a few cases.
  - Tip of thumb on shoulder test (demonstrate how to do it). Middle segment or mesomelic shortening may be there in Turner, so thumbs may not reach the shoulder.
  - Gait: DDH may be an association in Turner
- View from the side: look for
  - Micrognathia
  - Lordosis
  - Kyphosis
  - Scoliosis
- View from the back:
  - Neck: Standing at the back, look at the back of neck for short neck, webbing, low hair line, etc.
  - Spine: Have the child bend forwards to touch the toes, to detect scoliosis.
- Skin:
  - Pigmented nevi, haemangioma, lymphedema (in newborn).

General Examination

Vitals: Do not forget to record UL and LL BP because coarctation of aorta is a common association.

Hand to Head and Head to Toe Examination

- Nails: May be dysplastic, or hyperconvex.
- Pulse: Radio femoral delay (coarctation in Turner); bradycardia (in hypothyroidism).
- BP: Hypertension in Turner with coarctation.
- Head
- Eyes:
  - Look for slant of eyes.
  - Partial ptosis (Noonan); Squint; Epicanthic folds (rarely).
  - Fundus: Changes due to hypertension.
- Mouth:
  - High arched palate; Caries teeth (risk of endocarditis).
  - Micrognathia.
- Ears:
  - Low set in Turner, Noonan. Ear could be malformed and rotated.
  - Hearing impairment is common (could be conductive, sensorineural or mixed).
  - Try to visualize tympanic membrane for any perforation (be sure to use otoscope) as eustachian tube block and otitis is common.
- Neck:
  - Webbed neck (pterygium colli).
  - Low posterior hairline (Turner, Noonan); short neck. Goitre may be seen in hypothyroidism.
- Chest:
  - Broad shield like chest with widely spaced hypoplastic or inverted nipples (Fig. 6.92, p 117).
  - Pectus excavatum.
  - Scars of heart surgeries.
  - Full CVS examination.
- Abdomen:
  - Surgical scars (may have got gonads removed surgically to prevent danger of malignancy).
    Note: Gonads are removed only for those who have mosaic karyotype with retained Y chromosome (45X, 46XY). For XO Turner, the streak gonads need not be removed.
  - Hepatomegaly (CCF secondary to hypertension).
  - Splenomegaly (infective endocarditis).
  - Palpable enlarged kidney (hydronephrosis).
- Back: Scoliosis/kyphosis/lordosis
- Genitalia:
- *Tanner staging*:
- Lower limb:
- Oedema of hands and feet is a manifestation at newborn period, not later
- Rarely short metatarsals
- Differential diagnosis: Various causes of short stature (see p 449).

Investigations

- Karyotyping (45X, see Fig. 26.13, p 590).
- Thyroid function test (as hypothyroidism is a treatable cause of short stature).
- Cardiology evaluation (coarctation of aorta, bicuspid aortic valve).
- Ultrasound evaluation of abdomen (dysgenetic hypoplastic gonads; horse shoe kidney).
- Management: See p 518.

The students are advised to read "Manual of Pediatric Practice" by the same author to equip themselves to answer the investigation and management related questions during examination.

CHAPTER 8

Signs and Symptoms in Systemic Examination

In this section, signs and symptoms referable to systems will be discussed.

VERTIGO

It is the feeling of objects going round and round (objective vertigo) or the patient himself revolving (subjective). It is difficult for children to identify vertigo. Frequent falling to one side, crying with closed eyes as if in terror, or suddenly clinging on to the mother as if in terror may be the evidences of vertigo (a close differential diagnosis of these symptoms is complex partial seizure).

Vertigo, which worsens on movement is likely to be labyrinthine in origin. The child may have a history of recent respiratory or ear infection in labyrinthine vertigo. Associated diplopia and other localizing CNS findings suggest intracranial pathology. Acute vertigo may also be due to toxins.

The usual causes are:

- Motion sickness
- Ear infections (mastoiditis); acute labyrinthitis, viral or bacterial
- Migraine
- Manifestation of temporal lobe epilepsy
- Benign paroxysmal vertigo of unknown cause
- CNS diseases like brain tumour
- Trauma to head/ear
- Following a seizure
- Drug induced (sedatives, antihistamines)

SEIZURES

- Febrile seizures (6 months to 6 years. Brief in duration, no neurological deficits after seizure)
- Intracranial problems:
  - Infections like meningitis, encephalitis, etc.
  - Vascular events like haemorrhage (vascular malformation or trauma), thrombosis, etc.
  - Space-occupying lesions like tumours, tuberculoma, brain abscess, etc.
- Encephalopathy:
  - Hepatic encephalopathy.
  - Hypertensive encephalopathy.
  - Metabolic encephalopathy: E.g., hypoglycaemia, hyponatraemia, uraemic encephalopathy.
  - Toxic encephalopathy: E.g., drugs (e.g., theophylline) and toxins.
- Epilepsy (Two or more unprovoked seizures)
- Neurocutaneous syndromes like tuberous sclerosis, Sturge-Weber syndrome, neurofibromatosis, etc.
- Structural abnormalities of brain like lissencephaly.
- Inborn errors of metabolism.
- Pseudoseizures are not uncommon. Here, there is no definite pattern known to be associated with seizure. It occurs only during the day time and when being observed. The child does not sustain injuries as they fall "carefully."

Tetany looks like tonic spasm, but here there is typical posturing of hands and feet, *carpopedal spasm* (p 216).

Points to be elicited in history in case of seizures

- Nature of seizure movements: Clonic, tonic, tonic-clonic, or myoclonic.
- Type of seizure: Partial or generalized or started as focal but generalized subsequently.
- Duration of seizure(s); in case of multiple seizures, how was the sensorium in between seizures.
- Whether associated with up rolling of eyeballs, frothing, loss of consciousness, involuntary passage of urine/stools during seizures, fall/ injury, etc.
- Pre seizure phenomena (aura): Aura or automatisms.
- Post seizure phenomena: Drowsiness, delirium, Todd's palsy.
- What could have precipitated the seizures (usual factors must be inquired into, like fever, trauma, missing drugs in epilepsy, loss of sleep, flickering lights, etc).

HEADACHE

- Enquire if it is frontal (eye strain), temporal (migraine), or occipital (tension headache). Migraine headaches may be unilateral (may switch from side to side), occur off and on, may have an aura and associated with nausea, vomiting and visual disturbances. There may be history of similar headaches in the past and in family members. Tension headache is bilateral, continuous and band-like pressing in quality. Nausea or vomiting is *unlikely* with tension head aches and it does not disturb sleep.
- Inquire if it starts in one place and spreads (more likely to be organic if it stayed in one place).
- Associated with vomiting (migraine, intracranial pathology).
- Family history of headache.
- Headache due to fever per se (occurs in viral illness, goes off once the fever is controlled).
- Associated photophobia (cerebral irritation like meningitis).
- Does coughing, stooping or straining (e.g., at toilet) make it worse (increased intracranial pressure).
- Enquire if it is worse early in the morning (brain tumour or abscess). The severity of headache increases progressively over days to weeks in intracranial space-occupying lesions. Early morning vomiting day after day may suggest intracranial tumour.
- Enquire if it is worse at the end of the day (visual problems/tension headache).
- Infected tooth or ear disease may be the cause of headache, many a time unilateral headache.
- History suggestive of sinusitis.
- Hypertension is an important but often neglected cause for headache.
- Hyperacute onset of very severe headache may indicate subarachnoid bleed.
- Small babies with headaches cannot express themselves and may only be irritable. Also it is interesting to note that frowning is more common in case of headache, whereas grimacing is more common with abdominal pain than headache (not an absolute rule).

ATAXIA

The usual manifestation is unsteady gait. It may be seen in any sick child or in the very young. Motor ataxia is due to muscle incoordination as in cerebellar lesions and sensory ataxia is due to loss of proprioception. Clumsiness of a small child should not be interpreted as ataxia.

Common Causes of Acute Ataxia

- Acute post-infectious cerebellar ataxia: This may follow viral respiratory or gastrointestinal infections. The common agents implicated are varicella, coxsackie, echo, etc.

Acute post infectious cerebellar ataxia occurs in isolation without any accompanying CNS symptoms or signs.

- Drug induced (e.g., anticonvulsants, antihistamines, alcohol, etc).
- Intracranial tumours (especially of posterior fossa or those with sudden bleed or rapidly progressive hydrocephalus), intracranial infections, hydrocephalus, etc.
- Miller-Fisher syndrome: This is a variant of Guillain-Barre syndrome. The syndrome consists of ataxia, areflexia and ophthalmoplegia. Note that there is only ataxia and not limb weakness.

  Note: Acute labyrinthitis may produce ataxia-like gait, but note that it is disequilibrium (and hence posture cannot be maintained) and not ataxia (usually there is a history suggestive of URI/ear infection).

Recurrent episodes of ataxia may be seen in (mnemonic—**HUPI**):

- **H**artnup disease
- **U**rea cycle disorders
- **P**yruvate dehydrogenase deficiency
- **I**ntermittent branched chain aminoaciduria/late onset MSUD
- Basilar artery migraine is another cause for recurrent ataxia (may have vertigo, headache, paraesthesia and hemiparesis).
- Multiple sclerosis also has to be considered.

Chronic Static Ataxia

- Post encephalitis
- Agenesis of cerebellar vermis (clinically present as ataxic cerebral palsy)
- Hydrocephalus (arrested hydrocephalus)

Chronic Progressive Ataxia

- Posterior fossa tumours (subacute rather than chronic)
- Ataxia telangiectasia
- Friedreich ataxia (look for loss of posterior column sensations, absent knee jerk, upgoing plantar, pes cavus and kyphoscoliosis)

COMA

- History of fever indicates infective aetiology (meningitis, encephalitis, cerebral malaria).
- History of poison. Fever may be one of the presenting symptoms of certain poisonings (atropine group like dhatura).
- History of trauma.
- History of bites or stings.
- History of sudden onset may point towards a vascular event.
- History of gradual progression to coma over many days suggests slowly progressive lesions like a brain tumour.
- Past history of diseases (diabetes, epilepsy, heart, liver or renal disease) may be a pointer to the aetiology.
- Look for jaundice (may be hepatic encephalopathy). Reye syndrome does not present with significant jaundice. Here, the evolution of the disease helps in diagnosis. (A child, apparently recovering from a viral illness starts repeatedly vomiting and slips into coma.)
- Blood pressure (hypertensive encephalopathy).
- Examine fundus for papilloedema (intracranial space-occupying lesion, TB meningitis, etc).
- Look for any rash (meningococcaemia).
- Look for meningeal signs (meningitis, subarachnoid bleed).
- Look for signs of impending herniation (decerebrate posturing, irregular respiration, dilated fixed pupils either unilateral or bilateral).

DIPLOPIA

- The child complains of double vision.
- Associated headache and vomiting: Increased intracranial pressure.
- Elicit history of head injury, if any.
- Buzzing in the ears: Labyrinthine involvement is likely.

- Ask and examine for weakness of other cranial nerves or motor weakness in other parts of the body.
- Is it vertical or horizontal separation diplopia? Ascertain the direction of maximum separation of the images, to find out the paralysed muscle (p 198).
- For all practical purposes, the outer image is always false and the images are most widely separated when looking in the direction of action of paralyzed nerve or muscle.
- Diplopia at the end of the day: Myasthenia.
- Diplopia present only during the movement of the eye in one direction indicates extraocular muscle paralysis.
- Refer to the discussion on squint p 197.

SYNCOPE

- Vasovagal syncope: Following prolonged standing (orthostatic), fright (e.g., fainting during blood letting).
- Cardiac: Aortic stenosis, hypertrophic obstructive cardiomyopathy, arrhythmia.
- Metabolic: Hypoglycaemia.
- CNS: May be a seizure manifestation.
- Trauma: Because of head injury or blood loss.

EPISTAXIS

Blood coming out via anterior nares is usually termed 'epistaxis.' In case of more posterior bleeds, the blood may get ingested (which may get vomited out as hemetemesis) or get coughed out from nasopharynx (hemoptysis).

- Trauma (usually trivial like nose picking)
- Rhinitis
- Foreign body (one-sided nasal bleed, usually associated with foul smelling nasal discharge)
- Polyps
- Diphtheria
- Hypertension
- Bleeding disorders (e.g., von Willebrand disease, ITP, leukemia, etc)

DYSPNOEA

This is the subjective sensation of respiratory distress. It is not synonymous with tachypnoea, which actually means a rapid rate of breathing. However, significant tachypnoea is usually associated with dyspnoea (also see p 285).

- Mild dyspnoea: Dyspnoea during more than average physical activity. For example, there is exercise intolerance or the child cannot tolerate play activities tolerated by normal children. There is no dyspnoea during average walking, etc (corresponds to Gr I of NYHA); see p 285.
- Moderate dyspnoea: Dyspnoea during normal physical activity like walking to school, etc (corresponds to Gr II of NYHA).
- Severe dyspnoea: Dyspnoea during rest or activities of daily living like walking to bathroom, etc (corresponds to Gr III and IV of NYHA grading).

Ask about the onset: Very sudden onset in case of pneumothorax, foreign body aspiration, acute laryngeal oedema of anaphylaxis, etc. Dyspnoea of asthma and cardiac disease worsens at night. Dyspnoea worsening within minutes of lying down is due to CCF and not asthma. Ask about its relation to exertion or other factors. Exertional dyspnoea may be cardiac or exercise-induced asthma.

Deep and rapid breathing (Kussmaul breathing) indicates metabolic acidosis. Shallow rapid breathing is seen in pneumonia, pleurisy, etc. Shallow slow breathing is seen in morphine poisoning.

- **Respiratory**: Asthma, pneumonia, pleural effusion, pneumothorax, etc. Associated fever and cough indicates infectious pulmonary problems. Here, the sputum is likely to be purulent. Dyspnoea associated with pain in the chest may indicate pleural pain. Inspiratory difficulty is more common with upper airway obstruction, whereas expiratory difficulty is more common with lower airway obstructive diseases like asthma. Upper airway causes of dyspnoea are laryngotracheobronchitis, epiglottitis, laryngitis (e.g., diphtheria), foreign body, etc.

- **Cardiac**: Orthopnoea may be due to CCF (dyspnoea on lying down), or paroxymal nocturnal dyspnoea (getting up at midnight fighting for breath). Orthopnoea occurs within minutes of lying down due to blood from periphery stagnating in atrium as the failing heart fails to pump it out effectively. Sputum is frothy pink in heart diseases that produces pulmonary oedema (e.g., mitral stenosis). Severe anaemia is another cause for cardiac failure.
- Neurologic: Nerve palsy or muscle weakness may produce dyspnoea. This may be seen in diaphragmatic or intercostal paralysis due to polio, Guillain-Barre syndrome, etc.
- Hyperventilation: E.g., aspirin poisoning, diabetic ketoacidosis, central neurogenic hyperventilation or psychogenic (like anxiety).
- Chest wall deformities, e.g., severe kyphoscoliosis, fracture rib, etc.

COUGH

Enquire about: Duration/mode of onset; dry or productive (assessment of the mother from the sound of cough as the child may not expectorate); paroxysmal or not; whether associated with chest pain or not; factors exacerbating cough: e.g., exertion, posture, night time, etc.

History of dramatic response to bronchodilators points towards asthma. Ask for presence of haemoptysis, family history of tuberculosis, bronchial asthma and hay fever. Ask for overcrowding, environmental pollution, parental smoking and smoky kitchen.

- Paroxysmal cough terminating in vomiting is classical of whooping cough, but may be seen in asthma as well. Whoop is due to forced inspiration though a narrow glottis following a bout of spasmodic cough.

  Sudden onset of paroxysmal cough in a child who was well till then strongly suggests foreign body aspiration. Unlike pertussis, the cough of chlamydia pneumonia is paroxysmal dry and staccato (short inspiration in between coughs). The most common age group affected is 4–16 weeks.
- Cough that causes chest pain may be because of pleurisy. Here, one may observe that the child is consciously holding back the cough.
- Cough related to exertion may be due to asthma or cardiac disease. Note that the cough starts *after* the child is a few minutes into the exertion or soon after the exertion is terminated and not during the initiation of exertion in exercise-induced asthma. Cough of asthma can be dry and "tight" (especially in the early phase); some children produce plenty of secretions and the cough sounds wet from the beginning itself.
- Postural variation of cough is seen in lung abscess, sometimes in bronchiectasis, postnasal drip, etc. Cough of postnatal drip gets worse on lying down. Throat clearing type of cough, especially at night may be indicative of postnasal drip.
- Nocturnal cough is seen in asthma, postnasal drip, gastro-oesophageal reflux, etc. Significant fever is *not* expected in these conditions. Paroxysmal nocturnal dyspnoea has cough as a component, but the dyspnea component is far more obvious and overshadows the cough.
- Croupy cough often with stridor is seen in laryngotra-cheobronchitis. Harsh barking cough (simulated to the "bark" of a seal), worse at night, and hoarse voice are characteristic of LTB. The usual history of LTB is that the child goes to sleep with a mild rhinitis, gets up at night with stridor, cough and hoarseness. Brassy cough (with metallic tone) may also be seen in LTB (specifically thought to be due to tracheitis). Whoop is seen in pertussis. Note that small infants may slip into

apnoea after a paroxysmal cough rather than an effortful whoop.

- Aphonic cough (bovine cough) is seen in vocal cord paralysis. Bovine cough is the one which does not have the explosive nature.
- Irritation by foreign body or wax in ear can cause cough (reflex cough due to vagal stimulation).
- Pressure from enlarged lymph nodes either because of tuberculosis or leukaemia can cause cough.
- Drug-induced cough: It is seen in ACE inhibitor therapy.
- Psychogenic cough totally disappears at night. Short dry very loud honking cough, present only while awake is characteristic of psychogenic or habitual cough.

Note: Cough receptors are situated in airways and not in alveoli. So alveolar consolidation can occasionally present without cough. However, in small children almost all pneumonias are bronchopneumonia and hence pneumonia without cough is unusual (p 370).

If the child is bringing out sputum, enquire about its colour, and quantity.

- Productive cough is seen in bronchitis, pneumonia, bronchiectasis, lung abscess, etc. Sputum is purulent in pneumonia, lung abscess, etc; pinkish frothy in pulmonary oedema; blood-stained in mitral stenosis, bronchiectasis, etc; greenish in pseudomonas infection of cystic fibrosis. Very foul smelling sputum may be seen in lung abscess, bronchiectasis, anaerobic infections. Sputum in asthma is thick, viscid and whitish. Rusty sputum is seen in the resolution phase of pneumonia (the colour is due to degraded blood). Dry cough is seen in pleurisy, upper respiratory infection, interstitial lung disease, early stage of asthma, etc.
- Copious amount of sputum is seen in lung abscess and bronchiectasis.
- Three-layered separation of sputum (in the container) is described in bronchiectasis.

HOARSENESS

- Prolonged crying or shouting.
- Laryngitis (e.g., diphtheria, laryngotracheobronchitis, etc).
- Trauma due to intubation.
- Hypothyroidism.
- Steroid inhalation for prolonged periods (due to myopathy induced by steroids).

STRIDOR

- Stridor is usually inspiratory; can be expiratory (when narrowing is severe or narrowing is in lower trachea).
- Determine the quality of the voice; hoarseness or weakness implies glottic involvement.
- Examine the neck and chest for signs of increased work of breathing.

Causes

- Congenital laryngeal stridor: Usually starts a few days after birth (2 weeks or so), the child being comfortable despite the noisy respiration.
- Congenital lesions like web, vascular ring, etc.
- Infections: Croup, epiglottitis, diphtheria, retropharyngeal abscess, etc.
- Foreign body impaction in large airways, larynx, trachea, etc.
- Compression by thyroid.
- Others: Angioneurotic oedema, hypocalcaemic tetany, micrognathia, vocal cord paralysis, etc.

Noisy breathing: Snoring originates in the upper airways, at oro-nasopharynx. During sleep, the muscles become lax and vibrate with breathing to produce the snoring sound. Stridor is a continuous harsh inspiratory sound due to extrathoracic obstruction of airways; rarely when the obstruction is at the subglottic region or trachea, there may be expiratory component also, but as long as the predominant component is inspiratory stridor, the whole thing is called stridor only, not wheeze. Grunt is a short episodic expiratory sound, because of partially closed glottis during expiration. Rattle is the coarse, irregular inspiratory sound heard in patients almost dying; here the air passing through the stagnant secretions of upper airway or throat produces this rattle, which is palpable by hand placed over the neck or anterior chest.

HAEMOPTYSIS

Frothy material with bright red blood is *coughed out* in haemoptysis; non-frothy darker blood is *vomited out* in haematemesis.

Points to be Noted in History

History of cough; history suggestive of tuberculosis in the family; history suggestive of rheumatic fever (mitral stenosis can have haemoptysis); history suggestive of any bleeding diathesis; bad odour in the breath (lung abscess, bronchiectasis, etc); foreign body aspiration.

Infections

- Pneumonia
- Tuberculosis
- Bronchiectasis
- Lung abscess

Trauma

- Lung contusion
- Foreign body

Cardiovascular Cause

Mitral stenosis, pulmonary hypertension, pulmonary arteriovenous malformation, pulmonary oedema of any cause.

Miscellaneous

- Haemorrhagic disorder
- Leukaemia
- Anticoagulants
- Collagen vascular disease
- Goodpasture's syndrome
- Ruptured AV fistula
- Lung fluke (*Paragonimus westermani*) infestation

Haemoptysis without Pulmonary/Cardiac Involvement

Upper airway bleeding mistaken for haemoptysis like:

- Epistaxis
- Oral or nasopharyngeal trauma
- Acute tonsillitis
- Gingivitis

8

HAEMATEMESIS

This means vomiting of frank blood or altered blood ("coffee-ground"). Melaena indicates significant blood loss and may persist for a few days after haematemesis has stopped. Melaena without haematemesis points towards the origin of bleed from below the level of pylorus.

History

- Enquire about blood clots in vomitus, giddiness or syncope following the episode, which indicates heavy loss.
- History of epigastric pain (acid peptic disease).
- History of bleeding diathesis (bleeding from other sites).
- History of drug ingestion (e.g., aspirin, other NSAIDs, steroids).
- History of liver disease (cirrhosis, portal hypertension).
- Whether preceded by a series of vomiting (Mallory-Weiss syndrome).
- History of neonatal umbilical catheterization or intra-abdominal infections (e.g., appendicitis) in the past (both can predispose to extrahepatic portal hypertension by thrombus blocking the vessels).

- Spurious haematemesis: swallowed blood in the vomitus (e.g., blood from epistaxis, which was swallowed); coloured drinks ingested recently.

Causes

- Oesophageal: Oesophagitis, oesophageal varices.
- Gastric: Gastric ulcer, duodenal ulcer, gastritis due to NSAID, Mallory-Weiss syndrome.
- Liver: Portal hypertension, liver cell failure (bleeding due to coagulation failure). Vomiting fresh blood in copious quantity in a child who has no significant past history often suggests extrahepatic portal hypertension.
- Septicaemia (due to DIC).
- Swallowed blood (e.g., throat).
- Bleeding disorders.

Difference between Haematemesis and Haemoptysis

Haemoptysis is usually preceded by cough. The blood in haemoptysis is bright red, frothy and mixed with sputum. In haemoptysis, the pH is alkaline. In contrast, haematemesis is associated with vomiting, coffee ground colour and acidic pH (naturally as it has been in contact with gastric acid). Coffee ground colour points towards a slow bleeding for a few days. Dark red blood with clots indicates recent profuse bleeding (e.g., bleeding oesophageal varices).

Portal hypertension is the most common case of haematemesis kept for examination. Hence, a brief discussion on portal hypertension is given below.

Portal hypertension can be intrahepatic or extrahepatic. Intrahepatic may be assumed in presence of evidence of chronic liver illness or abnormal liver on clinical examination or history of jaundice.

- Ask for history of neonatal umbilical catheterization (portal thrombosis and hence extrahepatic portal hypertension); sources of portal pyaemia like appendicitis (may cause thrombosis); persistent respiratory problems (α_1-antitrypsin deficiency or cystic fibrosis); drugs and toxins (e.g., aflatoxin; drugs like aspirin may precipitate haematemesis); history of jaundice; psychiatric illness (Wilson); joint pain and rashes (autoimmune diseases and autoimmune hepatitis).
- Assess growth: Growth retardation is likely in chronic hepatic causes of portal hypertension.
- Enquire about vaccination like hepatitis B.
- Family history of consanguinity (Wilson, GSD type IV, α_1 antitrypsin deficiency, cystic fibrosis, etc).
- Look for signs of chronic liver disease and evidence for deficiency of fat-soluble vitamins like A, D, E or K (see p 406).
- Tachycardia, etc, associated with acute bleed may not be there if the child is already on β-blockers.
- A diagnosis of extrahepatic portal hypertension is justified when a child presents with haematemesis, the first episode usually at around 5–6 years of age or later, having no history or physical examination findings to suggest a liver disease.

DIARRHOEA

Ask about the onset, duration and progress.

Onset: Very acute onset could be food poisoning, so ask about food intake in the immediate past.

Duration: Duration of diarrhoea help to decide whether it is acute diarrhoea (usually <7 days), persistent diarrhoea (>14 days) or chronic diarrhoea. (The term chronic diarrhoea is reserved for non-infectious prolonged recurrent diarrhoeas like inflammatory bowel disease, celiac disease, malabsorption. etc.)

Progress: This should include inquiry into the quantity (large volume or small volume), quality (just watery or mixed with stool particles, blood/

mucous, foul smell, etc) and frequency of stools (help to assess possible dehydration), and associated symptoms.

Appearance of Stool

- Watery stools with increased flatulence and *perianal excoriation* suggests lactose intolerance.
- Watery large volume stools is likely in secretory diarrhoea (e.g., cholera, enterotoxigenic *E. coli* and other toxin-mediated diarrhoeas; rota virus diarrhoea is a combination of secretory and osmotic diarrhoea and the stool is watery; cholera stool is typically described rice-water stool).
- A greasy, bulky, foul-smelling stool that is difficult to flush is seen in fat malabsorption syndromes (steatorrhoea).
- Bloody stools indicates acute invasive diarrhoea (dysentery); rarely intususception (red-current jelly like bright red blood, sausage-shaped mass lateral to umbilicus, and exhausting cry in an infant of age group 6 months to 1 year). Also see hematochezia (p 160).
- Associated abdominal pain and tenesmus with blood in stools, if acute, suggests dysentery and if chronic, suggests inflammatory bowel disease, amoebiasis, etc. **Note**: Tenesmus is the painful urgency to pass stools.
- Pea soup stool is seen in typhoid.
- Green stools do not have specific significance, except that it indicates rapid GIT transit so that bile comes out before having had the time to get absorbed.

Associated Problems

- Vomiting, fever, abdominal pain, etc are to be specifically asked for. Worm infested children may pass worms also during diarrhoea (enhanced intestinal peristalsis brings the worms out).
- Decreased urine output indicates severity of dehydration. Hence, always ask for urine output in diarrhoea cases.
- Abdominal distension (hypotonia of malnutrition, hypokalaemia).
- Weight loss indicates chronic diarrhoea (always think of HIV in chronic diarrhoea with weight loss).
- History of rectal prolapse is common in whipworm colitis, cystic fibrosis and malnutrition when diarrhoea occurs. Loss of fat from ischiorectal fossa in malnutrition compromises support to the rectum & hence the prolapse.
- Antibiotic-induced diarrhoea and food allergy (cow's milk, soy, wheat, etc) must be kept in mind and inquired into.
- Severe malnutrition per se may cause diarrhoea. Unabsorbed bile salts in the gut act as an irritant and cause secretory diarrhoea. Poor epithelial regeneration in PEM may cause osmotic diarrhoea due to unabsorbed food in the gut.
- In coeliac disease, the diarrhoea starts a few months after introduction of wheat-containing weaning foods: i.e., in the second half of infancy.
- Look for acrodermatitis (around orifices), as zinc deficiency causes diarrhoea (acrodermatitis enteropathica). Perianal excoriation may also be found in lactose intolerance.
- Specifically ask for diet during diarrhoea. There are beliefs that child must be fasted during diarrhoea.

DARK STOOLS/BLOOD IN STOOLS

Dark stools and melaena may not be synonymous. Dark stools may be because of altered blood (melaena), oral iron intake, colouring agents in foods (e.g., some chocolates, grape juice), etc.

Fresh blood in stools is called haematochezia (see below) and is due to blood from near the rectum, e.g., fissure in ano (here there is linear staining on the sides of formed stools; mucus may not be there). History of constipation and severe pain during defaecation are seen in fissure in ano, but will not be there in bleeding, say due to polyps of colon. Blood *with mucus* or tenesmus is expected in invasive diarrhoea, amoebiasis, ulcerative colitis, etc. Severe intermittent colicky pain along with red stools in infants may be due to intussuception. Meckel's diverticulum and Henoch-Schonlein purpura are also associated with pain abdomen and blood in stools.

HAEMATOCHEZIA AND MALENA

Hematochezia is *fresh* blood in stools, whereas melaena is *altered* blood in stools (tarry stools). Ask for the duration, frequency, associated symptoms, etc. Haematochezia usually occurs in lower GI bleed. Melaena indicates bleeding proximal to the ileum. However, massive bleed proximal to the ileum may occasionally come out as fresh blood itself if it is not staying long enough there to get altered to black colour. Polyps and haemorrhoids are causes of fresh per rectal bleeding, but are very rare in childhood.

Streaking of stools with fresh blood and painful defaecation indicates anal fissure.

ABDOMINAL DISTENSION

- Abdomen of toddlers are normally protuberant. In grown-up children, it may be part of their obesity.
- Hypotonia (PEM, rickets, hypokalaemia, etc. Here, there may be visceroptosis also, causing liver and spleen to become palpable without actual enlargement.)
- Ascites (e.g., cirrhosis, nephrotic syndrome, etc).
- Massive organomegaly (e.g., massive spleen in thalassaemia, Gaucher disease, etc).
- Paralytic ileus (especially common following diarrhoea).
- Surgical abdomen (e.g., peritonitis).
- Chronic constipation (e.g., Hirschsprung disease).

ANOREXIA

- Physiological: This is common beyond infancy. This is because of deceleration of growth velocity and the baby acquiring the skill of locomotion for exploring the environment so that food becomes less of a priority for the child.
- Acute or chronic illnesses
- Hepatitis
- Uraemia
- Hypothyroidism (decreased metabolism and activity, so less need for food)
- Drugs
- Malignancy
- Depression

POOR FEEDING

Poor feeding is not always due to anorexia. Hence, it is considered in a separate heading here. If the child is gaining weight adequately, the complaint of poor feeding is likely to be just a reflection of maternal anxiety.

Excessive sweating and interruptions in feeding due to tiredness may indicate cardiac failure. Weak suck may be due to neuromuscular disorders, like Werdnig-Hoffman disease. Feeding problem in cerebral palsy can be due to problems of coordination of sucking and swallowing, gagging due to pseudobulbar palsy, excessive tongue thrusting, etc. Nasal regurgitation can occur as a normal phenomenon in vomiting, but as a feeding difficulty it may be part of cleft palate, palatal weakness, etc. Choking during feeding may be due to tracheoesophageal fistula.

DYSPHAGIA

This is the difficulty in swallowing.

- Is it due to obvious causes like local lesions, tonsillitis, etc.
- Ask for history of ingestion of caustics like acid or alkali.
- History of dog bite because it could be hydrophobia.
- Food seems to stop in the upper portion in palatal paralysis and lower portion in scleroderma.

- Swallowing difficulty is more with solids than liquids in mechanical obstruction like strictures (it is easier for liquids to bypass a mechanical obstruction); swallowing difficulty with liquids is more in neurological/muscle weakness (because of poor propulsive movements). In a neurological dysphagia like bulbar or pseudobulbar paralysis, one may have to ask for dysphagia, nasal regurgitation and a history of "fluids getting into the head" by which patients mean aspiration.
- Painful dysphagia (odynophagia) is seen in oesophagitis.

VOMITING

Nausea is the unpleasant sensation to vomit often associated with increased salivation. Retching is the intense urge to vomit, involving contractions of involved muscles.

Enquire whether the vomiting is projectile or not, frequency, content, whether bilious or not, its relation with food, and other associated symptoms. Persistent non-bilious vomiting in a 2–3-week-old infant suggests congenital hypertrophic pyloric stenosis; bilious vomiting in newborn suggests a more lower obstruction like duodenal atresia. Bilious vomiting may occur with paralytic ileus also. Many drugs can cause GI upset and vomiting. So ask for history of drug intake. History of loss of weight indicates the severity of vomiting. History of viral infection/aspirin intake should be elicited (Reye syndrome). Early morning projectile vomiting with headache suggests increased intracranial tension. Persistent vomiting and failure to thrive starting from introduction of specific foods in the neonatal period or later suggests inborn errors of metabolism or specific food intolerances (renal tubular acidosis will be a close differential diagnosis for this combination symptoms of failure to thrive and vomiting). Gastroesophageal reflux, migraine, hepatitis, meningitis, etc, are other causes of vomiting.

History

- Enquire about the frequency. Severity is indicated by dehydration (in acute) or loss of weight (in chronic).
- Enquire about the urine output (decreased urine output may be due to associated dehydration).
- Enquire whether it is associated with diarrhoea. Diarrhea and vomiting often go hand in hand.
- Enquire about urinary symptoms (fever and vomiting may be the presentation of UTI).
- Enquire about vertigo and ear symptoms. Vomiting and vertigo are the characteristic features of labyrinthitis.
- Look for jaundice: Vomiting is very common in infective hepatitis.
- Enquire about its association with headache, which is expected in migraine.
- Enquire about its association with cough: Post-tussive vomiting is common after paroxysmal cough in pertussis and asthma.
- Enquire about the time of the day: Early morning vomiting is seen in intracranial space-occupying lesions. Do not forget pregnancy as a cause in an adolescent!
- Enquire about antecedent symptoms: Abdominal pain indicates intestinal problems; headache indicating ICSOL, meningitis or migraine. Projectile vomiting, without antecedent nausea is supposed to be characteristic of a central nervous system cause (one finds it more commonly in textbooks rather than in patients with CNS disorders! Hence students must not discard CNS cause because the vomiting is not projectile).
- Contents of vomitus: Mention if it is food particles, blood, bile, etc.
- History of drugs: Drugs such as digoxin, theophylline, aspirin, iron, metronidazole, etc, can induce vomiting.
- Make sure it is not rumination when the child has recurrent vomiting but remains well despite vomiting. Rumination is the repeated

8

regurgitation of food into the mouth and then chewing and swallowing it.

- One must not overlook surgical causes for vomiting like intestinal obstruction or peritonitis.

JAUNDICE

Ask the child to look down and out, and look at the upper lateral margin of sclera (bulbar conjunctiva) in good daylight to detect subtle jaundice. Bile pigment has got affinity for elastic tissue and hence skin and sclera become pigmented in jaundice. In carotenaemia, sclera is not stained yellow.

Concentrated urine, haematuria, haemoglobinuria and drugs like rifampicin can cause highly coloured urine that may be confused with jaundice. Other areas to look for, especially in newborn, are soft palate, palm, sole, undersurface of tongue, etc.

Greenish–yellow jaundice, acholic (pale) stools, high coloured urine and itching suggests obstructive jaundice. Lemon yellow jaundice, yellow stools, normal coloured urine while passing (hence called acholuric jaundice) and no itching is suggestive of haemolytic jaundice. Jaundice in family members suggests hereditary (e.g.: congenital haemolytic anaemia, Gilbert's syndrome) or infectious (e.g., hepatitis A) causes. History of jaundice in neighbourhood and water source are important in hepatitis A.

History of jaundice in the neonatal period, blood transfusions, history of abdominal surgery (gallstones), history of similar disease in the family, etc, suggests haemolytic anaemia (especially hereditary spherocytosis). Jaundice with dark urine points to intravascular haemolysis (e.g., black water fever of falciparum malaria). Intake of hepatotoxic drugs like anti-TB drugs, valproic acid, etc, should also be considered as causes for toxic hepatitis. Carotenaemia is rare; here sclera is not coloured.

History

- Present from birth and progressively increasing in severity may be biliary atresia or the so-called neonatal hepatitis syndrome (these become a differential diagnosis only in a small infant).
- Presence of anaemia along with jaundice points towards haemolytic problem. Ask for family history of haemolytic diseases, history of treatment for gallstones, surgery for splenectomy or transfusion requiring anaemia—all pointing towards haemolytic anaemia that is familial. Family history of jaundice or psychiatric illness may be forthcoming in Wilson disease.
- Age of onset: Many conditions have typical age of onset.
- Colour of stool: Jaundice with clay-coloured stool suggests obstructive jaundice like biliary atresia or obstructive phase of infective hepatitis.
- Colour of sclera: Lemon yellow in haemolytic jaundice, greenish yellow in obstructive jaundice.
- Colour of urine: Dark urine suggests cholestasis. Dark urine is unlikely in haemolytic jaundice.
- Fever: Usually fever abates by the time jaundice gets established in uncomplicated viral hepatitis.
- Anorexia and vomiting: Expected in viral hepatitis.
- Itching: Itching with jaundice suggests obstructive cause for jaundice or obstructive phase of infective hepatitis. Scratch marks, if present, must be mentioned during case presentation.
- Abdominal pain: May indicate pain due to hepatic enlargement or gallstones.
- Drug ingestion: Drugs like anti-TB drugs may cause hepatitis.
- Source of water, history of injections or blood transfusions, to know the source of infection in infective hepatitis.

Ask for any contact with a jaundice patient.

- Playing in rat-infested premises: Consider leptospirosis. Jaundice plus red urine must make one highly suspicious of leptospirosis.

ABDOMINAL PAIN

This is the most misdirecting symptom in paediatric practice. Enquire about the site of pain, intensity, character of pain, mode of onset (all colics start abruptly), aggravating/relieving factors (like relief or aggravation with food, position, etc), radiation, associated symptoms (like dysuria, vomiting, diarrhoea, etc).

Painful abdomen that is worse on pressure is due to inflammations (peritonitis, appendicitis, etc). Pain that is relieved on pressure is due to intestinal colic.

- History of intermittent cry that exhausts the child, in an infant who has been started weaning, along with bleeding P/R ("red currant jelly") suggests the colicky pain of intussusception.
- Associated diarrhoea may indicate enterocolitis (shigella, salmonella, yersinia, campylobacter, etc). History of previous abdominal surgeries may point towards adhesions as the cause of pain.
- History suggestive of food poisoning may be sought.
- Recent introduction of any new food items must be asked for; it could be food allergy producing the pain.
- Ask for history of rashes; Abdominal pain may be a presenting symptom of Henoch-Schonlein purpura.

Organic vs Non-Organic Pain

Periumbilical pain is of intestinal origin. It may be just non-organic or organic due to various diseases of small intestine, worm infestation, etc.

The characteristics of such non-organic abdominal pain are:

- Periumbilical in location; does not disturb the child's sleep and play.
- Of very short duration (a few minutes).
- Pain periods may cluster for a few days and then pain-free periods for many weeks.

Signals Indicating that the Pain may be Organic

- Pain that awakens the child
- Organomegaly
- Weight loss
- Pain location other than periumbilical
- Extraintestinal manifestations (e.g., arthritis may indicate inflammatory bowel disease; altered sensorium following abdominal pain may indicate seizure, migraine, porphyria, etc). 8

Significance of Pain in Different Quadrants of Abdomen

- Epigastric pain: Retrosternal burning, aggravated by lying down and by acid foods like lemon juice may indicate acid peptic disease (peptic ulcer). Ask for relation of pain to food intake. Will need investigation for *Helicobacter pylori* (antibody in blood). Epigastric pain radiating retrosternally upwards suggests gastroesophageal reflux and oesophagitis. Epigastric pain that is worse on lying down and relieved by sitting up suggests hiatus hernia or pancreatitis.
- Right hypochondrial pain may be hepatic in origin, like hepatitis. Cholecystitis and cholelithiasis may present with recurrent colicky right upper quadrant abdominal pain, which may radiate to the back, right scapula, arm or neck. Fatty foods exacerbate symptoms. In between episodes of pain, the child will be asymptomatic. However, one must remember that gall bladder disease is very rare in children, and when it occurs, may be associated with chronic haemolytic anaemia, prolonged total parenteral nutrition, etc. Transient biliary sludging due to ceftriaxone may also produce similar pain.

Other causes of upper abdominal pain include referred pain of pneumonia, pancreatitis, etc. Pain of pancreatitis tends to radiate towards the back.

- Periumbilical pain is discussed above.
- Pain in the lumbar region may be renal in origin. Pain, which starts in the loin, radiating to the groin and sometimes towards the genitalia and inner thigh indicates ureteric colic (although it is popularly called renal colic, it is ureteric colic, to be more precise).
- Right lower quadrant pain may be related to appendix, caecum, etc. Pain, vomiting and fever, usually in that order, with pain being maximally localized to McBurney's point indicates acute appendicitis. Mesenteric adenitis per se is not considered a cause of abdominal pain. If it does cause pain, it may be periumbilical or in the right iliac fossa.
- Left lower quadrant pain may be related to faecal impaction/chronic constipation, inflammatory bowel disease, etc.
- Suprapubic pain may originate from the bladder (cystitis).
- Abdominal pain with a palpable mass: roundworm mass, chronic constipation, tuberculous abdomen, intussusception, etc. Intussusception is an acute event, where the child will be having an exhausting intermittent colic followed by another colic a little later. The child will be totally tired. The stool is typically described as "red currant jelly," which actually looks like a slightly diluted blood in colour. To one side of umbilicus a mass may become palpable. Rectal examination may find the tip of telescoping intestine.
- Psychogenic: This may be assumed when a precipitating factor can be identified, e.g., school phobia.
- When no organic or psychogenic factors could be identified, it is loosely termed "functional abdominal pain."

Other organic causes of abdominal pain include:

- Faecal impaction (chronic constipation).
- Parasitic infestation like helminthiasis, giardia.
- Henoch-Schonlein purpura (occasionally abdominal pain may precede purpura by 1–2 weeks).
- Infections like yersinia, tuberculosis.
- Pneumonia of lower lobe (referred pain).
- Diaphragmatic pleurisy, pericarditis.
- Diabetic ketoacidosis.
- Pain of abdominal wall may be due to herpes zoster, local inflammation, etc. In herpes zoster, look for rash, limited to specific dermatomes.
- Hernias, with some amount of obstruction.
- Migraine ("abdominal migraine").
- Porphyria.
- Allergic: Children get abdominal pain along with urticaria.
- Bezoars: It is the accumulation of eaten foreign materials (e.g., hair) in the stomach.
- Infantile colic, in infants less than 3 months, usually in the evening hours (no specific cause and no specific treatment).
- Sickle cell crisis.
- Lead poisoning (recurrent abdominal pain; usually a history of pica is obtainable).

CONSTIPATION

Constipation is passage of the stools less frequently than is normal for that particular child, especially if the stool passed is hard and the act is painful. Assess whether it is true constipation by considering the frequency and consistency of stools. Ask for soiling of underclothes. In chronic constipation, there may be encopresis, i.e., liquid stools may bypass the solid stool to come around it to soil the clothes. Abdominal examination may reveal palpable stool mass.

Causes of Constipation

- Hirchsprung's disease: Here, constipation is present from birth.

- Breastfed infants also may have constipation; for some strange reasons, constipation in breastfed infants starts around 6 weeks of age and not at birth!
- Onset with the introduction of cow's milk points towards cow's milk as aetiology.
- Problem of constipation starting at around 10–18 months of age: Functional withholding (? toilet training pressures).
- Disturbance in routine emptying time (e.g., entry to kindergarten).
- Dietary history: Too much non-fibre food may be a cause.
- Codeine group of drugs used for cough may cause constipation.
- Hypothyroidism may cause constipation.
- Fissure in ano: Painful defaecation and blood-streaked hard stools gives clue to the diagnosis.
- Prolonged immobility may cause constipation.

PICA

Enquire about the age at onset. Look for evidence of anaemia, helminthiasis, lead toxicity (e.g., abdominal pain, lead line of gum), etc. Look for any history that may contribute to emotional imbalance.

OBESITY

- Exogenous (dietary) obesity: Dietary history will give a clue. Usually, height is also advanced. If the child is short and obese, it is not simple obesity but pathological one.
- Endocrine: Cushing syndrome, hypothyroidism (p 540–541).
- Syndromes: Prader-Willi syndrome, Laurence-Moon-Biedl syndrome (p 515).
- Drugs like sodium valproate.

HALITOSIS

- Local causes: Dental caries, gingivitis, sinusitis, tonsillitis, retained foreign body nose, drying up of mouth (e.g., fasting, antihistamines), etc.
- Lung: Lung abscess, bronchiectasis.
- Metabolic: Fetor hepaticus of hepatic failure, acetone odour (similar to smell of nail polish remover) of diabetic coma, ammoniacal odour of uraemia, etc. Chronic constipation is also thought to contribute to halitosis by producing methane gas, which gets excreted in breath.

ISOLATED HEPATOMEGALY

Define the degree of enlargement of the liver by measuring the distance it extends below the right costal margin in the midclavicular line. 8

Causes of isolated hepatomegaly are enumerated below (**Note**: Remember that causes of hepatosplenomegaly may at times present as isolated hepatomegaly).

- Fever with hepatomegaly may have an infective aetiology. Examples are hepatitis, typhoid, tuberculous, pyogenic liver abscess, amoebic liver abscess, hydatid cyst, etc. Hepatitis and abscesses produce painful hepatomegaly.
- Anaemia with hepatomegaly may be due to sickle cell anaemia with autosplenectomy; severe anaemia of any cause can cause cardiac failure and hence hepatomegaly.
- Metabolic disorder: Glycogen storage disease types III, VI, IX may present with isolated *asymptomatic* hepatomegaly. Other metabolic disorders to be considered are other glycogen storage diseases, galactosaemia, tyrosinaemia, Wilson disease, α_1-antitrypsin deficiency, etc.
- Fatty liver: Kwashiorkor, steroid therapy.
- Cirrhosis (before the liver shrinks there will be a stage of firm hepatomegaly).
- Tumours: Primary tumours are hepatoblastoma (usually in toddler age) and hepatocellular carcinoma (may follow hepatitis B infection that occurred years earlier). Secondary deposits are also possible.
- CCF
- AV malformation

The following is a brief discussion on von Gierke's disease (glycogen storage disease type Ia):

- Short stature
- Rounded face ('doll's face')
- Hepatomegaly but no splenomegaly
- Kidneys may be enlarged
- Hypotonia
- Normal mental development if hypoglycaemia is prevented.
- Management involves frequent feeds.
- In Pompe's disease (GSD type II), there is cardiomegaly and myopathy (hypotonia and hyporeflexia) in addition to hepatomegaly.

ISOLATED SPLENOMEGALY

Define the degree of enlargement by measuring the maximum distance it extends below the left costal margin.

- Infective: Viral (e.g., IMN), bacterial (e.g., typhoid, TB, septicaemia) or parasitic (malaria, toxoplasma).
- Haematological: Haemolytic anaemia, congenital (e.g., thalassaemia, spherocytosis) or acquired (acquired autoimmune haemolytic anaemia).
- Malignancy: Hodgkin's, leukaemia, etc.
- Metabolic: Gaucher's disease.
- Portal hypertension.
- Connective tissue disorders like SLE, juvenile rheumatoid arthritis, etc.
- Splenic cyst or haemangioma.
- Miscellaneous: Iron deficiency anaemia (rarely causes splenomegaly), SLE, juvenile rheumatoid arthritis, etc.

HEPATOSPLENOMEGALY

Note: Enlargement of liver and spleen may be in varying proportions depending on the aetiology. This aetiology related predominance of organomegaly must be taken into account while deciding the priority of differential diagnosis.

Hepatosplenomegaly with Pallor (Anaemia)

- Infections:
  - Viral: Congenital infections in newborn.
  - Bacterial: Disseminated TB, infective endocarditis, typhoid, septicemia, leptospirosis.
  - Protozoal: Malaria, *kala azar*.
- Haematological: Haemolytic anaemia:
  - Congenital: Thalassaemia, sickle cell anaemia, hereditary spherocytosis.
  - Acquired: Autoimmune haemolytic anaemia.
- Malignancy: Leukaemia, lymphoma
- Metabolic: Wilson, Gaucher, Niemann-Pick disease
- Collagen vascular disease: SLE, JRA.
- Miscellaneous: Hypersplenism due to long standing splenomegaly, osteopetrosis.

Haemolytic anaemia is the first possibility. It presents rather as splenohepatomegaly. Family history of haemolytic anaemia, early age of onset (clinical detection around 6 months of age), repeated transfusions and haemolytic facies point towards congenital haemolytic anaemia. These findings are absent in the acquired variety, which may start following a febrile illness or as part of lymphoma. Coombs test will be positive in autoimmune haemolytic anaemia.

Hepatosplenomegaly with Icterus (Jaundice)

- Infections:
  - Viral: Viral hepatitis, infectious mononucleosis. Jaundice in disseminated TB is more likely to be due to anti-TB drugs than TB disease; obstruction by lymph node causing jaundice is more of a theoretical possibility. Neonatal hepatitis/biliary atresia in newborn; obstruction by choledochal cyst in newborn.

  - Bacterial: Septicaemia, leptospirosis
  - Protozoal: Malaria, *kala azar*
- Haematological: Haemolytic anaemia (congenital/acquired).
- Malignancy: Icterus may be because of obstruction by lymph node or extensive metastasis.
- Metabolic: Galactosaemia, α_1-antitrypsin deficiency, cystic fibrosis, etc.
- Cirrhosis: Jaundice occurs in late stages only. This is especially true in Indian childhood cirrhosis.
- Drugs: E.g., ATT, antimetabolites, anticonvulsants.

Hepatosplenomegaly with Jaundice and Anaemia

- Infective: Malaria, *kala azar,* disseminated TB.
- Haematological: Congenital (thalassaemia, sickle cell anaemia, hereditary spherocytosis) or acquired (autoimmune haemolytic anaemia).
- Wilson disease.

Haemolytic anaemia, congenital or acquired, is the first possibility. When associated with fever, malaria also becomes an important consideration. Wilson disease has a low-grade haemolysis and hence can present with this combination.

Hepatosplenomegaly with Fever

- Here, infections are the most probable cause.
  - Viral: Infectious mono nucleosis.
  - Bacterial: Typhoid fever. Widal test and clot culture will confirm the diagnosis.
  - Protozoal: Malaria (history of travel to endemic areas should strengthen the suspicion; blood picture will show the malarial parasite); kala azar.
- Malignancy: Leukaemia, lymphoma.
- Collagen vascular diseases like SLE (will have other manifestations of SLE), systemic onset JRA.

Hepatosplenomegaly with Lymphadenopathy with or without Fever

- Infection: IMN, HIV, disseminated TB, etc. Congenital infections in newborn
- Malignancy: Leukaemia, lymphoma, histiocytosis (histiocytosis is not truly a malignancy).
- Collagen vascular disease: SLE, JRA.
- Drugs: Phenytoin.

In this scenario, a malignancy like leukaemia is the possibility. Bleeding tendency and bone pain give additional clue. Blood picture and bone marrow examination will confirm the diagnosis. Lymphoma is the second common malignancy. 8

Infectious mononucleosis: Blood picture will show more than 20% atypical lymphocytes. Sore throat, rashes, lymphadenopathy, etc, may be present. It is said that epitrochlear lymph node is enlarged commonly in IMN.

Tuberculosis: History of contact with an adult case, matting of the nodes if present, Mantoux test, X-ray chest, and fine needle aspiration of the nodes or biopsy will confirm the diagnosis.

Hepatosplenomegaly with Bleeding Manifestations

- Infective: Viral haemorrhagic fevers like dengue; septicaemia. Congenital infections in the newborn.
- Haematological: Thalassaemia (petechiae secondary to hypersplenism due to big spleen).
- Malignancy: Leukaemia, lymphoma.
- Collagen vascular disease: SLE.
- Various causes of massive splenomegaly, which in turn produce hypersplenism.
- Metabolic: Gaucher, Niemann-Pick disease (bleeding is secondary to bone marrow replacement by storage cells).

Hepatosplenomegaly with Ascites

- Cirrhosis
- Abdominal or disseminated TB
- CCF
- Malignancy

Hepatosplenomegaly with Mental Retardation and Odd Facies

- Example is Hurler.

RENAL ENLARGEMENT: CAUSES

Unilateral Renal Enlargement

- Hydronephrosis
- Renal cyst
- Tumours (of kidney/suprarenals): Wilms' tumour, renal cell carcinoma, neuroblastoma, phaeochromocytoma

Bilateral Renal Enlargement

- Polycystic renal disease: The infantile form is autosomal recessive in inheritance and is associated with cystic disease of other organs, especially the liver (so look for liver enlargement); the adult form is autosomal dominant.
- Hydronephrosis: In boys, consider posterior urethral valves. Other causes include neurogenic bladder, e.g., children with spina bifida, or vesicoureteric reflux.
- Wilms' tumour (may be bilateral in 10%).
- Tuberous sclerosis (due to renal angiomyolipoma or polycystic kidneys).
- Glycogen storage disease type I.
- Amyloidosis (rare in children).

HYPOGONADISM (DELAYED PUBERTY)

1. Constitutional delay (history of delay may be elicitable in parents also).
2. Hypogonadotropic hypogonadism (low FSH, LH):
   - CNS: Congenital anomalies, intracranial tumours (craniopharyngioma), infiltrations (e.g., Langerhan cell histiocytosis X), irradiation, traumatic.
   - Primary gonadotropin deficiency (hypopituitarism).
   - Chronic systemic diseases: Chronic renal failure, gluten enteropathy, cystic fibrosis.
   - Malnutrition, anorexia nervosa.
   - Syndromes: Kallmann, Prader-Willi, Frolich.
   - Miscellaneous: Hypothyroidism, hyperprolactinaemia.
3. Hypergonadotropic hypogonadism (high FSH, LH): It is due to dysfunction of end organs of sex hormone production.
   - Turner (female), Noonan, Klinefelter (male).
   - Anticancer therapy (e.g., cyclophosphamide).
   - Damage due to orchitis.
   - Vanishing testes syndrome (testes that has vanished in fetal life, possibly due to vascular insults).
   - Sex hormone biosynthesis defects.
   - Infiltration and autoimmune disease of gonads.

PURPURA

Purpura is a general term for skin bleeds. When it is minute, we call it petechiae and large ones are called ecchymosis. Petechiae (<2 mm), purpura (2–10 mm) and ecchymosis (>10 mm) do not blanch on pressure.

- Infections: Viral (e.g., dengue) or bacterial (septicaemia, meningococcaemia, endocarditis, etc).
- Thrombocytopenia due to increased destruction; E.g., idiopathic thrombocytopenic purpura, haemolytic uraemic syndrome, disseminated intravascular coagulation, Kassabach-Merritt syndrome, hypersplenism, etc.
- Thrombocytopenia due to decreased production; E.g., aplastic anaemia (including Fanconi, TAR syndrome, acquired due to

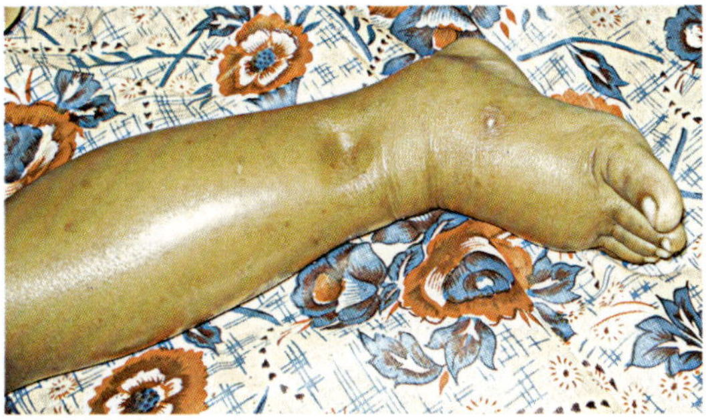

Fig.8.1 Pitting oedema of leg

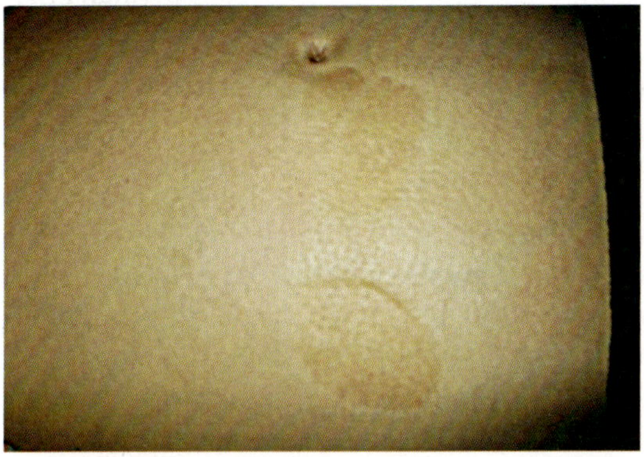

Fig.8.2 Abdominal wall oedema is demonstrated by pinching or pressing with stethoscope.

drugs/infections, etc), bone marrow infiltration by malignant cells as in leukaemia.

- Patelet function abnormalities: E.g., Bernard-Soulier disease, Glanzmann thrombasthenia or treatment with aspirin.
- Vasculitis: E.g., Henoch-Schonlein purpura.
- Collagen disorders: E.g., SLE.
- Drugs: Drugs producing thrombocytopenia or platelet function abnormality.
- Scurvy.

OEDEMA

Oedema is looked for by pressing just above the malleolus on lower tibia (Fig. 8.1); presacral area and scalp may show oedema in bed-ridden patients. As per the present WHO SAM guidelines, oedema of malnutrition is looked for by pressing on the dorsum of foot. Check for periorbital puffiness, pedal oedema, sacral oedema, oedema back of skull (especially in bed-ridden nephrotic syndrome patients), abdominal wall oedema, etc.

Acute or gradual in onset: Acute onset is seen in angioneurotic oedema, localized oedema may be due to trauma or allergy.

The causes of oedema are listed below:

- **Cardiac**: Cardiac failure produces dependent oedema. May have CVS-related symptoms like exertional dyspnoea, cyanosis, etc. In bedridden patients, expect sacral oedema. Severe anaemia also produces oedema due to "high-output cardiac failure." Also see discussion on p 287.
- **Renal**: Usually oedema first appears on the face, e.g., nephritis, nephrotic syndrome. Look for scrotal oedema (especially common in nephrotic syndrome). Renal oedema is worse in the morning. It is worth remembering that oedema is not a feature of chronic renal failure till the very late stages.
- **Hepatic**: Ascites is relatively common in cirrhosis. May have previous history of jaundice, e.g., cirrhosis with portal hypertension. ***Note***: Ascites is also common in nephrotic syndrome but is uncommon in glomerulonephritis and uncomplicated kwashiorkor. In cirrhosis, ascites precedes oedema of other parts, whereas in nephrotic syndrome ascites follows oedema of other parts.
- **Nutritional**: One may get a clue from the nutritional history, e.g., kwashiorkor, anaemia, beriberi. Anaemia and beriberi cause oedema due to cardiac failure. Oedema of kwashiorkor is due to hypoproteinaemia. Oedema due to excess or improperly diluted ORS leads to oedema of sodium retention.
- **Allergic**: May have associated urticaria and pruritis. Remember that angioneurotic oedema may not have accompanying pruritis or urticaria. Allergic oedema often recurs.

8

- **Endocrine**: Myxoedema. Periorbital puffiness is usually seen initially. In adults, pretibial oedema is said to be common. Cushing's syndrome and excess exogenous steroids are causes for oedema.
- **Localized oedema** (e.g., trauma, filariasis, venous thrombosis, varicose vein, allergic, etc). Milroy disease is congenital lymphoedema, confined usually to the legs. Superior vena cava obstruction produces localized oedema of face, many times associated with dilated veins and non-pulsatile engorged JVP.

Non-pitting oedema is extremely rare, may be due to infiltrations, filariasis, tumour, etc.

Early oedema may make its appearance felt by increased shininess of skin compared to the normal side.

Anasarca: This is the term used to denote generalized gross oedema.

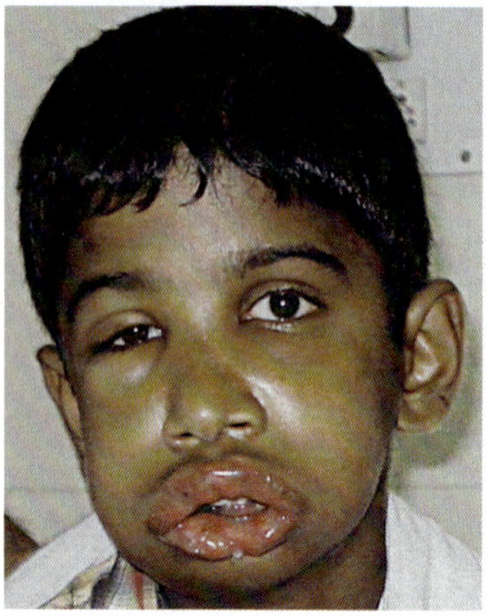

Fig.8.3 Allergic oedema

HYPERTENSION

Rule of Thumb

Normal systolic BP = 90 + 2x (x = age in years)

The most common cause of persistent hyper-tension in adults is essential hypertension (no obvious cause is found). However, the chance of having a secondary cause for hypertension is quite high in children and one must rule them out before stamping a diagnosis of essential hypertension.

The usual causes of hypertension can be associated with vessels to kidney, kidney & urinary outflow, 3 layers of adrenal cortex and adrenal medulla:

- Coarctation of aorta
- Renal artery stenosis
- Renal parenchymal disease (nephritis)
- Obstructive uropathy
- Hyperaldosteronism, usually due to an adenoma
- Cushing syndrome
- Congenital adrenal hyperplasia (11-β hydroxylase deficiency)
- Neuroblastoma
- Phaeochromocytoma

CHEST PAIN

Idiopathic and musculoskeletal chest pain are the most common. Pleurisy, pericarditis, pleurodynia (viral infection), costochondritis, trauma, herpes zoster, GERD, malignant deposits (e.g., sternal tenderness in leukaemia) are some of the causes. Pleural pain is catching pain, which recurs at the same phase of inspiration and expiration. Referred pain of upper lobe pneumonia may cause meningismus and lower lobe pneumonia may cause abdominal pain, with or without chest pain.

Pulmonary infarction in sickle cell anaemia and subdiaphragmatic abscess are rare causes of chest pain. Tender hepatic enlargement in hepatitis may cause lower chest pain, especially when the lower chest is percussed (see p 285). A detailed account of chest pain can be found in "Manual of Pediatric Practice" by the same author.

CRYING

- Shrill cry: CNS problem like meningitis.
- Cat-like cry: Cri-du-chat syndrome.
- Weak cry: Neuromuscular disorders like spinal muscular atrophy or in a very sick child.
- Crying on handling: Meningeal irritation, septic arthritis, fractures, other painful lesions anywhere, scalded skin syndrome (because

here skin is very tender), congenital syphilis, scurvy, etc.

- Hoarse cry: Laryngitis, hypothyroidism, epiglottitis, foreign body in larynx, vocal cord weakness, etc.
- Excessive cry in a small infant can be due to idiopathic infantile colic, hunger, blocked nose, ear ache, acute pain (intussuception, torsion testes, obstructed hernia, etc), post vaccination (DPT), etc.

FEVER

History

- Was the onset sudden (infection, *dhatura* poisoning, etc) or present for the past so many days (collagen disorders).
- High fever (severe infections, collagen diseases) or low-grade fever (minor viral infections)?
- Are there associated chills and rigor (indicates very rapid rise of temperature from the baseline)? Is there history of convulsions with fever? (central nervous system infection or febrile fits)
- Any recent vaccinations?
- Does the child sweat profusely when the fever subsides? (particularly seen in malaria). In the rare condition of anhidrotic ectodermal dysplasia, the child does not sweat at all.
- Was the fever intermittent, remittent or continuous? (p 40–41)

Usual Causes of Fever

- Infection: Bacterial, viral, spirochaetes, parasites
- Vaccination, especially DPT
- Malignancy
- Autoimmune, like SLE, systemic onset rheumatoid arthritis
- Inflammatory bowel disease
- Tissue injury: Trauma, burns, etc
- Drug fever

History and Examination

One should ask or look for cough, ear discharge, pyoderma, rashes, jaundice, urinary symptoms, arthralgia, travel to endemic areas of specific diseases and contact with fever cases. One should examine for hepatosplenomegaly, lymphadenopathy, jaundice, chest signs, meningeal signs and heart murmurs. Ear and throat also must be examined (see discussion p 418).

The diagnosis is often difficult in persistent fever. The logic in any diagnostic work up is: think of typical presentation of a common disorder; if nothing fits in, think of an atypical presentation of a common disorder; if still nothing fits in, think of typical presentation of an uncommon disorder. Lastly, if ever, think of atypical presentation of an uncommon disorder. 8

PAIN

- Pain away from organ of origin: Retrosternal pain in pericarditis; abdominal pain in lower lobe pneumonia, knee pain in hip disease.
- Colicky intestinal pain is usually around the umbilicus and is relieved by holding the abdomen. Colicky pain due to intra-abdominal inflammatory process will be aggravated by this manoeuvre (e.g., appendicitis).
- Pain of rheumatoid arthritis is worse in the morning and gets better as the activities progress.
- Pain of pleurisy gets worse on cough and deep inspiration.
- Headache of increased intracranial tension gets worse on cough and straining.

ENURESIS

History

- Is it during the day (likely to be organic) or at night only (most often due to physiological delay in bladder control)
- Was it that the bladder control was achieved once and then lost? (likely to happen in case

of stress like birth of a sibling or urinary infection, etc). If the child never attained bladder control, a detailed neurological examination is warranted (specifically look for evidence of menigomyelocele, tuft of hair in the back, sensations, etc).
- Is there family history of enuresis? (common in non-organic nocturnal enuresis)
- Is the urine volume increased or small volume is passed frequently? (the former indicates increased urine production like diabetes mellitus or diabetes insipidus or excessive water intake. The latter may indicate psychological urge like before exams or cystitis, urethritis, etc).
- Chronic renal failure and sickle cell anaemia will result in polyuria (due to defect in tubular concentration ability) and hence enuresis.
- Compulsive water drinking also results in polyuria and hence it should be probed in history.

POLYURIA

- Excess water intake
- Diabetes mellitus
- Diabetes insipidus
- Chronic renal failure
- Renal tubular acidosis
- During the phase of disappearance of oedema (e.g., polyuric phase of acute nephritis)

OLIGURIA

The causes may be prerenal, renal or postrenal.
- Prerenal: Hypotension, dehydration, burns, haemorrhage, etc.
- Renal: Acute nephritis, nephrotic syndrome, etc.
- Postrenal: Obstruction to urine flow like posterior urethral valves, phimosis, neurogenic bladder, etc.

HAEMATURIA

Haematuria may originate anywhere from glomerulus to urethral meatus. Cola-coloured urine indicates glomerulonephritis. Bright red colour indicates that haemorrhage is in bladder, urethra, etc. Blood stain only at the beginning of micturition means it is from urethra. Pain during the act of micturition may mean urethritis or rarely passage of small stones. Pain of renal colic is severe and not confined to the act of micturition.

Kidney

- Glomerulonephritis (post-streptococcal, HSP, SLE, etc)
- Pyelonephritis
- Haemolytic uraemic syndrome
- Stones
- Trauma
- Tumour (Wilms')

Ureter

- Calculus
- Trauma
- Tumour

Bladder

- Cystitis
- Tumour
- Stone
- Trauma
- Schistosomia

Urethra

- Foreign body
- Calculus
- Trauma
- Urethritis

Systemic

- Bleeding disorders
- TB
- Infective endocarditis (microscopic haematuria, not gross haematuria)
- Drugs: Anticoagulants, platelet inhibitions
- Exercise (very rare)

PALLOR

The term pallor is used here as a synonym of anaemia (though rarely it may indicate other conditions like shock). Anaemia is the reduction of haemoglobin concentration and haemocrit below the lower limit of normal for that particular age group. As an approximation, a haemoglobin level below 11 g/100 mL can be taken as anaemia in childhood. Even moderate anaemia (6–8 g/100 mL) can remain asymptomatic if it is slowly developing. The major causes of pallor are:

Decreased Production

This may be due to:

- Bone marrow failure: Aplastic anaemia may be either congenital (Fanconi's syndrome) or acquired (drug induced, infection induced, etc).
- Nutritional: Most common cause is iron deficiency. Deficiencies of folic acid, vit. B_{12}, etc, are rare causes of anaemia.

Increased Loss

This may be due to:

- Blood loss: Blood loss due to bleeding occurs in trauma, hookworm infestation, recurrent bleeding as in portal hypertension, etc.
- Haemolysis: Destruction of RBCs within the body occurs in haemolytic anaemia (congenital haemolytic anaemia like thalassaemia or acquired ones like autoimmune haemolytic anaemia).

Clinical Clues to the Differential Diagnosis

- *Leukaemia*: Pallor, fever, pain, bleeding tendency, hepatosplenomegaly and lymphadenopathy; 4Ps, see p 437. Blood film shows blast cells and bone marrow examination will confirm the diagnosis.
- *Aplastic anaemia*: Pallor and bleeding tendency without significant hepatosplenomegaly or lymphadenopathy. Blood film shows pancytopenia (see p 430).
- *Congenital haemolytic anaemia*: Suggestive family history, haemolytic facies, and mild icterus (see p 431-432).
- *Iron deficiency anaemia*: Suggestive age group and dietary history, gradual onset pallor without hepatosplenomegaly and lymphadenopathy (see p 430).
- *Intravascular haemolysis*: This occurs in conditions like G6PD deficiency and falciparum malaria. Acute onset pallor with red urine (haemoglobinuria). Pink colour of serum (separating after clotting) points towards the intravascular haemolysis.
- *Chronic illness*: Gradual onset pallor with other signs of the specific illness. Chronic renal failure is an example.
- *Haemorrhage*: Acute onset pallor along with blood loss as in case of trauma or coagulation disorders.
- *Acquired haemolytic anaemia*: Acute onset pallor with mild icterus. A positive Coombs test strongly favours this diagnosis. There may be an offending infection, systemic disorder or drugs.

8

Note

- Nutritional anaemia is unlikely below 6 months of age, except in cases of very low birth weight babies and children born to very anaemic mothers.
- Family history of anaemia may be obtained in congenital haemolytic anaemia. History of anaemia/jaundice/splenectomy/gallstones, etc, may point towards congenital haemolytic anaemia. Remember that certain congenital anaemias are X-linked, e.g., G6PD deficiency must not be diagnosed in a girl.
- Anaemia of thalassaemia presents clinically near 6 months of age (as the HbF comes down).
- Goat's milk consumption may predispose to megaloblastic anaemia.
- Malnutrition/pica/chronic infections/hookworm/drugs, etc, may cause anaemia.

- Drugs may produce haemolytic anaemia (e.g., primaquine in G6PD deficiency), bone marrow depression (e.g., chloramphenicol) or megaloblastic anaemia (phenytoin, folate antagonists, etc).

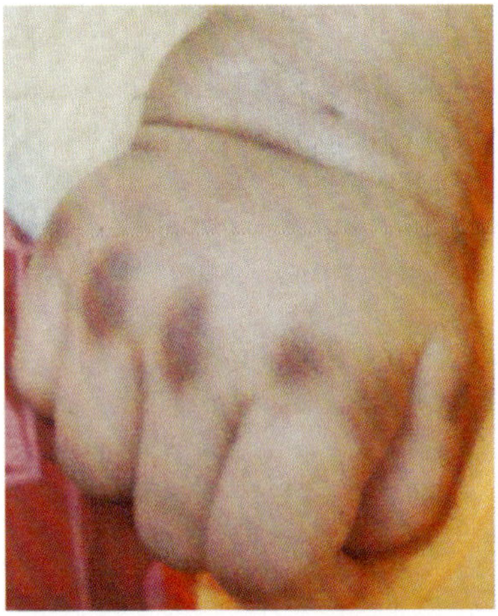

Fig.8.4 Hyperpigmentation of knuckle may be seen in various conditions like Addison disease, B_{12} or folic acid deficiency anaemia. The pigmentation shown here is from a rare syndrome and not megaloblastic anaemia.

BLEEDING

- Purpura, ecchymosis, etc, in a *well* child point towards a platelet disorder (e.g., ITP) or vascular disorder (e.g., Henoch-Schonlein purpura where purpura is localized to the outer aspect of leg and thigh). Recurrent epistaxis in a well child is usually due to local cause (like nose picking, foreign body, bleed from "Little's area," etc), but may be rarely due to von Willebrand's disease. Nose bleed also can be due to hypertension and retained foreign body. Most common cause of bleeding gums is poor dental health, but very rarely may be a manifestation of scurvy.
- Purpura, ecchymosis, etc, in a sick child could mean DIC, leukaemia or other serious infections like meningococcaemia.
- Bleeding into muscles and joints in a well child usually point towards congenital coagulation disorders like haemophilia.

Investigations in the case of bleeding are best read from p 435–438. Haemoptysis, haemetemesis and haematochezia are discussed separately in this chapter (p 157–160).

FAILURE TO THRIVE

FTT refers to the growth velocity below the 3rd percentile or a change in growth that has crossed two major growth percentiles within a short period of time (major percentiles are 90, 75, 50, 25, 10, 5, etc). Conventionally children < 3 years or maximum up to 5 years of age are included in the definition of FTT. Non-organic FTT with no known medical cause is common <5 years of age. One must remember that FTT may have both organic and non-organic components in its aetiology.

Confirm FTT by Measurement

Weight decreased, height decreased, head circumference decreased—"Primordial dwarf"

- Intrauterine insults
- Genetic or chromosomal anomalies

Weight decreased, height decreased, head circumference normal

- Constitutional delay
- Endocrinopathies
- Long standing FTT due to systemic diseases

Weight decreased, height normal, head circumference normal

- Recent energy deprivation or acute illness

The causes of FTT may be:

1. Problems of availability of food: Poverty, food fads, religious restrictions, ignorance, etc.
2. Food is available but food intake is a problem: Examples would be anatomical defects (e.g., cleft palate), pseudobulbar palsy, etc.

3. Food is available and eaten but is lost: Examples would be vomiting (e.g., congenital hypertrophic pyloric stenosis), diarrhoea, GERD, etc.
4. Food is eaten and reaches the intestine, but is not absorbed: Malabsorption syndromes, inflammatory bowel disease, coeliac disease, short bowel syndrome, etc. Bulky, foul-smelling stools point towards malabsorption. Wasted child with protuberant abdomen, with symptoms starting from the age of weaning (introduction of wheat) point towards coeliac disease.
5. Food that is eaten is absorbed, but is used up due to increased demand, leaving hardly anything for body building.
   - Endocrine: Hyperthyroidism, diabetes mellitus, diabetes insipidus, growth hormone deficiency, etc. Polyuria, polydipsia and weight loss are the likely presenting symptoms of diabetes mellitus. Midline abnormalities, microphallus, etc may be noticed in growth hormone deficiency.
   - Cardiac: Long-standing congestive cardiac failure of any etiology.
   - Respiratory: Long-standing pulmonary problems like cystic fibrosis, poorly controlled asthma, etc.
   - Hepatic: Cirrhosis, chronic active hepatitis.
   - Renal: Chronic renal failure, renal tubular acidosis.
   - Haematological: Chronic illnesses like thalassaemia, malignancies.
   - GIT: Chronic diarrhoea, GERD, coeliac disease, inflammatory bowel disease.
   - CNS: Cerebral palsy, mental retardation, myopathy, etc (due to swallowing difficulty and possibly neglect of the child).
   - Chronic infections: Tuberculosis, HIV, worm infestations, etc.
   - Metabolic: Inborn errors of metabolism (look for history and typical features suggestive of inborn errors of metabolism).
6. Food that is eaten is absorbed and is used up properly, but the body has inadequate potential for growth. Examples are syndromes of inadequate growth potential like the Seckel syndrome, IUGR baby, chromosomal anomalies, etc. History of previous neonatal deaths, antenatal infections, dysmorphic features, etc, may point towards chromosomal anomalies, perinatal infections, etc. Emotional deprivation is another example of a situation of failure to use the absorbed nutrients due to "endogenous shutdown."

SHORT STATURE

Aetiology

Variations of Normal

- Familial short stature (The child is short at birth, remains short as a child, and becomes a short adult like his/her parents.)
- Constitutional delay (The child has normal length at birth, grows up normally for a few months and then the growth falters to a slow rate; has delay in onset of puberty, but finally becomes an adult of normal height. Usually a history of similar growth pattern in childhood may be obtained in parents.)

Pathological Short Stature

1. **Disproportionate short stature**
   - Achondroplasia (short limbs). Increase in US/LS ratio suggests short lower limbs.
   - Vertebral anomalies (short trunk or short neck as in Klippel-Feil syndrome).
2. **Proportionate short stature**
   - ***Prenatal onset***: The history shows that the child was small at birth and continued to be small as he became older. Sometimes, history suggestive of intrauterine insults may be obtained. Dysmorphic features of syndromes may be identifiable.
     - Intrauterine growth retardation (ask for birth weight and length).

8

  - Chromosomal anomalies.
  - Certain syndromes (look for suggestive features/dysmorphism). Examples are Russell-Silver, Turner, Prader-Willi, etc.
- *Postnatal onset*:
  - **Malnutrition** (get detailed dietary history and look for any features of nutritional deficiency)
  - Chronic diseases of organ systems:
    - Infections: Tuberculosis, malaria, etc.
    - Endocrine: Hypothyroidism (discussed in p 452), diabetes mellitus, growth hormone deficiency (midline face defects, normal intelligence), Cushing's syndrome (obesity, moon face, striae), etc. Note that hypothyroidism can present as short stature without any other manifestation. Long standing rickets may be an occasional cause of short limbs, because of compression of weak ends of long bones. Cretins may retain infantile proportions compared to age-related peers due to slow growth.
    - Haematologic: Anaemia, thalassaemia.
    - Cardiac: Persistent cardiac failure.
    - Respiratory: Poorly controlled bronchial asthma, cystic fibrosis.
    - Renal: Chronic renal failure, renal tubular acidosis (may have history of polyuria and polydipsia).
    - GIT: Cirrhosis, malabsorption (large bulky stools in malabsorption; wasted child with protuberant abdomen in coeliac disease).
  - Emotional deprivation syndrome: It is as though the pituitary is shut down for some time. The child prefers to sit alone, avoids eye contact and is not interested in surroundings. Both weight and height will be less.
  - Iatrogenic: Steroid therapy (ask for drug history).

In chronic systemic disorders and malnutrition, height and weight are affected, i.e., children with chronic illness and malnutrition are short with failure to thrive.

In endocrine disorders like hypothyroidism, Cushing's or growth hormone deficiency, weight is preserved and, in fact, the child may be obese and short. Children with syndromic short stature also may be obese and short (e.g., Prader-Willi, Laurence-Moon-Biedl, etc).

If height charts are provided, the child's height may be plotted and projected in the graph to see the predicted adult height of the child. It may be compared with the mid parental height.

Thumb to shoulder test: Have the child touch the tip of the thumb to tip of shoulder. It overshoots the shoulder in proximal segment shortening (rhizomelic shortening), which is seen in achondroplasia (see Figs. 22.4, 22.6).

Investigations to be Done

- Routine blood, urine and stool.
- Renal function tests.
- Tests depending on involvement of other systems.
- X-ray for bone age.
- Thyroid function test.
- Karyotyping in Turner's syndrome or other dysmorphic syndromes.
- Growth hormone assay and follow-up with growth monitoring every 3 months. Normal child should gain 4–6 cm per year.

Quick Inspection in Short Stature

- Make a general inspection: Note any dysmorphism, disproportions, neck, hairline, nutritional status, etc.

- Look at the upper limbs: Fingernails, short 4th metacarpal, palms, carrying angle, etc.

Also read short stature from p 449.

TALL STATURE

- Familial
- Cerebral giantism
- Precocious puberty (tall compared to age matched peers during precocity, but ultimate height is less than the peers due to early fusion of epiphysis)
- Klinefelter syndrome
- Marfan syndrome

FLOPPY INFANT

Please see p 265.

Floppiness may be due to:

- **Central causes**: Neonatal brain insults like hypoxia, intracranial bleed, intracranial infection, hypoglycaemia, etc, may present as a floppy neonate. Hypotonia of chromosomal disorders like Down's syndrome is also thought to be central in origin. Hypotonic cerebral palsy is a rare entity where the usual progression of cerebral palsy from hypotonic to dystonic to spastic stage gets arrested at the initial hypotonic stage itself. It is a severe type of cerebral palsy with gross retardation of the child. Although hypotonic, the reflexes will be exaggerated and plantar response will be upgoing. Most of these children ultimately become spastic late in life.
- **Spinal cord**: Birth injuries causing spinal cord injury are rare. Although the child will be hypotonic initially, it will later become hypertonic and hyper-reflexic.
- **Anterior horn cell**: Werdnig-Hoffman disease (alert baby with hypotonia, absent reflexes and tongue fasciculations; may get a history of decreased fetal movements during pregnancy), polio (in yesteryears), some enteroviral infections, Pompe disease (hypotonia, cardiomegaly, hepatosplenomegaly).
- **Neuromuscular junction**: Myasthenia gravis, infantile botulism, drugs (hypermagnesaemia, aminoglycosides). Remember that if the mother is affected, the child can have neonatal transient myasthenia due to transplacental transfer of acetylcholine receptor antibodies.
- **Peripheral nerve**: Guillain-Barre syndrome, familial dysautonomia, congenital sensory neuropathy (rare).
- **Muscles**: Muscular dystrophies, congenital myotonic dystrophies, congenital myopathies (central core disease, Nemaline myopathy), polymyositis, glycogen storage disease (Pompe), carnitine deficiency, etc. Myopathies: Hypotonia and hyporeflexia (but not absent reflexes). Benign congenital myopathy: This is a diagnosis of exclusion. Hypotonia may be inconvenient as it causes joint hyper-mobility. It may persist into adulthood.
- **Miscellaneous**: PEM, rickets, Prader-Willi, Ehlers-Danlos, cretinism, malabsorption, etc.

8

DEVELOPMENTAL DELAY/REGRESSION

- Predominant speech delay: Hearing problem, autism, dyslexia, histidinaemia.
- Predominant motor delay: Benign hypotonia, motor deficits like cerebral palsy (e.g., hemiplegic CP), neuromuscular disorders like myopathy.
- Global delay that is non-progressive (the child is achieving milestones but at a later date than expected; child has not lost any achieved mile stones): Intrauterine infections, cerebral palsy (perinatal insults), cerebral malformations, dysmorphic syndromes, chromosomal disorders. One must look for stigmata of described chromosomal disorders or dysmorphic syndromes.
- Global delay that is progressive (child was developing normally, has slowed down in development and ultimately stopped achieving milestones and has actually lost some of the milestones already achieved):
  - Coarse facies: Hypothyroidism, mucopolysaccharidosis.

- Macrocephaly: Hydrocephalus, Alexander or Canavan disease.
- Cutaneous markers and hair: Neurocutaneous syndromes, Menkes kinky hair syndrome.
- Visceromegaly: Mucopolysaccharidosis, Niemann-Pick, galactosaemia, etc.
- Adrenal failure: Adrenoleukodystrophy (look for hyperpigmentation).
- Exaggerated startle response: Tay-Sachs disease.
- Myoclonus: Older child who was till then normal, developing intellectual deterioration and myoclonus may be subacute sclerosing panencephalitis.
- Handwashing movements: Female child who was normal initially, develops stereotyped handwashing movements and autistic features may be having Rett syndrome.
- Self mutilation: Lesch-Nyhan syndrome.
- Fundus abnormalities: Optic atrophy (white matter degeneration), cherry red spot (gray matter degeneration).

Do not forget environmental and emotional deprivation as an important cause for development delay. Hence. relevant history must be obtained.

Developmental lag is expected in prematurely delivered children, and they take a few months before they catch up with peers in both growth and development.

Autism also presents with delayed development and very poor socialization. It is a disorder in which the child gets preoccupied with inanimate objects without socializing with people around.

Features of Grey Matter Degeneration

- Intellectual deterioration
- Seizures
- Retinal changes, like retinitis pigmentosa and cherry red spots. Retina is part of "nerve cells" (i.e., grey matter).
- Examples of grey matter degenerative diseases are Tay-Sachs disease, GM_1 gangliosidosis, Sandoff disease, Menkes kinky hair disease, Rett syndrome, etc.

Features of White Matter Degeneration

- Spasticity
- Ataxia
- Optic atrophy (optic nerve is part of white matter)
- Examples of white matter degenerative diseases are metachromatic leukodystrophy, adrenoleukodystrophy, Krabbe's disease, etc.

Many diseases have features of both grey and white matter disease. The compartmentalization is possible only early in disease. Later, predominance of white or grey matter degenerations become too blurred to detect.

RECURRENT OR PERSISTENT PNEUMONIA

Recurrent pneumonia is differentiated from persistent pneumonia by the radiological clearance in between two episodes of pneumonia. The usual causes that must be suspected are:

- Inadequately controlled bronchial asthma.
- Bronchial obstruction by foreign body, lymph node, etc (recurrent pneumonia involving the same site).
- Congenital heart disease (left-to-right shunt lesions).
- Bronchiectasis (get high resolution CT scan done).
- Gastroesophageal reflux.
- Immune deficiency disorders.
- Ciliary motility disorders (diagnosis is by ciliary beat frequency of nasal scrapings measured under electron microscope).
- Cystic fibrosis (sweat chloride >60 mEq/L).
- Alpha-1 antitrypsin deficiency.
- Congenital abnormalities like pulmonary sequestration syndrome.
- Lung involvement secondary to systemic diseases like SLE.
- Anaemia and lung involvement may point towards pulmonary haemosiderosis.
- Unusual lung involvement like that encountered in HIV (*Pneumocystis carinii* or lymphoid interstitial pneumonia of HIV).

CHAPTER 9

Central Nervous System : Part–I

HIGHER MENTAL FUNCTIONS

Suffice to assess whether the child recognizes people around, realizes the place, time, etc; normal interaction with parents should obviate any further inquiries on this aspect. Emotional/behavioural disturbances and intellectual disturbances may be obtained from history. Deteriorating school performance is a good guide of intellectual deterioration in slowly progressive disorders.

Consciousness

It is the state of awareness.

Levels of Consciousness

- **Drowsy**: The child is sleeping but arousable by ordinary stimulus or a loud call. Once awake, the child responds *appropriately without further stimulation*, but goes to sleep again if left alone.
- **Stupor**: The child responds *only* to a strong noxious (painful) stimulus. The child localizes the pain and tries to remove the noxious stimulus (so it is a *cerebral* response and not just a reflex one). Soon after the removal of the stimulus, the child slips to sleep. The child may awaken from stupor, but is more likely to be restless or delirious.
- **Obtundation**: This is a stage between drowsiness and stupor. Here, the child may be awakened by a strong stimulus other than pain (e.g., a loud call with simultaneous shaking). The child will have *cerebral* response but may be very confused and hence the responses may be inappropriate.
- **Delirium**: This is an agitated confusional stage, sometimes with hallucinations and delusions. The child responds incoherently and many times violently. The response may continue without the child slipping back to sleep easily. A stuporous child when awakened with a noxious stimulus may go back to sleep when the stimulus is removed or may become delirious.
- **Light coma** or semi coma: In coma of any grade, there is no *cerebral* response to stimulation. In light coma, the child may be kept aroused as long as a noxious stimulus is being applied. The response is non specific, like moaning, movements of limbs, etc, but the child cannot localize pain and no directed attempt is made to remove the noxious stimulus (so the response is reflex and not cerebral).
- **Deep coma**: The only response to noxious stimulus may be decortication or decerebration.
- **Flaccid coma**: No response whatsoever, and there is total flaccidity with no reflexes.
- It is not that all patients will go through all these stages on their way to coma. In general, there are two main routes to coma. One route is characterized by *increased neuronal excitability* where there is delirium, seizure, stupor and coma (e.g., encephalitis, hepatic encephalopathy, etc). The other route is characterized by *decreased neuronal excitability* where

there is progressive lethargy, obtundation, stupor and coma (example would be sedative poisoning). Many a time, there will be overlapping of these two.

Glasgow Coma Scale

This scoring is not very useful for one-time examination of a patient, as in case of students' case presentation. Serial scoring of Glasgow coma scale helps in serial monitoring of the child with altered sensorium (most useful in head injury rather than medical illness). Thc chart below shows the scoring system for children. The one for infants is slightly different.

Recording AVPU for serial monitoring is more practical in clinical settings.
A: Alert
V: Responds to verbal stimulus
P: Responds to painful stimulus (record the type of response, see below)
U: Unresponsive

Painful stimulus: Apply a noxious stimulus (usually supraorbital ridge compression) and observe the response. Purposeful withdrawal away from pain or speech indicates preserved cortical function. Decorticate posturing in response to pain indicates lesion at the level of thalamus. Decerebration in response to pain indicates high pontine or midbrain lesions. Total flaccidity with no response to pain indicates lower pontomedullary lesions.

Asymmetric response indicates focal neurological deficits like hemiplegia.

Coma vigil: This was a term of yesteryears, usually used in terminal typhoid fever patients. The patient is in coma, but the eyes remain open, with random head and limb movements. But there is no voluntary movement or communication in response to command. To an observer, the patient appears alert, as the eyes are open, but there is no response to any external stimuli.

Locked-in syndrome: Here, the patient is awake but cannot perform any movement except certain eye movements. But for these eye movements, the patient may be mistaken to be in true coma. Some patients learn to communicate by eye movements. Usually, they can open their eyes and move eyeballs up and down on request. The brain lesion possibly spares the reticular activating system. The site of lesion is the ventral ponsbilaterally.

Contents of Consciousness

Delusion: They are fake beliefs that cannot be changed even by evidence to the contrary.

Hallucinations: They are false impressions from organs of special senses without them being really present, e.g., flashes of light, hearing voices, etc. Flashes of light may be seen as aura in migraine.

Eye opening (E)	Verbal response (V)	Motor response (M)
4. Spontaneous 3. To call 2. To pain 1. None	5. Normal 4. Sentences but not fully oriented 3. Words only 2. No words, only sounds 1. None	6. Normal 5. Localizes pain 4. Withdraws to pain, no proper localization 3. Decortication 2. Decerebration 1. None

Total maximum score possible: E+V+M = 15. Minimum score is 3, not zero.

For intubated patients, modified GCS score with Grimace response or a newer score FOUR- Full Outline of Unresponsiveness Score (Eye response, Motor response, Brainstem response, Respiration) may be used.

Illusion is the mistaken interpretation of what one sees. Magicians do all their tricks by cleverly hiding certain things, thus creating illusion in the audience. If one mistakes a rope for a snake, it is an illusion. So in illusion, there is actually something, but it is interpreted wrongly. This differentiates illusion from delusion.

Dementia: It is an acquired disorder of cognitive function, usually with decline in intellect, memory and personality in the presence of normal sensorium. The usual causes are tumours, encephalitis, SSPE, multiple minute infarctions due to vasculitis (e.g., SLE), heavy metal poisoning, chronic dialysis, old age, etc. In dementia, the patient is aware of his loss of memory, whereas in Alzheimer, the patient is not aware of his disability.

Amnesia: Inability to recollect past events and/or new ones. It is common after head trauma.

Amnesia is the loss of memory of past events. Retrograde amnesia is loss of memory for remote events, whereas anterograde amnesia is loss of ability to recollect newly learnt material. To test the former, the child may be asked about some past events. To test the latter, the child may be shown for a minute, a few familiar articles that interest him (like animals, birds, etc) and asked to recollect them after 5 min.

Orientation in time, space and person: One can ask the child where he is now and is it morning or evening, etc.

Attention: Attention should be tested before testing memory, speech etc. It is tested by digit repetition test. Normally at 6 years can repeat 5 digits and by 10 years can repeat 6 digits.

Memory: Immediate memory is tested by telling the child a word or two and asking the child to repeat it. Short-term (recent) memory is tested by asking the child what he has taken for breakfast, etc. Also test the long-term memory (of remote events).

Intelligence (Calculation and Abstract thinking) is the ability to apply prior knowledge successfully to a new situation and to use reason in solving problems.

Questions must be in accordance with the level of education of the child or level of development expected at that age. For example, a 6-year-old child may be requested to do a simple addition. One may have an assessment depending on the school performance as well. For a younger child, assessment of milestones of development gives a rough idea of intelligence.

9

Speech

Speech or language is not just talking. It involves the higher cortical function for language, muscles of articulation for articulation, and voice production for phonation. Speech is a function of dominant hemisphere. Left brain is dominant in all right handed persons and almost 70% of left handed persons. Speech should be assessed for Comprehension, Fluency, Repetition, and Naming.

The **sensory speech** involves two elements, i.e., comprehension of spoken words (auditory speech) and comprehension of words that one sees (visual speech). Thus, auditory speech is understanding the speech one hears and visual speech is understanding the written speech.

Motor speech consists of two elements, talking and writing. Broca's area of the frontal lobe controls spoken speech production and hence may be having controlling connections with areas representing mouth, tongue, lips, etc. Written speech has a different area in the frontal lobe, which may have control over cortical areas representing the hands and fingers.

Dysphasia is the defect in speech function due to damage to cortical centres of the dominant hemisphere. Near total absence of speech (comprehension or production of language in written or spoken form) may be termed as **aphasia**.

Motor or expressive aphasia is when one cannot have fluent talk (only a few words or inappropriate words) or fluent writing as the child normally was having before the illness.

Speech may be agrammatic and telegraphic but the comprehension remains good, e.g., the child understands a picture as tiger, but cannot find the word tiger, and instead goes about describing it as an animal that roars, lives in forest, etc. One must clearly have an understanding of normal developmental lags in children before making comments on aphasia.

Sensory or receptive aphasia (Wernicke's Aphasia) is failure of comprehension of spoken words or written words. They can go on talking fluently many words but the examiner understands it is not the reply expected for his question. There won't be any repetition. There will be neologism, paraphasisas. Autistic children go on talking such nonsense.

In sensory aphasia, the child does not understand your question but in reply goes on with fluent meaningless talk so that you know the child has not picked up the meaning of what you have put to him. In motor aphasia, you can see that the child has understood what was told to him and he is desperately trying to bring out the right reply but is not getting words for it. Thus, *impaired comprehension but fluent talk* is the hallmark of sensory aphasia, whereas *non-fluent talk with retained comprehension* is the hallmark of motor aphasia.

Conductive Aphasia is the loss of repetition with preserved comprehension and output. It is due to lesion of the Arcuate fasciculus.

Nominal Aphasia is inability to recall the name of an object but can go on talking about its use, parts etc. It is due to a lesion of the angular gyrus.

Word deafness: Inability to understand the meaning of words that are heard.

Word blindness: Inability to understand the meaning of words that are seen.

Global aphasia is when both sensory and motor speech are affected.

Before diagnosing aphasias, one has to make sure that the child has adequate hearing/vision and there are no motor problems interfering with speaking/writing.

In all the aphasias, the site of lesion is the cortex. Although subcortical aphasia is a known entity, it is the field of the neurologist and the student of paediatrics need not be unduly worried about it.

Dysarthria is the disorder of articulation. Here, the content of speech is normally meaningful, but sounds odd due to poor articulation. Lips, tongue, palate, pharynx, etc, are involved in the process of articulation. Lip sounds are tested by asking the child to say "ma, ba, pa," etc, tongue sounds by "ta, da," etc, and palate/pharyngeal sounds by "ga." Disorders of articulation may occur because of muscle disorders affecting muscles of articulation or disorders of nerves supplying these muscles (VII, X, XII) or affection of cortical centers or corticobulbar pathways controlling the nuclei of these nerves (X, XII). The most common cause of dysarthria is LMN lesions such as Guillain-Barre syndrome, polio, myopathies, etc, which produce nasal twang due to palatal paralysis. XII nerve palsy produces faulty articulation of sounds that need the tongue for their production. VII nerve palsy produces faulty production of sounds that require the lips for their production. Lesions of cortical centres causing dysarthria are rare because the concerned cranial nerves have bilateral innervation. An example of UMN dysarthria ("spastic dysarthria": slurred, thick, slow, indistinct speech) is cerebral palsy with pseudobulbar palsy. Here, defective articulation is associated with "effortful" phonation and the gag reflex is exaggerated ("speaking with hot potato in mouth").

Staccato speech: During speech, there are intermittent, explosive loud syllables with undue stress; seen in cerebellar disease.

Scanning speech: The individual syllables are pronounced clearly, with long pauses in between, seen in cerebellar disease, i.e., Sc-aa-nn—ing, , Thi-ru-va-na-ntha-pu-ra-m.

Speech in extrapyramidal lesions: This is low volume monotonous speech.

Phonation or production of sounds is by the larynx and the muscles of articulation modify these sounds to different meaningful sounds. ***Dysphonia*** is the disorder of voice production. It may occur due to paralysis of laryngeal nerve, vocal cord nodules, oedema of larynx, etc. Sound (voice) production can be affected by paralysis of respiratory muscles, and also because of insufficient air available for phonation (e.g., emphysema, Guillain-Barre syndrome, poliomyelitis, etc).

Dyslexia is one of the spectrum of specific learning disorders of developmental origin, where the child has difficulty to master reading skills despite having normal intelligence (developmental reading disorder).

Dysgraphia: Inability to write properly.

Echolalia: Involuntary repetition of words or phrases (which the examiner tells) without knowing their meaning (like an echo). It may be seen in autism.

Apraxia: Inability to accomplish previously learned and performed complex motor activities, even though motor system, sensory system, coordination and understanding are relatively intact. It occurs when there is parietal lobe dysfunction.

Agnosia: Inability to comprehend verbal or symbolic language even though the sensory pathways and sensorium are intact. It is due to lesions of the parietal lobe or occipital lobe. Eg. Finger agnosia, asteriognosis.

Emotions: Look for evidence of emotional incontinence, e.g., in chorea. Patients with psuedobulbar paralysis (here the lesion is UMN) have incontinence of emotion, laughing or crying on slightest provocation. They have inability to stop emotions at will.

Handedness must be inquired if relevant. Here, note that even left handed children may be compulsorily trained to use their right hand for writing and hence beware not to get fooled by asking the child which hand he uses to write. Ask which hand he uses to comb his hair or throw a ball.

GAIT AND STANCE

Stance is the way a person stands and gait is the way a person walks. While the child is standing, look for kyphosis, scoliosis, lordosis and the distance between feet (normal distance between the feet while standing is no more than 2 inches at the level of medial malleolus). Persons with cerebellar disease have a wide-based stance. Now ask the child to stand with feet close together and look for any unsteadiness. If not unsteady, ask the child to close the eyes and look for unsteadiness while the eyes are closed (Romberg sign-test for posterior column). Next ask him to walk normally. Look for arm swing, pelvic tilt, lurching to one or both sides, length of steps, any asymmetry and associated movements of upper limbs. (shoulder and the armswing).

Finally, make him walk in tandem steps and observe the Pelvis.

Important Notice: Gait is a function of a combination of many nervous system faculties including motor, sensory (including the joint sense), vestibular, cerebellar and cortical functions. Hence, gait is discussed here under higher functions. However, there are many medical teachers who would like gait to be discussed under the examination of motor system. Although one can argue for or against this, it is best that the student follows his/her teacher's protocol. (Refer Pg: 584) Abnormal types of gait include the following.

Hemiparetic Gait

The arm is adducted and internally rotated at shoulder; the elbow is flexed; the forearm is semi-pronated, and the wrist and fingers are flexed. Hemiplegic arm does not have the automatic swinging on walking. In the lower extremities, in mild cases the only indication of paresis may be that the ball of the patient's shoe may be worn out more on the affected side. In significant hemiplegia, the lower limb is slightly flexed at hip, extended at knee with plantar flexed and inverted foot.

In severe cases, the hand may be clenched; the knee is held in extension and the ankle is plantar flexed, making the paralyzed leg functionally longer than the other. The patient therefore circumducts the affected leg while walking.

In hemiplegia, the flexors of hip, knee and dorsiflexors of ankle are weak. Thus, the foot remains plantar flexed; to avoid dragging of foot on ground, the sensible option is to raise the foot high. However, the gait cannot be high stepping because of hip flexion weakness; the weakness of foot extension will keep the foot plantar flexed and this tends to cause the patient to catch the toe on the ground when walking and may cause trips and falls. The solution for the patient is to tilt the pelvis up and to swing the whole lower limb sideways in a circular movement when walking so as to clear the toes off the ground (circumducting gait). During the swinging phase of circumduction, there is a slight lateral flexion of trunk to the unaffected side and hyperextension of hip. Wear pattern of the child's shoes give a clue to the dragging toes. (Fig.9.1)

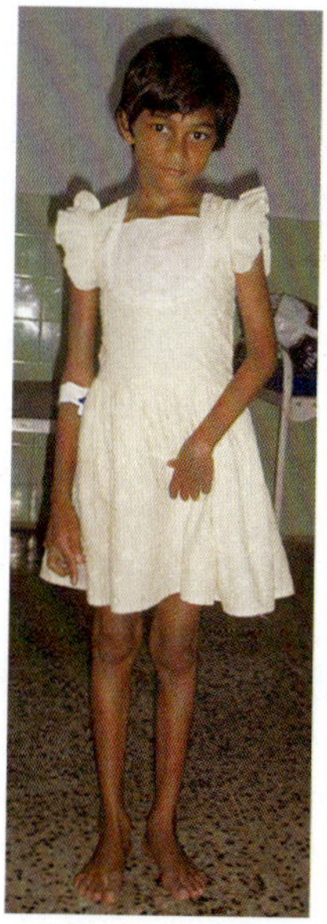

Fig.9.1 Hemiplegia: Typical posture of a hemiplegic child.

Ataxic Gait

In ataxia, the patient spreads the legs apart to provide a wider base of support to compensate for the imbalance while standing or walking. In severe cases, patients stagger as they walk; walk with reeling, uncoordinated steps, like an intoxicated individual. The heel-to-toe or tandem walking manoeuvres and standing on one leg will uncover subtle forms of ataxia.

Ataxia results from lesions of the cerebellum and may be isolated or may be associated with other cerebellar findings. When the lesion is unilateral (cerebellar hemisphere), the patient may veer to the side of the lesion; in bilateral cerebellar involvement, the patient may fall to either side. When the lesion is in the midline (flocculonodular lobe) associated nystagmus is expected.

In vestibulitis also the patient may sway towards the abnormal side. Here, the nervous system examination will be otherwise normal.

Shuffling Gait

There is a difficulty or hesitation in initiation of steps (start hesitation). Once the patient starts walking, he does so with short shuffling steps. In some patients, the steps (albeit short) and pace may vary with a tendency to accelerate (festinating gait) as he/she walks. Both types are seen in Parkinson's disease, which anyway is a very rare disease of childhood. The associated movements of upper limbs are absent. In short, the characteristics of shuffling gait are small steps, stooped posture, shuffling and festination.

High-stepping Gait

High-stepping gait is commonly seen in LMN foot drop (e.g., nerve palsy following gluteal IM injection). In high-stepping gait, the individual takes high steps (as if climbing a flight of stairs) while walking on a level surface. In this peculiar gait pattern, the patient is stepping high to avoid the toes dragging on the ground with each step. Unlike hemiplegia, here the hip and knee flexors are normal and thus can lift the leg higher than normal; hence there is no need for circumduction.

High-stepping, Slapping Gait, Stamping Gait (De-afferentation)

High-stepping stamping gait is seen in posterior column lesions and peripheral neuropathies when the position sense is impaired (especially while walking in the dark when the visual feedback is no longer compensating for the loss of position sense). As the patient puts the feet down one by one, they stamp the ground (heel touching the ground first, the front part of the foot then slaps or stamps down on the ground), hence the description of a foot-slapping gait. The patient does not have an idea of where in space his legs are, and hence raises legs higher than necessary. Similarly when bringing down the feet also the patient is not having an idea when the leg is going to touch the ground and hence the slapping on the floor (floor is reached unexpectedly before the downward velocity of leg can be reduced). When we raise the foot from the ground it is somewhat dorsiflexed and when it is going to touch the ground again, the foot goes to a bit plantar flexion to make toes touch the floor first. In loss of proprioceptive sensation, the patient cannot anticipate when the foot is going to touch the floor and hence this plantar flexion for toes to touch floor first does not occur. Hence, the heel touches ground first. One can compensate for this by visual feedback, but normally we walk looking straight ahead and not looking at the foot.

The **Romberg test** will be positive in deafferentation. Ask the patient to stand upright with the feet together and eyes closed. Normally, the proprioceptive feedback will keep the subject upright and steady. In deafferentation the patient becomes unsteady (see p 207,223). 9

High-stepping gait can also be the result of the functional elongation of the legs due to bilateral foot drop, but here the toes hit the ground first and not the heel. In addition, the gait abnormality of foot drop does not increase while walking in the dark.

Spastic or Scissoring Gait

In this condition, both the legs are held in adduction at the hip and the thighs rub against each other as the patient walks; spasm of the inner thigh muscles also occurs. If the spasm is severe, with each advancing step the knees tend to slide over each other like the blades of a pair of scissors. The knee is extended, foot plantar flexed and the child walks on tip toes. This is typically seen in diplegic cerebral palsy.

Waddling Gait

There is exaggerated lumbar lordosis; the patient walks on a broad base, tilting the pelvis abnormally downward. It may be seen in muscle diseases. A similar gait is seen in neglected congenital dislocation of hip (developmental dysplasia of hip).

When we stand with weight bearing on one leg, the gluteus medius of that side pulls the pelvis down to stabilize the hip, which means the opposite side of hip is a bit raised. When gluteus

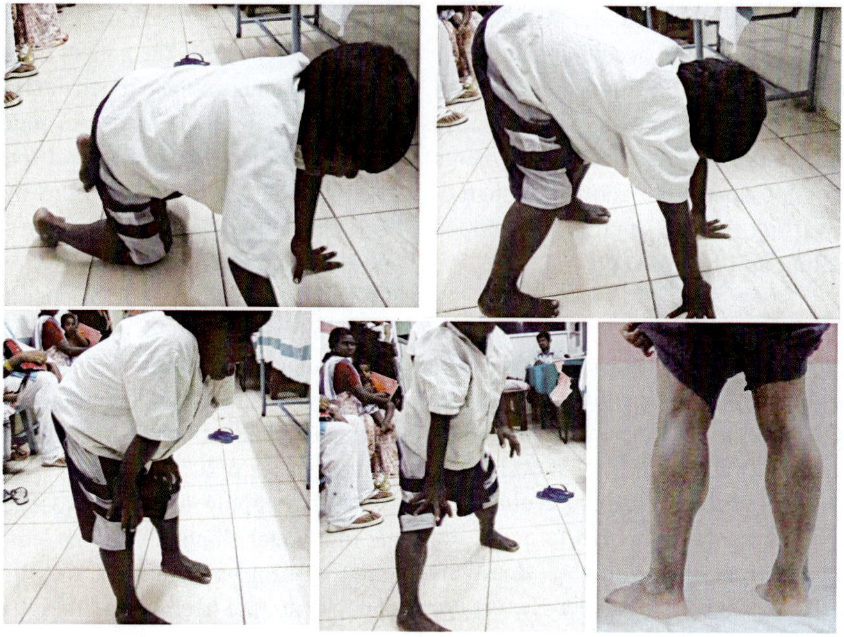

Fig.9.2 Gower sign *(Courtesy Dr Guruprasad)*

medius of weight bearing side is weak, it cannot put down the pelvis of same side, so much so, the opposite pelvis drops (opposite of what would have happened had there been no weakness). When there is bilateral weakness of gluteal muscles, this tilt happens alternatively to produce waddling.

Gower's sign, seen typically in Duchenne muscular dystrophy, occurs when the patient attempts to stand up from the squatting posture; he characteristically assumes a quadruped posture, and then climbs up on his own thighs using his arms to do so before he assumes the erect posture (Fig. 9.2).

CRANIAL NERVES

Cranial nerves I to XII must be examined. However, examination need not be in that order. The nerves affected must be tested first to avoid tiring the child during crucial parts of examination. Cranial nerves I, II and VIII are purely sensory. Cranial nerves III, IV, VI, XI and XII are purely motor. V, VII, IX and X have both motor and sensory functions. Lower part of face, XI, XII have cortical control from the opposite hemisphere only. All the other cranial nerves have bilateral cortical control.

Olfactory Nerve (1st nerve)

Olfactory nerve testing is difficult in children and is also not useful as it is not affected in most of the neurological disorders. The most common cause for poor smell perception is rhinitis or blocked nose! Each nostril must be tested separately using familiar substances like asafoetida, coffee powder, etc preferably with the child's eyes closed; chocolates or chewing gums to which the child is more familiar is better in younger ones. Pungent substances like ammonia must not be used as it stimulates pain fibres carried by V nerve and the child perceives it even when the sense of smell is lost. In Kallman's syndrome, there is anosmia, obesity and hypogonadism. Perception of smell indicates an intact olfactory pathway and identification of the smell indicates and intact cortical centre. Olfactory discrimination can be tested from 5 years onwards.

Optic Nerve (2nd nerve)

Testing is to be done for acuity of vision, field of vision and colour vision. In addition, one must examine the fundus and the pupils.

1. Acuity of Vision

It is not enough to ask if vision is OK; because even total loss of vision in one eye may go unnoticed until each eye is tested separately. In older children, distant vision can be objectively tested by Snellen's chart and an estimate of near vision can objectively obtained by getting the child to read Jaeger eye chart. Other printed material can be used as bedside tool for near vision. If acuity of vision is very low, test if the child can see finger movements, held in front of the eyes. If even this cannot be seen by the child, test if he can perceive the light, by moving a lighted torch in front of the eye.

E test for illiterates may be used for 3 years and older children but since it requires the child to tell to which directions the lines of E point to, it may not be suitable for a small child. Instead, the child can be shown letters or pictures of animals/bird on screen and asked to take from the tray given to him, the matching plastic letter or animals/bird shapes similar to the one shown on the screen. If the visual acuity improves with a pin hole test, the visual impairment is due to refractive errors.

In small infants, blink response to bright light, visual following of red balls, etc can be used. In cerebral palsy, fixing and following may be acquired late due to delayed CNS maturation rather than optic nerve problem.

Menace reflex: Here, we test the defensive eye blinking reaction of the child by moving the examiner's fingers suddenly and threateningly towards the patient's eyes. This is used in uncooperative patients whose vision is suspect.

Nyctalopia: This is poor vision in darkness. May be seen in vitamin A deficiency, retinitis pigmentosa, etc. Albinism may be one of the reasons.

Hemeralopia: This is day blindness, meaning vision is poor in good light. It may be detected in rare disorders like congenital cone dystrophy and some disorders of macular degeneration.

2. Field of Vision (Fig. 9.3, 9.4)

Objective method is perimetry (Bjerrum's screen is used for formal testing). It can also be tested by the confrontation method. The examiner sits or stands in front of the patient about 3 feet away. Ask the patient to look straight at the examiner's eyes and bring the moving fingers of both hands of examiner from the periphery of field of the vision inwards to the centre from four quadrants, starting from just outside the examiner's field of vision in each quadrant. The patient is instructed to say 'yes' when he sees the examiner's fingers. This is a quick and practically useful technique. But ideally both eyes should be tested separately. For examining the patient's right eye, the left one is kept closed by a patch or hand and the patient is instructed to look straight into the examiner's left eye. The examiner's right eye is kept closed. Now bring moving the fingers towards the centre from the periphery from nasal side, temporal side, superior side and inferior side to mark all the quadrants, the examiner's field of vision remaining as a normal control. In a young child, one may test menace reflex from all quadrants to see whether the field of vision is grossly normal.

Scotoma: This is a defect or hole in the field of vision. It may be noted in optic neuritis or retrobulbar neuritis. But the most common situation of its occurrence is during an attack of migraine. Concentric constriction of field of vision may occur in retinitis pigmentosa.

9

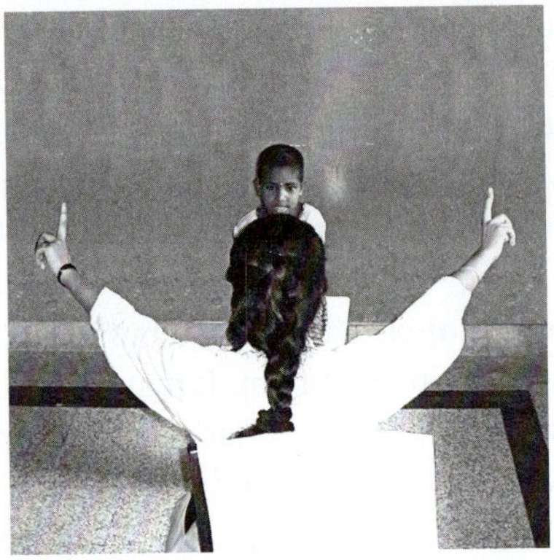

Fig.9.3 Field of vision (quick method)

Hemianopia: One half of the visual field is lost. The child may repeatedly bump into the obstacles on one side.

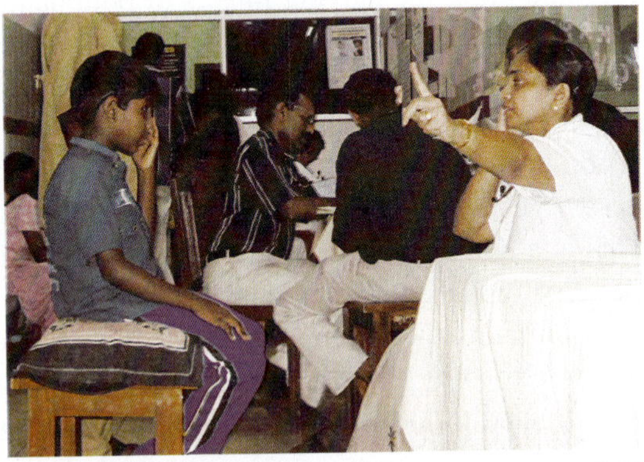

Fig.9.4 Field of vision (Confrontation method): The ideal method of testing the field of vision is shown in this picture. Note that the examiner and the child are at the same height level (child's chair has pillows to elevate him to the level of examiner) and that the examiner's fingers are well stretched out to the periphery. However, in children it is always advantageous to use the quick method where both sides are tested simultaneously.

- Hemianopia is usually homonymous hemianopia, meaning same part of the visual field is affected on each side (e.g., loss of nasal field of vision in one eye and temporal field of vision in the other eye).
- Heteronymous hemianopia means loss of either the nasal or temporal field of vision in both eyes. For example, bitemporal hemianopia occurs in tumours of pituitary gland (craniopharyngioma) due to its pressure over the optic chiasma.
- Congruous hemianopia: This will be obvious only on formal charting of visual fields. Thus, it is an area of interest to the ophthalmologist, not paediatrician. The outline of visual field loss is exactly similar in both fields of vision and occurs in lesions posterior to the lateral geniculate body, e.g., optic radiation.
- Incongruous hemianopia: The outline of visual field loss in both fields are different. The lesion is more anterior, e.g., in the optic tract or chiasma.

Detailed testing for hemianopia is not practical in children, but is of importance in adult medicine. The interested student may refer to *Hutchison's Clinical Methods* for more details (Ref. 4).

3. Colour Vision

Ishihara's test is used for formal testing. For clinical situations, one may give coloured objects and ask the child to name the colour. 3–4-year-old child will be able to say three colours. Red–green deficiency is the most common congenital colour blindness. Drugs like ethambutol produce blue–green impairment.

4. Fundus

Examination of the fundus is also a must. The postgraduate student must look at the fundus of as many children as possible, whether it is relevant or not; only by seeing a large number of fundi, the student will get familiarized with normal appearance and its variations.

To circumvent pupillary constriction due to light reflex, reduce the illumination of the room before examining the fundus. The examiner holds the scope in his right hand and uses his right eye to examine the patient's right eye. Then walk around the bed to the left side for examining the left eye. Leaning across the patient to examine the left eye is uncomfortable and also prevents the child from fixing at distant objects. Also trying to use the wrong eye result in nasal collision of patient and the doctor! It is best to use a mydriatic drug for examining the fundus (after pupillary reflexes are examined, because after mydriasis pupillary reflex becomes meaningless). Ask the child to look at a distant object and not at the ophthalmoscope. In case of smaller children, ask the mother to stand behind the examiner and make some interesting movements like protruding tongue off and on. The child is instructed to look at mother and tell when she is protruding the tongue. So the child voluntarily looks away from the ophthalmoscopic light and makes it easy for the examiner to see the fundus. If the child is still not keeping the eye stationary and is moving it, the best way is to keep the ophthalmoscope still and as the child moves off and on, the fundus comes into view momentarily and take that opportunity to have a view of the fundus. For infants, let the baby suck on a nipple and if it is keeping its eye open, this is the best possible opportunity to have a look at the fundus.

First look for the red reflex by shining the ophthalmoscope from a distance and then advance closer to the eye. Normal fundus is orange red in colour. If the disc does not come into view on examination, trace vessels to the point of their convergence where the disc comes into view. Examine the disc, vessels, macula and the periphery. Note the colour of disc, clarity of edges and the size of depression at the centre (optic cup at the middle of the disc; it looks yellower than the rest of the disc).

The optic disc is pinkish yellow with well-defined margins. Look at the vessels that enter/leave the disc. The veins are wider and darker. Note if the vessels are continuously visible as they enter the disc or appear to disappear (a break in continuity) before reappearing again. Note whether the curves of vessels are smooth and gradual or acute and tortuous. Note the points of crossing of vessels each other; note if one vessel appears to obliterate the other. Look for any haemorrhages (if present, note its shape and relation to vessels); look for any exudates. Inspect retina and see if there is any deviation from uniformity of colour at any place. Finally ask the patient to look at the light to bring macula into view (since looking straight to light will bring on papillary constriction, examination for macula generally needs mydriatics).

The Disc

The medial border of the disc is normally less well defined compared to the temporal (colour is less pale than temporal, so the demarcation from background retina is less clear). Temporal border is yellower than the nasal border and hence stands out sharp against the background of orangish retina. Venous pulsation may be normally seen, and it is best appreciated as the veins enter the optic nerve head. Venous pulsations may be induced by gentle pressure over the eyeballs. Venous pulsations are due to the compression of the veins with each arterial pulsation. The arterial pulsation increases the pressure within the eyeball and hence the compression of the veins, which are compressible (but arteries are not). In papilloedema, the pressure is already raised so that the veins are constantly kept compressed and hence there is no venous pulsation. The physiological cup (optic cup) will be obliterated in papilloedema. The upper and lower margins of disc also become indistinct like the nasal margin; temporal margin is the last to become blurred.

The Vessels

The arteries are narrower and less dark-red compared to veins. Arteries may show a central reflecting line ("silver wire") due to the light reflecting from the rounded arteries (veins are flatter and hence this line is not seen). Variable lumen size (wide and narrow) throughout the course is typical of long standing systemic hypertension. Also, thickened (sclerotic) arteries of systemic hypertension will compress the veins at the point of crossing, obliterating them for a short distance. Engorged tortuous veins ("serpent like") may be seen in papilledema.

The continuity of the vessels appears to be interrupted ("disappear") at the disc margin in case of papilledema; or hump of vessels entering and leaving the disc becomes prominent. This is due to the elevation of the disc. If the power of the ophthalmoscope lens needed to be changed to visualize the vessels over the disc compared to the other areas of the retina, then it may be assumed that the disc is elevated. Thus, the evidence of papilloedema are disappearance of venous pulsations, obliteration of physiological cup, engorged tortuous veins, narrowed arteries and merging of the optic disc with surroundings or its actual elevation from the surrounding. In addition, the area covered by disc enlarges, margins become indefinable; irregular radial red streaks may appear to give disc an "angry" appearance. Still later, haemorrhages/ecchymosis may appear. In addition, white streaks and patches of exudates appear near the disc margins, spreading outwards to macula to give the described appearance of "macular star" or macular fan of exudates; this macular fan the author has seen only in one child in the past 30 years, in a case of malignant hypertension in pheochromocytoma.

Visual acuity is not affected in papilloedema till very late. However, objective testing of visual field will show that the blind spot is enlarging. Papilloedema is seen in brain abscess, intracranial tumours, severe hypertension, pseudotumour cerebri, etc.

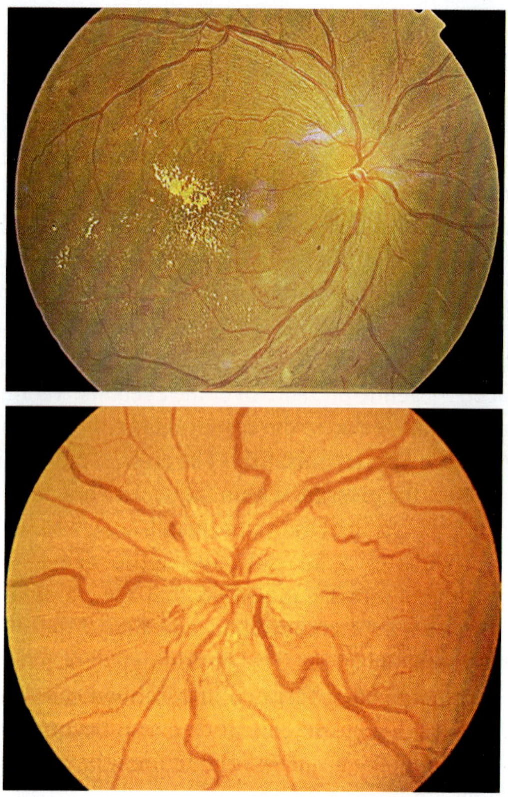

Fig.9.5 Papilloedema. In addition to papilloedema, fundus at the top shows changes of long standing hypertension (cotton wool spots and macular oedema)
(Courtesy: Dr Anitha Balachandran).

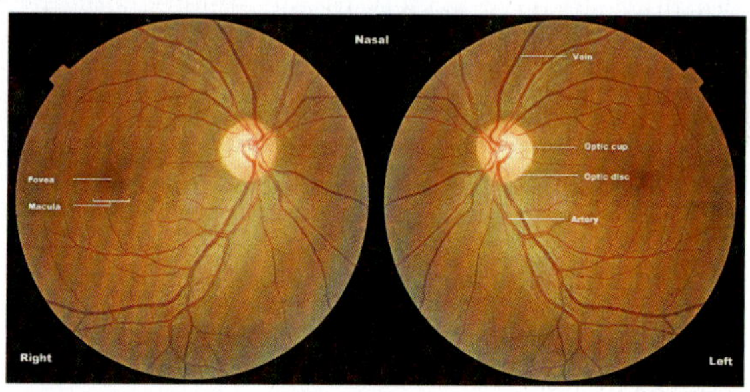

Fig.9.5a Normal fundus

Stages of Papilloedema (Frisen scale)

Stage 0 -	Normal optic disc
Stage 1 -	Very early papilloedema with obscuration of nasal borders of the disc only, without elevation of disc borders
Stage 2 -	Early papilloedema with obscuration of all borders with a complete peripapillary halo.
Stage 3 -	Moderate papilloedema with elevation of all borders with increased diameters of the optic nerve head, with obscuration of vessels at disc margins and peripapillary halo with finger like extensions.
Stage 4 -	Marked papilloedema with elevation of entire nerve head and total obscuration of segments of major blood vessels on the disc.
Stage 5 -	Severe papilloedema with obscuration of all vessels and obliteration of optic cup with macular exudates.

The Retina

Examine the periphery of the fundus for chrorioretinitis, choroid tubercles, haemorrhages, exudates, etc. Haemorrhages may be linear streaks along the vessels or larger ecchymosis. Small pin head dots are seen in diabetic retinopathy (microaneurysms). Exudates are discussed above. Often for visualizing the periphery, mydriatic is essential. Chorioretinitis is seen in toxoplasmosis, rubella, CMV, etc. Choroidal tubercles are seen in miliary tuberculosis (they are rounded, slightly raised and yellowish at centre). Retinitis pigmentosa is seen in some neurodegenerative diseases where it appears like the histopathology appearance of bone corpuscles (Fig. 6.57, p 102). Phakoma is a collection of glial cells appearing in retina as a white plaque; may be seen in tuberous sclerosis, neurofibromatosis, etc. "Cherry red spot" is to be looked for in macula. Macula is a dark orange area lateral and slightly below the disc. Fovea is an area from where a bright light reflex is obtained. For examining the macula, ask the child to look directly into the ophthalmoscope. Cherry red spot is seen in storage diseases like Tay-Sachs disease, Niemann-Pick disease, sialidosis, etc. Note that the cherry red spot appears more like a dark brown spot rather than a red spot (as is seen in the Fig. 9.7).

Optic Atrophy

Pale yellow (almost white) disc is due to optic atrophy; the disc stands out dramatically against the background of orangish retina. There will be reduced number of vessels; the number of vessels that cross the disc margin is reduced to 7 or less (normal adult standard is 10) (Kestenbaum sign). These are the usual findings in primary optic atrophy. Primary optic atrophy is due to local lesions in optic nerve, retina, etc or certain familial disorders like Leber's optic atrophy.

Optic atrophy is said to be secondary or consecutive optic atrophy when it follows long standing papilloedema. Here, the disc appears dirty, grayish with irregular and indistinct margins (the architecture of optic nerve head is lost due to the insult). In contrast, in primary optic atrophy the disc is pale yellow with sharp margins (the architecture of optic nerve head is well maintained).

Myopic Fundus

Myopic disc appears very pale and large. It is best to obtain opinion of ophthalmologist. Examining through patient's own spectacles gives the most accurate information.

Hypermetropic Fundus

The disc is small and may appear reddish so that the edges may appear indistinct as it merges with surrounding reddish retina. Vessels are normal.

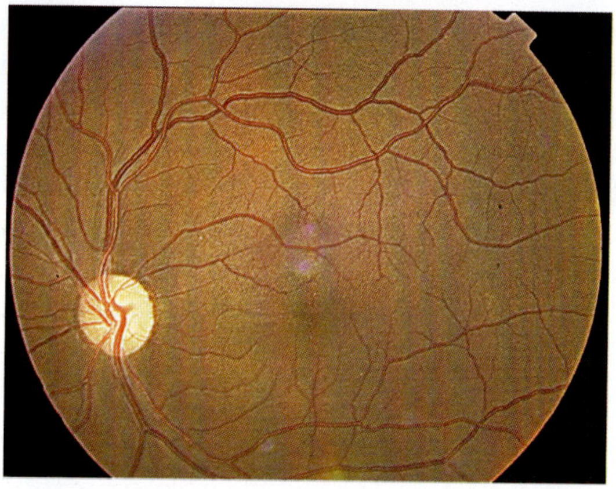

Fig.9.6 Optic atrophy *(Courtesy: Dr Anitha Balachandram)*

Glaucoma

The optic cup is very large (almost making one suspect whether the cup is the disc itself).

Papillitis

Clinical findings are consistent with papilloedema but less remarkable; there is marked loss of vision and pain during movement of eyeballs. Papillitis is almost always unilateral. Papillitis could either be due to inflammation or demyelination.

Retrobulbar Neuritis

The patient is blind but the fundus examination fails to reveal any abnormality. "Neither the doctor nor the patient sees anything!"

Pseudopapilloedema

It is the anomalous elevation of optic disc without having papilloedema. By fundus examination, it looks like mild papilledema but without vessel engorgement or symptoms. The appearance may remain static throughout life. This term should not be confused with pseudotumour cerebri, where there is true papilledema due to actual increase in intracranial pressure.

Drusen disc, due to some proteinacious deposit near the nerve head (colloid bodies or Drusen bodies) during the developmental process is a common reason for pseudopapilloedema. The shapes of discs of two sides may be different if they can be made out. The Drusen affected one may be oval in shape, and the fundus is not angry looking unlike papilloedema.

Foster Kennedy Syndrome

This is mentioned here only on theoretical interest. One will never see it in a life time! A strategically positioned tumour in posterior inferior frontal region can cause optic atrophy on the same side by compression and papilledema on the other side by venous obstruction.

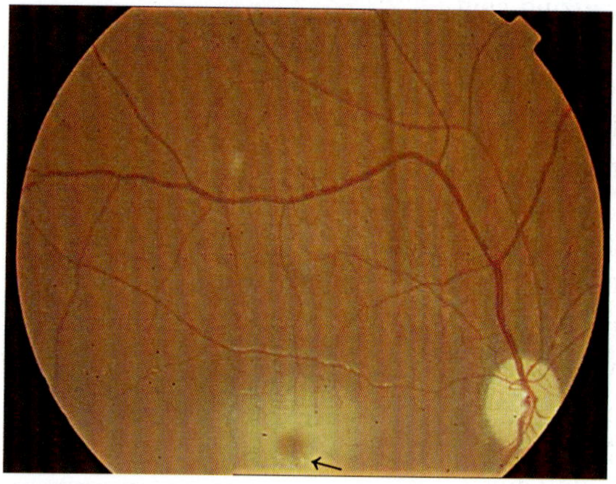

Fig.9.7 Cherry red spot

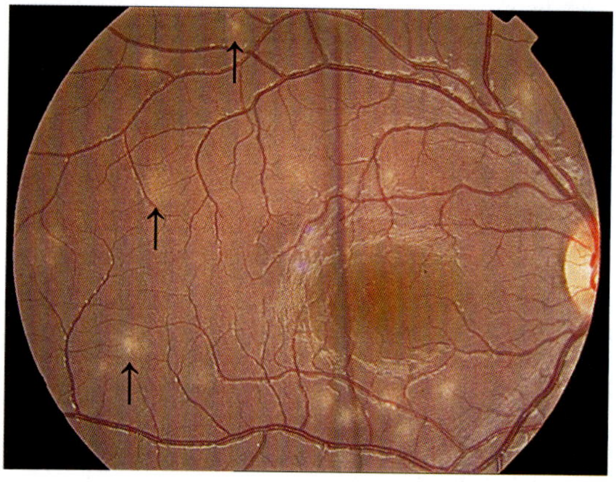

Fig.9.8 Choroidal tuberculosis

5. Pupil

It is discussed along with the third nerve.

Nerves III, IV and VI

The functions of these nerves are so closely related that it is best considered together. They control all external ocular muscles. Autonomic nerves running in relation to these nerves and the V nerve regulate pupillary muscles.

Abducens Nerve (VI): Supplies the lateral rectus (mnemonic: "LR6"). The nerve has a long intracranial course so that it may get involved in generalized disturbances like cerebral oedema (false localizing sign). VI nerve palsy produces convergent strabismus, meaning that since abduction is weak, the eye remains adducted. Attempts to look laterally produces diplopia as the affected eye cannot turn laterally (also see Fig. 24.93).

Trochlear Nerve (IV): Supply superior oblique (mnemonic: "SO_4"). The left trochlear nucleus and nerve supply the right superior oblique and vice versa (it is because the nerve crosses before exit).

Weakness due to IV nerve palsy/nuclear agenesis may be congenital. In case of congenital, the child adjusts with head tilt towards the opposite shoulder to eliminate a vertical deviation of two images from the two eyes; thus will never be noticed or symptomatic unless specifically looked for. Acquired IV nerve palsy is very rare. Most clinicians may not have seen one themselves. The most common cause of acute fourth nerve palsy is head trauma causing transient stretching of the nerve. Lax superior oblique tendons is another cause for presentation like IV nerve palsy.

The diplopia gets worse when the affected eye looks toward the nose. The contribution of the superior oblique muscle to downward gaze is greatest in this position. Common activities requiring such a convergent gaze are reading and walking downstairs. In Fig. 9.14 (p 197), the adduction and internal rotation of left eye is less than the right eye when looking at a pen kept at nose level. This is suggestive of IV nerve paralysis (see p 197).

Oculomotor Nerve (III): Supply all other extraocular muscles, except lateral rectus and superior oblique. It also supplies the levator palpebrae superioris and serves as an efferent for the pupillary reflex. Paralysis causes divergent strabismus. See discussion below (see Fig. 24.92).

The nerves III, IV & VI route through the cavernous sinus on their way to the muscles and hence ophthalmoplegia can occur in cavernous sinus thrombosis.

- *Tests to be performed*: III, IV and VI nerves are usually tested together. Examine for ptosis, pupils, squint and nystagmus. Also test for pupillary reaction to light and accommodation. Look for eye movements in all directions and convergence. Ask for diplopia. Make a note of exophthalmos (protruded eyeball) or enophthalmos (recessed eyeball), if present.

  After examining the pupils, the student must be able to localize any abnormality of the pupil detected as due to local cause, autonomic cause or cranial nerve nucleus involvement. In case eye movement abnormality is detected, the problem could be localized to muscular problem, cranial nerve lesion, cranial nerve nuclear lesion or supranuclear control. Although nystagmus is looked for, it must be borne in mind that it is closely related to vestibular function and hence this should be considered before localizing the lesion.

1. Ptosis

Compare the proportion of cornea covered by the upper lid in both eyes to identify ptosis. If pupil is at least partly covered by the lid, there is definite ptosis. The causes of ptosis are congenital, paralysis of 3rd nerve, paralysis of cervical sympathetics (i.e., Horner syndrome. Here, the ptosis is partial and is due to the weakness of tarsal muscles of upper lid), myasthenia gravis, myopathies involving eye muscles, local inflammation of the eye, etc. In myasthenia, on prolonged fixation, the lid will droop progressively, but after a blink it may get restored to normal. In ocular myopathy, the ptosis is fixed and head is often held extended in an attempt to see under the drooping lids. In case of III nerve palsy, look for wrinkling of forehead, which may point towards the child attempting to keep the eyes open by frontalis action (Fig. 9.9). In such cases, one may try to fix the frontalis by a hand on the head and see if ptosis now becomes obvious. In case of sympathetic paralysis, the child may still be able to elevate the lid voluntarily but left alone again droops to partial ptosis.

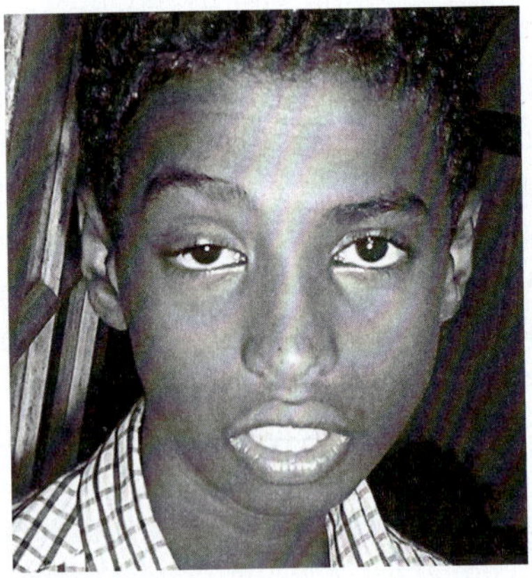

Fig.9.9 Ptosis partially compensated by right frontalis action.

2. Eye Movements

- The eye movements are complex due to the involvement of more than one muscle in individual movements. Hence to test each muscle, the position at which a single muscle is producing an action without the help of other muscles is to be selected. Thus, when the eye is abducted, superior and inferior recti act as pure elevators or depressors (recti abducted for testing. Mnemonic: "rab for test"). It is easy to remember that the reverse is true for the obliques; the superior and inferior obliques are pure depressors or elevators when in adducted position.

  The action of ocular muscles: the muscles paired below act as a pair for the movements indicated.

  Lateral rectus (VI nerve): Moves the eye horizontally outwards; Medial rectus (III nerve): moves the eye horizontally inwards.

  Superior rectus (III nerve): elevates the eye when it is turned outwards; Inferior oblique (III nerve): elevates the eye when it is turned inwards.

  Inferior rectus (III nerve): depresses the eye when it is turned outwards; Superior oblique (IV nerve): depresses the eye when it is turned inwards.
- The testing of extraocular muscles may appear complex, but it really is very simple and takes practically no time. Look for ptosis. Ask the child to look to the right. Now his right lateral rectus and left medial rectus are tested. Then from this position ask the child to look up. Now his right superior rectus and left inferior oblique are tested. Then ask the child to look down. Now his right inferior rectus and left superior oblique are tested. Similarly, test on the other side, and finish the testing by

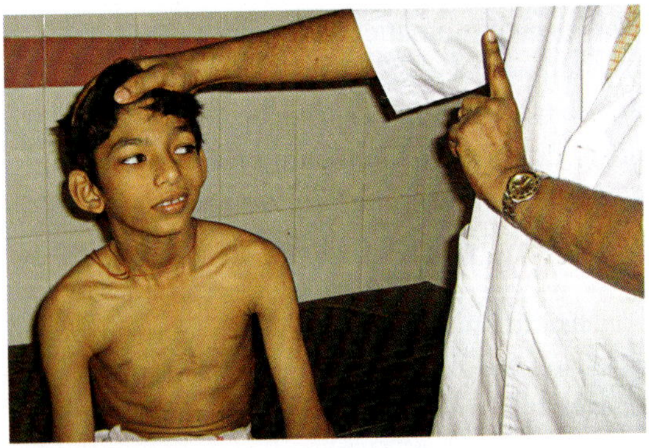

Fig.9.10 Testing for extraocular muscles on left side individually. Note that the head is fixed to avoid inadvertant head movements.

asking the child to look at a distance and then shift his look quickly to a finger kept near the nose; this tests the convergence.

- Some clinicians prefer another method; they start with testing of accommodation, followed by asking the child to follow the object that he moves around in the direction shown in Fig. 9.12.
- For patients in coma, one can test ***Doll's-eye movement*** or oculo-cephalic response to find out if the eyeball is moving in various directions. Rotate the head from side to side and observe the eye for conjugate movement in opposite direction. Neck flexion produces upgaze and extension produces downgaze. Doll's-eye movement shows that the brainstem is intact.
- If coma is deep, doll's-eye movement may not be obtained. So one may try ***cold calorie test***. The head is elevated 30° to the horizontal and cold water is instilled into the external auditory meatus. The response in a conscious patient is nystagmus with its slow phase towards the irrigated ear (brainstem response) with a rapid corrective jerk in the opposite direction (cerebral hemisphere correcting the deviating eye). The reverse of this is expected when one irrigates with warm water. The fast component of nystagmus in a normal conscious child is remembered by the mnemonic, COWS—cold opposite warm same (see p 239).
- **Supranuclear palsy**: Lesions of the cortex or midbrain (supranuclear palsy) cause gaze palsy without paralysis of individual ocular muscles.

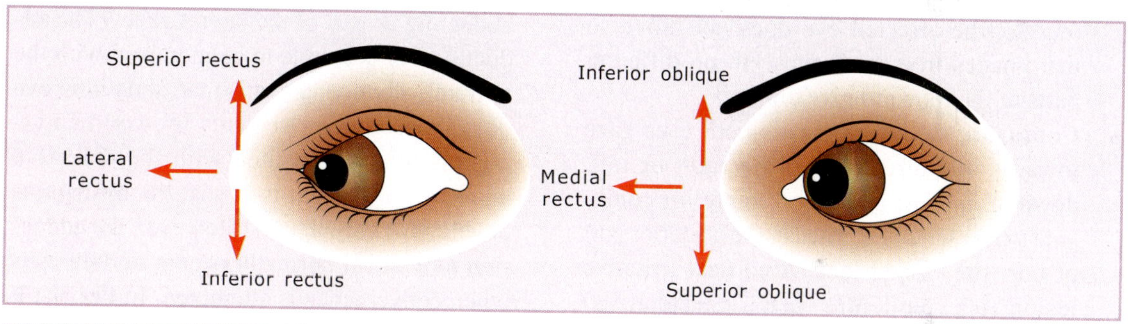

Fig.9.11 Eye movements

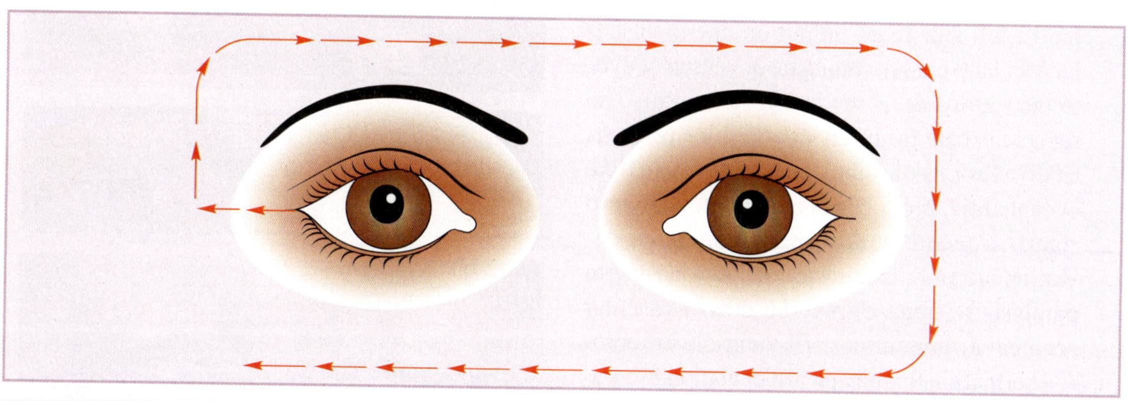

Fig.9.12 Direction of movement of the object to test all extra ocular muscles

Gaze palsy means paralysis of movement of *both* eyes in one direction or other. In supranuclear palsy, there is no *diplopia* ("double vison"), as it is the gaze to one direction that is lost. Hence if one eye is not moving, there is corresponding immobility of the other eye also so that both eyes are in corresponding parallel axes and so there is no diplopia. If the child can cooperate, ask him to fix his eyes on a particular object while the examiner turns his head passively; in supranuclear palsy, the eyes will move throughout their full range on reflex fixation, even though voluntarily the child cannot do so. The presence of diplopia localizes the lesion to the nucleus or infranuclear location (LMN lesion). Thus, if there is weakness of one extraocular muscle, when one is looking towards the direction of action of that muscle, the affected eye does not move so that images from both eyes fall on different parts of the retina to give diplopia.

- **Conjugate deviation** means both eyes gaze towards one direction, to the right or left, down or up. The centre for control of conjugate movements is situated at the posterior part of opposite frontal lobe. A cortical irritative lesion (e.g., epileptic focus; encephalitis) causes conjugate deviation of eye to the opposite side (mnemonic: CIA, meaning cortical irritative away). A cortical destructive lesion on the left side (e.g., infarction due to vascular accident) causes conjugate deviation of eyes to the same side as the lesion (left side). The reverse is true for brain stem lesions (e.g., irritative lesions of right side of brain stem, like encephalitis, produces conjugate deviation to right). Upward or downward conjugate deviation are rare. Downward deviation (due to paralysis of upgaze) may be due to vascular accident or tumour near III ventricle or tentorial herniation. Fixed upward deviation is commonly due to drug side effect (oculogyric spasm due to metoclopramide).
- **Internuclear connections**: For conjugate movements to take effect, the nuclei of III, IV, VI nerves of both sides are connected to each other by fibres running through the medial longitudinal fasciculus at brain stem, which also contains fibres connecting vestibular nuclei. Of course, conjugate movements may have a central control from frontal lobe (see discussion on conjugate deviation above) and possibly occipital lobe.
- **Internuclear ophthalmoplegia**: Since the medial longitudinal fasciculus is essential for coordinating conjugate movements, a lesion in the medial longitudinal fasciculus will cause dissociation of conjugate movements. In the usual scenario, there is weakness of adduction of the eye on the side of lesion of MLF and nystagmus of the opposite eye, which is abducting as part of the lateral gaze. (The adducting eye is unable to be in unison with the normally abducting eye; so the abducting eye does corrective movements by way of nystagmus to come in tune with the defective adducting eye. That is to say, the nystagmus develops in normal eye.) However, the adduction movement normally occurs in both eyes when convergence is attempted. In Fig. 9.13, on looking to right, the ocular deviation to right

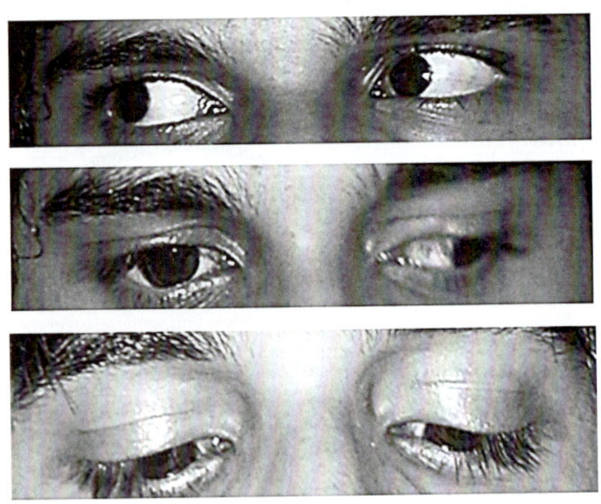

Fig.9.13 Internuclear ophthalmoplegia

is normal in both eyes. On looking to the left, the adduction of right eye is defective and the eye may somewhat turn downwards on attempted adduction; lateral movement of left eye, which occurs simultaneously as part of conjugate movement, causes marked nystagmus of left eye. On looking to the tip of nose, both eyes adduct as part of convergence.

- **Skew deviation**: One eye is up and out, whereas the other looks down and in; i.e., vertical dysconjugation of eyes.
- **Exophthalmos** is the protrusion of the eyeball. It may be due to retro-orbital lesions, craniostenosis, or Graves disease (here it is bilateral and may be associated with lid retraction; if sclera is seen above the iris, then there is lid retraction). It is unlikely to be due to neurological lesions. Assess protrusion of the eyes by looking down on the eyes from above and behind the patient's head. Unilateral exophthalmos can still be due to thyroid disease, but more likely are orbital or retro-orbital neoplasms or granulomas. In cavernous sinus thrombosis, there is exophthalmos, ptosis and oculomotor palsy. **Enophthalmos** is retraction of the eyeball. It may be seen as a congenital anomaly (maldeveloped eye), in Horner's syndrome and in severe dehydration.

3. Squint

It is the lack of parallelism of visual axes (see Figs. 24.92 & 24.93). There are two types of squint, paralytic and concomitant.

- **Paralytic squint**: Paralysis of one or more extraocular muscles causes paralytic squint. When looking towards the direction of action of the paralyzed muscle, there is limitation of ocular movement in that direction so that images from two eyes fall on different parts of retina, causing diplopia. However, there is no squint when looking in directions where the paralyzed muscle does not have its action. It is to be noted that uniocular diplopia (diplopia when one eye is closed) is always due to local causes like opacities in the lens/cornea, astigmatism or dislocated lens.
Diplopia of neurological origin manifest when both eyes are open (in neuroparalysis only one image is formed from each eye and hence only one image falls on the retina when the other eye is closed).
- **Concomitant squint**: Here, squint is present in all positions of eyes. When the fixing eye is covered, the squinting eye can move in all directions, in full range. There is no double vision as the defect has been there since early years (at birth or below 5 years) and brain has learned to suppress the image from the squinting eye. In fact, that is the greatest danger, the brain ignoring the image from squinting eye, so that the squinting eye becomes amblyopic (see p 198).
- **Convergent squint**: Here, the eyeballs are turned inwards. It is a paralytic squint due to paralysis of the lateral rectus, due to VI nerve palsy. An apparent convergent squint is normal in the first few months of life, possibly due to the fact that medial rectus is stronger or child is trying to look at close point bringing accommodation into play. Refractory errors also may cause a convergent squint as the child tries excessive accommodation. This will disappear once the child starts wearing glasses.
- **Divergent squint**: It is a paralytic squint, usually due to third nerve palsy. Third nerve palsy causes divergent squint (due to unopposed action of lateral rectus), dilated pupils and ptosis (Fig. 24.92).

9

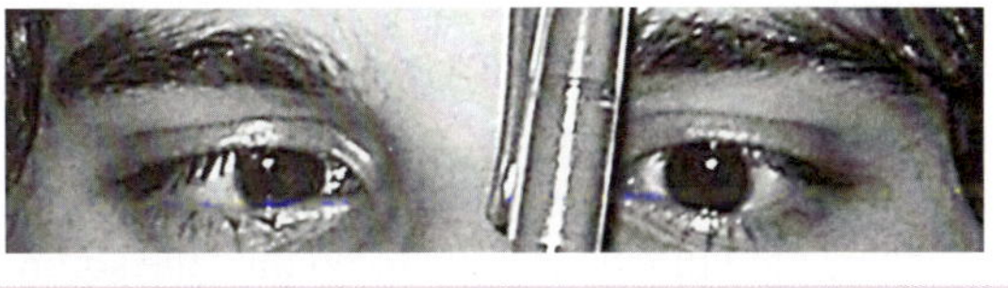

Fig.9.14 IV nerve palsy

- Trochlear nerve supplies superior oblique muscle whose function is looking down and in. Palsy of the superior oblique muscle (IV nerve palsy) causes inability to turn the eye down and in. We do not look down and in usually and hence visible squint is rare. Double vision while walking downstairs is the classical symptom that will clinch the diagnosis. An isolated right superior oblique paralysis results in exotropia to the right (divergent squint), causing confusion with III nerve palsy. The lack of ptosis and/or pupillary involvement allows easy distinction of the exotropia of IV nerve paralysis from that seen in III nerve paralysis.
  Note: Even when squint is not very apparent on clinical examination, if the child complains of diplopia, there is every possibility that there is a subtle squint and so look for it meticulously. If there is still difficulty, try the following. Ask the child to follow your fingers in different directions and find out at which position the double vision is maximum. Then find out which eye is to be covered to obliterate the outer image. It is because at maximum diplopia, the outer image is formed by the defective eye. Also look for a head tilt, which may be there to compensate for diplopia.
- **Cover-uncover test**: Ask the child to look at a distant object. Cover one eye and observe the uncovered eye for any movement. If the uncovered eye moves, it means that the uncovered eye is now fixing, which in turn means that it was the covered eye that was fixing when both eyes were open and the uncovered eye was squinting without fixing. In the Fig. 9.15, the patient is looking ahead but the left eye is squinting (turned inwards). However, when the good eye is covered, the squinting eye is forced to fix for the patient to continue viewing the object. To do this, the squinting eye moves to take up the central position. This is concomitant squint. In paralytic squint, the squinting eye cannot move when the good eye is covered. The movement of the squinting eye when the normal eye is fixing (uncovered) is primary deviation. The movement of the normal eye when the squinting eye is forced to fix (by covering the normal eye) is secondary deviation. Primary and secondary deviations are of equal magnitude in concomitant squint. In paralytic squint, the secondary deviation is greater than the primary deviation (extra effort to move the paralysed eye causes excess conjugate movement of normal eye).

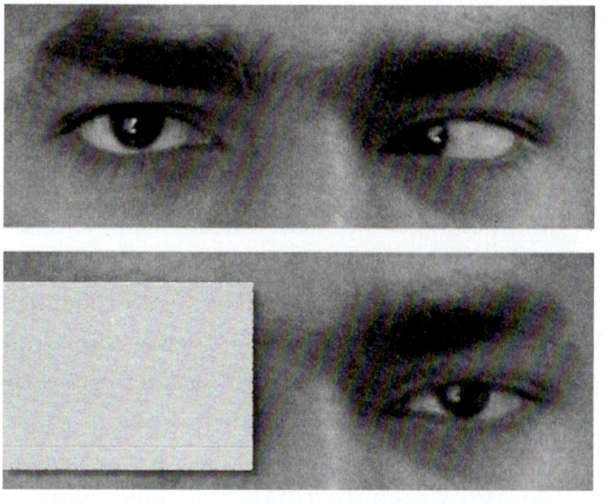

Fig.9.15 Concomitant squint

Diplopia

- Diplopia may become manifest even before a neurological examination can reveal weakness of ocular muscles. The images fails to fall on the corresponding areas of two retinae.
- The false image is less clear or less distinct.
- Displacement of false image may be vertical or horizontal or both.
- Separation between the true and false image is greatest (the false image is farthest) in the direction in which the weak muscle has its action.
- Method of testing:

- Cover one eye with red transparent glass.
- Move an object in various directions as described under testing of extraocular muscles.
- Ask if the patient sees one object or two.
- If two, whether the two images lie side by side or one above the other. If exactly side by side, medial or lateral rectus is weak. If one above the other, superior/inferior oblique/recti are involved.
- Which of the images (nearer one or farther one) is red?
- At which position of the eye there is maximum displacement of the images? If maximum displacement occurs when looking to the left and up, the pair of muscles involved is the left superior rectus and the right inferior oblique (see p 194). To know which of the two muscles of this pair is at fault, ask the patient which of the two images is farthest, the red one or the white one. If the red glass were over the left eye and on looking to the left and up the red image is the farthest, then the muscle moving the eye upwards while looking to the left is at fault, that is superior rectus. In this scenario, if the white image were the farthest, then right inferior oblique would be at fault (it is the duty of right inferior oblique to focus the image from right eye).

4. Nystagmus

The eye instead of fixing, oscillates when trying to fix. Nystagmus is normal at extremes of lateral gaze in normal subjects. Contrary to popular belief, nystagmus is not a diagnostic sign of cerebellar disease. It can occur in defective vision, vestibular disturbances (vestibular nuclei or its central/peripheral connections), brainstem dysfunction, etc.

Method of examination: Hold an object like pencil in front and ask the child to look at that. Move the pencil to left, right, up and down (while looking down, hold eyelids up by hand to visualize any nystagmus) and maintain that position for a few seconds to look for nystagmus. On lateral deviation, extreme lateral deviation and prolonged lateral deviation can cause nystagmus due to strain (when the strained eye drifts medially there is a rapid corrective movement that manifest as nystagmus).

By convention, the direction of nystagmus is described according to its fast component (see COWS under cold calorie test, p 239). But it is always more informative to give a full description; e.g., on looking to the right there is fine nystagmus with its fast component to the right.

9

- **Horizontal nystagmus**: To and fro oscillation in the horizontal plane with slow component in one direction and fast component in the opposite direction. It is the most common type and occurs in vestibular and cerebellar lesions.
- **Vertical nystagmus** is rarer but can occur in brainstem problems like brainstem encephalitis, syringobulbia, compression from cerebellar tumours, tonsillar herniation, Arnold Chiari malformation, etc but by far the most common reason is drug toxicity, examples being phenytoin, phenobarbitone, etc. This is not a nystagmus on looking up or down but a nystagmus where oscillation in up-down direction, no matter what the position of eye. Depending on which direction the fast component goes, it is termed up-beat or down-beat nystagmus (up-beat is far more common).

  Mnemonic: Visualize cerebellum and brainstem. Brainstem is a vertically placed structure and so vertical nystagmus; Cerebellum is a horizontally placed structure and so horizontal nystagmus!
- **Rotary nystagmus**: It is seen in labyrinthine disorders (imagine the rotating feel of labyrinthitis, you will not forget the type of nystagmus). It is occasionally seen in a congenitally blind child. More common in the blind child is pendular nystagmus where, to and fro movements are equal (see p 194). If the student

can imagine a blind man trying to localize things by to and fro and rotary movements of his hand, then the student will not forget the type of nystagmus in the blind.

- **Optokinetic nystagmus**: It is elicitable in the normal person. The classic example is a child looking out of the window from a moving bus. When the child follows the objects outside (like the trees), the eye slowly moves to follow that object till it disappears, and then suddenly the eye is pulled back to the opposite direction in a quick corrective action. Thus, there is a slow and rapid component of this nystagmus. In clinical setting, optokinetic nystagmus is elicited by making the child look at a rotating drum with black and white stripes. Usually in all nystagmus, the rapid corrective jerk (rapid component of nystagmus) is produced by the frontal cerebral cortex and lesions here may abolish it. As the eye deviates, the cerebral cortex identifies it as wrong and quickly pulls back to the normal position to produce the rapid jerk.
- In **pendular nystagmus** of visual defects (macular abnormalities, chorioretinitis, high infantile myopia, albinism, etc), there is no rapid component as there is no visual impulses going in for the cortex to identify the eye movement as wrong. Nystagmus in a visually handicapped child is basically because the eye is not fixing at anything and hence wandering. Pendular nystagmus is oscillation to either side of midline, of equal amplitude, but of variable speed (speed increases on trying to fixate).
- **Opsoclonus**: It is rapid, chaotic multi-directional eye movements seen classically in metastatic neuroblastoma. When this rapid jerky movements are only in horizontal plane, the term 'occular flutter' is used.

5. Pupils

Sphincter pupillae is supplied by the III nerve and dilator pupillae is supplied by the cervical sympathetics.

- **Constricted pupil (miosis)** is seen in morphine poisoning, organophosphorus poisoning, pontine haemorrhage, Horner's syndrome, etc. Mnemonic of pupils in coma: **M**id size pupil in **M**idbrain lesions and **P**in point pupil in **P**ontine lesions. But the most common cause of bilateral constricted pupil is normal variation! For example, in deep sleep or sedation the pupil may remain constricted. In addition to the above mnemonic, interruption of sympathetic anywhere can cause dysfunction of dialator pupillae muscle and hence small pupil. Sympathetic pathway may get interrupted anywhere from hypothalamus to brainstem to upper thoracic spinal cord, sympathetic ganglia, sympathetic fibres and plexus along the carotids and the sympathetic running along the ophthalmic division of V cranial nerve.
- **Dilated pupils (mydriasis)** are seen in optic nerve paralysis, third nerve paralysis, diphtheria (due to ciliary nerve damage), etc. But the most common cause of dilated pupil is mydriatic eye drops! Sympathetic stimulation as in fear can also cause dilated pupils. Parasympathetic paralysis also cause dilated pupil. Parasympathetics have their origin at pre-tectal nuclei and Edinger Westphal nucleus in midbrain, travel along with III cranial nerve to ciliary ganglion in the orbit. Unilateral dilated pupil may be because of third nerve damage due to brain herniation (of course, mydriatic eye drops is a more common cause for unilateral dilated pupil). In very early stages of herniation, there may be irritation of nerve to produce constricted pupil transiently and once the third nerve gets dysfunctional due to compression, the pupil gets dilated.
- Fibres from the retina relay in Edinger-Westphal nucleus of both sides, so that the pupillary reflex and accommodation will be bilateral even if only one eye is stimulated.
- **Accommodation**: Ask the child to look at a distant object and then suddenly look at the

finger kept near the nose. Observe the constriction of both pupils and convergence (adduction) of both eyes medially.

- **Direct light reflex**: This is tested by showing light to a pupil, bringing it slowly from the lateral side to see the reaction of pupils clearly. If the light is shown from the front, accommodation response also may act and hence the importance of showing light from the lateral side for testing light reflex. Look at the other eye for consensual light reflex, which is the constriction of the other pupil.
- In lesions of the afferent pathway (optic nerve), when light is shown to the affected eye, there is no direct or consensual light reflex and the pupil remains dilated. However, when light is shown to the normal eye, there is normal direct light reflex of normal eye and normal consensual light reflex on the affected eye. This is because the consensual light reflex is mediated by the efferent limb (III nerve), which is intact in the affected eye.
- **Swinging light test** for afferent lesions (optic nerve): When light is shown alternatively to one eye and to the next, normally the pupil to which light is shown will constrict. But if there is an afferent lesion in the right eye, when light is shown to the right eye, there is no reaction to any eye as the stimulus is not conveyed to brain. But when light is shown to the left eye, both eyes constrict as a result of direct and consensual reaction, respectively. Now take the light to the right eye, and alas! You will find the right eye goes on dilating in spite of light being shown to it (Marcus Gunn pupil). This is because the right eye, which had constricted by consensual reflex just a moment ago is now dilating to its normal position, uninterrupted by the light shown to it, the light shown being not perceived because of optic nerve lesion.
- In lesions of the efferent pathway (oculomotor nerve), when light is shown to the affected eye, there is no direct light reflex on that eye (pupil remain dilated), but will have consensual light reflex in the *opposite* eye.
  This is because the normal optic nerve from the affected eye carries impulses to E-W nucleus (common for both sides) and efferent goes to oculomotor of both sides. Since the oculomotor is normal in the opposite eye, one gets the consensual light reflex there. As the oculomotor is not intact in the affected eye, the direct reflex cannot occur in the affected eye. When light is shown to the normal eye, consensual light reflex cannot occur in the affected eye, again because the oculomotor is not intact.
- It may be noted that most of the time there is no total palsy of nerves and hence these reflexes will be sluggish rather than totally absent in the above mentioned situations.
- Argyll **R**obertson **P**upil: **A**ccommodation **R**eflex **P**resent and **P**upillary **R**eflex **A**bsent. [Mnemonic : ARP-read forward & backward]. It is classically described in neurosyphilis but may be found in encephalitis as well. The site of lesion is debated, but since syphilis is known to affect multiple sites, tectum of midbrain and ciliary ganglion may be the probable candidate sites.
- Myotonic pupil (Holmes-Adie): Pupillary reaction is very slow. In fact, pupil reacts better to accommodation than light. There is exaggerated response to minute doses of methacholine eye drops. The site of lesion is possibly ciliary ganglion.
- ***Oculomotor apraxia***: The patient cannot turn his eyes independent of head movement; so to look to one direction he has to turn the head, not just the eyes alone; it may be seen in ataxia telangiectasia.
- ***Saccades***: These are voluntary rapid eye movements trying to fix at different targets. Instruct the patient to rapidly fixate alternately on two widely separated targets. Test the saccade movements in horizontal, vertical, and oblique

9

directions. Observe for the time to initiate saccade and the velocity of saccade movements.

- ***Pursuit***: These are smooth tracking movements by the eyes to keep the object of interest centred on the retina. Hold the head of patient still and ask him to follow the swinging stethoscope. Normal eyes will keep up with the swinging stethoscope.

III Nerve Nucleus

The postgraduate student may be required to know details of oculomotor nerve nucleus, especially when the patient has a partial third nerve involvement.

The oculomotor nucleus is located in the dorsal midbrain at the level of the superior colliculi. This is a compound nucleus and not a simple one. The components of oculomotor nucleus complex include two midline structures and two lateral ones as shown in the diagram (Fig. 9.16). The oculomotor nucleus complex receives bilateral cortical innervation and has connection with cerebellum and brainstem nuclei.

Fibres destined for levator palpebrae muscle (see Fig. 9.16) and the pupillary sphincter (from Edinger-Westphal nucleus) come from the midline unpaired nuclei. The fibres for the superior rectus arise from the contralateral nucleus and cross over to innervate the muscle.

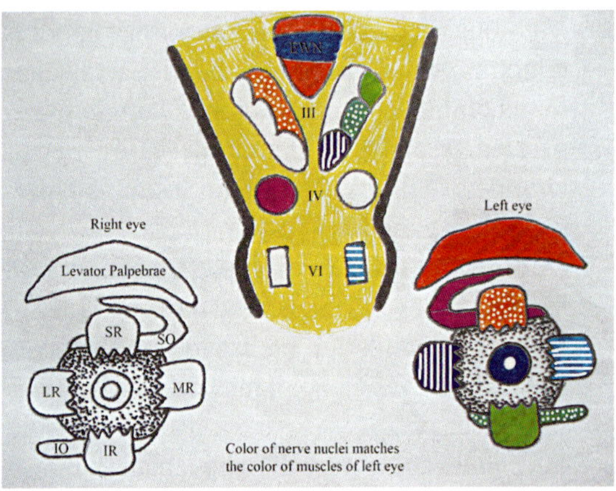

Fig.9.16 III nerve nucleus at the top and two eyes with extra ocular muscles at the bottom *(Drawing by Dr Binoy Stephen)*.

The fibres for the inferior and medial recti, and inferior oblique arise from the ipsilateral oculomotor nucleus. Sixth nerve nucleus has ipsilateral innervation, whereas the IV nerve crossover to innervate the opposite side.

Trigeminal Nerve (V Nerve)

The child is asked to clench the teeth hard and the contractions of the masseters and temporalis are palpated over the cheek and temple. He is asked to open the mouth and asked to try to deviate the jaw to either side against resistance. Sensory loss over the ipsilateral face and weakness of the muscles of mastication are expected in paralysis of fifth nerve.

- When mouth is opened wide, the jaw deviates to the paralyzed side if there is paralysis. This is because the action of each pterygoid muscle (supplied by V) is to push the jaw to the midline. So when one side is paralyzed, the jaw moves to the paralyzed side, being pushed over by the pterygoid muscle of the healthy side. Naturally, if the child is asked to move the jaw laterally against resistance, the movement to the side opposite to paralysis is weak. Difficult to comprehend? Pterygoid muscle, which is to bring the jaw to midline is the one that must act when one tries to move the jaw to the opposite side. If this is paralyzed on one side, movement of the jaw in the opposite direction is weak (refer to an easy mnemonic under the discussion of XII nerve, p 209).
- In case of bilateral paralysis, the jaw droops and the jaw movements are weak to either side. However, one must remember that even unilateral paralysis of V is rare, leave alone the bilateral paralysis.
- Test for jaw jerk. Let the child's jaw sag a bit, place a finger below lower lip and tap it in a downward direction with percussion hammer.

There may be a palpable or observable upward jerk. Absent jaw jerk has no significance as many normal people have absent jaw jerk.
It is exaggerated, even to the extent of jaw clonus in UMN lesions above the level of pons.

- Also look for corneal reflex (afferent is trigeminal) by stroking at the limbus with a cotton strand.
- Corneal reflex: If there is no response to touching the cornea on one side, it could be due to sensory (V) or motor (VII) problem. In V nerve lesions, there will be no eye lid blinking on either side when the abnormal side is stimulated; and a normal blink from both eyes when the normal side is stimulated. In VII nerve lesion, there will be no blink response on the side of facial paralysis, no matter which side is stimulated; and there will be a blink response on normal side when the abnormal side is touched.
  Important: Loss of corneal reflex may be the first sign of cerebello-pontine angle tumour.
- Test for sensations over the face. Testing over the forehead & upper part of side of nose; cheeks & upper lips; and chin & anterior part of tongue tests ophthalmic, maxillary and mandibular divisions, respectively. Note that the skin over the angle of jaw is supplied by cervical segments, and not V nerve.
- Note: Trigeminal nerve nucleus has a descending tract, which may extend down to the spinal canal as far as C2. Thus, in lesions like syringomyelia involving the upper cervical segments, one may find sensory blunting of the face (pain and temperature) although the lesion is in the spinal cord.
- Fibres supplying lacrymal and salivary glands from the facial nerve travel through the branches of V nerve.
- The causes of V nerve palsy include brainstem glioma, cerebellopontine angle tumour (acoustic neuroma), demyelination, cavernous sinus thrombosis, etc.
- Lesions of V nerve in peripheral locations are not seen in clinical situations. In cavernous sinus thrombosis, ophthalmic & maxillary divisions of V nerve (usually sensory deficits) may be involved. Tumours of cerebellopontine angle involve V, VII and VIII nerves and cerebellar outflow tracts.

Facial Nerve (VII Nerve)

Facial nerve: For clinical purposes, facial nerve proper and nervus intermedius are considered as one entity. N. intermedius carries secretory fibres to lacrymal gland (via greater petrosal nerve) and to salivary gland (chorda tympani); chorda tympani also carries taste sensation from anterior $2/3^{rd}$ of tongue.

On inspection, note any asymmetry of wrinkles of forehead or nasolabial fold while talking/smiling and spontaneous blinking. Assess motor functions by requesting the child to perform manoeuvres described later in this section.

A lower motor neuron lesion of the nerve, results in complete lack of ipsilateral facial movements (both upper and lower parts of face are involved); the nasolabial fold on the paralyzed side is obliterated; the face draws to the *opposite* side as the patient smiles (due to the action of muscles of normal side). Eye closure is impaired, and the ipsilateral palpebral fissure is wider. LMN facial palsy is the result of interruption of common final pathway anywhere from nucleus to muscles.

Useful points for localization in LMN VII palsy: If VI nerve also is involved, lesion could be in pons. Hemiplegia, if present, will be on the opposite side. (crossed hemiplegia)

If V and VIII nerves are also involved, lesion is at cerebello-pontine angle.

If taste, salivation and tears are affected, lesion could be between brainstem and departure of chorda tympani nerve in middle ear. Distortion of sound due to stapedius palsy will also be associated.

9

If taste and salivation are affected, but tear production is normal, lesion is in middle ear, after the departure of superficial petrosal branch, but before the departure of chorda tympani.

Usual paralysis of VII is only motor; in which case the site of lesion is likely to be either nucleus or compression at facial canal.

Damage to VII in the parotid gland (e.g., iatrogenic) results in some muscles of face being paralyzed (usually those in upper part of face), whereas others are not.

In unilateral upper motor neuron lesion, *only the lower half of the face is paralyzed.* This is because the lower part of the face has supranuclear control from the opposite hemisphere only. (Most of the other cranial nerves and the upper part of face have got bilateral cortical innervation so that just one hemisphere dysfunction cannot produce UMN palsy of these cranial nerves; also see p 209). However, please note that some involvement of eye closure can occur in UMN also and hence take into account the condition of the patient before committing to whether it is UMN or LMN. For example, in a case of hemiplegia, if facial palsy is on the same side, UMN facial is most likely.

Localization of LMN Facial Palsy

- If it is a nuclear palsy (i.e., facial nerve nucleus is involved), it will be LMN but generally there will be associated pyramidal signs or involvement of adjacent nerve nuclei like V or VI.
- Isolated LMN facial palsy has its site of lesion in an extracranial location (unlikely to be nuclear involvement). The most common cause is Bell's palsy where the site is somewhere near the stylomastoid foramen (Fig. 9.16a). Here, LMN facial palsy without sensory involvement and without hyperacusis is expected as the chorda tympani and nerve to stapedius have branched out before the facial nerve reaches the stylomastoid foramen.
- Facial nerve also carries parasympathetics to the salivary and lacrymal glands. Lacrimation may be absent when the lesion is in the geniculate ganglion. Taste will be affected if the lesion is before the chorda tympani nerve has branched out. Hyperacusis is likely if the lesion is proximal to nerve to stapedius.

Method of Testing

- Raise the eyebrows (frontalis muscle). Keep a hand of the examiner over the scalp of the child to block the occipital head of occipitofrontalis helping this movement (optional). Occipital head is supplied by the posterior auricular branch of VII.
- The child shuts the eyes tightly and the examiner tries to open it (orbicularis oculi). Subtle differences between the two sides may be made out by noting the ability to bury the eyelashes on tight closure of eyes.

Bell's phenomenon: In case of LMN VII palsy, if the child attempts to shut the eyes, the eyeball will roll upwards (this upward movement of eyeballs is a normal phenomenon but is made obvious by the inability to close the eyes in case of VII nerve palsy). The orbicularis oculi and superior rectus contract together producing the upward movement of eyeball with closure of eyes

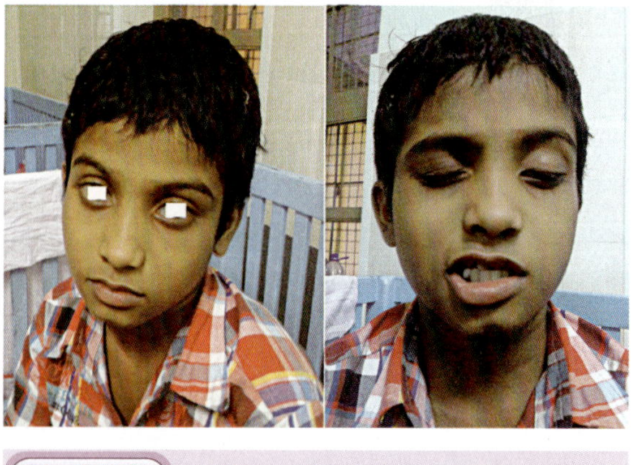

Fig.9.16a LMN Facial Palsy

normally (oculofacial synkinesis). When orbicularis is weak, the superior rectus overacts producing an exaggerated upward movement of the eyeball. This does not happen in UMN lesions as there is no muscle paralysis. Thus, it is useful in differentiating bilateral UMN and LMN lesions of facial nerve.

- Ask to show the teeth (say "eee"; demonstrate to the child what he is expected to do) and observe any deviation of angle of mouth. This deviation of angle of mouth must not be confused with the congenital absence of depressor anguli oris muscle where only the lower lip goes down (the lower lip of normal side goes down, whereas that side with absent muscle remains as such). It is first noticed in infancy when the baby cries or smiles (asymmetric crying facies).The condition is cosmetically insignificant as the infant gets older (as the muscle does not contribute significantly to facial expression in childhood/ adulthood. Compare the nasolabial folds on both sides. It will be obliterated in the paralyzed side.

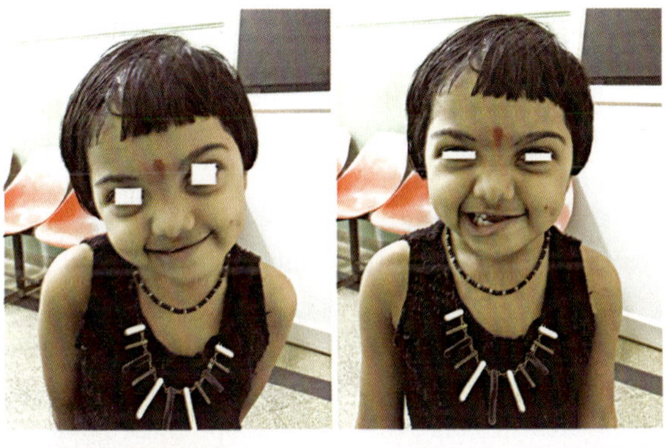

Fig.9.16b Depressor Anguli Oris muscle hypoplasia

- Ask to pout the lips (like whistling) so as to kiss a pencil held in front (orbicularis oris).
- Blow the cheek with the mouth closed (buccinator); slightly press the cheek with fingers to see if air is retained on slight pressure.
- Evert the lower lip forcefully to pull up the skin of neck (platysma) (Fig. 9.17). Another method is to ask the child to show his teeth and open the mouth wide at the same time; this will make platysma stand out.
- Ask for any hyperacusis.
- Test the taste of the anterior 2/3rd of tongue. It is difficult in children (and often not necessary). The tongue is pulled out and kept outside the mouth while different substances are kept on the tongue (about 2 cm from the tip) for the person to indicate the taste by writing or pointing to the appropriate tastes written on paper. The mouth is rinsed before the next substance is kept. Usually sweet (sugar), salt (common salt), sour (vinegar) and bitter (quinine) are tested in adults, but the latter two are not tolerated by most children. All other tastes are not exactly tastes but "flavours," which require intact sense of smell to appreciate (next time you get a blocked nose with common cold, appreciate how different all flavours appear; also flavours are best appreciated at the moment of swallowing and not when it is put on the tongue, because in pharynx, nasopharynx communicates to give access to smell).

  Use of galvanic current to give a metallic taste for testing sense of taste is only experimental (electrogustometer) and not used in clinical examination.

Regarding secretory functions, it is best to ask the patient rather than any manoeuvre. Of course one can use a split lemon to get good salivary secretion, which can be observed by asking the child to raise the tip of tongue to visualize flow from maxillary gland.To assess tear production Schirmer test can be done.

9

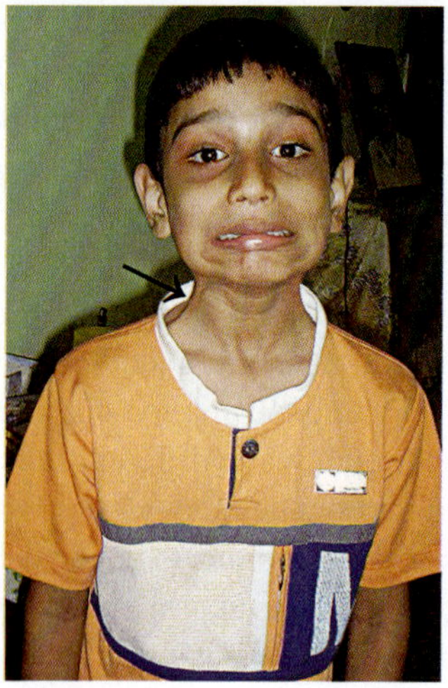

Fig.9.17 Platysma

Bilateral LMN facial palsy may occur in Guillain-Barre syndrome, leprosy, etc. Bilateral UMN facial palsy may occur in certain cerebral palsies associated with pseudobulbar palsy.

Emotional facial palsy: Deviation of mouth on smiling, which disappears while voluntarily says "eee" is called emotional facial palsy; this occurs rarely in deep seated lesions of opposite thalamus or its connections to frontal cortex. Bilateral emotional paralysis may be seen in Parkinsonism.

Vestibulocochlear Nerve

Auditory Nerve

The cochlear nerve carries impulses from hair cells of organ of Corti to the chochlear nucleus in pons. Most fibres cross, run in lateral lemniscus to the medial geniculate body and then to the superior temporal gyrus; however, there is transmission of uncrossed fibres as well so that unilateral nerve deafness due to cortical lesion is unlikely.

The examiner can compare the acuity of hearing of the child with that of himself. One can use a watch to see if the child can detect its ticks. However, it is worth noting that the modern quartz watches do not emit enough sound. Also inquire about any tinnitus (often deafness is accompanied by tinnitus, especially in sensorineural deafness).

Conductive deafness is usually due to wax or damage to tympanic membrane. Sensorineural deafness (called perception deafness or nerve deafness) is due to the lesions of cochlea or auditory nerve or its central connections.

- **Rinne's test**: In normal ear, air conduction is better than bone conduction. Place the vibrating tuning fork (512 Hz or 256 Hz) near the ear (Ref. 4). When the child ceases to hear, it is placed over the mastoid. The child will not normally hear it now. If he can hear it now, it means that the bone conduction is better than air conduction, meaning there is some block to air conduction like blocked ear canal or middle ear disease (negative Rinne test). This is called conductive deafness. In nerve deafness, both air and bone conduction are diminished proportionately so that Rinne's test gives normal pattern. This is positive Rinne test (normal ear has positive Rinne).
- **Weber's test**: A vibrating tuning fork is placed over the forehead in the midline. Normally, it is equally heard in both ears. In nerve deafness, the sound is better heard on the normal side. In conductive deafness, the sound appears to be better heard on the side with conductive hearing loss. This feeling is because the bone conduction reaches the blocked ear "unopposed," whereas in the normal ear the bone conducted sound is modified by the interference of the air conducted sound.
- If deafness is present, aroscope must be used to look for wax or middle ear diseases.

Causes of Perception Deafness (nerve deafness)

- At cochlear level: Meniere's disease, drug toxicity, otosclerosis, etc.
- At nerve level: Drug toxicity, meningitis, cerebellopontine angle tumour, etc. C-P angle tumour will involve V and VII nerves in addition, which is of localizing value.

- At brainstem level: Pontine lesions, vascular, tumour, etc.

Audiometry is used for objective recording of hearing loss. High tone hearing loss is seen in nerve deafness and low tone hearing loss in middle ear diseases.

Vestibular Nerve

Vestibular nerve carries impulses from semicircular canal, saccule and utricle to the vestibular ganglia on the main trunk of nerve and then to the vestibular nucleus in the medulla. Vestibular nuclei have connections with cerebellum, III nerve via medial longitudinal fasciculus, nuclei of upper cervical nerve, spinal cord and the temporal lobes.

Vertigo and nystagmus especially on head movement is suggestive of labyrinthine dysfunction. (Vertigo is the hallucination of movement of one's self or one's surroundings.)

- Calorie test is used to assess vestibular function (see p 239).
- The **Romberg test** is classically described for proprioceptive deficiency, but it also evaluates vestibular control of balance and movement. When standing with the feet placed together and eyes closed, the patient tends to fall toward the side of vestibular hypofunction. When asked to take steps forward and backward, the patient progressively deviates to the side of the lesion (see p 185, 223).

  The Romberg test also may be positive in patients with polyneuropathies, but these individuals do not fall consistently to one side, as do the patients with vestibular dysfunction. One should remember that slight swaying with eyes closed may be normal in a small child, especially if that is the only abnormality.

Glossopharyngeal and Vagus (IX and X)

Functions of these two nerves together are:

- Carry general sensations from pharynx, tonsils, soft palate and posterior one-third of tongue.
- Carry taste sensation from posterior third of tongue (only IX nerve).
- Motor supply to palatal and pharyngeal muscles.
- Motor supply to vocal cords (only X nerve).

These two nerves are usually tested together.

- Nasal regurgitation of fluids and nasal twang of voice may indicate palsy of these nerves. Dysphagia, choking while feeding, dysphonia and dysarthria are the other presenting symptoms. Cough will lose its explosive sound. Hoarse voice may indicate vocal cord paralysis; nasal twang indicates palatal paralysis. 9
- Note the position of the uvula. It is in the midline normally. In case of paralysis of X, it deviates to the normal side when the child says Ahh (i.e., it moves to the side opposite to the one that is paralyzed). Also observe the posterior pharyngeal wall, which also moves towards the normal side (to the side opposite to the one that is paralyzed).
- Arching of palate is by a movement away from the midline due to muscle contraction. So when one side is paralyzed, the palate moves toward the opposite side due to the pull of normal side. There will be little movement on the affected side (Fig. 24.95). In case of bilateral palatal palsy, the palate remains immobile when saying 'Ahh.'
- **Gag reflex**: Tickle the posterior pharyngeal wall with a spatula or a throat swab. Tongue retraction and elevation and contraction of the palate and pharyngeal musculature in response to touching the posterior wall of the pharynx, tonsillar area, or base of the tongue are the expected normal responses. The afferent is IX and the efferent X. Theoretically, there will be diminished gag reflex plus the child will not appreciate the sensation of touch of the spatula in case of isolated IX palsy. In case of isolated X palsy, the child appreciates the touch but

fails to produce the gag reflex (palatal elevation). It is practically impossible to test this in small children. Fortunately, there are practically no clinical situations where there will be isolated palsy of X or IX without involvement of the other. Palatal reflex is the elevation of the soft palate (and in case of contralateral paralysis, ipsilateral deviation of the uvula) on stimulation of the soft palate. In clinical practice, one need test only the gag or palatal reflex. Here, one can easily differentiate UMN and LMN palsy. In UMN, there is exaggerated gag reflex, but diminished volitional movement of palate while saying Ahhh. In LMN, both these are diminished.

- **Sensory testing**: Testing the taste sensation of the posterior third of tongue (IX nerve) is difficult even in adults and is not attempted in children (ideally tested with galvanic current). General sensation of posterior third of tongue is also via the IX nerve and hence testing of general sensations will suffice in case testing of sensation becomes necessary. Sensation of the soft palate and pharyngeal wall are also under IX nerve.
- **Bulbar palsy**: This is the LMN palsy of nerves originating from the bulb (medulla). Jaw jerk and gag reflex are lost. There will be pooling of saliva in the throat, dysphagia, dysarthria, nasal regurgitation of fluids, etc. In most clinical situations, it means palsy of IX and X although they are not the only nerves from the bulb (9–12 nerves are bulbar in origin). Examples of conditions causing bulbar palsy are polio, Guillain-Barre syndrome, etc (see Fig. 24.95).
- **Pseudobulbar palsy**: This is the UMN palsy of nerves originating from the bulb (medulla). It is due to the interruption of bilateral supra nuclear (corticobulbar) pathways. Other UMN signs like pyramidal signs or symptoms suggestive of cortical involvement like emotional lability can be seen. Jaw jerk and gag reflex are exaggerated. It is seen in quadriplegic CP. The tongue may be small and spastic and there may be dysarthria/dysphagia.
- Unilateral paralysis of the recurrent laryngeal branch of vagus results in hoarseness of voice, but phonation remains possible. Bilateral paralysis results in stridor (both cords remain immobile in mid abduction; phonation may not be possible).
- Motor part of the IX nerve is not tested clinically but it does have motor supply; IX nerve supplies the stylopharyngeus muscle, but cannot be tested independently.

Possible lesions:

- Unilateral pure motor paralysis: Poliomyelitis, diphtheria, botulism.
- Unilateral sensory loss (i.e., only IX affected): As an isolated finding, this is not found in clinical situations.
- Unilateral motor plus sensory loss: Lesions at medulla like vascular accidents, syringobulbia, tumours, etc.
- Bilateral UMN paralysis: Pseudobulbar palsy.
- Bilateral LMN paralysis: Bulbar palsy of various causes; poliomyelitis, toxins, etc.

Accessory Nerve (XI Nerve)

- Trapezius muscle is tested by shoulder shrugging against resistance. In case of paralysis, there will be drooping of shoulder on the affected side, and the scapula may drop to a lower level. Total weakness of trapezius is unlikely as part of trapezius is supplied by cervical nerves.
- Sternomastoid is tested by asking the child to turn to one side or other against resistance (Fig. 9.18). In case of weakness of the muscle, the child cannot turn the head away from the affected side against resistance. (Try the test on yourself and see that sternomastoid of one side contracts to move the head away from that side.) Both sternomastoids can be tested

together by asking the child to flex the head against the resistance applied to the underside of chin. Or, rest a hand on child's forehead and ask him to bend his head forwards; both sternomastoids will stand out together and can be compared.

Bilateral LMN paralysis involving XI nerve may be seen in poliomyelitis, spinal muscular atrophy, etc. Poliomyelitis may cause unilateral LMN palsy as well. Clinically significant UMN palsy involving XI nerve alone is not seen.

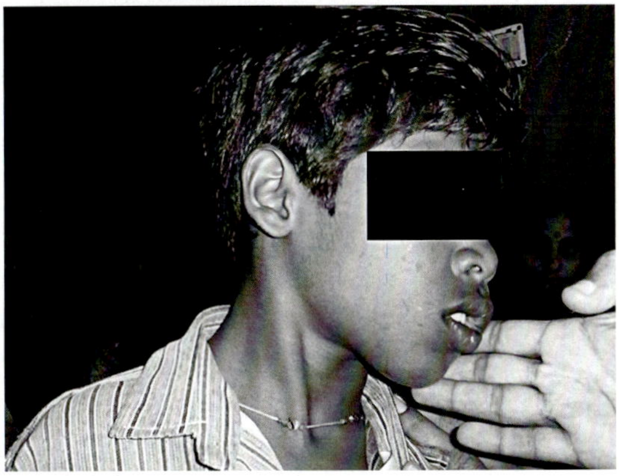

Fig.9.18 Testing the sternomastoid

Hypoglossal Nerve (XII Nerve)

- XII nerve contains only motor fibres.
- Look at the tongue resting on the floor of mouth to visualize fasciculations (not by protruding the tongue or crying). Fasciculation of the tongue may be noted in Werdnig-Hoffman disease.
- Atrophy of the affected side of tongue may be noticed in LMN paralysis of one side (Fig. 24.97).
- In UMN lesions, the tongue is spastic, thin, pointed and without atrophy. One may easily appreciate spastic and flaccid tongue by palpating with a gloved finger.
- Ask the child to protrude the tongue. It deviates to the paralyzed side (Fig. 24.97). This is easy to understand. Just imagine that both halves of the tongue move towards the midline on protrusion, and each side balances the other side when one protrudes the tongue. So when one side is paralyzed, the normal side pushes the tongue to beyond the midline towards the paralyzed side.
- In case of bilateral paralysis, the tongue is greatly reduced in size and there is difficulty in protruding the tongue out of mouth and difficulty in speech (both these are nearly unaffected in unilateral lesions). This should not be confused with a short frenulum holding back the tongue tip, in which case the tip curves downwards on protrusion.
- Test the lateral movement of tongue inside the mouth and compare its relative strength by palpation over the cheeks. Ask the child to say la la to look for tongue movements.
- Persistent dimple on percussion of tongue may be seen in myotonia.
- Mnemonic (rule of 17): There is always confusion whether muscle contraction causes movement to the same side or opposite side when a cranial nerve of one side is paralyzed. All students are familiar with facial palsy (VII) and know that the mouth deviates to the opposite side in case of VII nerve paralysis. X nerve also causes deviation of uvula to the opposite side in case of paralysis. Note that VII plus X makes 17. Paralysis of XII and V causes deviation to the same side; again note that XII and V add together to give 17, thus making an easy mnemonic. Another mnemonic is SOOS, meaning same - opposite - opposite - same, in the order 5, 7, 10, 12.
- Note that in VII and V nerve palsies, there may be an apparent deviation of tongue due to deviation of angle of mouth or deviation of jaw, respectively. This should not be interpreted as XII nerve palsy.

9

- In contrast to most other cranial nerves, hypoglossal and accessory nerve nucleus have cortical pyramidal control from opposite hemisphere only (see p 203).

Unilateral or bilateral LMN palsy of XII may be seen in poliomyelitis, syringomyelia, etc. Unilateral UMN palsy of tongue may be seen in association with hemiplegia; bilateral UMN palsy of XII may be part of pseudobulbar palsy.

MOTOR SYSTEM

Bulk of Muscles

Assess the three "S": the size, shape and symmetry of a muscle. The presence of atrophy, hypertrophy, abnormal bulging or depression in a muscle is an important diagnostic finding in the presence of different muscle diseases or abnormalities. Hypertrophy occurs with commensurate strength from use and exercise. On the other hand, hypertrophy with weakness is seen commonly in Duchenne muscular dystrophy. The shape also may be altered when the muscle or tendon is ruptured.

Atrophy is more marked in LMN lesions compared to UMN lesions.

The muscles are measured, using a measuring tape. A point is chosen on the muscle, which is at a measured distance from a bony point (e.g., 7 cm above olecranon); make sure that you are measuring around a point that represents the maximum bulk of the muscle. Note that a minimal difference between the sides is common, e.g., the right side is larger in right-handed individuals.

Tone of Muscles

Muscle tone is the resistance offered by the muscles to passive stretch. The muscle may be hypotonic or hypertonic.

Hypotonia is defined as decreased tone. History suggestive of decreased tone include floppiness, baby slipping through when held by axilla, excessive range of movements, etc. Hypotonia may be seen in lower motor neuron lesions, spinal shock stage of UMN lesions and some cerebellar lesions. Rheumatic chorea has hypotonia as a component but all other extrapyramidal lesions have hypertonia.

Hypertonia may manifest as spasticity or rigidity.

History suggestive of spasticity include difficulty in changing napkins/cleaning perineum (adductor spasm), tendency for scissoring of lower limbs, toe walking, etc.

- Pyramidal lesions result in spasticity that may manifest as a clasp-knife phenomenon (i.e., resistance to passive movement initially with sudden giving way, usually toward the completion of joint flexion or extension). Subtle spasticity can be made out by *rapid* supination–pronation movements and looking for a sudden "supinator catch" during the movement. A point worth noting is that spasticity is more easily made out during rapid movements. In case of infants with spasticity, evaluation of angles also will give an idea of the tone. Examples of such angles are adductor angle, popliteal angle, scarf sign, etc (see p 22–24).
- Rigidity refers to the increased tone associated with extrapyramidal lesions; it may result in a cogwheel (rigidity with interruptions, possibly rigidity associated with tremor) or lead-pipe (uniform) resistance to passive movement. Cog wheel rigidity is best made out at wrist, that too in the first moments of testing. It is argued that cog wheel rigidity can occur without tremor, in which case one should assume that agonist-antagonist muscles alternatively gives way, off and on.

  Note: In rigidity, the tone is uniformly increased in both the agonist and antagonist muscle groups. In spasticity, although the tone is increased in both the muscle groups, tone will be more in one of the muscle groups (antigravity muscles). Pyramidal hypertonicity is more evident in the flexors & pronators in upper limb and extensors & adductors in lower limb.

- Spasticity is velocity dependant and is prominent with rapid passive movement by the examiner. Rigidity is length dependant and is elicitable always, and is more prominent with slow passive movement by the examiner.

Tone is assessed by:

- Observation of position at rest: The posture of a hypotonic infant with an LMN lesion is characteristic, with abduction and external rotation at the hip joints and flexion at the knee, producing a frog leg posture. The upper limbs are abducted at the shoulder with flexion at the elbow and the hands beside the head. In case of infants, one can hold them by their axilla. They tend to slip through if hypotonic. If spastic they will not slip through and there will be scissoring of lower limbs during this procedure.
- Palpation of muscles: The muscle is palpated for the feel of the muscle; the muscle normally feels firm. Atrophied muscle has the feel of loose cloth; spastic muscle feels hard. In pseudohypertrophy of Duchenne, involved muscles feel rubbery.
- Passive movements: The limbs are moved passively at each joint to assess the tone. (But in usual clinical practice, each and every joint is not tested; rather upper and lower limbs are grossly tested in a few joints.) Contractures, if any, can also be detected during the passive movements. *Upper limb*: One may try shaking the hand at the wrist holding at distal forearm and look for the extra range of mobility of the hand. Roll the hand round at the wrist and assess the tone. Also try rapid supination–pronation movements to assess the tone. *Lower limb*: The lower limb is flicked up at the knee joint in a supine child; the lower limb normally lifts off the surface and remains in the air for a fraction of a second or so and then comes down and moves along the surface of the cot. The hypotonic limb drags along the surface of the cot rather than remaining momentarily lifted off while flicking. The spastic limb, remains in the air longer than normal when flicked up. The rigid limb hangs in air even longer.
- In small infants, tone can be assessed by different angles. The normal values differ based on the age. Angles are not assessed beyond 12 months of age. The head must be kept in the midline as turning to one side changes the tone. Some of these angles are:
  - **Scarf sign**: In the supine infant, the upper limb is pulled across the chest holding the flexed elbow. Elbow does not cross the midline in infants less than 3 months of age.
  - **Heel to ear manoeuvre**: Lift both the legs of the supine infant without lifting the pelvis from table and try to bring it to the ear.
  - **Adductor angle**: In the supine infant, the hips are abducted by holding onto the extended knee. The adductor angle is the angle between the thighs. It is less than 75° below 3 months of age.
  - **Ankle dorsiflexion**: It is the angle between the dorsum of the foot and the anterior aspect of leg when the foot is dorsiflexed on to the anterior aspect of the leg (see p 468).
  - **"180° flip method"**: Refer to p 256, 528.

9

Power (whenever possible grade the power)

Power is the force that can be voluntarily generated. Muscle power is tested for groups of muscles moving various joints. Before testing power, always look for tenderness and contractures of muscles and joints. Fix the proximal joints to avoid trick movements by the uninvolved muscles. The child is allowed to do the movement completely (e.g., flexing the elbow) and then the examiner tries to oppose the movement. One will get better cooperation from the child by this technique. The goal of testing is to know which part is involved and to what extent; whether it is predominantly proximal or distal or both.

Grading of Muscle Power

0 Absent voluntary contraction
1 Feeble contractions that are unable to move a joint (muscle contraction may be seen or felt)
2 Movement with gravity eliminated
3 Movement against gravity
4 Movement against partial resistance
5 Full strength

- LMN lesions cause total loss of motor power as all the impulses need the final common pathway of LMN to reach the muscle. In UMN lesions, the power and tone are not totally lost.
- The cortical control is for movements and not for individual muscles and hence in UMN lesion there is paralysis of movement. In LMN lesion, there is paralysis of individual muscles innervated by the nerve or anterior horn cell concerned.
- It may be noted that the terms paraplegia, hemiplegia, etc, are used conventionally to denote pyramidal damage and hence should not be used for LMN paralysis. For example, lower limb weakness due to polio should not be called paraplegia. Diplegia is used conventionally to denote paresis of both lower limbs in cerebral palsy. Here, the term 'paraplegic cerebral palsy' should not be used.
- Most authorities use the term 'paralysis' and 'paresis' interchangeably but some use the term paresis for partial weakness and paralysis for total weakness.
- Predominant proximal muscle weakness is a feature of muscle disease. It is indicated by difficulty in getting up from sitting position, combing hair, etc.
- It is easy to make out significant weakness by simple tests, which are not too very formal. For example, the patient may be asked to stand on one leg, stand on tip toe (S1), stand on heel (L5), stand on everted feet, stand with feet close together with eyes closed, jump, hop, etc.

For upper limb, one may ask the child to write, use a cup, cap a pen, etc.

History and Findings Suggestive of Specific Weaknesses

- In case of weakness, ask for the onset, progression and symmetry of weakness.
- Suggestive of LMN lesion: Wasting, hypotonia and fasciculations.
- Suggestive of distal muscle weakness: Difficulty in hand manipulations like buttoning the shirt, opening the cap of a bottle, making a bolus of food, writing, etc. For the lower limb, difficulty in holding the chappal in place (slipping of chappals) is the history obtained in distal weakness.
- Suggestive of proximal muscle weakness: Difficulty in combing the hair, difficulty in taking objects from a height. In case of combing of hair, it is the difficulty in raising the arm above the head that is to be looked for and not the fine distal movements involved in combing proper. In case of lower limb, observe for the difficulty in getting up from sitting position, climbing up and down the stairs, etc.
- Suggestive of axial muscle weakness: Difficulty in getting up from lying down posture and turning over in bed.
- Suggestive of pyramidal weakness: Distal weakness is more than proximal, and it is usually characterized by inability to do fine skilled movements. Toes grazing the ground while walking, dragging of the limb while walking, etc.
- The patient is asked to extend and raise both the arms in front of him as if he were carrying a book. The patient is asked to keep his

arms in place while he keeps his eyes closed and counts to 10. Normally, their arms remain in place. If there is UMN weakness of the upper limb, the upper limbs will pronate and may fall.

In psychogenic weakness, the limb falls without pronation.

Testing of Muscle Groups

(Testing of individual muscles is discussed in the next chapter, p 240).

- Neck: Extend and flex the neck against resistance offered at occiput and chin, respectively.
- Movements at shoulder: Abduct and elevate the arm beyond 90° against resistance offered at mid arm. Flex (bring towards the chest) and extend the arm.
- Movements at elbow: Flex and extend the forearm against resistance. Test supination and pronation against resistance.
- Movements at wrist: Let the child make a fist with hand; now the child is requested to flex and extend at wrist joint against resistance.
- Grip: Ask the child to grasp examiner's finger with the examiner trying to pull it off. When done simultaneously on both sides, the power can be compared in unilateral weakness.
- Intercostal muscles: Splint the abdomen below the costal margin with the examiner's hands. This restricts the movement of diaphragm and hence if intercostals are weak there will be increasing dyspnoea now.
- Diaphragm: Here, splint the chest by encircling the chest with examiner's hand; dyspnoea will increase if diaphragm is paralyzed.
- Upper abdomen: Ask the child to raise the head and chest in supine position without arm support.
- Lower abdomen: Ask the patient to raise his extended legs without arm support.
  Beevor sign: This is seen with bilateral lower abdominal wall paralysis that results in upward deviation of the umbilicus when the patient tries to raise his head and sit up from the supine position.
- Movements at hip: Ask the supine child to raise the extended leg off the couch against resistance offered at thigh.
  Adduction/abduction of hip, gravity eliminated and against resistance, may be tested with the child supine. In case of marked weakness, gravity eliminated flexion/extension movements of hip may be tested with the child in side position (easy to visualize that flexion/extension in side position eliminates gravity). Abduction against gravity also is tested with the child in side position (p 242). Extensors of hip are tested against gravity and resistance with the child in prone position. Hip rotators can be tested by externally or internally rotating the lower limb against resistance offered at side of foot (p 465).
- **Hoover's sign**: Ask the supine patient to raise one leg while the examiner places his hand below the other heel. Normally, as one leg is raised, there is an involuntary pressure on the other heel. If the limb that is being raised is weak, extra pressure is felt at the normal heel as the patient is making an extra effort to raise the weak limb. This is a useful sign to detect subtle weakness of lower limb. In case of malingering psuedoparalysis, there will not be any pressure felt on the hand kept beneath the normal limb simply because the child is not trying to lift the affected limb at all!
- Movements at knee: Test knee flexion and extension. Gravity eliminated movement is tested in side position.
- Movements at ankle: Test dorsiflexion, plantar flexion, inversion and eversion against resistance. Gravity eliminated testing, if needed, may be done by changing the position of the limb.

Myotonia: The contraction of muscle persists even after the voluntary effort has ceased. The child will have difficulty in releasing a handshake. (Assess myotonia when releasing after the very first grip. After repeated attempts, the myotonia eases off and hence may be missed.) One may percuss over the thenar eminence to find that there is a persistent contraction of muscle resulting in the thumb raising up and holding. Or one may percuss the tongue to find that the dimple persists for sometime. Also shake hands with parents. One may be able to demonstrate myotonia in parents in case of myotonic dystrophy. Postgraduate students must make it a habit to test for myotonia in mother of floppy baby with suspected myopathy.

Coordination of Movements

Coordination of movements can be tested by the finger–nose test, heel–knee test, gait, etc. Perfect coordination requires intact sensory system, vestibular system and cerebellar system. Before commenting on coordination, appropriate allowance must be given to the weakness, if any, due to pyramidal, extrapyramidal or LMN lesions. Coordination can be tested reliably only when the muscle power is greater than 3.

INVOLUNTARY MOVEMENTS

All involuntary movements disappear during sleep, except hemiballismus and myoclonus.

Tremor

- Tremor is the rhythmic involuntary oscillatory movements. This is tested for by asking the child to keep the hand outstretched with the fingers spread apart. Tremor is normal in anxiety, but nowadays the most common cause is the use of salbutamol. Thyrotoxicosis and drug withdrawal are rare causes of tremor.
- **Intention tremor**: Tremor is exaggerated by voluntary movement, especially towards reaching the target. It is seen in cerebellar lesions.
- Pill rolling movement of Parkinsonism is also considered a type of tremor (rest tremor).
- Titubation is the tremor (up and down oscillatory movement) of the head. It is seen in lesions of the vermis of the cerebellum.
- **Asterixis**: Asterixis is a sudden brief loss of postural tone. It is considered a tremor. Here, the child is asked to stand with his hands outstrectched held in dorsiflexion at the wrist and the fingers extended. There may be a sudden flexion movement (flap) at the wrist (the hand drops) and/or metacarpophalangeal joints, followed by voluntary corrective extension movement. It is found in hepatic failure.

  Asterixis is not really specific for liver failure, but it helps in early detection of drowsiness of encephalopathy. Visualize a drowsy child being asked to stand with outstretched hands. Within a short while, his hands will drift down; the same thing will happen even if you are asked to do the same while feeling sleepy! This is possibly because the drowsy brain does not properly process the proprioceptive information from the periphery.
- Infantile tremor syndrome is seen in malnourished children.

Chorea

Sudden, jerky, involuntary, non-repetitive, quasipurposive movements. The most common cause is Sydenham's chorea of rheumatic fever where the lesion is supposed to be at the caudate nucleus. It is exaggerated by emotion and voluntary movement but disappears during sleep. The child tries to mask the abnormal movements by merging it with voluntary movements making it look like quasi-purposive. Hypotonia and emotional lability are associated features of *rheumatic* chorea.

Signs in Chorea

- **Milk maid sign**: Ask the child to grasp the examiner's fingers. Alternate squeezing and relaxing of the child's fingers will be felt by the examiner's fingers.

- **Pronator sign**: Ask the child to hold the extended upper limbs above the head with palms facing each other. The hands tend to pronate.
- **Jack in box sign**: Ask the child to protrude the tongue and keep it outside. The tongue goes on moving in and out of mouth.
- **Hung up knee jerk**: This is because of a choreic movement coming during elicitation of the stretch reflex. Naturally 'hung up' phenomenon is not demonstrable with every elicitation of knee jerk.

Athetosis

This is the continuous slow writhing involuntary movements of the extremities, but all the other characters are similar to chorea. In fact, it is usually associated with chorea, so that it is called choreoathetosis. It may be seen in rheumatic fever, extrapyramidal type of cerebral palsy, etc. The lesion is said to be at putamen. Athetosis may also be found in degenerative diseases involving the CNS (Wilson disease, Hallervorden-Spatz disease) and as a sequel to encephaliltis.

Ballismus

This is the sudden violent flinging movement around the proximal joints, usually confined to one side (hence called hemiballismus). The site of lesion is the subthalamic nucleus. It may be seen in association with chorea and athetosis.

Dystonia

It is sustained muscle contraction in abnormal postures. It may be seen in extrapyramidal type of cerebral palsy. The site of lesion is said to be the same as athetosis. In fact, dystonia is a maintained posture seen in athetosis but without the writhing movements. Oculogyric crisis due to drug over dose (e.g., metoclopramide, phenothiazine, etc) is a dystonic reaction of ocular and neck muscles.

Myoclonus

This is a sudden jerk of a limb or muscle group. Myoclonus can be epileptic or non-epileptic. Sleep myoclonus is normal in newborns. Hiccough is in fact a diaphragmatic myoclonus.

Sudden extension myoclonus (as though pulled from back with a string) is typically seen in subacute sclerosing pan encephalitis (SSPE). Myoclonus with sudden dropping of head and flexion movement of arms (salaam seizure) is seen in infantile spasm.

Minipolymyoclonus (Fasciculatory Tremor)

This is a term applied to describe the tremor-like movements seen in the small joints of the hand in Kugelberg-Welander disease. Unlike Werdnig-Hoffmann disease, here the degeneration of anterior horn cells is quite gradual giving a chance for re-innervation from adjoining areas; this may be producing the minipolymyoclonus (which in fact are fasciculations).

Fasciculation

Twitching of muscles after exercise, especially after isometric exercise is normal. Fasciculation and fibrillation are seen in anterior horn cell disease like Werdnig-Hoffman disease. It is looked for with the tongue resting inside the mouth (fibrillation can be clinically seen only in tongue). Fasciculations can be induced by hyperventilation, exercise (especially isometric) and by tapping of the muscle.

Tics

Tics are stereotyped repetitive movements confined to particular muscle groups. It is a habit spasm and is suppressible voluntarily for a short time. It is common in children. Tourette syndrome is a combination of multiple motor and vocal tics, hyperactivity and coprolalia (obscene language).

Cramps

It is the painful involuntary contraction, usually

of calf muscles. It is seen due to exertion, electrolyte imbalance, exposure to cold, deficiency states (like calcium, B complex), etc.

Tetany

This is carpopedal spasm. It is due to hypocalcaemia, which may be induced by alkalosis (e.g., hyperventilation producing respiratory alkalosis). An attack of carpopedal spasm can be precipitated by applying the pressure of inflated BP apparatus when there is hypocalcaemia (Trousseau's sign). The other sign described in hypocalcaemia is Chvostek's sign (tapping facial nerve in front of the external auditory meatus produces brisk contraction of facial muscles).

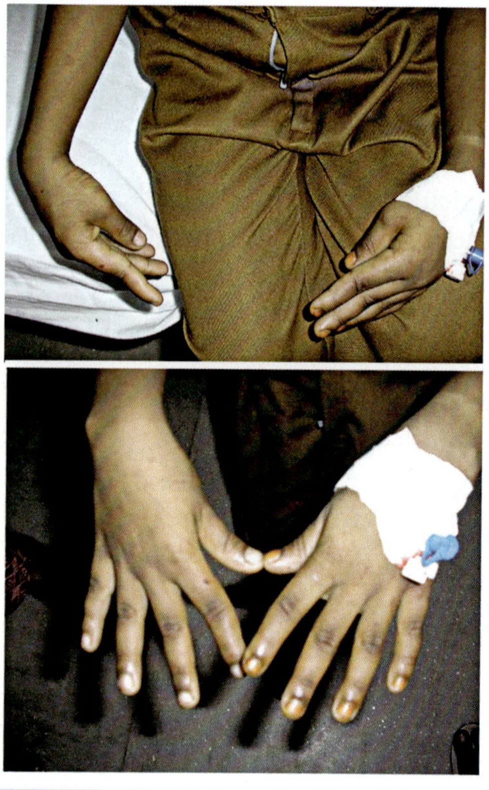

Fig.9.19 Tetany: The first picture shows tetany and the second one shows improvement following IV calcium.

"***Associated movements***" are normal involuntary movements (e.g., swinging of arms while walking). In fact, its absence is what is abnormal (seen in extrapyramidal lesions).

REFLEXES

Superficial Reflexes

- **Corneal/conjunctival reflex**: The corneal and conjunctival reflexes can be elicited by gently touching the edge of the cornea or conjunctiva, respectively with a sterile wisp of cotton with the child looking to one side. The normal response is bilateral winking. Absence of such a response implies V or VII paralysis. There should be no confusion between these two nerve palsies as in VII palsy the voluntary eye closure is affected, which is normal in V palsy. Blinking of only one eye suggests weakness of the VII nerve on the side that does not wink.
- It is not desirable that many students elicit corneal reflex with cotton wool. At least there is some chance of damage to cornea, especially in the inexperienced hands. An alternative method is blowing gently over the cornea of one eye protecting the other eye with your hand (to avoid stimulating both eyes together). The wind blown is a safe stimulant for corneal reflex.

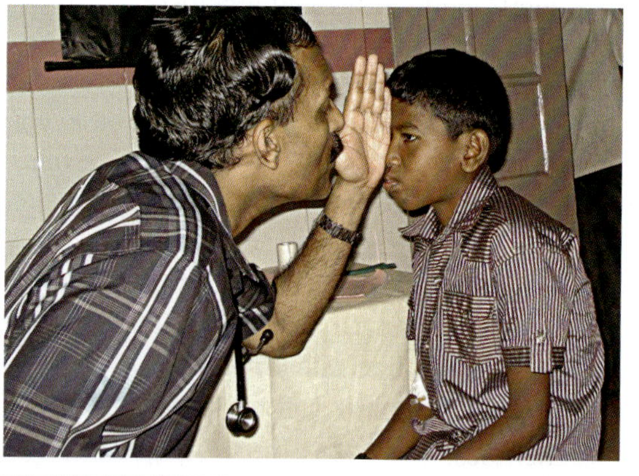

Fig.9.20 Testing for corneal reflex by blowing air

- **Palatal and pharyngeal reflexes** are also superficial reflexes. They are discussed earlier under cranial nerves (p 191).
- **Abdominal reflex** (T6–T12): The abdominal wall is stroked below the costal margins from the *lateral to the medial* side. This is repeated below the umbilicus also. This elicits contraction of the muscles of the anterior abdominal wall. The abdominal wall should be kept completely relaxed during the procedure. Abdominal reflexes may be lost in cortical lesions also, because these reflexes have long arcs going even up to the cerebral hemispheres. Thus, abdominal reflexes may be lost due to LMN lesions affecting T6–T12 or UMN lesions.
- **Cremasteric reflex** (L1): This reflex is elicited by drawing a line along the medial thigh and watching the movement of the testis. A normal reflex is elevation of the ipsilateral testis. As per same reason discussed earlier, cremastric reflex also may be lost in UMN lesions.
- **Anal reflex** (S3, S4): Elicited by gently stroking the perianal skin. It results in puckering of the anal orifice.
- **The plantar (Babinski) reflex** (S1): This Fig.9.21 reflex may be elicited in several ways, each with a different name. The most commonly performed manoeuvre is stroking the lateral aspect of the sole with a sharp object (blunt object is preferred in children). It is best not to take the stroke too much medially into the anterior sole as this may bring in the plantar grasp. The normal response is plantar flexion of the great toe, which is considered an absent (negative) Babinski sign. Dorsiflexion of the great toe suggests an upper motor neuron lesion and is referred to as a positive Babinski sign. Dorsiflexion of the big toe also may be associated with fanning out of the other toes, as described in Babinski's original description, but is not a necessary accompaniment of all abnormal responses. When the response is confusing, do it gently, increase the noxiousness only if there is no response to gentle stimulation. If the first response is extension of the big toe, take it as significant, irrespective of whatever movement the other toes show. When one gets up-going and down-going plantar (and not a consistent response) as one does it repeatedly, see if the technique is correct. If so, decide democratically! If plantar is up-going more times than down-going, take it as significant up-going plantar. And above all, correlate with the clinical condition the patient is having. And it is not that all pyramidal lesions should have up-going plantar invariably. In fact, long-standing lesions like cerebral palsy may occasionally have down-going plantar response. In spinal cord transection, while eliciting plantar, flexion of the knee and hip may rarely occur in the paretic leg with urinary and faecal incontinence. This is referred to as the "mass" reflex stimulation anywhere below the level of lesion (not just sole) can produce mass reflex (p 262). Total absence of any response may indicate absence of cutaneous innervation in the S1 segment or loss of motor innervation in the L5 segment ipsilaterally. Plantar response may be extensor in small infants till they learn to walk well. It may be extensor in deep sleep and deep sedation.

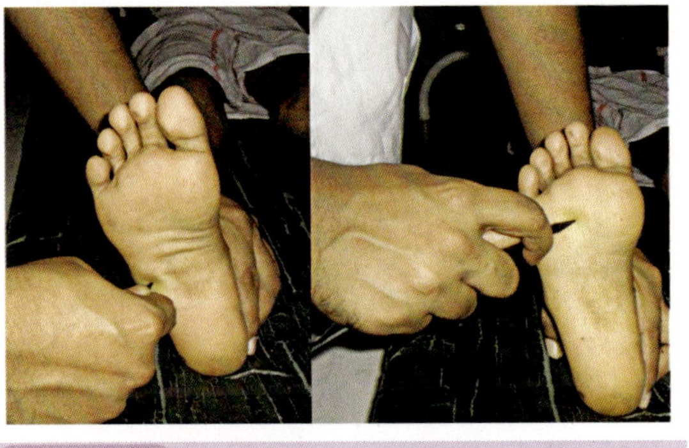

Fig.9.21 Plantar reflex showing extensor response (+ve Babinski sign)

9

The other methods described to elicit the extensor toe response in cases of organic disease of the corticospinal reflex paths are:

- *Chaddock's reflex*: When the lateral malleolar skin area is stimulated with a light stroke, extension of the great toe occurs.
- *Oppenheim's sign*: Apply firm pressure over the upper anteromedial surface of tibia with thumb and index finger and look for extension of toes.
- *Gordon's sign*: Squeeze the calf muscles and note the response of the great toe. Fanning or extension is considered abnormal.
- These alternative methods of eliciting the reflex tells us that the area from where the reflex can be elicited is quite large, meaning the possibility of a more extensive lesion.

Rossolimo's sign: On tapping the pulp of the patient's toes, there is flexion of the toes in pyramidal lesion. Note that the positive response is flexion of toes. Not a popular or validated sign in clinical medicine.

Deep Tendon Reflexes

If the deep tendon reflexes are not elicitable, examine after ***reinforcement*** (Jendrassik manoeuvre). Examples are clenching of teeth, pulling of flexed fingers, forcefully adducting thighs, etc. By this, the basal tone of muscles are increased so that it is easier to obtain the reflex.

Table 9.1 Tendon reflexes & their spinal roots

Reflex	Spinal roots
Jaw jerk	Trigeminal
Biceps	C5, C6
Supinator	C6
Triceps	C7
Knee	L2, L3, L4
Ankle	S1

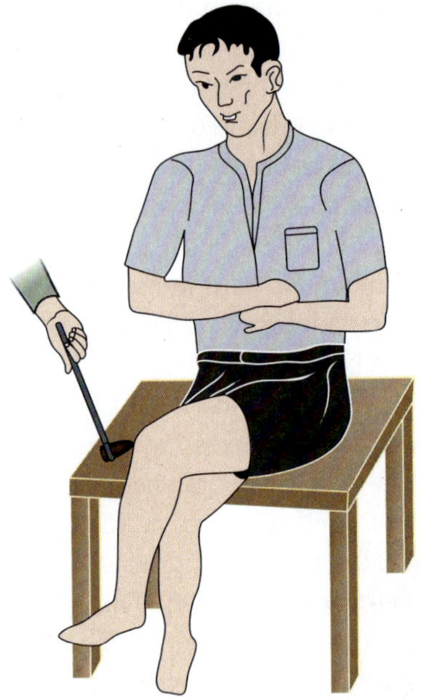

Fig.9.22 Knee jerk after reinforcement

The magnitude of reflexes varies with the different reflexes tested and this must be borne in mind before committing that a reflex is abnormal. For example, knee jerk in many children is normally also brisk (grade 3). Less than six beats may be taken as ill-sustained clonus.

- **Jaw jerk**: This is elicited by placing the examiner's index finger on the patient's lower jaw (with mouth slightly open) and then striking it with the reflex hammer. Normal jerk is just visible. An exaggerated reflex indicates the presence of a lesion above the pons (bilateral supranuclear lesion). Absent reflex is likely in trigeminal nuclear and trigeminal nerve lesions. Bilateral supranuclear lesion causing exaggerated jaw jerk is expected in quadriplegic cerebral palsy.

Table 9.2 Grading of deep tendon reflexes

Score	Reflexes
0	Absent (0)
1	Sluggish or present only with reinforcement (+)
2	Readily elicited (like normal ankle jerk) (++)
3	Brisk without evidence of clonus (like normal knee jerk) (+++)
4	Associated with clonus (++++). Here, one may mention if it is associated with sustained or ill-sustained clonus

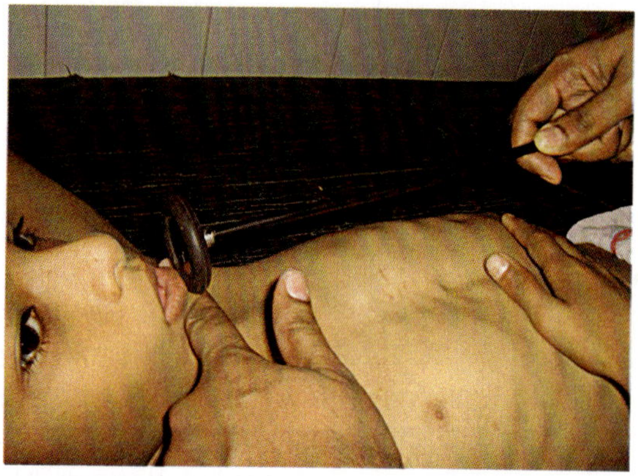

Fig.9.23 Jaw jerk

- **Biceps jerk**: With the child's arm semi-flexed at elbow resting on the examiner's forearm, strike over the examiner's thumb placed over the biceps tendon.
- **Supinator jerk**: Strike at the styloid process of radius in semi-pronated forearm (Figs. 9.25, 9.26).
- **Triceps jerk**: With the arm semi-pronated and flexed at elbow, pull the arm across the chest of the patient and then strike the triceps tendon just above the olecranon. Another position for elicting the triceps jerk is shown in Figure 9.28.

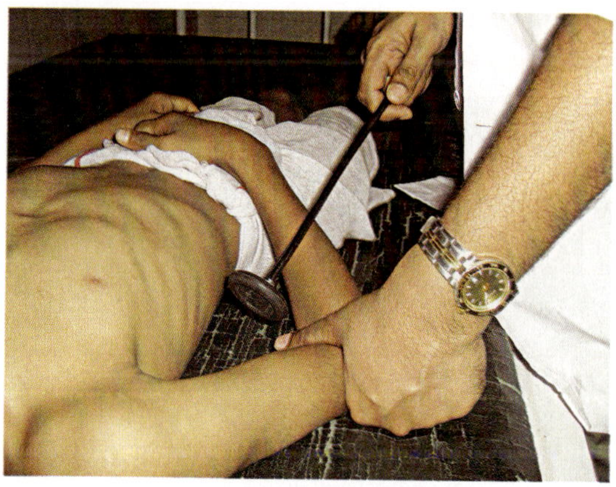

Fig.9.24 Biceps jerk

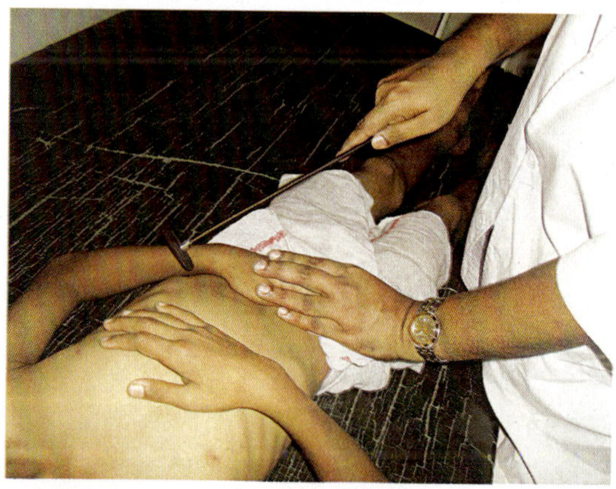

Fig.9.25 Left supinator jerk

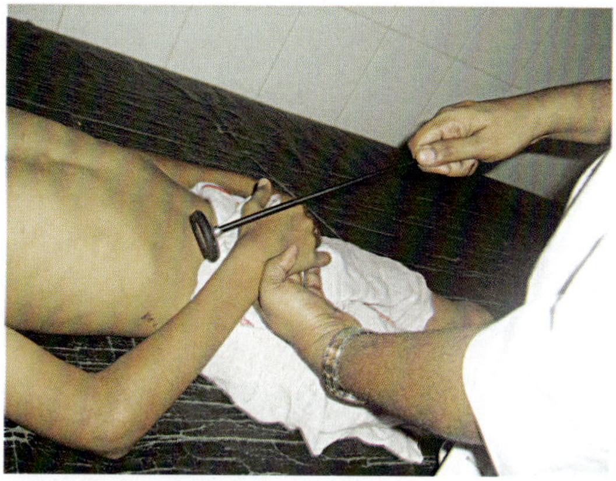

Fig.9.26 Supinator jerk

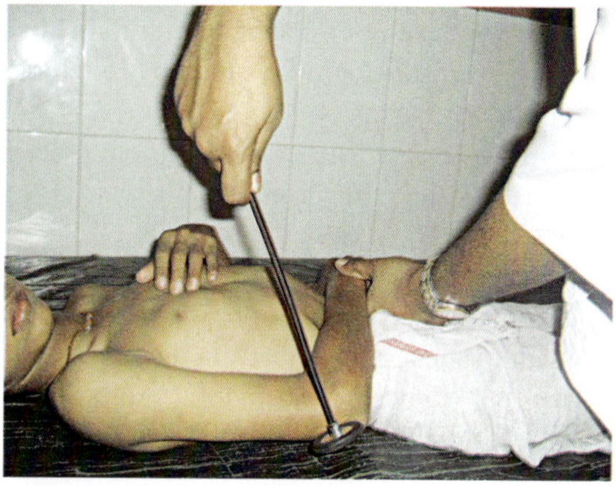

Fig.9.27 Triceps jerk in supine patinet

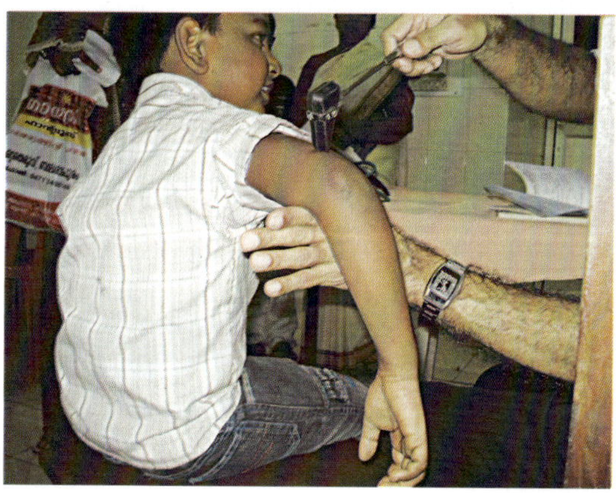

Fig.9.28 Triceps jerk

- **Knee jerk**: This can be elicited with the child sitting with his legs hanging or supine with the examiner's hands below the knee to raise it slightly above the bed (Fig. 9.29). In UMN lesions, make sure to look at the other leg also while eliciting the knee jerk. An adduction of the other leg while eliciting the knee jerk is called adductor spread of knee jerk, meaning that the reflex has spread even to the other limb, in turn pointing to a significant UMN lesion.

  When the knee jerk is very much exaggerated, it becomes elicitable even when struck down the anterior aspect of tibia rather than the conventional position. This is especially seen in spastic cerebral palsy. If the reflex is exaggerated, look for the **patellar clonus** by suddenly pushing down the patella by thumb and index finger and maintaining the downward pressure.
- **Ankle jerk**: If supine, rotate the hip externally, partially flex the knee, dorsiflex the ankle to make it feel just tight and then strike the Achilles tendon with a hammer. Also try to elicit **ankle clonus** by dorsiflexing briskly, holding the leg by knee. If not obtained, ask the child to push the feet on the examiner's hand to make the tone correct and try again (Fig. 9.30).

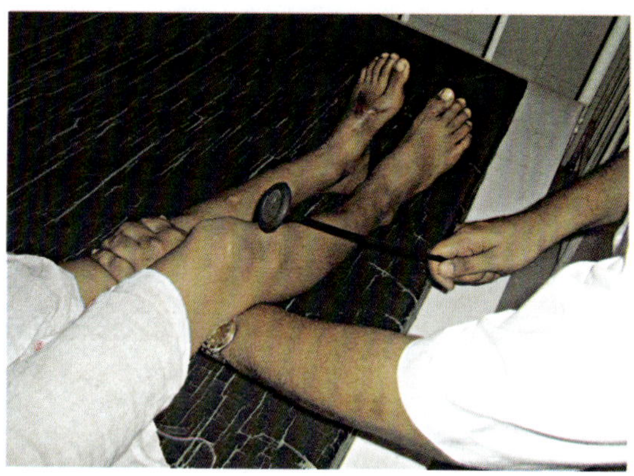

Fig.9.29 Knee jerk

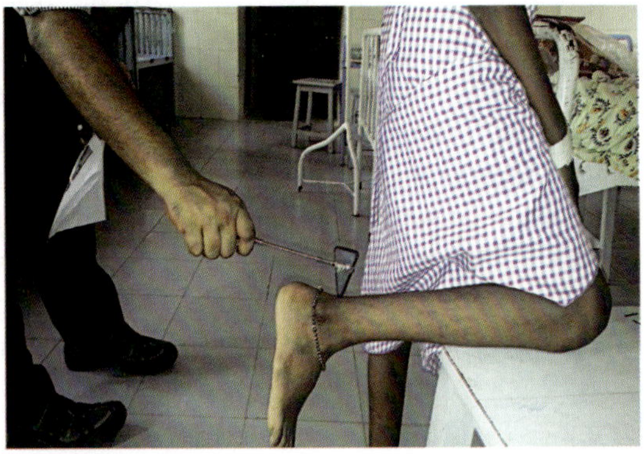

Fig.9.30 Method to elicit ankle jerk to demonstrate delayed relaxation in hypothyroidisum.

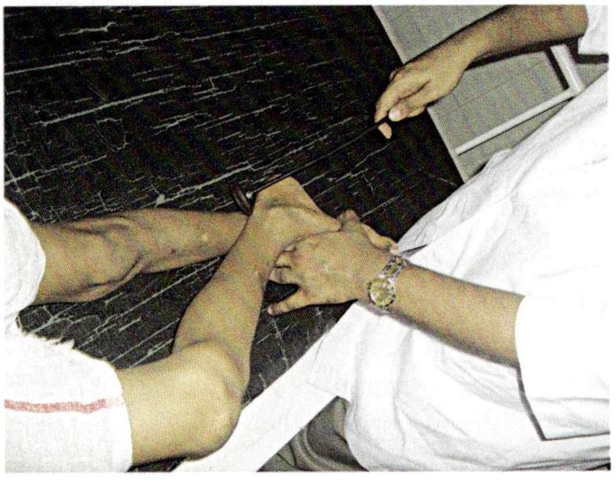

Fig.9.31 Right ankle jerk

It is easier to elicit the clonus if the dorsiflexion movement is combined with a slight eversion movement at ankle. More than six oscillations, qualify to be called as sustained clonus. Child "standing" on 90° flexed knee on a chair is also a good position to elicit ankle jerk.

One may fail to elicit exaggerated reflexes in the following situations:

- Severe contractures.
- Severe spasticity. In these situations, some clues may be obtainable. For example, even though knee jerk is not elicitable one may see a cross adductor response in the other limb: the telling evidence that it is a highly exaggerated reflex.
- Neuronal shock in UMN lesions (here the upgoing plantar will give valuable clue).
- When the child is voluntarily keeping the limb stiff, often out of fear. Diverting the attention of the child may help relax muscles.

Autonomic Nervous System

It consists of sympathetic and parasympathetic. Origin of the sympathetic is thoracolumbar (T1–L2), whereas origin of the parasympathetic is craniosacral (through cranial nerves 3, 7, 9, 10 and sacral segments S2–S4). Both these systems are under control of the hypothalamus.

9

Indicators of Abnormalities of the Autonomic Nervous System

- Postural fall of BP (suggestive history is giddiness while getting up from lying position).
- Skin: Excessive or less than normal sweating; flushing or pallor of skin; piloerection; oedema
- Pupillary immobility.
- Retention or incontinence of urine or faeces.
- Bronchospasm.
- Plenty of saliva or scanty thick saliva (most often demonstrable in animal experiments than humans).
- Penile erection without obvious cause (adults).

SENSORY SYSTEM

Terms to Describe Sensory Phenomena

- Paraesthesia: Sensations of spontaneous origin like pins and needles, numbness, etc, without an actual stimulus.
- Anaesthesia: Loss of all sensations (numbness).
- Hyperaesthesia: Exaggerated perception of sensations, usually seen in transverse myelitis at the level of lesion. The fastest method to detect hyperaesthesia is to run a blunt pointed

object from the area of sensory dulling upwards to the normal area. If there is hyperaesthesia, the child will cry out in pain as the stimulus reaches the border of these two zones.

- Root pain: Spontaneous severe pain radiating down to the periphery along the root. The pain is increased by coughing, sneezing, etc.

While examining the sensory system, the patient's eyes must be closed and the patient is directed to verbally respond to appreciation of sensations. But decide judiciously: small children may become uncooperative when asked to close their eyes.

Lateral Column Sensations

Fibres conveying sensations enter the spinal cord via posterior root and terminate within the posterior horns within 2–4 segments higher on the same side. After synapsing, the fibres crossover to the opposite side and ascend in the lateral spinothalamic tract to thalamus and then to the parietal cortex. The arrangement of fibres in the tract is opposite to what is found in the posterior column (see discussion below under posterior column). The primary modalities of sensation are light touch, pain and temperature.

- **Light touch**: Light touch is tested by touching the skin with a wisp of cotton or tissue; corresponding areas of both sides must be compared.
- **Pain**: This is tested by a blunt pin. To detect hyperaesthesia, draw the pin from the anaesthetic area to the normal area and watch for a wince on patient's face as the area of hyperaesthesia is reached.
- **Temperature**: Temperature can be tested by touching the patient's skin with two test tubes, one with warm water and after an interval with cold water; compare the identical areas of the two sides and also to a benchmark like the patient's own forehead (assuming sensation there is normal). Hot water is avoided as it may stimulate pain fibres; use only warm water. Pain and temperature sensation are specifically lost but other sensations preserved in syringomyelia (dissociated anaesthesia). Pain and temperature sensations ascend exclusively in lateral spinothalamic tract, whereas crude touch ascends in anterior (ventral) spinothalamic tract.

Posterior Column Sensations

Fibres conveying sensations from one side of the body ascend in the posterior column of the same side, enter and synapse at nucleus gracilis and nucleus cuneatus and then cross over to the opposite side and terminate in the thalamus. The distribution of fibres in the posterior column is as follows. The lower limb fibres are most medial (inner) and the upper limb fibres are most lateral. This knowledge has implications in localization of spinal lesions. It is not difficult to remember if one visualizes that as the posterior column ascend up, more and more fibres from upper parts of the body join the tract so that the lower limb fibres that were there initially in the tract become medial to the fibres joining the column later. Applying the same logic, one can visualize the fibre arrangement in lateral column as well. In the case of the lateral column (spinothalamic tract), the fibres entering the lateral column cross over to the other side before ascending further. So the lower limb fibres have crossed over and occupied the most lateral position on the other side; as the tract ascends up, more and more fibres from upper parts of the body join and cross over to the other side. However, this can only be medial to the lower limb fibres that have already crossed and occupied the lateral-most position on the opposite side.

- **Vibration**: Vibration is tested using a tuning fork, preferably with a frequency of 128 Hz; compare the two sides and also with the same body part of the examiner (as normal control). When the child stops feeling the vibrations, remove the tuning fork and see if the examiner can still appreciate the vibration, meaning that the child has reduced perception of vibration. For testing vibration, bony points are used like malleoli, tibial tuberosity, iliac spine, head of ulna, elbow, etc. The test has meaning only in an older child who can volunteer reliable information.

- **Joint/position sense (proprioceptive sensations)**: Certain impulses from muscles, joint, etc, are not consciously perceived but are carried to the cerebellum via the posterior columns and spinocerebellar tracts for necessary automatic body adjustments in space. One finger of the patient is held by its side by examiner's fingers (do not hold the finger by its upper and lower sides because the difference in pressure will be used to say the position rather than using the joint sense). Keep the eyes of the child closed and move the patient's finger up and down a few times and then is brought to a halt. Now ask the patient whether the finger is directed up or down. Before starting the test, the child must be demonstrated what is meant by up or down. The examiner may also test by placing one limb of the child in a particular position and asking the child to keep the other limb in the same position with the eyes closed.
- **Romberg's test**: This is a test for position sense (also see p 185, 207). On standing with the eyes closed and the feet together, the patient with a posterior column dysfunction classically sways to the point of falling down. This sign may also be positive if the patient has a significant vestibular dysfunction. It must be remembered that slight swaying with eyes closed may be seen in normal young children. History of losing balance and falling while washing face (temporary loss of visual compensation for loss of proprioception) is suggestive of loss of posterior column sensation.
- **Pressure** (deep pain or pressure touch): Pinching the tendo Achilles will elicit deep (pressure) pain. Squeezing muscles also serves same purpose.

Cortical Sensations

The cortical sensory system includes the somatosensory cortex and its central connections. This system enables the detection of the position and movement of the extremities in space (i.e., kinaesthetic sensation), size and shape of objects (i.e., stereognosis), tactile sensations of written patterns on the skin (i.e., graphaesthesia), and tactile localization and tactile discrimination on one or both sides of the body.

- Position sensation is tested with the patient's eyes closed. The examiner moves various joints, being sure to hold the body part in such a way that the patient may not recognize the movement simply from the direction in which the patient may feel the pressure from the examiner's hand. It is a posterior column sensation, but requires cortex for its interpretation. One can have some interesting theoretical work up on this. That is, if vibration is perceived but not joint position, it means a lesion above the thalamus, i.e., vibration can be perceived at the thalamic level but for recognition of joint position, cortex also is needed. Fortunately such a difficult clinical scenario does not arise even rarely!
- Stereognosis is tested by placing some familiar object (e.g., ball, cube, coin) in the patient's hand while his/her eyes are closed and asking the patient to identify the object. Inability to recognize the object by its size or shape is referred to as astereognosis. Ability to recognize a substance by its texture also may be tested by giving paper, cloth, metal, etc, to a child with his eyes closed.
- Agraphaesthesia is the inability to recognize letters or numbers written on the patient's skin.
- **Tactile localization**: Ask the child to locate where he has been touched.
- **Two-point discrimination**: An ordinary compass can be used to touch two points simultaneously. Even as little as 0.5 cm will be perceived in the fingertips, whereas in the legs as

much as 3–4 cm only may be perceived normally. Parietal lobe is supposed to be the site for two-point discrimination.

- **Sensory inattention**: When the corresponding parts on two sides of the body are touched simultaneously, the child fails to recognize touch on the affected side, but when touched individually, touch on both sides are perceived. This is supposed to be a sign of opposite parietal lobe involvement.

It is worth noting that total sensory loss is not possible with cortical lesions, as many sensations are perceived at the thalamus itself.

Sensory Dermatomes

A rough idea of distribution of sensory dermatomes is helpful in case of a child with sensory deficits.

Sensory supply of trigeminal nerve—ophthalmic, maxillary, mandibular divisions, is shown in Fig. 9.32.

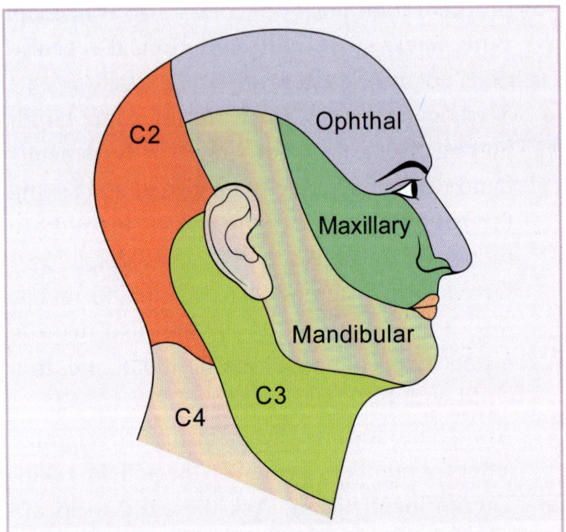

Fig.9.32 Trigeminal (sensory) *(Drawing by Dr Binoy Stephen).*

- C1 has no cutaneous supply, but it supplies the meninges.
- C2: Occiput, ear lobe, etc.
- C3: Side of neck behind the ear.
- C4: Around the shoulder.
- C5: Lateral arm up to the elbow.
- C6: Lateral forearm up to thumb.
- C7: Middle finger (mnemonic: remember C7 as the most projecting spine and C7 supplies the most projecting or the longest finger!).
- C8: Medial (ulnar side) of forearm.
- T1: Medial side of elbow and upwards.
- T2: Axilla (it is easy to remember the upper limb innervation if one visualizes C4–T2 as sweeping the arm progressively from shoulder through the lateral side, then to the medial side and ending in the axilla).
- T3–T8: Chest.
- T8 will be approximately at the costal margin.
- T10 will be approximately at the umbilicus.
- T12 will be approximately at the pubis.
- L1: Below the inguinal ligament.
- L2: Thigh (anterior aspect).
- L3: Knee (mnemonic: Remember the knee as a junction of three bones and hence L3!).
- L4: Medial aspect of the tibia in the anterior leg.
- L5: Lateral aspect of the anterior leg.
- S1: Sole (mnemonic: S1 supply sole, we all have only one soul!).
- S2: Back of thigh.
- S3, S4: Around the anus.

CEREBELLAR SIGNS

Cerebellar signs are partially discussed along with the examination of motor system. In cerebellar disease, the side of the lesion is the same as that having the deficit (i.e., a left-sided lesion produces left-sided deficit).

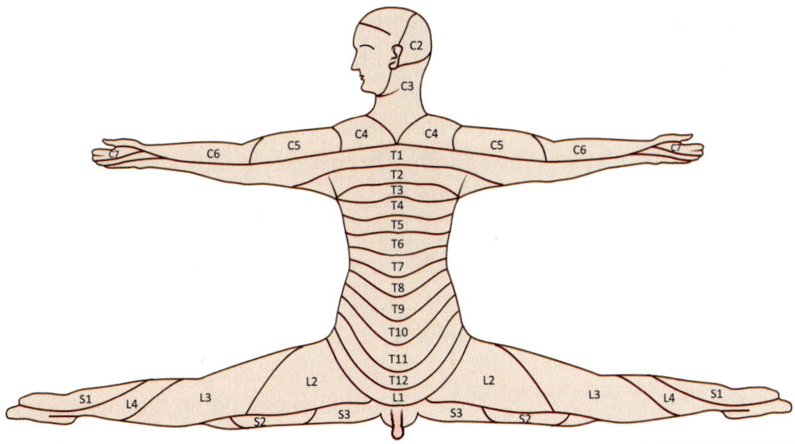

Fig.9.33 Innervation *(Drawing by Dr Binoy Stephen).*

Cerebellar signs are listed below (arranged from head to foot):

- Nystagmus, gaze evoked. The fast component is towards the side of lesion.
- Dysarthria (staccato, slurred, or scanning speech): Scanning is slow dragged out speech as though scanning. Staccato speech has undue stresses at points where stress is not to be used (see p 182).
- Titubation or head nodding (rhythmic oscillation of head on trunk).

Upper Limb

- Finger–nose test (dysmetria), can use finger-to-finger test also.
- Dysdiadochokinesia (inability to carry out rapidly alternating movements): This may be tested by asking the child to pat one hand with the other hand with rapidly alternating supination–pronation movements.
- **Rebound phenomenon**: The patient pulls the forearm against resistance from the examiner. The examiner suddenly releases his resistance keeping his other hand near the face of the child to prevent the rebound of the child's hand injuring the child's own face. In cerebellar disease, the child's hand fails to get arrested immediately after release of resistance and flies up with considerable force.
- **Intention tremor**: May be tested by the finger–nose test. As the fingers are nearing the target, there is exaggerated tremor. The child should fully extend and abduct the arms to about 90° and then touch the tip of his nose with the finger and then the examiner's finger. Intention tremor can be made out in the heel–knee test also (place heel over the opposite knee and slide down along the shin).
- **Dysmetria and past-pointing** (inability to stop intended movement at the correct place): This is tested by the finger–nose test where the finger may overshoot the nose or strike the nose with undue force because the distance is wrongly assessed by the child.
- **Dyssynergia** (incoordination): There is difficulty in smoothly carrying out complex movements. Rather the movement will have to be broken down into individual components for the child to perform it.
- **Trunk**: Truncal ataxia (ataxia in sitting position, cannot sit without support). Truncal ataxia is seen in lesions of midline cerebellar structures.

Lower Limb

- **Gait ataxia** (swaying to either side which is better appreciated on tandem walking). Gait ataxia is discussed under the heading "gait" (p 183). Limb ataxia can be made out with the child standing with outstretched arms. Limb ataxia is seen in lesions of cerebellar hemispheres.
- **Tandem walking**: The patient is asked to walk normally and in tandem. In the latter, the patient is asked to walk in straight line placing one foot immediately in front of the other (i.e., heel to toe). A tendency to sway or fall to one side indicates ataxia, suggesting cerebellar dysfunction. In sensory ataxia, the child walks fairly well with the eyes open but sways to fall when the eyes are closed as sensory input from eyes no longer compensates for the loss of posterior column sensations like position sense. In unilateral cerebellar disease, the patient sways towards the side of lesion.
- **Heel–knee test**: The child is asked to place the heel of one foot on the knee of the other leg and then to move the heel down over the tibia.
- **Pendular knee jerk**: The jerk elicited (with the child sitting in a chair with legs hanging) does not stop soon but goes on oscillating. Usually more than three swings are taken as significant to call it is pendular.
- Hypotonia with retained reflexes.
- The Romberg test evaluates the proprioceptive deficiency (posterior column sensation); it is not a test for cerebellar function (p 185, 207, 223).

SIGNS OF MENINGEAL IRRITATION

Nuchal rigidity or ***neck stiffness*** is tested by placing the examiner's hand under the patient's head and gently trying to flex the neck. Undue resistance implies diffuse irritation of the cervical nerve roots due to meningeal inflammation. In uncooperative children to differentiate between voluntary resistance and true neck stiffness, bring the child to the edge of the bed and let the head hang over the edge of the bed. It is a very uncomfortable position for the child and hence he no longer resists flexion of neck, but true neck stiffness will persist (see p 116, column 2).

Brudzinski neck sign is flexion of both knees during the manoeuvre to test nuchal rigidity. This indicates diffuse meningeal irritation in the spinal nerve roots.

Kernig's sign is elicited by flexing the hip and knee on one side to 90° while the patient is supine and then extending the knee further with the hip still flexed at 90° (Fig. 9.34). This results in stretching of spinal nerve roots of lower limbs that are already compressed by inflamed meninges. Hamstring spasm results in pain in the posterior thigh muscle and difficulty of knee extension. Normally, knee extension of about 135° is possible without any pain. With severe meningeal inflammation, the opposite knee may also flex during the test (***Brudzinski leg sign***).

Testing for neck stiffness in the sitting position will bring out subtle neck stiffness. This is because in sitting position (in bed) with extended legs, the nerve roots are already stretched so that minimal further stretching is enough to bring out pain and spasm.

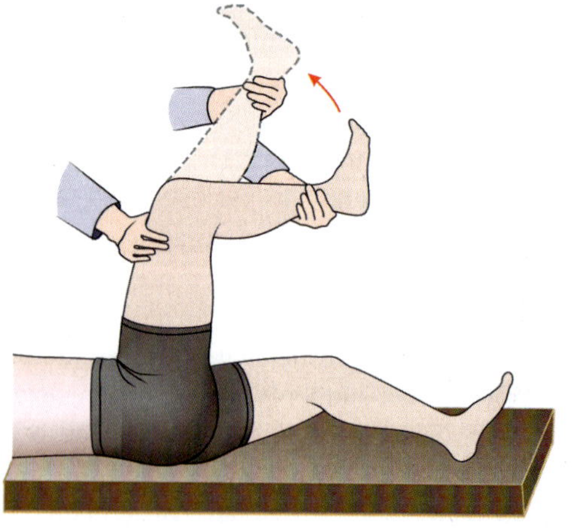

Fig.9.34 Kernig's sign

Neck rigidity may be seen in meningitis, subarachnoid haemorrhage, tetanus, herniation of brainstem (possibly due to the stretching of dura), meningism (e.g., upper lobe pneumonia), local painful lesions (here lateral movements are also likely to be restricted), etc.

Tripod sign: When the child is asked to sit in bed with extended legs, he does so by flexing the knees and supporting himself with his hands placed far behind him in bed (this is to avoid flexing the spine, which will be painful due to paraspinal muscle spasm) and the neck extended. It is classically described in the preparalytic stage of polio, but may be seen in severe meningeal irritation also. However, when the *prone* child is brought to the edge of the bed with the head hanging outside the edge of the table, the head hangs down limp in polio (neck flop), whereas in meningitis the child tries to prevent head flexion over the edge of the table as there is no neck flop here and neck flexion causes pain.

SKULL AND SPINE

MacEwen Sign or Cracked-pot Sign

A cracked pot sound on percussion of the skull is obtained when there is suture separation, usually due to increased intracranial pressure. This is elicited by percussing with a finger on parietal eminence and listening by placing the ear or stethoscope to the scalp a little away or on the other side of head. It is elicitable in hydrocephalus or any other causes of increased intracranial tension of some duration (only a long standing increased ICT will allow suture separation).

It may be normally elicitable in small children if their skull bones have not yet fused.

Cranial Bruit/Carotid Bruit

Auscultate for a bruit. Usual sites looked for are over the anterior fontanel, orbit and temporal region. Intracranial bruit can occur in 10–15% of normal children, especially over the temporal area. Conditions associated with cranial bruit are fever, anaemia, thyrotoxicosis, loud cardiac murmurs, etc. Arteriovenous malformations and vein of Galen malformation are possible causes for pathological bruit.

Transillumination of the Skull

- Transillumination of the skull is done in case of macrocephaly in young infants.
- Use a torch with a black rubber rim around the lighted end.
- Apply the rim of the torch firmly to infant's scalp in a dark room.
- A halo of up to 2 cm in the frontal area and 1 cm in the occipital area is accepted as normal in young infants.
- This is an important screening procedure in macrocephaly, subdural effusion, subdural haematoma, hydrocephalus, hydranencephaly, porencephaly, etc.
- In hydranencephaly, where the brain is replaced with a fluid-filled bag, the skull as such glows when transillumination is done (Fig. 9.35).
- Impaired transillumination is expected in case of caput succedaneum, cephalhaematoma, scalp oedema, thick black hair and lack of dark adaptation of the examiner.
- Transillumination may not occur if the cortex is thicker than 1 cm.

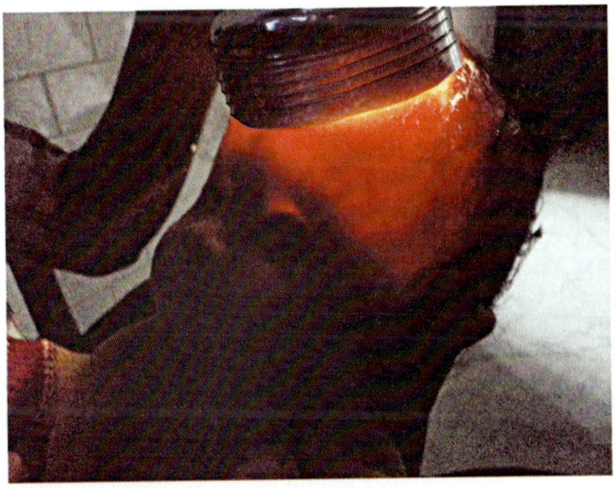

Fig.9.35 Transillumination of skull

- Isolated suboccipital transillumination may suggest dilatation of the IV ventricles in Dandy-Walker syndrome.

Spine

- Look for percussion tenderness over the spine. Look for gibbus, dimple, tuft of hair or congenital deformities or scoliosis.
- Look for **peripheral nerve thickening**: Just above the elbow (ulnar nerve), neck of fibula, are the usual sites. Peripheral nerve thickening is seen in Hansen's disease, hereditary motor sensory neuronopathy type III (Dejerine Sotta's disease), etc.

CHAPTER 10

Central Nervous System : Part–II

LOCALIZATION OF LESIONS IN NERVOUS SYSTEM

For localization of lesion in CNS, history is as important as physical examination. The first step is to localize the lesion to an anatomical site.

Anatomical Diagnosis

- Is the lesion upper motor neuron (UMN) or lower motor neuron (LMN)?
- If it is an UMN lesion, is the lesion in the brain or in the spinal cord?
- If the lesion is in the brain, is it in the cortex, subcortex (corona radiata), basal ganglia, internal capsule, midbrain, pons, medulla or cerebellum?
- If the lesion is in the spinal cord, which level of the spinal cord is involved?
- If the lesion is LMN, which structure is involved, anterior horn cell, the radicles, the peripheral nerve, neuromuscular junction or the muscle?

Aetiological Diagnosis

One must think of the aetiology after making an anatomical diagnosis. This is best ascertained by the mode of *onset* and *progression* of disease. Think of the aetiology in a classified approach as congenital, traumatic, inflammatory (including demyelination), vascular, degenerative, neoplastic and others (like toxic, metabolic, etc).

Onset

Ascertain the speed of onset of the symptom—was it acute, subacute or insidious?

- *Acute onset*: May be due to demyelination or stroke (vascular accident).
- *Subacute onset*: Infection, inflammation.
- *Insidious onset*: Tumours, degenerative diseases, etc.

Progression

Ask for the course of illness. Is the deficit recovering, progressing, static or waxing and waning?

- **Congenital**: Present from birth. In cerebral palsy, the insult occurs to a growing brain and the insult is not progressive. So the symptoms also do not progress. That is, the child will achieve milestones (may be after some delay) and will not lose achieved milestones. However, unexpected worsening can occur in cerebral palsy also following a seizure or development of hydrocephalus.
- **Vascular**: In a vascular accident, there is maximum deficit at onset (i.e., within about 72 hrs of onset) and then gradually the child recovers.
- **Demyelinating**: Sudden onset, progresses for sometime and then recover partially or completely. Example is Guillain-Barre syndrome. Waxing and waning or intermittent progression is characteristic of multiple sclerosis. In multiple sclerosis, there is progression with each episode of exacerbation, i.e., the child will improve after each episode, but the

recovery falls short of pre-exacerbation neurological status.

- **Degenerative**: The onset is slow and progression gradual. There is loss of acquired milestones. As small children are growing fast and attaining milestones, it is possible that in some cases milestones are achieved even with the progression of the disease so that one may find only a delay in developmental milestones rather than regression of milestones. This should not mislead the student into missing the progressive nature of the disease. On follow-up, these children will be found to lose the acquired milestones.
- **Neoplastic**: Symptoms in tumours are slow in onset and gradual in progression. Sudden worsening of symptoms can occur even in a tumour when there is bleed into it or when hydrocephalus develops.

UPPER MOTOR NEURON LESIONS

The UMN lesion may be a pure pyramidal lesion or may involve damage to tracts other than the corticospinal tract.

In UMN lesions, power is slightly reduced but movement is severely impaired, due to alteration of tone.

A pyramidal lesion is characterized by:

- **Hypertonia and hyperreflexia** (postgraduate students may note that hypertonia is not due to pyramidal tract involvement per se but rather due to involvement of the parapyramidal tracts. The classical cerebral lesion is a combination of involvement of the pyramidal tract and the parapyramidal tracts like the tectospinal, the reticulospinal and the vestibulospinal tracts). The hypertonia in pyramidal lesion is described as clasp knife spasticity.

  On passively moving the involved limb, one encounters an initial increase in resistance followed by an abrupt give way.
- **Spastic paralysis**: Some power in the limb will be retained unless the lesion is acute and severe in which case, the patient will be in a state of "neuronal shock." Weakness is predominant in the distal muscles and compromises skilled movement. The muscle bulk is preserved and atrophy if present, will be late and mild. Involvement of muscles is also characteristic. If one can visualize a hemiplegic patient and understand that he assumes that posture due to the action of stronger muscles, one can easily understand the pattern of involvement in pyramidal lesions. The abductors of the shoulder, extensors of the elbow, extensors of the wrist, flexors of the hip and dorsiflexors of ankle are weak (Fig. 9.1, p 185).
- Positive Babinski's sign.
- A reduction in the superficial reflexes.

The Distribution of Muscle Weakness in UMN Lesion

In an UMN lesion, there is a particular pattern of muscle weakness seen resulting in a predictable position of the limbs.

In the upper extremity, the shoulder is adducted, internally rotated, the elbow and wrist flexed. When the upper limb is held out in front of the body, classically one observes a pronator drift, the limb going into pronation due to the relative supinator weakness. In the lower extremity, it is kept extended, with plantar flexon at the ankle while supine. On standing hip & knee are slightly flexed due to plantar flexed foot causing apparent lengthening. It is not due to stronger hip flexors.

Features of Lesions in Different Levels of the Brain

- **Cerebral cortex**: Evidence of cortical involvement is altered sensorium, seizure or intellectual deterioration like dementia. Hemiplegia, if present, is not dense.

  In a cortical lesion, the motor deficit is on the opposite side and usually affects the face and arm more as their area of representation in cortex is large. Aphasia is more likely in the left (dominant) hemispheric lesion. Patients with right hemisphere lesions may have visuospatial problems.

- **Frontal lobe**: Social disinhibition, motor aphasia, appearance of primitive reflexes like grasp reflex, etc.
- **Parietal lobe**: Cortical sensory loss is evident in a cortical lesion involving the parietal lobe. Apraxias, losing the way to one's house, inability to calculate, etc, are possible. (***Note***: Apraxia is the inability to do a known act despite comprehending the command and in spite of the absence of any weakness; or the inability to do a series of tasks (on command) despite being able to do each segment individually.) Hemiparesis is very subtle as only a few fibres of the pyramidal tract arise from the parietal lobe. In fact, many times a slight asymmetry of the sides is picked up rather than weakness. In the picture shown (Fig. 10.1), the difference in size of two thumbs placed side by side, picked up the hemiplegia rather than any gross weakness. Parietal lobe functions may be remembered by mnemonic, CLAP (Calculation, Language, Appreciation of size, shape, weight and texture and Planned movement).

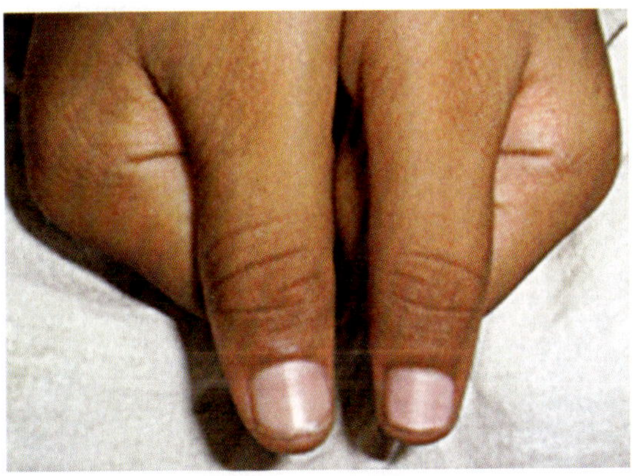

Fig. 10.1 Comparison of thumbs in hemiplegia (congenital)

- **Temporal lobe**: Hallucinations (auditory, visual, olfactory or gustatory), complex partial seizures, sensory (Wernicke's) aphasia.
- **Occipital lobe**: Bilateral lesions result in cortical blindness (blindness despite normally reacting pupils and normal fundus).
- **Subcortical lesion (corona radiata)**: Clinically appears like cortical lesion but convulsion and altered sensorium may not be there. Hemiplegia when present may be more dense than cortical lesion, involve the face, arm and leg more uniformly, because the pyramidal fibres converge as they descend so that more fibres tend to get affected in a given lesion. The sensory loss is more evident in a subcortical lesion, but note that the primary modalities of sensations are "perceived" at the thalamus itself.
- **Internal capsule**: Contralateral *dense* hemiplegia is expected as the fibres are closely packed. Hemi-anaesthesia and homonymous hemianopia may be there. Seizures and altered sensorium are absent.
- **Thalamus**: Contralateral mild hemiparesis with hyperalgesia. Hemisensory loss may be there.
- ***Note***: 3rd and 4th cranial nerve nuclei are in the midbrain, 5th to 7th in the pons and 9th to 12th in the medulla. For lesions at or below the midbrain, there is contralateral hemiplegia and ipsilateral cranial nerve palsy. Contralateral hemiplegia is because the pyramidal tracts decussate only lower down in the medulla (see below). For lesions above the midbrain, hemiplegia and cranial nerve palsy (if present) are of the same side.
- **Midbrain**: Ipsilateral third nerve palsy with contralateral hemiplegia (Weber's syndrome).
- **Pons**: Ipsilateral 6th/7th nerve palsy and contralateral hemiplegia (Millard-Gubler syndrome).
- **Medulla**: Ipsilateral 12th nerve palsy and contralateral hemiplegia (medial medullary syndrome).

10

When the lesion is in the brainstem, the cranial nerve is affected on the side opposite the hemiplegia (crossed hemiplegia), the crossed upper motor neurons to the cranial nerve having ended at the cranial nerve nucleus, and the pyramidal fibres are yet to decussate.

- **Extrapyramidal**: In a disease affecting the brain, movement disorders like chorea, athetosis, ballism or dystonia is in favour of extrapyramidal lesion. A parenchymal lesion is more likely here (e.g., due to vasculitis of TB meningitis), since a compressive lesion is highly unlikely to affect the deep-seated basal ganglia.

Decorticate and Decerebrate Postures

- Decorticate rigidity: Arms are flexed at the elbows and wrists; shoulder is adducted and legs are extended.
- Decerebrate rigidity: Arms are extended at the elbow and flexed at the wrist; shoulders are adducted and internally rotated; forearm is pronated; legs are extended at knee and ankle.

An upper motor lesion above the level of the red nucleus when severe and extensive, results in a decorticate posture with the thumb in the fisted position, the forearm pronated, the elbow flexed and with the lower limb in extension and the foot in inversion. When the lesion is below the level of the red nucleus, but above the origin of the vestibulospinal and the reticulospinal tracts, the upper extremity will be in pronation and extension, lower limb in extension and the neck in extension (decerebrate posture).

The red nucleus output reinforces the antigravity flexion of the upper extremity. When its output is eliminated, the unregulated activity of the reticulospinal and the vestibulospinal tracts reinforce the extension tone of both the upper and lower limbs. If you have difficulty in recollecting the positions in decerebration and decortication, use the following association. The word 'decerebration' has so many "e." So the posture in decerebration is extension!

Appearance of Latent Reflexes

A pyramidal lesion may unmask certain latent reflexes.

- **The finger flexion reflex**: The examiner places his middle and index finger across the tips of the patient's slightly bent four fingers and lightly taps his own fingers with a percussion hammer. Flexion of the four fingers and distal phalanx of the thumb can be seen.
- **Hoffman's sign**: The distal phalanx of the patient's middle finger is grasped firmly between the examiner's thumb and index finger. Flick the middle finger of the patient downwards with the other thumb forcing a sudden flexion of the distal phalanx.

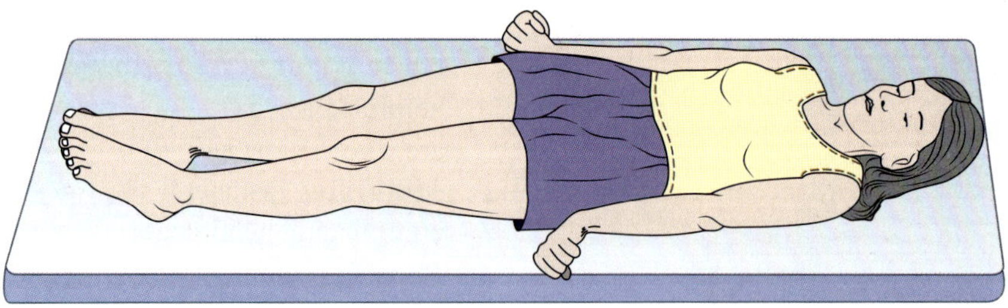

Fig.10.2 Decerebrate posture

In pyramidal lesion, tips of all fingers flex and the thumb flexes and adducts.

- **Tromner's sign**: The examiner holds the distal phalanx of the patient's partially flexed middle finger between his thumb and index finger. Tap the volar surface of the distal phalanx with the middle finger of the other hand of examiner. Response is same as in Hoffman's sign. In Tromner's, the examiner is extending the child's distal phalanx, whereas in Hoffman's the examiner flexes the child's distal phalanx.
- **Wartenberg's sign**: The patient flexes his four fingers and pulls against resistance offered by the examiner's flexed four fingers. The thumb adducts, flexes and moves inward in a pyramidal lesion (in a normal individual, the thumb remains nearly immobile at its initial position or it extends).

Primitive Reflexes

Reappearance of these neonatal reflexes signifies diffuse cerebral damage, particularly of the frontal lobes (hence the term "frontal lobe release" signs).

- **The sucking reflex**: Gently touch the corner of the mouth with the index finger; this elicits a reflex sucking.
- **Snout reflex**: Keep a finger on the upper lip and tap lightly on it. Puckering of lips will be seen if the reflex is positive.
- **The grasp reflex**: Stroking the palm between the thumb and index finger causes the patient to grasp your finger.
- **Palmomental reflex**: On scratching the thenar eminence, there is reflex contraction of the muscles of the chin (ipsilateral mentalis).
- **Glabellar tap**: Tap repeatedly over the glabella (above the root of nose). Normally, the eyes close with each tap but cease to do so with about 3–5 taps. The eyes continue to blink with each tap until you stop tapping, if the patient has a bilateral UMN palsy (e.g., pseudobulbar palsy).

Features of Lesions in Different Levels of the Spinal Cord

Here, there will be nothing to suggest involvement of brain, i.e., there will be no altered sensorium, no seizures, no cranial nerve palsy, etc. The face is spared. Hence, the lesion may be assumed to be in spinal cord.

- When UMN signs are present in both the upper and the lower limbs, the lesion is somewhere before the LMN leaves the spinal cord to innervate the upper limbs. Therefore, the lesion has to be high cervical, probably between C1 and C5. Atlanto-axial dislocation is possible in Down's syndrome, mucopolysaccharidosis, etc, and hence look for physical findings suggestive of these conditions. Also look for suggestions of craniovertebral anomalies like short neck, torticollis, restriction of neck movements, etc. Loss of pain and temperature sensations over the face may localize a lesion to C1–C2 (if it is spinal lesion) as this finding is due to the involvement of descending tract of trigeminal nerve.
- When there are UMN signs in both the lower limbs, with LMN signs in both the upper limbs, the lesion is somewhere where the spinal nerves innervating the upper limbs leave the CNS; i.e., the lesion is probably at the region C5–T2. Sensory level and reflexes help to further localize the lesion. If the biceps jerk is absent but triceps jerk is exaggerated (and also exaggeration of finger flexion), the lesion is at C5. When the supinator jerk is elicited, if elbow flexion is absent, but there is exaggeration of finger flexion (inversion of supinator jerk), the lesion is at C5, C6. Refer to notes on inverted reflexes.
- When there are UMN signs in the lower limbs and the upper limbs are normal, the lesion is somewhere in the spinal cord above the point where the nerves innervating the lower limb leave the spinal cord and below the region of the cord with innervation of the upper limbs.

The lesion is likely between T2 and L1. The sensory level and loss of abdominal reflexes in different quadrants help to further localize the lesion.

- When there are LMN signs in both the lower limbs with no other signs, the lesion involves the region of the spinal cord that innervates the lower limbs. The lesion has to be between L1 and S2 (if the lesion is in the spinal cord, it has got to be in the stage of spinal shock to be confused with a LMN lesion). This lesion has to be further localized, as to whether the lesion has affected the spinal cord and the cauda equina, or whether the lesion has affected only the cauda equina. This differentiation is mainly based on bladder and bowel involvement, the symmetric lesion and presence or absence of radicular pain. Asymmetry of involvement and root pain argues in favour of a cauda equina lesion.

Inversion of Reflexes

This may help in localization of lesions in certain circumstances. All movements are a combination of agonist and antagonist action. So when one of these is missing, the other action will be seen. Examples are:

- **Inverted biceps reflex**: On eliciting the biceps jerk, there is no flexion of elbow, but instead there is extension of the elbow due to the action of triceps, the antagonist muscle of elbow flexion. This is seen in lesion at C5, which cuts off supply to biceps but supply to triceps is intact.
- **Inverted supinator reflex**: On eliciting the supinator jerk, there is no flexion of the elbow but instead there is brisk flexion of fingers. Lesion is at C5, C6.
- **Inverted knee reflex**: On eliciting the knee jerk, there is flexion of the knee (hamstring action) instead of the expected extension. The lesion is at L3, L4.

Glove and stocking anaesthesia is found in peripheral neuritis. This is because the pathology starts from the end of the peripheral nerve and the longest nerves to the lower limbs are affected first. When the sensory impairment reaches the legs, the upper limbs start getting affected.

Saddle anaesthesia: Loss of sensation in the perianal area and in the upper part of both posterior thighs is seen in conus medullaris lesion. Saddle anaesthesia, if present in a cauda equina lesion, is likely to be asymmetrical (it is unlikely that the nerve roots of cauda equina are affected symmetrically bilaterally).

Sacral sparing: This is the preservation of sensations of S3, S4 while there is loss of sensations at higher level. It indicates an intrinsic cord lesion like syringomyelia (the sacral fibres are outermost in spinothalamic tract and will be spared in compression from within).

Note: In case there is any loss of sensation, mention if there are any trophic ulcers or not.

Types of Spinal Lesions

Spinal cord lesions can be broadly classified as non-compressive myelopathy and compressive myelopathy. In non-compressive myelopathies, the onset is very gradual, progression is very slow, there is no sensory level and there is no involvement of bladder. Example of a non-compressive myelopathy is hereditary spastic paraparesis, which rarely presents in paediatric age group.

Compressive myelopathy can be classified as a compression from within the spinal cord (intramedullary) or compression from outside the spinal cord (extramedullary). Extramedullary lesions can be further classified as extramedullary intradural and extramedullary extradural.

- **Intramedullary lesion** (syringomyelia): Early bladder (and rarely rectal) sphincter involvement (bladder fibres are near the centre of spinal

Table 10.1 Comparison of extramedullary and intramedullary lesions of the spinal cord

	Intramedullary	Extramedullary
Root pain (Radicular pain)	Absent	Present
Symmetry of weakness	Symmetric	Asymmetric
LMN signs at level of lesion (e.g., muscle atrophy)	Common	Unlikely
Bladder involvement	Early	Late
Dissociated sensory loss	Present	All sensations affected
Trophic changes	Early	Late
Sensory involvement	Descending	Not

cord), dissociated sensory loss (pain and thermal fibres being affected as they cross and make themselves vulnerable to lesions in the centre of cord), relative symmetry of the sensory involvement (as the lesion is spreading out from centre), a descending pattern of sensory involvement (because the upper limb fibres are medial and lower limb fibres lateral in spino-thalamic tract), an indistinct upper level of sensory involvement, absence of radicular pain, marked muscle atrophy at the level of lesion and trophic skin changes are all signatories of an intramedullary lesion (e.g., syringomyelia).

- **Extramedullary lesion**: Root pain, definite sensory level and late involvement of bladder are characteristic of extramedullary compressive myelopathies. Rarely, motor irritative phenomena like fasciculations may be found, which are unlikely in intramedullary lesion. Spasticity is more marked in extramedullary lesion compared to the intramedullary one. Extramedullary compressive lesions can be located intradurally or extradurally.
  - Extramedullary **intradural** lesion: Early onset unilateral radicular pain (early as the roots get irritated while passing through the dural space; unilateral as the lesion starts from one side or other), spasticity, slow onset of sensory loss, late bladder affection (bladder fibres are near the centre of the spinal cord, away from the site of lesion) and little or no atrophy are characteristically seen in an extramedullary intradural lesion. Example is neurofibroma, which grows within the dura and compresses the cord from one side.

    Brown-Sequard syndrome: In theoretical or experimental transection of the cord, pyramidal weakness on the ipsi-lateral side and spinothalamic sensory loss on the opposite side are expected. A similar situation can arise in compression due to a extramedullary intradural lesion.
  - Extramedullary **extradural** lesion: The features of extramedullary intradural lesion will be there but in addition there is deformity of the spine (gibbus) and increased pain on pressure on the vertebral spine, paraspinal muscle spasm, etc. Cord compression is relatively symme-trical unlike the extramedullary intradural lesion where there is marked unilaterality. Imagine the example of an extramedullary extradural lesion (TB spine). Compressing from the back causing relative symmetry.

Transverse Myelitis

A sharp sensory level on the abdomen or chest below which there is dulling of all sensations is characteristic of transverse myelitis. There may be a band of abnormally heightened sensory perception in a band like area over the chest or abdomen (drag a pencil along the body from down upwards and when the band of hyperaesthesia is reached, the child winces). A girdle sensation or a girdle pain may be there. There will be weakness of the limbs below the level of lesion, which is distal and affects the fine movements more than proximal movement (as in any other UMN lesion). The weakness tends to be more or less symmetric and the symmetry depends on the extent of spinal cord involvement. Bladder affection accompanies a cord lesion (rarely bowel also), due to the involvement of the autonomic fibres in the cord. A history of hesitancy or overflow incontinence must be sought.

The spinal shock state is a clinical curiosity, where an UMN lesion resembles a LMN lesion. It results from severe damage to the spinal cord, often complete transection. It is due to the sudden removal of the descending control on the lower motor neuron, which makes the LMN nonfunctional temporarily. It may last from 24 hrs to up to a month. The typical clinical features are flaccid paralysis and areflexia. However, the plantar response may be extensor although it may fail to produce any response at times. Flexor plantar response is highly unlikely.

When the spinal shock recovers, the deep tendon jerks appear and they will be exaggerated. Muscle tone reappears. The bowel or bladder dysfunction will resolve.

Spinal Segmental Level vs Vertebral Level

There are 8 cervical segments, 12 thoracic (dorsal), 5 lumbar, 5 sacral segments and one coccygeal segment in a spinal cord. Since the spinal cord is shorter than the vertebral canal, the spinal segments do not correspond to the vertebra overlying it. A rule of thumb to find out the spinal segments corresponding to the vertebra is given here.

Vertebral body	Spinal cord level
Cervical vertebra	Add 1
1–6 dorsal	Add 2
7–9 dorsal	Add 3
10th dorsal	L1 and L2
11th dorsal	L3 and L4
12th dorsal	L5 and sacral segments

Spinal levels according to muscle group involved

L1-	Hip Flexors
L2-	Hip Adduction
L3-	Knee Extension
L4-	Foot Inversion (minor- ankle dorsiflexion)
L5-	Ankle dorsiflexion, Foot eversion, Extension of big toe (EHL).Hip Abduction
S1-	Plantar Flexion,Hip extension (minor)
S2-	Knee flexion

BLADDER DYSFUNCTIONS

- Hesitancy: There is difficulty to initiate the act of micturition. It takes a lot of time and effort to begin micturition.
- Precipitancy (urgency): The patient cannot hold on for sometime once the bladder sensations are triggered.
- Retention: Bladder is full but cannot void.
- Dribbling: Constantly wetting the dress by drops of urine coming out.

Cortical or Uninhibited Bladder

Since the pons is the coordinating centre for *detrusor sphincter synergia*, any lesion above the pons will have a coordinated detrusor-sphincter action and complete involuntary emptying occurs as in case of the newborn. There is no danger of vesicoureteric reflux (VUR) and hence it is referred to as *"safe bladder."*

When there is a lesion at the paracentral area of frontal lobe, there may be evacuations at socially unacceptable situations like a newborn (social incontinence). Since the arc up to the pons is intact, the bladder emptying is complete, with no residual urine and no detrusor sphincter dyssynergisia. Associated frontal lobe symptoms like dementia are possible.

Spinal or UMN or Hyperreflexic Bladder

Any transection above the sacral cord but below the pons will cause spinal bladder (e.g., transverse myelitis).

During the acute spinal shock stage, the bladder remains toneless with a large volume of urine and overflow incontinence (thus at this stage it looks like LMN bladder). When the tone recovers, the spinal reflex arc slowly brings back the detrusor contractions, which may force open the contracted sphincter periodically to cause dribbling.

As the acute stage passes off, the bladder becomes *hypertonic* with *small capacity,* which empties suddenly and *reflexly* with the help of the spinal centre ***(automatic bladder)***. The pontine centre will facilitate micturition only when a critical volume of urine accumulates in the bladder. However, the spinal centre has a lower threshold so that it fires more frequently (hence small capacity bladder). Since the connection with the coordinating centre (pons) is lost, there is no guarantee that the sphincter will open when the detrusor contracts and hence there will be residual urine. Contraction against a non-relaxing sphincter may induce back pressure and reflux of urine up the ureter (VUR). This leads on to infections and thus damages the upper urinary tract. Hence, UMN bladder is referred to as *"unsafe bladder."* There will be no bladder sensations in transverse myelitis, as the afferents cannot reach the thallamus or the cortex.

LMN or Areflexic Bladder

The bladder remains *areflexic* with *huge capacity* and high residual volume that will predispose to infections.

Sensory denervated bladder: This is described in diabetic neuropathy in adults and is uncommon in a child. Here, the sensory limb is lost and hence there is no bladder sensation. There is dribbling incontinence with large bladder volumes. Since the motor limb is normal, the patient may be able to void by straining in a timetable manner even if there is no bladder sensation. The total emptying of bladder may not materialize as the bladder is too flabby.

Motor paralytic bladder: The motor limb is damaged. Bladder sensation is appreciated, but the patient voluntarily cannot void. This causes an areflexic bladder with urinary retention and overflow incontinence. As the sphincter yields, manual compression can empty the bledder. This may be transiently seen in Guillain-Barre syndrome or poliomyelitis.

Autonomous bladder: When there is a combined involvement of both sensory and motor limbs almost totally, and hence the local vesical plexus takes over and functions as an autonomous bladder. This can never empty the bladder completely. There is no sensation of bladder fullness and there is continuous dribbling (dribbling incontinence) with high residual volumes even after evacuation. Such situations are seen in cauda equina lesions and spina bifida where the LMN connections to the bladder are damaged.

The student who is not well versed with bladder dysfunctions, is advised to read "*Manual of of Pediatric Practice*" by the same author.

LOWER MOTOR NEURON LESIONS

LMN lesions are characterized by wasting, hypotonia and hyporeflexia.

1. Flaccid paralysis (hypotonia): The limb that is affected does not offer any resistance to passive movement. This is due to the loss of the stretch reflex.
2. Areflexia or hyporeflexia: This is again due to the interruption of the stretch reflex pathway.
3. Atrophy: Early and marked.

Anterior horn cell disease: Fasciculations (look at the tongue) with no sensory loss and gross wasting characterize an anterior horn cell lesion like spinal muscular atrophy. In several anterior horn cell diseases, there is wasting out of proportion to the weakness.

Root disease (radiculopathy): Pain is a hallmark of root disease and the radicular pain shoots down the limb, with at times paraesthesia and sensory dulling. Root pain increases by coughing and sneezing. The findings are usually asymmetric (affects only the myotomes and dermatomes supplied by the given radicle) with atrophy, weakness and sensory loss.

Peripheral nerve: In peripheral nerve affection due to polyneuropathies, there is distal symmetric weakness, atrophy and glove and stocking type distribution of sensory loss and paraesthesia. These findings will be in the distribution of the muscles innervated by a nerve, if it is a mononeuro-pathy (e.g., sciatic nerve palsy following gluteal IM injection). There is early atrophy of the muscles and sensory loss.

Neuromuscular junction: In neuromuscular junction disease, the weakness is usually proximal and symmetric, with fatiguability after exertion and diurnal variation as the hallmarks. With prolonged use, the muscle becomes weak and recovers with rest. Ptosis is the most common presenting symptom and in the initial stages ptosis may be asymmetrical, a point to be taken note of. The muscle tone is normal and deep tendon reflexes are preserved. Wasting is unusual. There is no sensory loss.

Muscle diseases: In muscle diseases, the weakness is proximal and symmetric, the muscle bulk is usually maintained till late in the illness, and sensory phenomena are absent. Deep tendon reflexes will be decreased proportional to the weakness.

Note

1. Weakness in LMN lesions is usually proximal more than distal. Exceptions are there like peripheral neuropathies. Rule of thumb: A patient with only proximal muscle weakness, or proximal more than distal muscle weakness in a limb is most likely having LMN weakness. In a patient with definite pyramidal weakness, if he has proximal muscle weakness more than distal, look for an additional LMN lesion.
2. Combined picture of UMN and LMN lesions is seen in spinal arachnoiditis, as in TB spinal arachnoiditis.

LOCALIZATION BY A RAPID NEUROLOGICAL EXAMINATION IN A COMATOSE PATIENT

- Normal brainstem reflexes and no lateralizing signs indicate bilateral diffuse cerebral hemispheric dysfunction. Possibilities are encephalitis, encephalopathy (hypertension, hepatic failure, hypoglycemia, etc), acute demyelination or poisoning. It can be a manifestation of any condition producing cerebral oedema.
- Normal brainstem reflexes with lateralizing signs indicate unilateral dysfunction. Infarction, tumours, brain abscess, haemorrhages, etc are the possible causes. Focal signs in postictal states will be transient.
- If brainstem reflexes are abnormal, it indicates compromise of brainstem function either directly or by herniation. It indicates an advanced stage of cerebral dysfunction.
- Papilloedema almost rules out metabolic/toxic coma as papilloedema is very rare in acute events like metabolic coma. Hypertensive encephalopathy and lead encephalopathy may be associated with papilloedema.
- Neck stiffness is seen in meningitis, meningism, and subarachnoid haemorrhage.
- Motor response: Apply a noxious stimulus (usually supraorbital ridge compression) and observe the response. Purposeful withdrawal away from pain or talking indicates preserved cortical function. Decorticate posturing in response to pain indicates subcortical or upper brainstem lesion. Decerebration in response to pain indicates high pontine or midbrain lesions (intercollicular level).

Total flaccidity with no response to pain indicates lower pontomedullary lesions. Asymmetric response indicates neurological deficits like hemiplegia.

- Normal pupils are expected in cortical and subcortical lesions. In midbrain lesions and in central herniation, non-reactive midsize pupils or slightly dilated ones may be seen (lack of reaction is because of interruption of the pupillary light reflex fibres). In pontine lesions and in metabolic coma, small reactive pupils may be seen. Pontine lesions interrupt the sympathetic pathways and hence the pin point pupils; they remain reactive to light but one may need a magnifying glass to appreciate it. Small pupils are also seen in organophosphorus or opioid poisoning. Small reactive pupils also may be seen in metabolic coma, some medullary lesions and transiently in early rostral-caudal herniation. Drugs usually produce a normal reactive pupil (except morphine, atropine, etc). Unilateral dilatation of pupil if not due to local application of drugs or third nerve palsy, is always due to a mass lesion producing herniation. Bilateral dilated pupils may be due to local mydriatic application, post-ictal stage, poisoning due to certain agents like *dhatura*, hypoxia, encephalitis, etc.
- **Cold calorie test**: Keep the head in the midline and raised to 30° (head tilt is to ensure that the lateral semicircular canal is horizontal). Ensure that the tympanic membrane is intact. Syringe 50 mL cold water at about 30°C into the external auditory canal with a tube for 30 sec and look for tonic deviation of eye to the same side, which indicates intact brainstem. This is followed by nystagmus with fast component to the opposite side. Nystagmus may be there for about 30 sec, then gradually decays away over next 2 min. After a rest of at least 5 min, the procedure is repeated with warm water (warm or cold water is either 7°C above or below the body temperature). Using warm water (44°C) elicits opposite response. Mnemonic: COWS; Cold Opposite and Warm Same side nystagmus (by convention, nystagmus is named after the direction of fast component). Abnormal response is obtained both in structural and metabolic lesions. When there is no response to the standard test, some clinicians use still colder water. Simultaneous bilateral cold water application results in slow phase down and fast phase up, whereas the reverse occurs if warm water is applied.
- **Doll's-eye manoeuvre** (oculocephalic reflex): Hold the eyes open, passively rock the head from side to side. At the extreme lateral position, watch for any movement of eyes (see p 195). Also do flexion and extension of neck and observe for eye movements.

BREATHING PATTERNS AND CNS LOCALIZATION

- **Cheyne-Stokes breathing**: Slowly increasing depth of respiration to reach a plateau, then decreasing to become apnoeic, only to restart the cycle all over again. Cheyne-Stokes respiration denotes severe bihemispheric damage. Cheyne-Stokes breathing is somewhat the normal breathing pattern arising from the brainstem centre. When the "smoothing effect" of this natural pattern by the hemisphere is lost, this pattern of breathing becomes clinically obvious.
- **Central neurogenic hyperventilation**: Patients with lesions in midbrain and upper pons exhibit hyperventilation.
- **Apneustic breathing**: It is characterized by a long inspiratory pause, during which air is retained for several seconds; it is seen in lower pontine lesions.
- In **Biot's breathing** the apnoeic periods are interposed with respirations of varying depth and varying irregularity. Another pattern in

Biot's breathing is abrupt apnoea alternating with four or five breaths of normal depth.

- **Ataxic breathing** is completely irregular in rate and rhythm and is usually seen in medullary lesions.

EXAMINATION OF MUSCLE POWER

The testing of muscle power is very important to assess the degree of weakness, the differential involvement of various groups of muscles, and in assessing the progress of the disease. The formal muscle testing is not always possible in young children, in delirious or uncooperative patients and in comatose patients. In these patients, noting the spontaneous or pain induced movement of the limbs and the asymmetry between the two sides can give important information.

Principles of Muscle Testing

- Always look for pain, tenderness or contractures in muscle, which may give a false impression of weakness. If there is pain or muscle contractures note that in your case record.
- Fix the proximal joint before testing a movement, because some movements can be mimicked by the action of muscles in the proximal joint (e.g., when testing pronation, if the humerus is not fixed, the rotators of shoulder may produce similar movement).
- For certain movements, synergistic action of other muscles is essential, e.g., in handgrip, wrist extension is a synergistic movement; if there is wrist drop, the handgrip may appear erroneously weak. In this case, make the wrist extend manually and then only test for grip strength.
- Muscle power can be tested in two ways—isotonic and isometric. In isotonic contraction, the child is asked to do a movement while the examiner tries to resist it. In isometric contraction, child is asked to keep the muscle contracted and the examiner tries to break it. This method is relatively easy to administer in children; e.g., the child is asked to keep the upper limb in a flexed position when testing biceps, and the examiner tries to break it.

Testing of muscle *groups* was discussed in the previous chapter (p 213). A short discussion on the method of testing of selected muscles is attempted here. Using the above principles all the muscles can be tested provided one knows the origin, insertion and the important function of the muscle.

As a ***quick screening*** test if the child is able to stand, walk, climb stairs, stand on one foot and jump normally, his lower limb muscle power is normal. If he is able to button his shirts, eat by himself, comb his hair, and carry weights above his head, his upper limb power is normal. If he can get up from bed without support and turn over, then his hip and paraspinal muscles are functioning well. Try to examine the weak muscles in detail, which can be determined from a good history.

- **Abductor pollicis brevis** (Supply: T1 via median nerve): The importance of this muscle is that this is the first one to become weak in carpal tunnel syndrome. Keep the hand over the table with palm facing upwards. Steady the fingers and abduct the thumb at right angles to the plane of fingers against resistance (Fig. 10.5).
- **Opponens pollicis** (Supply: T1 via median nerve): Keep the hand over the table. Ask the child to touch the little finger with the thumb, and oppose the movement by your fingers (see Fig. 10.24).
- **Interossei**: Palmar interossei adduct and dorsal abduct the fingers (mnemonic: PAD and DAB). Remember: the first dorsal interossei abduct the index finger and not the thumb. The interossei along with lumbricals flex the metacarpophalangeal and extend the interphalangeal joints.

(In claw hand, when the interossei and lumbricals are weak, the metacarpophalangeal joints are hyperextended and the interphalangeal joints are flexed.) Tested by trying to pull out a card held between fully extended fingers of the child (Another method see Fig. 10.10, 10.12).

- **Adductor pollicis** (Supply: T1 via ulnar nerve): Ask the child to adduct the thumb close to index finger (Fig. 10.6). The adductors of both hands can be compared by the *card test*. The child is asked to hold a card between the thumb and index finger of both hands and the examiner tries to pull off the card. If one adductor is weak, child uses the flexor pollicis longus to hold the card and there will be flexion of the thumb.
- **Flexors of fingers**: Ask the child to squeeze your fingers. Try to remove the fingers and assess the strength of grip. If the wrist extensors are weak, the examiner should assist in keeping the wrist extended. The flexion of distal interphalangeal joint is by flexor digitorum profundus and proximal IP joint is by flexor digitorum superficialis.
- **Flexors/extensors of wrist**: Fig. 10.19 22.
- **Biceps** (Supply: C5 via musculocutaneous nerve): Ask the child to flex the elbow completely keeping the forearm supinated (brachioradialis act as a flexor of elbow in midprone position and hence avoid pronation) and you try to extend the elbow (Fig. 10.7).
- **Brachioradialis**: (Supply: C5,6 via radial nerve): Ask the child to flex the elbow, keeping the forearm in the pronated position, against resistance (Fig. 10.8).
- **Triceps** (Supply: C7 via radial nerve): Ask the child to keep the elbow extended completely and keep it in that position. The examiner tries to flex the elbow (Fig. 10.18).
- **Supraspinatus** (Supply: C5 via suprascapular nerve): The first 30° of abduction of shoulder is by supraspinatus. While abducting the shoulder against resistance, palpate for the contraction of muscle (Fig. 10.16).
- **Infraspinatus** (Supply: C5 via suprascapular nerve): Patient flexes the elbow, holds the elbow to his side and then attempts to turn the forearm backwards against resistance (Fig. 10.11).
- **Rhomboids** (Supply: C5 via nerve to rhomboids): With hands on hips, the patient tries to force the elbow backwards. In Fig. 10.14, the rhomboids are not prominent, but the area where it is expected is marked by arrow.
- **Deltoid** (Supply: C5 via circumflex nerve): Middle fibres abduct the shoulder from 30 to 90°. Anterior and posterior fibres draw the abducted arm forwards and backwards, respectively. Patient is instructed to hold the arm abducted at around 60° against examiner's resistance (Fig. 10.9).
- **Trapezius**: Actions: Abduction of arm above 90°; shrugging of shoulders. When there is weakness of trapezius, there is drooping of shoulder, squaring (the rounded contour is lost) and winging of scapula (Fig. 10.17).
- **Pectorals** (Supply: C6,7,8 via lateral and medial pectoral nerves): Ask the child to raise the arms above 90° keeping the elbow extended and resist the examiner's attempt to separate the forearm (pectorals are adductors of shoulder). Place the hands on the hip and press inwards (tests sternocostal part) (Fig. 10.31).
- **Serratus anterior** (Supply: C5,6,7 via nerve to serratus anterior): The child is asked to push against a wall keeping the elbow flexed. In serratus weakness, there is winging of scapula (Fig. 10.15).
- **Latissimus dorsi** (Supply: C7 via nerve to latissimus dorsi): Easiest method is to ask the patient to cough while palpating the muscle to feel its contraction. Or keep the patient's arm abducted to above 90° and ask to adduct against resistance (this brings clavicular part of pectorals also into action) (Fig. 10.23).

- **Neck muscles**: Test for flexion, extension and lateral rotation of neck muscles (see p 463). Neck muscle weakness is prominent in polymyositis, dermatomyositis and in Guillain-Barre syndrome.
- **Abdominal muscles**: Ask the child to get up from supine posture without using the upper limb and feel for the contraction of muscle (keep the forearm crossed over the chest). When the weakness is confined to lower abdominal muscles, *Beevor's sign* will be positive (p 213). Keep the child's hand over the chest, and ask him to flex the neck forwards, the umbilicus will move up. To appreciate the movement better keep a ruler at the level of umbilicus.
- **Respiratory muscles**: Examine the movements of the chest. Look for paradoxical movements. Ask the child to count as much as possible without taking a breath (single breath count). Check for the power of intercostal muscles by splinting the abdomen and vice versa (p 213).
- **Flexors of hip**: Mainly psoas major. Ask the child to flex the hip against resistance keeping the knee flexed (Fig. 10.27).
- **Extensors of hip**: Keep the child prone. Ask him to raise the hip backwards against resistance. The knee should be kept flexed (Fig. 10.3). We can eliminate gravity by keeping the child in the lateral position and doing the same manoeuvre.

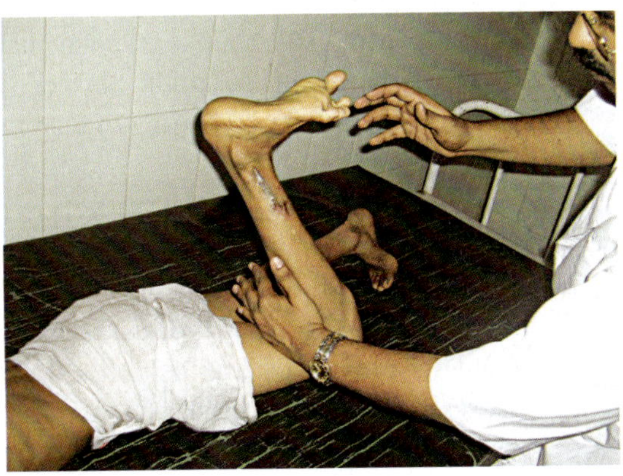

Fig.10.3 Hip extension

- **Adductors of thigh**: The child lies supine. Keep the limbs abducted (thighs wide apart) and ask him to move the limbs towards midline, the resistance being applied on the inner aspect of thigh (Fig. 10.38). Adduction against gravity is tested by keeping the child in the lateral position, the opposite limb is kept abducted, and the limb close to the ground is adducted upwards (not a comfortable position!) (Fig. 10.4).
- **Abductors of thigh**: Keep the child in supine position with the knees close together. Ask him to separate the thighs against resistance (Fig. 10.37). If you want to test against gravity, ask the child to abduct the limb upwards while lying in a lateral position. If the right abductors are to be tested, child should lie in left lateral position so that the right limb will be above.
- **Flexors of knee**: Keep the child prone; ask him to flex the knee against resistance. It can also be tested with the child supine (Fig. 10.35).
- **Extensors of knee**: Ask the child to keep the knee extended, and you try to break it by applying pressure on the leg. The hip should be kept flexed. If weak, you have to support the thighs (Fig. 10.34).
- **Dorsiflexion of foot**: Ask the child to press on your hand kept on the dorsum of foot (Fig. 10.33).
- **Plantar flexors**: Ask the child to kick on your hand kept on the sole of foot while you try to resist it (Fig. 10.36). Do not forget to fix the leg; otherwise, the movement can be imitated by the action of hip muscles.
- **Invertors**: You have to keep the limb in the inverted position and ask the child to keep it in the same position, while you apply resistance to inversion.
- **Evertors** are also tested in the similar manner by keeping the foot in everted position.

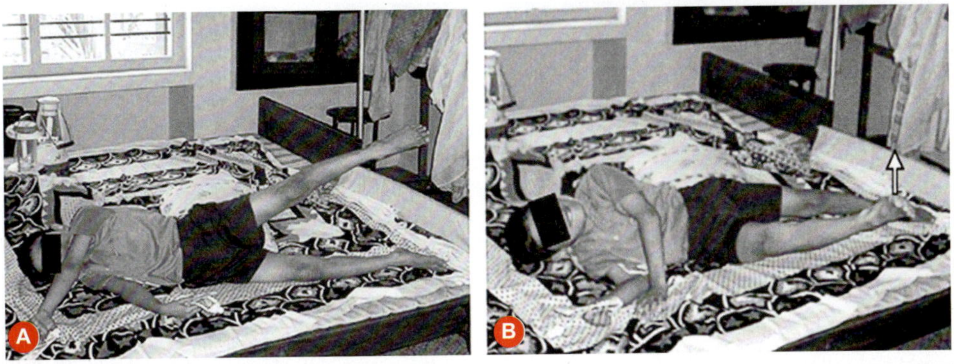

Fig.10.4 Abductors of thigh of left side (A) and adductors of right side (B)

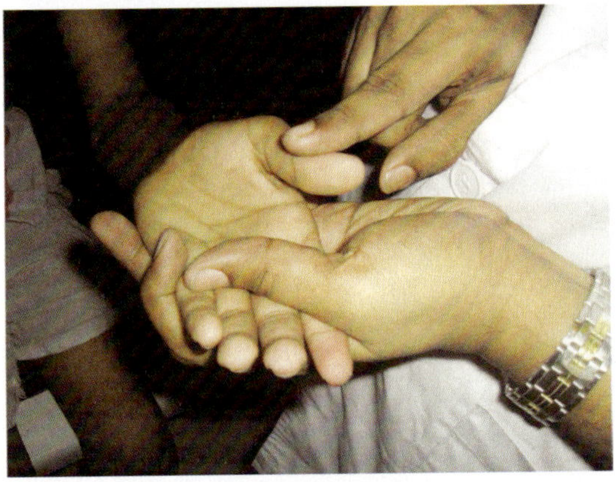

Fig.10.5 Abductor pollicis. Abduct against resistance in a plane perpendicular to palm.

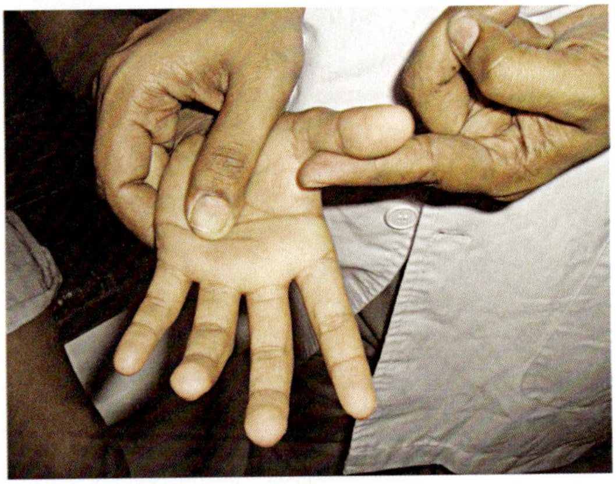

Fig.10.6 Adductor pollicis. Adduct thumb to the plane of palm in a perpendicular manner.

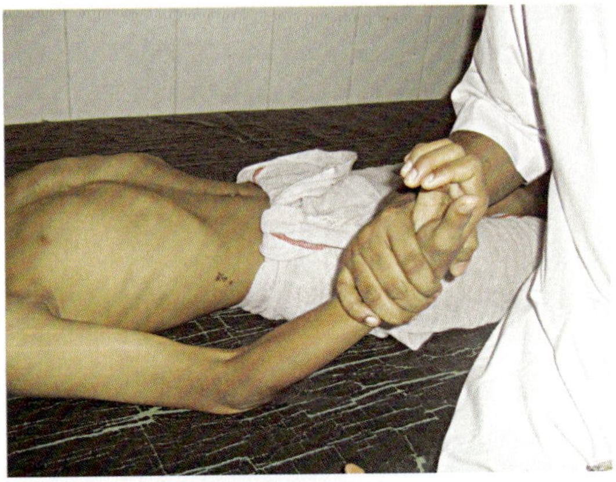

Fig.10.7 Biceps. Flexion of supinated forearm against resistance.

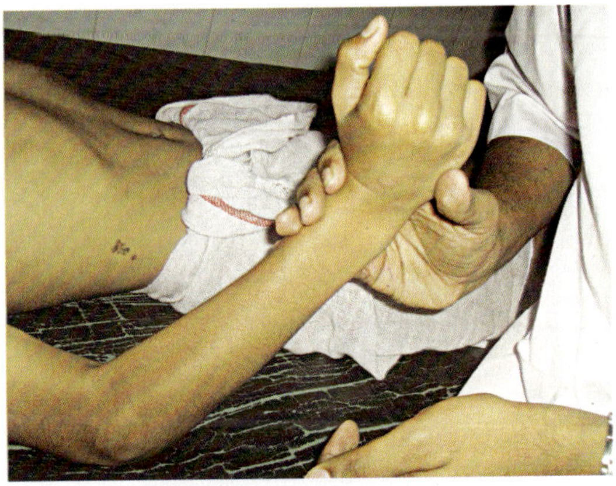

Fig.10.8 Brachioradialis. Flexion at elbow of semipronated forearm against resistance

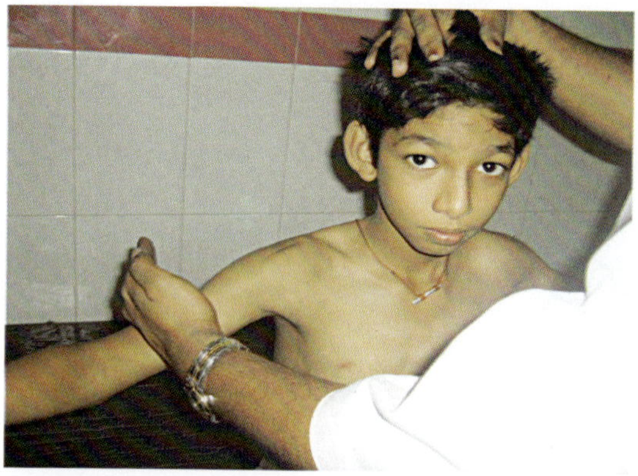

Fig.10.9 Deltoid. Abduct arm to 90° to thoracic cage against resistance

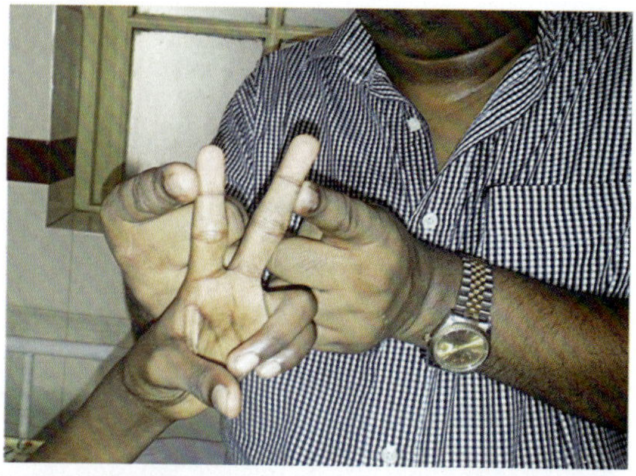

Fig.10.10 Dorsal interossei. Keep two fingers separated in 'V' shape & then try to adduct then against resistance.

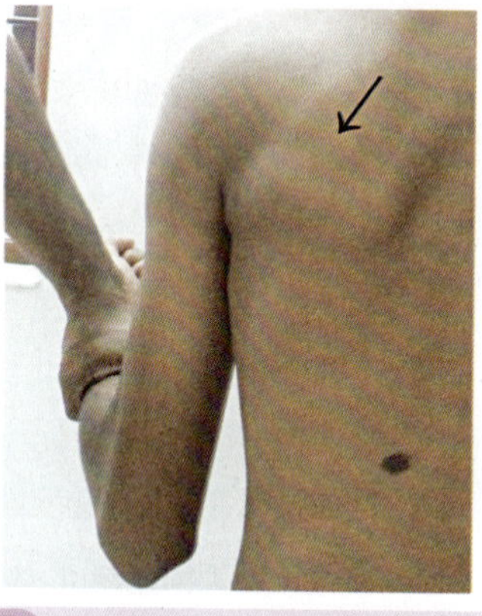

Fig.10.11 Infraspinatus. Extension of arm in a plane parallel to shoulder joint, against resistance.

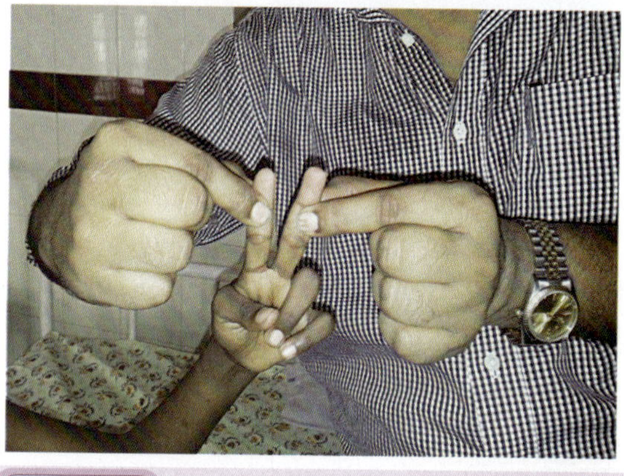

Fig.10.12 Palmar interossei. Try to separate two adjacent adducted fingers against resistance.

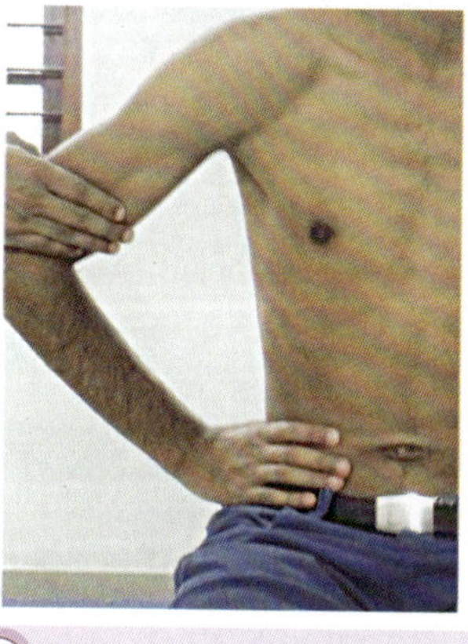

Fig.10.13 Pectoralis. Keep the hand over hip, try to rotate the arm towards the chest against resistance.

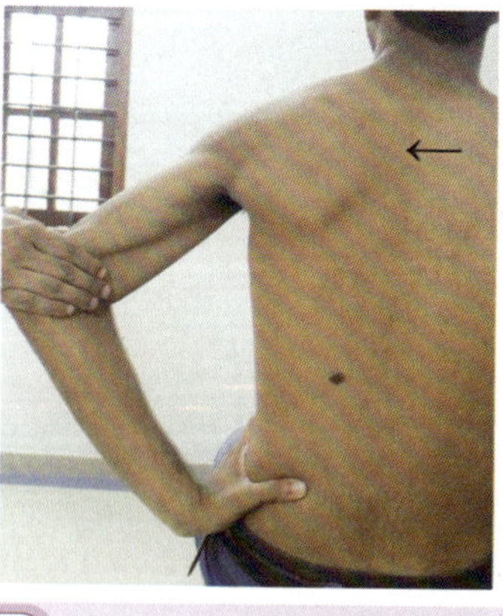

Fig.10.14 Rhomboids. Keep the hand over the hip, try to rotate the arm backwards against resistance.

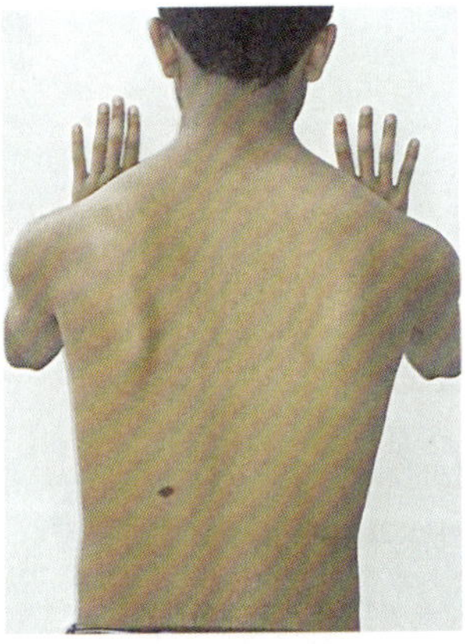

Fig.10.15 Serratus anterior. Push against the wall.

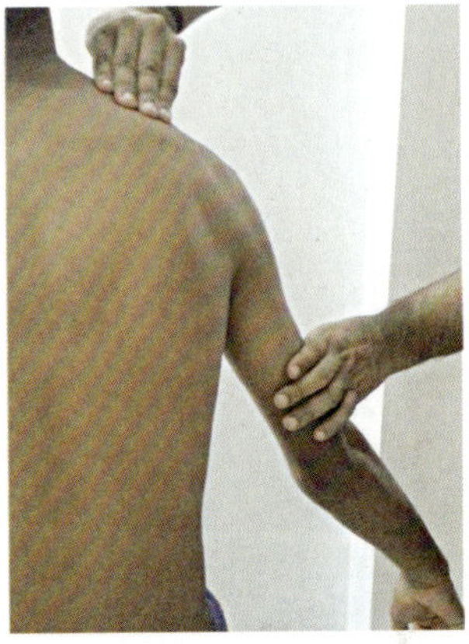

Fig.10.16 Supraspinatus. Abduct arm to 30° against resistance.

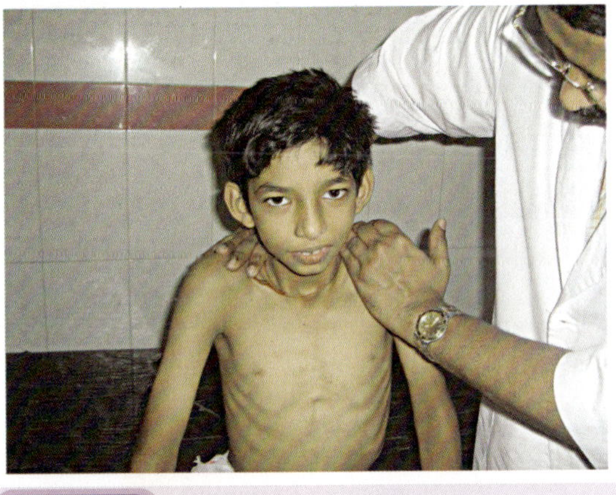

Fig.10.17 Trapezius

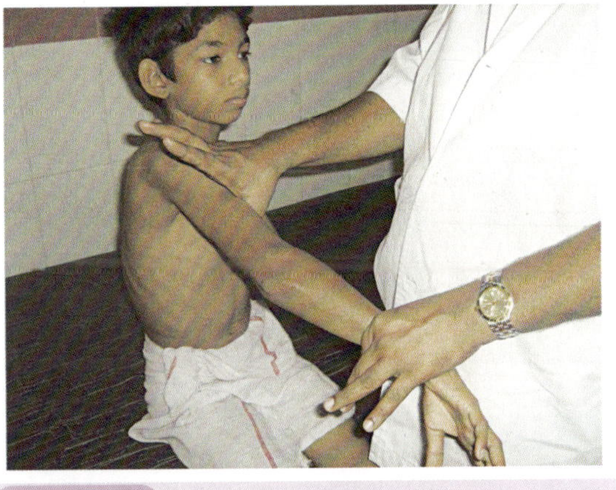

Fig.10.18 Triceps. Fully extend the elbow against resistance.

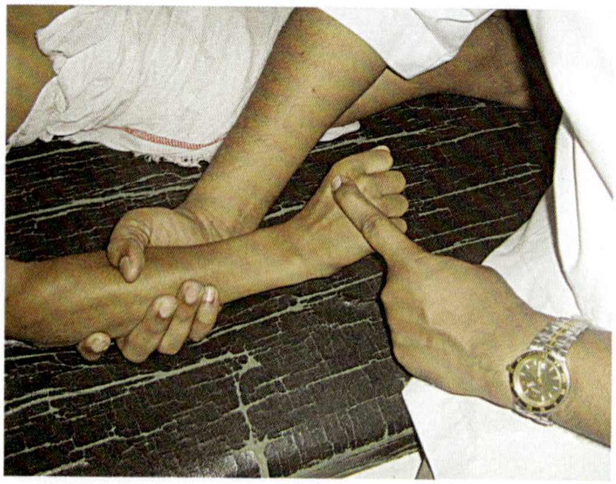

Fig.10.19 Wrist dorsiflexion. Extend the fisted wrist against resistance.

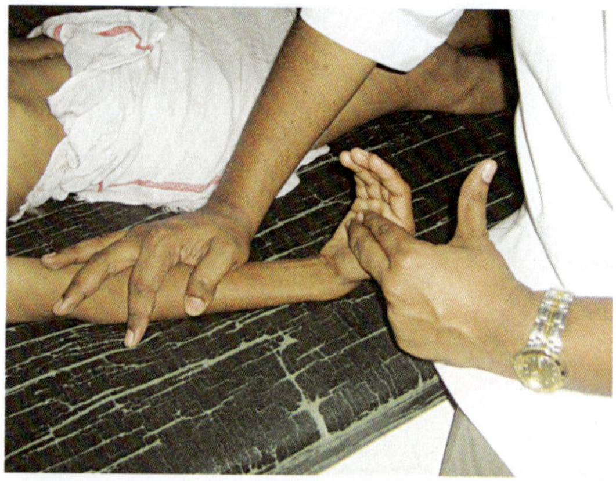

Fig.10.20 Wrist palmar flexion. Flex at wrist, the open hand against resistance.

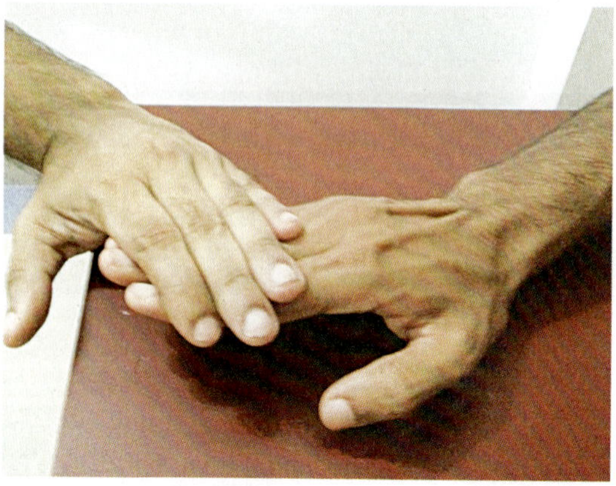

Fig.10.21 Extensor digitorum. Keep the fingers extended at M–P joint (with the forearm in line with the hand) against resistance.

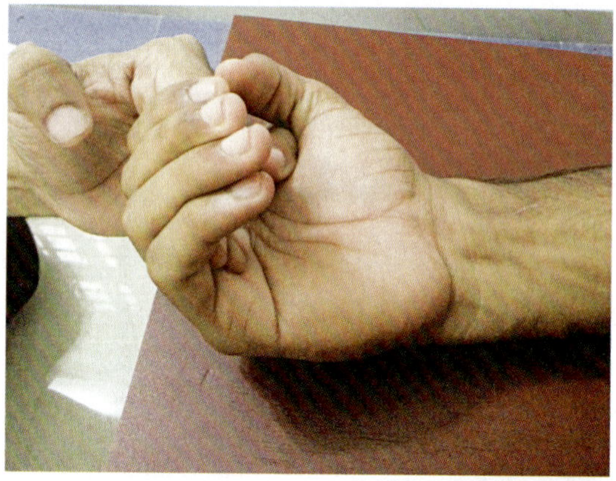

Fig.10.22 Flexor carpi muscle. The examiner resists patient's attempted flexion of wrist.

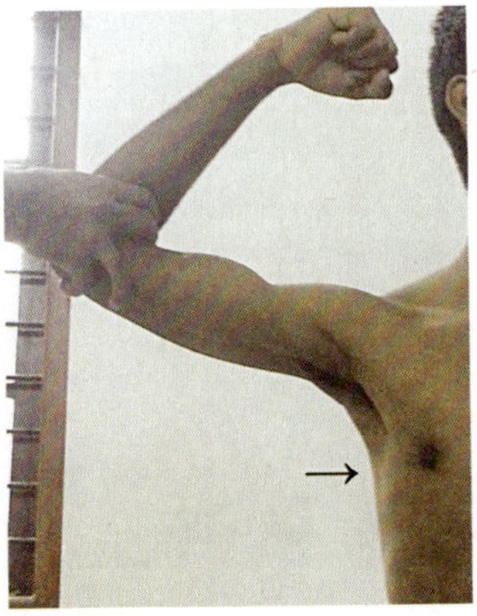

Fig.10.23 Latissimus dorsi. Resisting the patient's attempt to adduct the abducted arm.

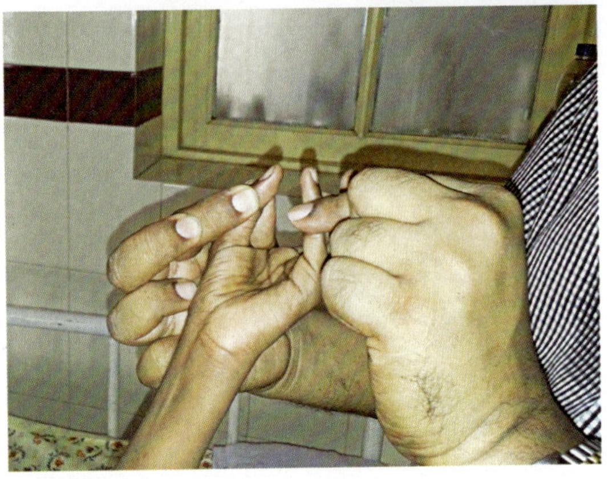

Fig.10.24 Opponens pollicis. Patient tries to touch the little finger with thumb against resistance.

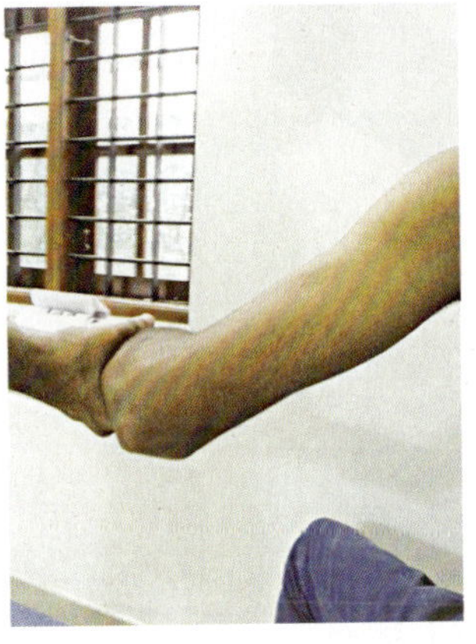

Fig.10.25 Triceps. Patient tries to extend elbow against resistance.

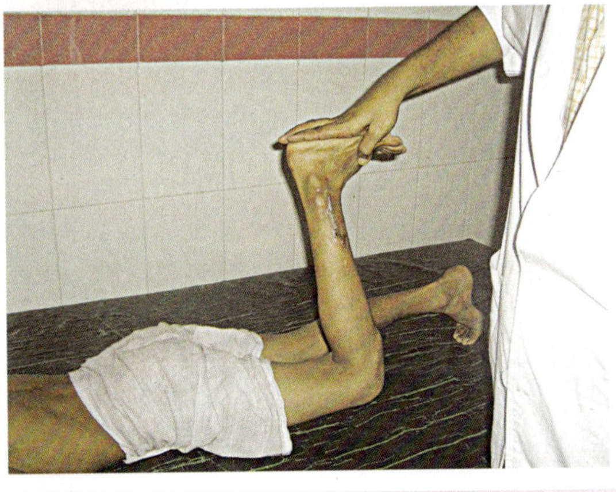

Fig.10.26 Extensors of hip. The patient tries to lift up the thigh.

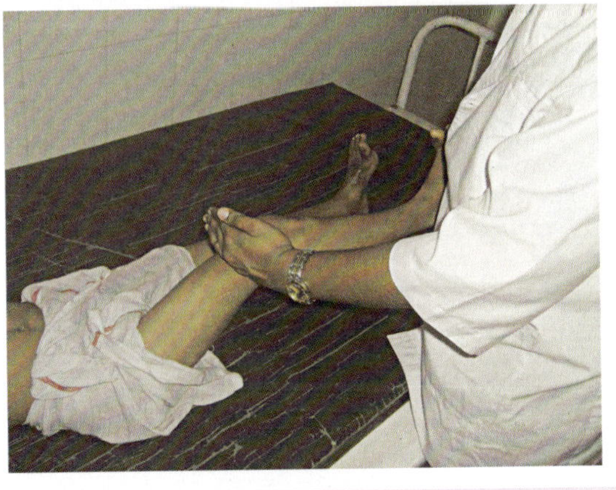

Fig.10.27 Hip flexors. Patient flexes hip against resistance.

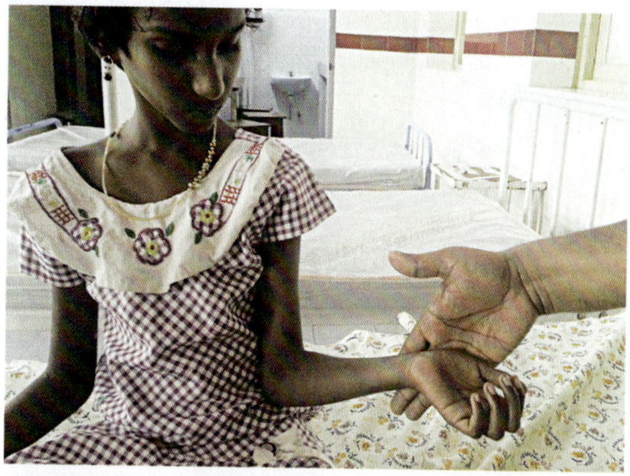

Fig.10.28 Lateral rotator of shoulder. Keep arm adducted to the body, keep forearm at 90° of try to rotate forearm laterally against resistance.

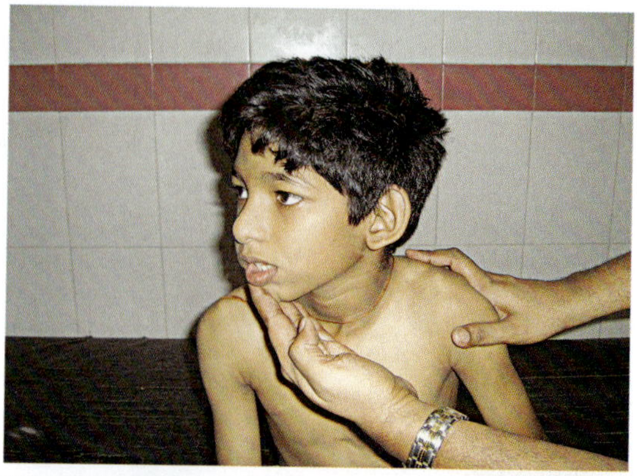

Fig.10.29 Left sternomastoid

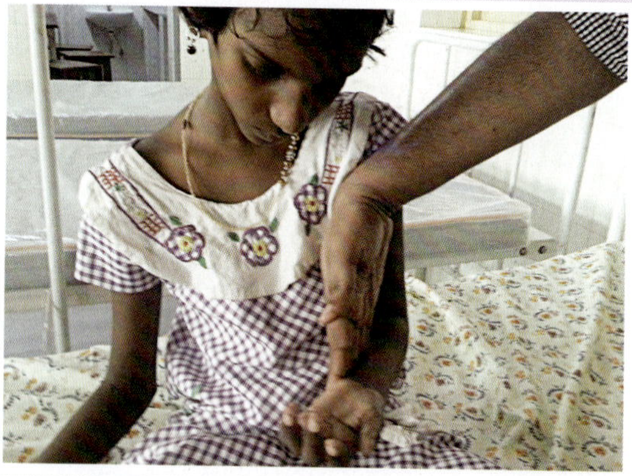

Fig.10.30 Medial rotator. Keep arm & forearm as in Fig. 10.28 & try to rotate forearm medially against resistance

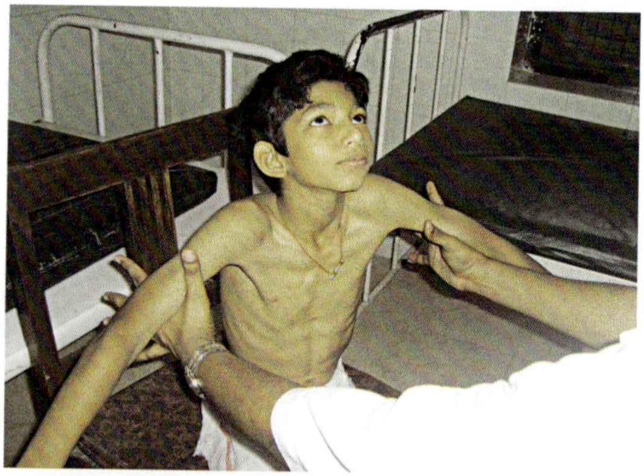

Fig.10.31 Pectoralis major, sternal head. Downward & inward movement against resistance.

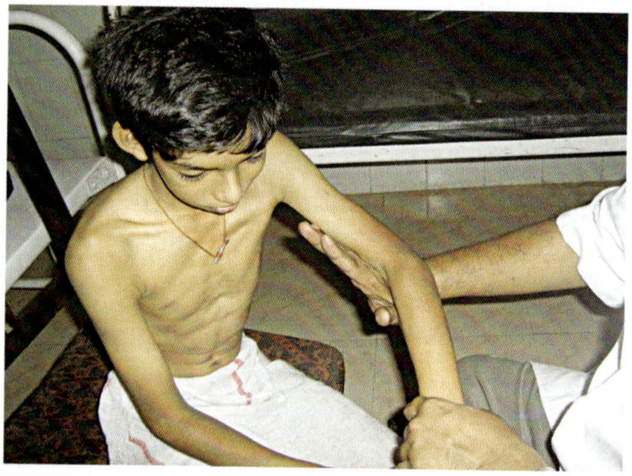

Fig.10.32 Clavicular head of pectoralis major. Here the movement is resisted horizontally.

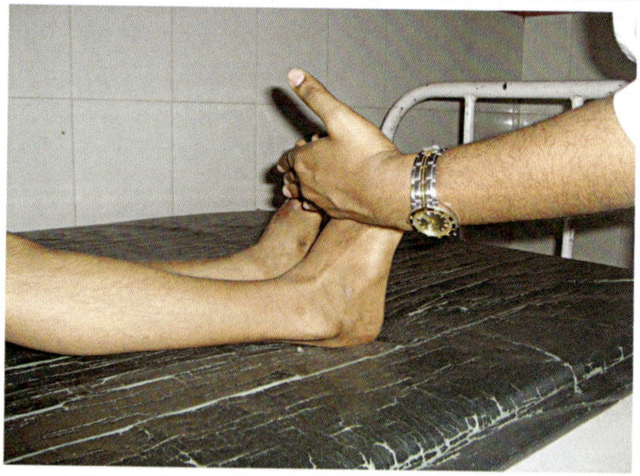

Fig.10.33 Dorsi flexors of foot

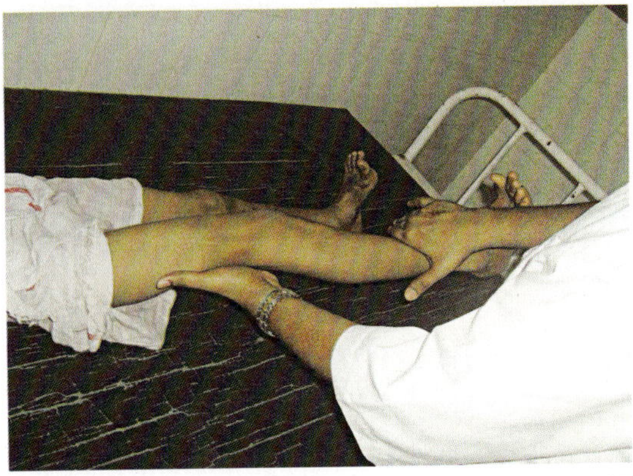

Fig.10.34 Extensors of knee. Extend knee against resistance.

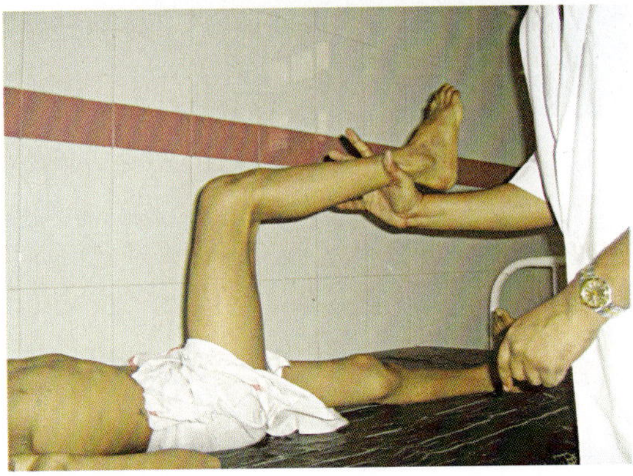

Fig.10.35 Flexors of knee. Flex knee against resistance with hip & knee kept at 90° flexion.

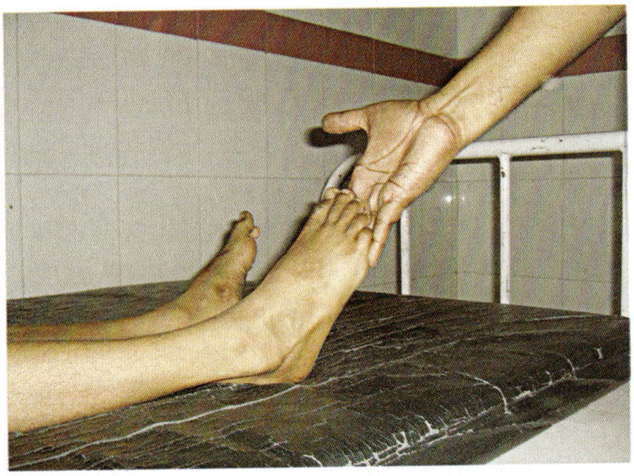

Fig.10.36 Plantar flexors of foot

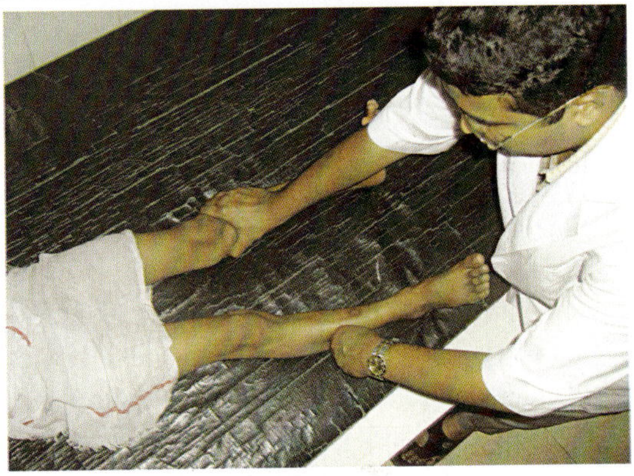

Fig.10.37 Testing abductors of right hip. Note that the opposite leg is kept fixed.

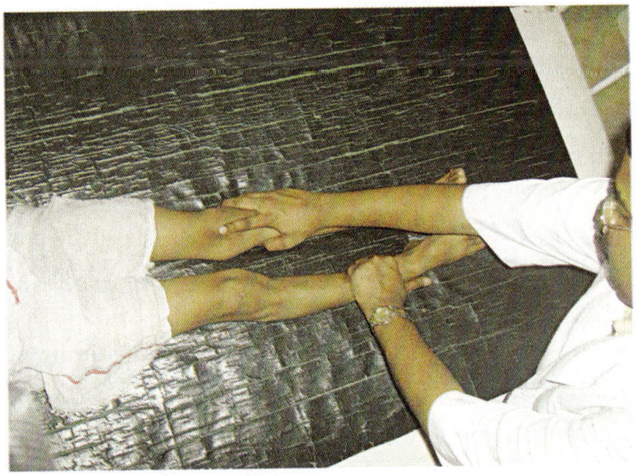

Fig.10.38 Testing adductors of right hip. The resistance can also be offered at the inner thigh rather than the legs. Note that the oposite leg is kept fixed.

Acknowledgement: Demonstoation of mucles testing is contributed by Dr Shahanaz Ahamed MD, DM (Neuro).

CHAPTER 11

Disorders of Nervous System: Case Sheet Formats

History

Common symptoms in children are developmental delay, seizures, aspiration of feeds, weakness, sudden loss of power, loss of previously attained milestones, increasing head size, etc.

- Altered sensorium: Preceding fever, history of trauma, drug or poisons and pre-existing diseases (like hypertension, liver or kidney diseases) must be inquired into.
- Seizures: Sometimes, it may be difficult to make out whether the event was seizure itself. Aura (rare), frothing from mouth, up rolling of eyeballs, loss of consciousness, bowel/bladder incontinence, etc must be inquired into. Seizure, whether it is focal or generalized, with or without preceding fever, history of trauma, drug or poisons and family history of seizure must be inquired.
- Weakness: Paralysis within minutes to hours may be CNS haemorrhage or thrombosis. In case of GBS, paralysis could be ascending or rarely descending, which must be made out from history.
- Abnormal movements.
- Other presenting complaints are discussed along with respective cases.

History of Onset, Duration and Progress

Onset, whether acute (maximum disability within minutes to hours, e.g., seizure, stroke), subacute (within days, e.g., infections), chronic (weeks to months, e.g., tumours, neurodegenerative disorders) or paroxysmal (event comes on and off, e.g., seizure episodes of epilepsy; migraine). In case of chronic disorders, ascertain from history, whether the course is slowly progressive, slowly improving or static. Any precipitating factors: e.g., a neurological deficit starting with a fall. Rarely, the fall itself may not have caused the deficit.

When memorizing the order of history taking in CNS symptoms, always remember the scheme for CNS examination (see p 2).

- History related to higher mental functions – Consciousness, orientation, memory, intelligence, speech, handedness, emotional state.
- History related to cranial nerves:
  - I – History of anosmia/parosmia.
  - II – History of problems in visual acuity, colour vision.
  - III, IV, VI – History of ptosis, squint, nystagmus.
  - V – Deviation of jaw, sensation over face, conjuctival/corneal sensation.
  - VII – Closing of both eyes, deviation of angle of mouth, drooling, difficulty in drinking with straw, taste sensation over anterior 2/3rd of tongue.
  - VIII – Hearing, vertigo, tinnitus.
  - IX, X – Nasal twang, good cough reflex, swallowing difficulty.
  - XI – Turning head to both sides, shrugging of shoulders.
  - XII – Tongue deviation, atrophy of tongue.
- History related to motor system – Weakness, floppiness/clumsiness, stiffness, atrophy/hypertrophy, involuntary movements.

- History related to sensory system – touch, pain, temperature, pressure, hyperesthesia, parasthesias.
- History related to bowel and bladder disturbance (bowel disturbance unlikely).
- History related to cerebellar function – Nystagmus, truncal ataxia, dysarthria, titubation, gait ataxia.
- History related to meningeal irritation – Headache, fever, neck stiffness.
- History related to raised ICT – Headache (usually morning), projectile vomiting, visual disturbance.

GROSS MOTOR FUNCTIONAL STATUS CLASSIFICATION (GMFS)

Level I:Walks without limitations but abnormalities detected on neurologic examination.

- Infants move in and out of sitting and floor-sit with both hands free to manipulate objects; crawl on hands and knees; pull to stand and take steps holding on to furniture. Motor mioestones may be slightly delayed.
- Children get into and out of floor-sit and chair sit to standing and walks without the need for support.in all settings; climb stairs without the use of a railing and perform gross motor skills such as running and jumping, but speed, balance and coordination are limited.

Level II: Walks with minimal adult help like holding the hand

- Infants maintain floor sitting but may need to use their hands for support to maintain balance, creep on their stomach or crawl on hands and knees, pull to stand and take steps holding on to furniture.
- Children floor sit but may have difficulty with balance when both hands are free to manipulate object but can chair sit with both hands free to manipulate objects.
- Movements in and out of sitting are performed with or without adult assistance, pull to stand on a stable surface, crawl on hands and knees, cruise holding onto furniture.
- Children walk indoors and climb stairs holding onto a railing or with assistance if there is no railing.
- Running and jumping, are poorly co ordinated.
- Children may walk with adult assistance,

Level III: Walks Using a Mobility Device which the child himself can operate.

- Infants maintain floor sitting when the low back is supported, roll and crawl forward on their stomachs.
- Children maintain floor sitting often by "W-sitting" and require adult assistance to assume sitting and creep or crawl as their primary methods of self-mobility and may pull to stand with help and cruise short distances.
- Children sit on a regular chair but may require pelvic or trunk support to maximize hand function
- Chair-Sit to stand and floor- sit to stand require physical assistance.
- Children walk with a hand-held mobility device (walker) and adult assistance for steering and turning and climb stairs.

Level IV: Walk with Powered Mobility devices & require adult ot operate the device.

- Trunk support is required for floor sitting, can roll to supine and may roll to prone.
- Children floor sit when placed, but are unable to maintain floor sit balance without use of their hands for support and frequently require adaptive equipment for balancing.

- Self-mobility for short distances is achieved through rolling, or crawling.
- Children sit on a chair but need adaptive seating for trunk control and to maximize hand function.
- Children move in and out of chair sitting with assistance from an adult or a stable surface to push or pull up on with their arms.
- They may walk for short distances at home with powered mobility or a body support walker with adult assistance.
- At school, outdoors and in the community children are transported in a manual wheelchair or use powered mobility.

Level V:No self walk Totally dependant on adult to carry along, with or without device.

- Infants are unable to maintain antigravity head and trunk postures in prone and sitting and require adult assistance to roll.
- Physical impairments restrict voluntary control of movement and the ability to maintain antigravity head and trunk postures.
- All areas of motor function are limited.
- Children have no means of independent movement and are transported in a manual wheelchair in all settings or may be carried by an adult.
- Some children achieve self-mobility using a powered wheelchair with extensive adaptations for seating and control access.

CEREBRAL PALSY

Background Information

Cerebral palsy is a motor/movement disorder due to a non progressive pathology of cerebral origin, which has resulted from an insult to the developing brain.

Aetiology

Mnemonic: **JAP-B** standing for **J**aundice, **A**sphyxia (**Note**: Only around 10% of CP can be directly attributed to intrapartum hypoxia), **P**rematurity (most common cause of CP), **P**renatal (IU infections, cerebrovascular accidents in utero, etc) and **P**erinatal problems (e.g., traumatic delivery, hypoglycaemia, etc) and **B**rain anomalies, either congenital (e.g., neuronal migration disorders) or acquired (encephalitis, meningitis. Yes, one can develop CP postnatally).

How do you differentiate CP from post-meningitic/encephalitic sequelae?

Post-meningitic/post-encephalitic sequelae: Children had previously normal development till the insult and the present state is a sequel of that insult.

If meningitis occurs in a developing brain (especially <2 years), there is always a dilemma whether to call it post-meningitic sequelae or CP. In fact, meningitis/encephalitis is considered as a very important postnatal cause of CP. As a rough guide, you can call these sequelae as CP if it had occurred during the developing stage of brain. After that, you may call them meningitis/encephalitis sequelae (provided the previous development was normal and antenatal and birth history cannot account for the deficits).

Types of Cerebral Palsy

- Spastic CP:
  - *Diplegic CP* (both lower limbs are affected)
  - *Hemiplegic CP*
  - *Quadriplegic CP (tetraplegia)*
  - Cerebral monoplegia and triplegia are exceptionally rare
- Extrapyramidal CP (dystonia and choreoathetosis in varying proportions)
- Cerebellar or ataxic CP
- Mixed CP:
  - *Ataxic diplegia*

- *Dystonia and/or choreoathetosis associated with various forms of spastic CP*

Chief Complaints

- C/o delayed milestones (noticed since when)
- Aspiration of feeds
- Seizure

History of Presenting Illness

- *Describe the present illness* in short (ODP of the acute event like seizure, aspiration, etc)
  - If no acute event is present, just mention that the child was admitted for evaluation of delayed milestones, and describe the achieved milestones in chronological order.
  - Describe positive history of any CNS symptoms, if present.
  - Sample statement: Since the *complaints started* at the age of __, I would like to start my history from __ age (if the delay in development was noticed by parents before 1 year, you may start HOPI from the newborn period or even antenatal period. Remember that if you start history from a particular age, e.g., 9 months, you should be sure that the child attained all milestones at appropriate ages till 9 months. In case of doubt, always start from newborn period. In history, the emphasis is to establish that the disease process is static and not progressively deteriorating, which means that the child will not lose any acquired milestones and achieve a few new milestones at a much later date than normal. The next emphasis is to have an idea of aetiology.
- *H/o aetiology:*
  - ***Antenatal history***
    - Age of mother
    - Consanguinous/non-consanguinous marriage
    - Treated for infertility (problems are more likely in such cases)
    - History of abortion/neonatal deaths
    - 1st trimester:
      - Per vaginum bleeding/spotting
      - Fever with rash/neck swelling
      - Drug intake/radiation
      - Folic acid tablets: When was it started
      - Hyperemesis (one of the causes is thought to be pyridoxine deficiency)
      - Jaundice/thyroid status
    - 2nd trimester:
      - Weight gain (if such history is available)
      - Gestational diabetes mellitus, pre-eclampsia
      - Iron, calcium tablets: whether taken
      - Quickening, fetal movements (decreased fetal movements can be due to hypotonia, increased fetal movements may suggest fetal seizures): when was it first appreciated
      - USG – oligamnious/polyhydramnious/IUGR/anomalies/twinning
    - 3rd trimester:
      - Gestational diabetes mellitus, pre-eclampsia
      - Bleeding per vaginum
      - PPROM, fever, UTI, foul smelling liquor, abdominal tenderness (risk of sepsis)
  - ***Birth history***
    - Term/Preterm (prematurity is the most common cause of CP)
    - Mode of delivery, birth weight, cried soon after birth or not.
    - Feeding problems/sucking
    - Passage of urine, meconium
    - Respiratory distress soon after birth (could cause hypoxic brain injury)

11

- NICU admission
- Jaundice: Phototherapy/exchange transfusion. Kernicterus can be related to extrapyramidal cerebral palsy
- Poor activity: Could be sepsis or hypoglycaemia; both increases the risk of CP. Symptomatic hypoglycaemia has 50% chance of brain injury.
- Seizures in neonatal period (could be hypoxic ischaemic encephalopathy, hypoglycaemia, IC bleed, meningitis, etc).

- ***Postnatal history***
  - Ask for course of child after NICU discharge.
  - After neonatal period – feeding, activity, weight gain, jaundice fever, irritability, seizures (meningitis/encephalitis).
- ***CNS history***
  - Higher functions: Good tone and activity makes normal higher functions likely.
  - Speech, hearing and communication
  - Cranial nerves: Swallowing problem, nasal regurgitation, etc are the most common cranial nerve problems in CP. The others are squint, visual problems and hearing problems. Sample questions would be: is there any change in behaviour or does the child cry when light is switched off? Does the baby startle if the door is slammed shut?
  - Motor system
  - Wasting/hypertrophy (if mother has noticed)
  - Stiffness/limpness; if noticed, UL versus LL; right versus left. Stiffness or floppiness is likely to be noticed if mother has another child before. Otherwise, grandparents notice this better. History of easy wearing out of tips of shoes indicates tip toeing due to spasticity.
  - Scissoring/difficulty in changing diapers (could mean adductor spasm).
  - Power – UL/LL, proximal versus distal; right/ left.
  - Sensations, bladder/bowel involvement (if such a history is available; usually none will be available).
  - Involuntary movements, if any.
  - Cerebellar signs.
  - Nystagmus, titubation, ataxia, intention tremor (try to get information from mother).
  - Features of increased intracranial pressure.

▪ *Early markers of spasticity in a case of development delay:*
Paucity of limb movements, stiffness, difficulty in changing diapers, increased irritability, limp, posturing, fisting, arching of back, tongue thrusting (on attempted feeding), choking, aspiration, abnormal eye movement (for all types of CP), commando crawl, bottom shuffling (for diplegia), early hand preference, splaying of hands on trying to reach objects, late sitting balance (for hemiplegic CP).

▪ *Associated problems:*
  - Seizures, increasing head size
  - Feeding difficulty, GERD, PEM, constipation
  - Visual and hearing problems
  - Bulbar dysfunction and hence aspiration of feeds
  - Carious teeth
  - Kyphoscoliosis
  - Hip dislocation
  - Malnutrition, vitamin D deficiency (no sun exposure)
  - Contractures, bed sores, recurrent RTI, UTI
  - Constipation due to immobility
  - Behavioral problems, aggressive behaviour, self mutilation. In grown up children, depression.

- *Treatment history:*
  Any long-term drugs (anti-epilectics, anti-spasticity), physiotherapy, surgery
- *H/o activities of daily living*: EDTA, eating, dressing, toilet, ambulation
  - How is feeding managed?
  - How toilet needs are managed?
  - Dressing: How much help needed?
  - Sleep
  - Behaviour with peers, emotional disturbances
  - Ambulation (can walk unassisted or with aids, wheelchair or bedridden)
  - Objectively, it is best assessed by giving the child common articles like cup, spoon, tooth brush, etc ask them to do the task. Ask them to undress and dress (if old enough).
- *Immunization*: Very likely to be incomplete.
- *Developmental history* in chronological order including vision, hearing, dentition (mention only if not described with the initial history).
- *Dietory history*: Intake is likely to be in-sufficient.

Family History

- History of neurological illness, seizures, development delay in siblings/family.
- Any sibling deaths, abortions in the family.

Socioeconomic History

- Impact of CP on parents and normal siblings. Disruption of family routines, financial considerations. Any social support received or aware of any such schemes.

General Examination

1. General comment: Comment on any obvious things like dysmorphism or particular posture (fisting, obligatory asymmetric tonic neck reflex, neck retraction or arching back, hemiplegic gait, etc).
2. Vitals
3. Anthropometry: Due to feeding issues, very likely to be malnourished. Head circumference: microcephaly is likely.
4. Objective assessment of development by the candidate. Comment whether this objective assessment tally with the elicited development history.
5. Head to foot examination
   - Head: Size, anterior fontanel, posterior fontanel, abnormal shape of skull, loss of hair (there may be localized alopecia of occipital region due to constant lying in that position).
   - Face: Any dysmorphism (chromosomal anomalies).
   - Eyes: Squint, dropping of lid, nystagmus, cataract, roving eye movements (due to blindness), chorioretinitis, vitamin A deficiency, optic atrophy (on fundus examination).
   - Ears: Deformity, low set.
   - Nose
   - Mouth: Deviation of angle, drooling, hygiene, pooling of secretions, dentition.
   - Chest – Rachitic changes, deformities.
   - Abdomen: Organomegaly, hernial orifices.
   - Genitalia: Any anomalies.
   - Limb:
     Deformity: Windswept (quadriplegia)/ folded wing (hemiplegia), callosity, limb size/length disparity (best appreciated by comparing thumbs or big toes side by side), vasomotor changes (hemiplegia), scissoring (diplegia, quadriplegia).
   - Palpate for tone. Keep head of baby in midline while assessing the tone.
   - Test passive range of movements to look for contractures (at least hip adductors and tendo-achillis must be evaluated for contractures).
   - Hip subluxation; contracture, if present, dynamic or fixed.
   - If the child can walk, observe the gait.

11

- For small infants, try 180° flip manoeuvre.
  - Supine: Any posture, like obligatory asymmetric tonic neck reflex (keep the head in midline). Turn head to side and see if the body follows.
  - Pull to sit by hands: Assess head lag and grasp.
  - Sitting: Assess sitting ability; whether the child can withstand lateral jolting.
  - Hold vertically holding under the axilla: Increased tone at axilla; lower limbs extended, scissoring; automatic walking when touched on top of table. Tilt sidewise to assess head righting.
  - Ventral suspension by supporting under the abdomen: Look for back arching. Bring the baby rapidly down to elicit parachute response (usually above 9 months) to detect asymmetry between the sides.
  - Prone in bed: Back arching, neck retraction.
- Power: Only a rough assessment will be possible in infants.
  Note asymmetry between the sides. If the child can lift the limb off the bed, power is > grade 3.
- Reflexes: Keep head in midline while eliciting reflexes.
- Skin: Neurocutaneous markers, bed sores, callosity.
- Spine
- Involuntary movements

Diagnosis: ___ year old child is a case of static encephalopathy; physiologic classification (spastic/hypotonic/choreoathetoid/mixed); topographic classification (diplegic/quadriplegic/hemiplegic/double hemiplegic); with functional grade (Gross Motor Functional Classification)_______ with/without convulsion with/without squint, visual defect, hearing deficit with a development age (mental/motor age) with PEM/LRTI/contractures, and the most probable aetiology being antenatal/natal/postnatal insult secondary to _______.

Investigations

- CT or MRI can localize the lesion (e.g., periventricular leukomalacia in diplegia; structural abnormalities of brain like neuronal migration disorders in quadriplegia; lesions at basal ganglia in extrapyramidal CP).
- Intrauterine infection screening.
- Investigations for associated problems: Seizures (EEG), hearing loss (audiometry/BERA), etc.
- Karyotyping in dysmorphic babies.
- Metabolic screening in case of affected siblings, or consanguinity.

Treatment of Cerebral Palsy

The cerebral pathology cannot be corrected. Hence, treatment of associated defects and optimum utilization of available motor functions are the aims.

Treatment of the Associated Deficits

- Seizures: Anticonvulsants.
- Visual problems (squint, refractory errors): Ophthalmology consultation; spectacles.
- Hearing loss (if present): Hearing aids and speech therapy.
- Early stimulation (visual stimulation, hearing stimulation, tactile stimulation, etc): Helps in better arborization between the neurons.

Management of CP

- Management is planned by a team of various specialists.
- Physiotherapy is to be done continuously at home and hence mother must get trained to do it.
- *Prevention of contractures*: During the day time, passive and active movements of joints through full range of motion. Splinting at night.

Adductor contracture: Carry the child on the loin side of the mother with one leg in front and the other leg behind. Keep a pillow in between the thighs during sleep.

- *Feeding*: Assisted feeding; nasogastric feeding; gastrostomy feeding, etc.
- Constipation: Stool softeners.
- *Drooling*: Anticholinergics; surgical repositioning of duct.
- *Hyperactivity*: Drugs like methylphenidate, atamoxetine.
- *Education*: Will need modifications at school environment depending on the disability or consider special schools.
- *Orthopaedic and neurosurgical measures*: Release of contractures; Selective dorsal rhizotomy can modify the lower limb hypertonia; Arthrodesis at the best functional position. Management of hip dislocation if any.
- *Spasticity*: Drugs useful are diazepam, baclofen, dantrolene sodium, etc. Trihexyphenidyl for dystonia. Injection of botulinum toxin to spastic muscles for relaxation of spastic muscles.
- *For activities of daily living*: EDTA, eating, dressing, toilet and ambulation.
- Wheel chairs for moving around; sitting type toilet to avoid the squat. Dress with press buttons. Computer, bells, etc for communication.
- Spastic societies, Cerebral palsy day,mobile apps for CP, and social security schemes. (Eg: in Kerala Ashwasakiranam).

It is desirable that the students read the management of CP from the 'Manual of Pediatric Practice' by the same author.

Questions

1. Define and classify CP.
2. Functional grades of CP.
3. Overview of CP management.

HEMIPLEGIA

- Presenting complaint: Paucity of right/left sided limb movement since ____
- History of presenting complaints
- Onset, duration and progress: Acute/subacute/chronic:
  - Sudden catastrophic onset (within minutes) in haemorrhage and embolism. Haemorrhagic: Sudden, progressive in minutes to hours, precipitated by stress/emotion, features suggestive of raised ICT (altered sensorium, vomiting, headache); neck stiffness (in subarachinoid haemorrhage); seizures are common. Embolic: Sudden, often precipitated by exertion; maximal deficit at the onset; seizures are common.
  - Acute onset (1–2 days) in pyogenic/viral meningitis, encephalitis, thrombosis, etc. Thrombosis: e.g., noticed on waking up; stuttering progression; seizures are rare.
  - Subacute onset (over many days) in TB meningitis, brain tumours, partially treated pyogenic meningitis, ADEM etc.
  - Chronic progressive hemiplegia in brain tumour, brain abscess, chronic demyelinating diseases; Chronic non-progressive hemiplegia in cerebral palsy.
  - Paraoxysmal in case of Todds palsy, migraine, etc.

Describe the evolution of motor weakness: Distribution of weakness as per history and whether improving/worsening since the onset.

Any clumsiness (falling to one side, drooping objects, spilling drinks, etc), any stiffness, any wasting noticed by parents, any involuntary movements.

- History to elucidate aetiology:
  - Haematological:
    - Prothrombotic conditions:
      - History of stroke in family, similar complaints in the past.

- Diarrhoea, dehydration (most significant in infants).
- History of facial puffiness, decreased urine output (nephro-tic).
- History of severe pain in hand, foot, abdomen (sickle cell anaemia, Fabry).
- Bleeding:
  - Bleeding in the past, rash/petechie in self or family.
  - Fever, bone pain, weight loss (leukaemia).
- Cardiac:
  - History of cyanosis, spell, squatting episodes (CCHD).
  - History of fever with chills, petechie, haematuria (IE).
  - History of arthritis, sore throat, fever (RHD).
  - History of cardiac surgery (prosthetic valve).
  - History of hypertension.
- Infection: Chicken pox (varicella vasculopathy), fever, TB (fever, weight loss, loss of appetite), otorrhoea, viral exanthems (HSV, mumps).
- Para-infectious – vaccination, viral illness.
- Connective tissue disorder – joint pain, rash (SLE).
- Drug intake – amphetamine, anti-platelet drugs.
- Head injury – fall, accidents, oral trauma [popsicle (ice cream on a stick) injury].
- History of skin lesions, developmental delay (neurocutaneous syndromes).

- *History of complications:*
  Bed sore, contracture, tongue bite, increase in head size, skin changes, bowel/bladder disturbance, hearing/vision.
- *Treatment history and course in hospital:*
  Any drugs – DOTS/IM injections, surgery (VP shunt), procedures done (lumbar puncture).
- *Activities of daily living: EDTA, eating, dressing, toilet, ambulation.*

Features suggestive of raised ICT: Convulsions, headache, vomiting, bradycardia, hypertension.

Birth History

- Preterm birth, traumatic delivery, birth asphyxia
- Bleeding
- Umbilical sepsis/catheterization (embolism)

Immunization History

Development History

Could bring out asymmetry of motor movements and motor development delay in case of hemiplegic CP.

Dietary History

Family History

- Similar complaints in parents/siblings (sickle cell anaemia, homocystinuria).
- Familial stroke: Fabry's disease, OTC deficiency, MELAS, Leigh's disease, sulphatase deficiency.
- Family history of epilepsy or migraine.

General Examination

General comment on consciousness, typical posture, if present (upper limb is flexed, adducted and semipronated; lowerlimb is extended, adducted and plantar flexed). Anything to suggest trauma (accidents or non accidental trauma in battered baby).

Ask the child to reach out for an object: there is abduction of arm, flexion of wrist, hyperextension and spreading out of fingers.

Vitals

- Pulse: Describe in detail the rate, rhythm ,volume, bilateral equality, any radio radial or radio- femoral delay and any special character, if present.

- BP: Hypertension may cause IC bleed; even in that case, hypotension may be seen in acute stage when in neuronal shock (measure in the non affected limb) or better to record 4 limb BP.
- Pallor: Malignancy, sickle cell anaemia, connective tissue disease; massive IC bleed (like AV malformation).
- Cyanosis: CCHD can cause cerebral thrombosis (<2 years) or cerebral abscess (>2 years).

Anthropometry

- Significant if Marfanoid habitus (in which case arm span and other signs, such as wrist and thumb sign have to be looked for). Marfanoid features may indicate homocystinuria.
- Look for any limb length discrepancy (possible in long standing hemiplegia).
- Head circumference.

Head to Foot Examination

- Anterior fontanelle may be bulging in case of raised ICT.
- Also auscultate over the eyes for bruit (because anastamosis of ICA and ECA branches occur in the orbital area).
- Eye: Ectopia lentis (in Marfan's and homocystinuria) (Fig. 6.54).
- Fundus: Look for bleed/choroid tubercles/ papilledema (indicating raised ICT)/Roth spots/ retinal angiomas (Fig. 9.5, 9.8).
- Pharynx: Look for trauma (accidental pencil trauma, which the child may have been biting or holding between the teeth).
- Ear discharge: May be a focus for brain abscess.
- Neck, axilla etc: Lymphadenopathy may be looked for, in which case Kochs becomes a possibility.
- Do not forget to palpate the carotids, one at a time and auscultate for bruit.
- BCG scar: TB meningitis is a common cause for neurological deficits including hemiplegia.
- Joint bleed (coagulopathies).
- Back: Look for pressure sores in chronic case; scoliosis (neurofibromatosis type I, spinal tumour), scars (excised tumour), tenderness (Pott spine).
- Look for palpable bladder.
- Skin: Look for neurocutaneous markers: Portwine stain (Sturge Weber syndrome may be associated with cerebral vessel abnormalities), haemangiomas; Rash (SLE); Petechiae (very low platelet count can predispose to IC bleed).
- Look for the markers of infective endocarditis.
- Skin vesicles: Herpes encephalitis can cause lateralized neurological deficits.

11

Examination of the Central Nervous System

Higher Mental Functions

Level of consciousness, behaviour, memory, speech and handedness.

Ask the child his name, school, parents name etc to assess dysphasia/aphasia (possible when dominant hemisphere is involved). Show the child pictures of animals he is familiar with and ask to name them.

Cranial Nerves

- 2nd nerve: Examine for homonymous hemianopia (may be present in hemiplegia when the site of lesion is internal capsule or above).
- 7th cranial nerve: Mention if UMN/LMN on same side/opposite side; this helps in localization of the lesion. UMN VII nerve palsy localizes lesion above pons. LMN VII palsy may localize lesion to pons. *Note*: If VII nerve palsy is on the same side of hemiplegia, it is most likely UMN.
- Other cranial nerves are to be examined as per CNS examination format: mostly unaffected in hemiplegia. Make sure you have examined 12th nerve.

Motor System

- Bulk: Mention wasting, if present. If so, document by measurement and comparison with the normal side. Limb length discrepancy may be useful in differentiating congenital and acquired hemiplegia.
- Tone: Clasp knife spasticity in the limbs (acute stage may be hypotonic); examine for pronator spasm (earliest sign in spasticity).
- Power: Assess and grade.
- Tests for subtle hemiplegia:
  - Unstable position of lower limb heightens the hemiplegic arm posture (Fog test). Examples are walking on heels, walking on inside of feet (everted) or outside of feet (inverted), etc. Sometimes walking on outside of foot is called Fog test and inside of foot as reverse Fog test.
  - Cover test: In infants, cover the face with a cloth and find which hand the child uses to remove the cover; if the child uses both hands, try to restrain them and see which hand has more power.
  - Ask the child to keep hands outstretched for 30 sec; the weak side drifts down.
  - The affected lower limb remains laterally rotated, so that the outside of foot touches the bed when supine.
- DTR: Exaggerated; look for clonus (both ankle and patella). Observe the opposite limb for adductor spread while eliciting the knee jerk (this is never normally present beyond 7–9 months of age).
- Superficial reflexes: Plantar gives extensor response; abdominal reflexes: lost in acquired hemiplegia, preserved in congenital hemiplegia.
- Co-ordination, gait (circumduction gait) and involuntary movements.
- Abnormal persistence of neonatal reflexes (asymmetric tonic neck reflex, grasp reflex); early hand preference point towards congenital hemiplegia.
- Sensory functions – Preserved normally. In case of time constraints, sensory testing can be avoided, except cortical sensations.
- In older children, assess cortical sensations. Hemiplegia due to parietal lobe lesions may show loss of cortical sensations; most of these are lost when the dominant hemisphere is involved. However, sensory extinction (sensory inattention) is demonstrable when either hemisphere is involved. Constructional apraxia occurs when non-dominant hemisphere is involved (ask the child to draw something which the child was able to draw before the illness; arts like drawing, music, etc are functions on non dominant hemisphere).
- If there is no involvement of higher functions and cranial nerves, then there is a possibility that the site of lesion is in spinal cord. In that case, sensory examination is a must.
- Cerebellar functions are normally preserved in hemiplegia.
- Skull and spine: No abnormal findings are expected.
- CVS: Look for any heart disease, especially congenital cyanotic heart disease, which allows emboli to bypass lung due to R to L shunt.
- Carotid bruit (moya moya, stenosis).
- Abdomen: Look for renal bruit.

Diagnosis

Cerebrovascular accident, right/left hemiplegia, with or without cranial nerve/other deficits, localization (cortical/subcortical/internal capsule), pathology (thrombus/bleed), aetiology (guess as per risk factors), complications, functional status.

The term 'double hemiplegia' is a confusing one: when there is involvement of all four limbs and upper limbs are more involved than the lower limbs (i.e., the typical distribution of hemiplegic weakness), it may be called double hemiplegia. If all the four limbs are involved more or less equally, it is called quadriplegia.

Investigations in Acute Hemiplegia (Stroke)

- CT, MRI.
- Routine blood counts and peripheral smear (leukaemia, polycythemia, thrombocytopenia, sickle cell disease).
- Test for sickling (sodium meta bisulfate), if indicated.
- ESR is high in collagen vascular diseases.
- ANA, ds DNA for SLE.
- Protein C, S, antithrombin C for hypercoagulable states.
- ABG, serum lactate, pyruvate (MELAS: mitochondrial cytopathy, encephalopathy, lactic acidosis and stroke).
- ECG, X-ray, echo including Doppler of heart and carotids. Blood culture if endocarditis is suspected.

Treatment of Acute Hemiplegia

- Thrombolysis within 3 hrs of the event is available in selected centres for adults; the same is not yet available in most centres for children.
- Treatment of meningitis if diagnosed so.
- Surgical correction of vascular anomalies (e.g., clipping of arteriovenous malformations).
- Surgical removal of tumours, if any.
- Correction of other specific problems: e.g., atrial fibrillation; hemoconcentration in sickle cell anaemia; treatment of endocarditis, etc.

Questions

1. What is stroke? Stroke is defined as an acute onset focal neurological deficit lasting >24 hrs of presumed vascular origin.
2. How to differentiate between acquired vs congenital hemiplegia?
3. How do you anatomically localize the lesion in stroke?
4. Note on moya moya disease.
5. Alternating hemiplegia of childhood.

PARAPLEGIA

Chief Complaints

Weakness of both lower limbs, sensory loss, radicular pain, bowel/bladder complaints (only bladder complaint will be there).

Onset, Duration and Progress

- Acute/subacute/chronic: Acute in case of transverse myelitis or trauma.
- Progressive (compressive; cord compression by tumour, etc). One limb getting affected after the other limb points towards compressive lesion expanding from one side.
- Improving (inflammatory, demyelination).
- Waxing, waning (some cases of demyelination).

CNS History

- Higher functions
- Cranial nerves – 2nd nerve for visual disturbance (optic neuritis in Devic's disease) 9, 10, 11, 12 – high cervical lesion
- Other motor symptoms
- Sensory – Hyperesthesia, paraesthesia (numbness, tingling, pins and needles), radicular pain, saddle anaesthesia, temperature sensation. In transverse myelitis, there is loss of sensations below the level, hyperaesthesia at the level of lesion and normal sensation above the level.

Autonomic: Bowel/bladder (detailed history); loss of sweating in the affected area; temperature difference between the normal and the affected parts.

Aetiology

- Trauma
- TB: Contact history; back pain, evening fever, weight loss
- Malignancy: Bleed, bone pain, fever, pallor.
- Infection: Viral illnesses, URI, diarrhoea, rash,
- Vaccination
- Poison: Lathyrism
- Insect bite: Tick paralysis

- Similar episodes in past: Multiple sclerosis
- Rash in dermatomal pattern: Herpes zoster
- Root pain: Radiating pain increasing on cough/ sneeze

  Note: Cerebral palsy with weakness of both lower limbs is conventionally called diplegia, not paraplegia. Other intracranial causes of paraplegia are parasaggital tumours, saggital sinus thrombosis, anterior cerebral artery occlusion, etc.
- History for complications – UTI, contracture, foot deformities, bed sores.
- Activities of daily living: (EDTA), eating, dressing, toilet, ambulation.

Family History

- Hereditary spastic paraparesis, TB.

General Examination

- Eye – Optic neuritis (neuromyelitis optica, i.e., transverse myelitis plus optic neuritis)
- Evidence of TB
- BCG scar
- Spine – Tuft of hair, sinus, mass, gibbus
- Skin – Cafe au lait spots (neurofibroma could cause compression)

CNS Examination

- UMN features in lower limbs in spinal lesions (however, first few days may have flaccidity due to spinal shock; at this stage also plantar will be upgoing).
- Flaccid paraplegia in LMN lesions (anterior horn cell or peripheral nerve).
- Sensory level.
- Bowel and bladder involvement: Bowel incontinence is unlikely. Regarding bladder, specifically ascertain whether it is retention, retention with overflow, whether bladder fullness sensation is appreciated, whether voluntary initiation of micturition is possible, etc.
- The lower limbs are generally kept in full extension (hip, knee and ankle); this is called paraplegia in extension. Most paraplegias are in extension because some extrapyramidal fibres remain intact to keep the extensor tone. However in spinal transection, extrapyramidal fibres are also disconnected so much so there is paraplegia in flexion. Here, there is mild flexion of thigh, knee and ankle. This flexor tone is provided by the spinal reflex arc. So when an area below the level of lesion is stimulated, one may encounter flexor withdrawal response mediated by spinal reflex arc; one may also encounter mass reflex due to spinal reflex arc resulting in limb withdrawal by flexion and at times associated with emptying of bowel and bladder. However, this withdrawal response is not seen in paraplegia in extension because spinal reflex arc gets overridden by the extrapyramidal control.

Diagnosis

Paraperesis, anatomical level – vertebral (extradural/intradural/intramedullary), aetiology (compressive/vascular/infective/demyelination), complication, functional status.

Questions

1. Types of neurogenic bladder
2. Anatomical localization of lesion
3. Conus medullaris and cauda equina syndrome
4. Hereditary spastic paraparesis
5. Pott's spine
6. Transverse myelitis

HYDROCEPHALUS

- Chief complaints – Increased size of head.
- Developmental delay features of raised ICT (vomiting, altered sensorium).
- History of presenting illness:

  In young infant, it is better to start with antenatal history

- Onset, duration and progress:
  - History suggestive of increased intracranial tension: Vomiting, headache, seizure, altered sensorium.
  - History of abnormal movements.
  - History of abnormal eye position & movement (sun-setting). (due to impingement of dilated suprapineal recess on the brainstem tectum)
- CNS history:
  - Higher function – sensorium, gait ataxia.
  - Cranial nerve including especially second and sixth (visual defect, squint).
  - Motor system including involuntary movements, and special emphasis on lower limb symptoms.
  - Sensory system.
  - Cerebellar system: Ataxia is likely. Also, titubation of head.
  - Raised ICT (if such history is not already elicited).
  - Bowel/bladder complaints.
- Aetiology:
  - Antenatal history: History of infection (toxoplasma, mumps).
  - History of drugs: Vit A, radiation.
  - Detection in AN US scan.
  - History of abortions.
  - Birth history: Preterm (IC bleed and later hydrocephalus)/dystocia/instrument (because of large head).
  - Postnatal history: Trauma, infection/sepsis, Koch's contact, increased hospital stay, swelling at the back (neural tube defects).
- Complications: poor feeding, functional impairment, stridor, shunt complications (infection/block); abdominal pain (shunt peritonitis), haematuria (shunt nephritis).
- Treatment history: Drugs, surgery; if surgery is done inquire whether there was improvement post surgery.

- Immunization history
- Developmental history – Delayed development/loss of milestones. Also elicit history regarding activities of daily living (ADL).
- Nutrition: Growth failure is likely. Hence, inquire for any feeding difficulties.
- Family history:
  - Siblings/family members
  - Koch's contact
  - Congenital aqueductal stenosis (X-linked recessive)
  - Measure parents' head circumference
- Socioeconomic: If beneficiary of any schemes, whether adopted family planning.

11

General Examination

Comment on the general level of alertness of the baby. Look for any obvious features of syndromes or neurocutaneous disorders. Note any titubation of head or truncal ataxia while the child is sitting.

Vitals (Cushings triad)

- Pulse: Bradycardia is likely if there is increased ICT.
- BP: Hypertension, if any, may be part of increased ICT.
- Respiration: Note the rate and depth.

Anthropometry

- PEM is likely in IU infection, inborn errors of metabolism, etc.
- Tall in Soto's. Short with short limbs in achondroplasia.
- Head circumference: Always measure twice or thrice to get two same values. Measure parents head if not done already.

Head to Foot

- Head:
  - Shape of head (view from different angles before commenting). Frontal bossing is very common in obstructive hydrocephalus (aqueduct stenosis will have

prominent frontal region and small posterior fossa). Parietal prominence in subdural collection or large porencephalic cyst. Dandy Walker malformation or post fossa cyst may have prominent occiput region. In Arnold Chiari, the occipital region has no bulge at all.

- Palpate fontanels, sutures and for shunts; anterior/posterior fontanel, other fontanel, sutural separation, dilated scalp veins. Assess AF tension, with the child sitting and not crying (otherwise tension may appear falsely elevated). In case of raised tension, look for craniotabes (if present, look for evidence of rickets also) and McEwan sign.
- If shunt is palpable, try to trace the shunt and see if broken or migrated; try to find out if shunt is working by pressing the bulb.
- Transillumination (see p 227).
- Auscultate for bruit over the eye balls, temporal fossa and retroauricular area (arteriovenous malformation involving vein of Galen may be a cause for hydrocephalus).
- Eyes: Any ptosis; nystagmus (may be present if hydrocephalus is due to brain tumour); sun-setting sign, squint (VI nerve palsy). Always look for upward movements and lateral movements of eyes, which are likely to be affected. Note that because of frontal bossing causing physical barrier, there may be a false impression of upgaze palsy when palsy is not there really.

- Face: Dysmorphism/coarse facies
- Limbs
- Spine – Evidence of dysraphism (neural tube defects) or scar of its surgical correction; scoliosis (in association with spina bifida, neurofibromatosis type I)
- Abdomen: Abdominal scar of VP shunt; organomegaly of storage disorders (MPS)
- Skin: Neurocutaneous markers
- CNS examination:

Higher Functions

- Sensorium, speech
- Cranial nerves – Special emphasis on optic nerve: includes visual acuity and field; field defect is likely in tumours; fundus for papilloedema in recent hydrocephalus or optic atrophy in long standing hydrocephalus; chorioretinitis in congenital toxoplasmosis; Cherry red spot and macrocephaly in Tay Sach.
- Pupil may be unreactive to light in a rare event of pressure by dilated III ventricle (Parinaud's syndrome; upgaze palsy is also due to the pressure of dilated III ventricle).
- Also examine nerves 3, 4, 6. Isolated 6th nerve palsy may be a false localizing sign due to raised ICT.
- Hearing may be impaired in post meningitis hydrocephalus and MPS.
- Limbs:
  Spasticity – lower limb > upper limb. In case of neural tube defects and some leukodystrophies, LMN signs of lower limbs instead of UMN.
- Gait:
  Because the fronto-ponto-cerebellar fibres goes around the cerebral ventricles, hydrocephalus may stretch it; so may have ataxia. In addition, Dandy Walker has cerebellar extension and hence may produce cerebellar signs
- Reflexes: Deep tendon reflexes superficial reflexes (corneal, conjuctival, abdominal and plantar) and neonatal reflexes (Moro, snout, grasp, palmo mental) are examined. Moro may be difficult to elicit as the head is large; try lowering the angle of head in relation to the body while continuously supporting the head.

- Lower limb reflexes will be exaggerated, except in case of neural tube defects.
- Sensory system: May be omitted except in case of spina bifida where sensory blunting may be obtained.
- Cerebellar signs may be present, especially in Dandy Walker malformation.
- Spine: Already discussed with general examination.

Diagnosis

— year old child with progressive increase in head size, with/without signs of raised ICT, with/without focal neurological deficit, with/without development delay, with/without seizures, diagnosis is hydrocephalus (communicating/non-communicating) probable aetiology being ——.

Causes of Macrocephaly

- Large bones:
  - Achondroplasia, rickets, congenital haemolytic anaemia
  - Localized bone swelling as in organized cephalhaematoma
- Large brain:
  - Sotos syndrome
  - Mucopolysachharidosis
  - Inherited metabolic disorder of white matter: Alexander, Canavan
  - Inherited metabolic disorder of grey matter: Tay Sach's disease
- Large CSF space: Hydrocephalus (aetiology, see box, p 265)

Investigations

- CT scan
- TORCH screen

Treatment

Medical: Acetazolamide; repeated LP as a temporary measure; a period of observation to see if the hydrocephalus gets arrested.

Surgical: Shunt surgery, most often VP shunt.

Questions

1. Hydrencephaly and megalencephaly
2. CSF production & circulation
3. Different shunt surgeries

FLOPPY INFANT

Keep in mind the following important possibilities:

- Werdnig Hoffmann disease (spinal muscular atrophy type I)

11

Communicating hydrocephalus

- Achondroplasia
- Basilar impression
- Benign enlargement of subarachnoid space
- Choroid plexus papilloma
- Meningeal adhesions following meningitis
- IC bleed or malignant infiltration

Noncommunicating hydrocephalus

- Aqueductal stenosis
- Post infectious obstructions
- X-linked
- Chiari malformation
- Dandy-Walker malformation
- Abscess, haematoma, tumours and neurocutaneous disorders
- Vein of Galen malformation

- Hypotonic stage of cerebral palsy (normal evolution of CP is hypotonic to dystonic to spastic cerebral palsy over a few months. In some cases, this evolution gets delayed to keep the baby hypotonic longer).
- Congenital myopathy
- Congenital muscular dystrophy and congenital myotonic dystrophy
- Myasthenia gravis
  Please read p 177 for classification.

Chief Complaints

- Weakness/limpness of all limbs
- Paucity of movements
- Delayed motor milestones
- Recurrent respiratory infections (aspiration due to floppiness)

History of Present Illness (HOPI)

- Age of onset (helps to categorize the type of SMA; botulism typically presents with sudden onset in an otherwise normal child)
  - Progressive/static
  - Ascending (GBS)/descending (botulism)
  - History suggestive of frog-like posture, weak cry, poor cough, feeding difficulties, regurgitation, fasciculation
- History suggestive of CNS involvement:
  - Higher functions: Usually normal; in late cases hypoxia-related CNS dysfunction may be expected.
  - Cranial nerves (deviation of angle of mouth, nasal regurgitation, etc).
  - Motor system: History suggestive of wasting, hypertrophy, involuntary movements.
  - Sensory system: If the baby comforts on touch, the baby is appreciating touch.
  - Bowel/bladder
  - Vision/hearing
- Aetiology:
  - History suggestive of antenatal fever, drugs, pregnancy-induced hypertension, labour complications like birth asphyxia, etc. Drugs like magnesium sulphate/anaesthetic agents given to mother can cause temporary floppiness in newborn baby. Hypotonic stage of CP may mimic floppiness.
  - History suggestive of icterus, phototherapy, exchange transfusion: Kernicterus.
  - History suggestive of constipation, neonatal jaundice, hoarse cry: Hypothyroidism.
  - History suggestive of drug intake in the baby: (e.g., aminoglycosides can cause neuromuscular blockade).
  - History suggestive of honey intake as prelacteals feeds: Botulism.
  - History suggestive of IM injections: Traumatic paralysis.
  - History suggestive of diurnal variation: Myasthenia.
  - History suggestive of facial features (myopathic facies), swallowing difficulty, choking: Myopathy.
  - History suggestive of in coordination, titubation: Cerebellar ataxia.
  - History suggestive of cardiac failure (Pompe's can have cardiac failure plus flaccidity).
- Complications:
  - Feeding problems, impaired functional ability, bladder/bowel problems, bed sores.
- Activities of daily living in older children.
- Treatment history and course in hospital (including physiotherapy and/or use of braces/splints).

Antenatal History

- When was quickening noted. Fetal movements may be inconspicuous if fetus is floppy.
- Decreased fetal movements, polyhydramnios, breech presentation.
- Birth: Trauma, asphyxia, seizures, cyanosis, respiratory distress, neonatal jaundice.

Immunization

Development

In a case of SMA gross motor and to a lesser extent fine motor development are delayed. Language, social, hearing and vision will be normal. If global developmental delay is there, it is more likely to be a case of hypotonic stage of CP rather than SMA.

Nutrition

Emphasize method of feeding (like if baby is getting feeds through palada as the baby is too weak to suck) and consistency of feeds.

Family History

- Consanguinity (e.g., SMA is autosomal recessive, myotubular myopathy is X-linked recessive).
- Other affected babies/intrauterine deaths/ abortions.
- Parents/siblings: See if the parents have got dysmorphic face or myotonia on handshake (myotonic dystrophy); alternatively the candidate may ask the parent to make a fist and open it a few times; they may find it difficult to open and close in quick succession. Any ptosis in parents (myasthenia).
- From history they may have difficulty in releasing hands on getting down from bus or they themselves may have noticed the difficulty in releasing things held in hand.
- Pescavus in the mother (HMSN: hereditary motor sensory neuropathy).
- History suggestive of myasthenia in the mother; can cause transient neonatal myasthenia.
- Enquire if they have adopted family planning measures. Will be useful for final counseling regarding further pregnancy.

General Examination

In general comment, its best to describe the decubitus:

1. Frog leg posture: Externally rotated at hip and slightly flexed at knee.
2. Jug handle (internally rotated shoulder).

- If the child is coughing/crying, assess whether normal or weak cough and hoarse cry or not.
- Child may be having feeding tube, oxygen tube, etc, which must be mentioned as such in general comment.

  Vitals: Remember, the respiratory muscles may be involved and hence the rate may be high and depth of breathing shallow. Look for diaphragmatic seesaw breathing in SMA.

11

Assessment of Growth (Anthropometry)

Gross deviations are unlikely.

Developmental Assessment

- 180° flip examination may be done in children less than 1 year (beyond that it may be difficult to do the different manoeuvres), see p 256.
- Assess in supine position: Posture of the child and quality of spontaneous movements.
- Pull to sit: Observe head lag.
- Sitting: Back rounded/straight; ability to sit unsupported; degree of head control.
- Suspend by axilla and then attempted weight bearing: Look for slip through sign due to weakness of shoulder girdle; lower limb scissoring; advanced weight bearing (because of spastic stiff lower limbs, the baby appears to bear weight on legs before the age a normal child could ever stand).
- Ventral suspension: Use the forearm/hand to support the body of child in prone position (rag doll appeareance: as all the limbs fall down due to hypotonia and baby lies in inverted U posture). If the neck appears retracted during this procedure, consider cerebral palsy rather than LMN floppiness.
- Put the child in prone position: Assess tone, posture and spine. Small infants may be as

sessed for his/her ability to raise himself/herself on his/her arms: place the baby prone, keep his/her hands on either side of shoulders with palm facing down to the bed and elbow flexed. This position helps the infant pull up on hands if he is able to do so.

- Amiel Tison angles may be assessed and mentioned if the same has been taught to the student (whether this assessment is needed depends on individual medical college protocol).

Head to Foot Examination

- Head:
  - Microcephaly in a case of cerebral palsy.
  - Macrocephaly in a case of meningomyelocoele (Arnold Chiari).
  - Flat occiput with localized loss of hair due to prolonged lying down in the same position.
- Face:
  - Myopathic facies (long drawn expression less face).
  - Syndromic: Down, Prader willi, Zellweger.
  - Doll-like facies (glycogen storage disease, i.e., Pompe).
  - Alert bright face (SMA).
  - Sleepy face due to ptosis (myasthenia).
- Eyes:
  - Cataract in Lowe's, Zellweger, congenital myotonic dystrophy
  - Ptosis
  - Opthalmoplegia
  - Examination for evidence of IU infection, as hypotonic CP may be a differential.
- Ear: Test for hearing (IU infection may be related to CP).
- Mouth
  - Triangular, fish mouth; i.e., inverted V shaped upper lip ("tented" upper lips).
  - Tongue: Macroglossia in Pompe.
  - Look for fasiculations:

    (Apart from tongue, fasiculations can be noted wherever the subcutaneous fat is minimal., e.g., deltoid region in an infant.
- Upper limbs: Position at rest, fisting (clues to cerebral cause of hypotonia are abnormalities of brain function, dysmorphic features, fisting of hands, brisk reflexes).
- Look for contractures.
- Small hands and feet in Prader Willi.
- Specifically look for poly mini myoclonus in older children with SMA (p 199).
- Chest: Note the shape: whether bell shaped (SMA); any splaying of lower ribs (SMA).
- Hernial orifices.
- Testis (whether descended). Hypotonia may be associated with delay or failure of descend of testes. Under developed genitals in Prader Willi.
- Lower limbs – Congenital dysplastic hip, club foot, hypertrophy (in case of certain myopathies).
- Look for contractures (contractures develop even in a hypotonic infant due to lack of movements).
- Spine: Look for markers of spinal dysraphism like tuft of hair/ lipoma); scoliosis.

Examination of the Central Nervous System

- Higher mental functions: Normal in SMA.
- Cranial nerves:
  - Unreactive pupils in botulism; 3, 4, 6 (ptosis, opthalmoplegia); 9, 10 (pooling of secretions, gag reflex, uvula movement).
  - In a young infant, observe feeding: effective suckling and swallowing indicates normal function of 5, 7, 9 and 10 cranial nerves.
- Motor system:
  - Wasting: Note if predominantly proximal/ distal and whether symmetrical.
  - Tone: Hypotonia (assess whether hypotonia is symmetrical).

- It is best to perform 180° flip manoeuvre if not already done in development assessment.
- Comment on any contractures or hypermobility of joints.
- Comment on any hip dislocation.
- Power: Assess and grade
  - Accurate grading is not possible in small infants. Suitable modifications of tests must be done, like tickling the feet and observe movement against gravity.
- In SMA, one may notice movements of fingers and toes although proximal muscles cannot make any movements.
- Examine for neck flop, respiratory muscles (by splinting diaphragm and intercostal muscles one at a time).
- Look for paradoxical respiratory pattern.
- Mention if there are any involuntary movements.
- In meningomyelocele, there is flaccid weakness (LMN) of lower limbs.
- DTR: Decreased or may not elicitable (older children do Jendrassik's manoeuvre before commenting "not elicitable").
  - If DTR is exaggerated in a hypotonic baby, it is not any of the LMN lesions; it has got to be a UMN lesion, e.g., cerebral palsy. In that case, proceed as for examination of cerebral palsy.
- Superficial reflexes and plantar are likely to be normal in most floppy babies.
- Look for persistence of primitive reflexes (likely to persist in hypotonic CP), see p 233.
- Sensory and cerebellar system are normal in SMA.
- Skull and spine.
- Other systems:
  - CVS: Look for cardiomegaly (Pompe).
  - Respiratory system: Likely to have respiratory infection due to aspiration.
- Abdomen: In case of myopathy, look for hepatomegaly. Hepatosplenomegaly may be detectable in IU infections (which may be one of the causes for CP).

Diagnosis

— month old infant, male/female, with slowly progressive/static weakness/floppiness of all 4 limbs, with no perinatal events, drowsy/alert baby, with preserved or diminished deep tendon reflexes Most likely diagnosis is ——. Also see p 536.

Investigations: CPK, NCV, karyotype, genetic study (SMA), echocardiography (Pompe).

ACUTE FLACCID PARALYSIS

When you approach a case of acute flaccid paralysis in a child, think of the following differential diagnosis:

1. Guillian Barre syndrome (p 531)
2. Transverse myelitis
3. Traumatic neuritis
4. Poliomyelitis

Also rule out – myasthenia, drug-induced paresis, infective (diphtheria), hypokalaemic/hyperkalaemic periodic paralysis, and botulism.

Chief Complaints

Weakness (1 or more limbs, usually lower limbs are involved).

History of Present Illness (HOPI)

- Onset, duration and progress (ODP)
  - Sudden/insidious
  - Static/Progressive
  - Duration
  - Initial involvement whether ascending (GBS) or descending (botulism)
  - Proximal v/s distal (distal in peripheral neuropathies)
  - Whether there is any diurnal variation (myesthenia); Any difficulty in getting up from squatting position (weakness of proximal muscles of pelvic girdle).
  - Symmetrical (GBS) or asymmetrical (polio) paralysis. Unilateral or bilateral. Patchy involvement is more in favour of polio.

Contiguous ascending or descending progression is in favour of GBS. Localized paralysis of only some parts in polio may lead to localized bulges in abdomen termed as **phantom hernia**.
  - History of pain (myalgia may indicate early phase of polio or myositis). Subjective pain sensations are possible in early stages of GBS as well.
- History on CNS symptoms:
  - Higher functions.
  - Cranial nerves: 7, 9, 10th nerve – GBS.
  - 3, 4, 6th – Miller Fisher variant of GBS.
  - Bulbar involvement.
  - Motor system – Tone, power, reflexes.
  - Sensory system – GBS, myalgia.
  - Cerebellar signs – Ataxia (Miller Fischer syndrome).
  - Autonomic involvement – Flushing, sweating, palpitations, postural hypotension.
  - Bowel/bladder: In polio, bladder paralysis is very transient and recovers. Motor paralytic bladder of GBS may last longer. Motor paralytic means the patient can appreciate bladder sensation but cannot voluntarily void.
- History on aetiology:
  - Fever at onset (in polio), fever 2–3 weeks prior (e.g., history of GI infections) in GBS
  - Diarrhoea: Hypokalaemic paralysis, GBS
  - Trauma
  - Rash: Herpes zoster; rash and fever preceding transverse myelitis
  - IM injection – traumatic neuritis, polio (provocative polio on IM injection if polio virus is already in circulation while getting injected)
  - Pica – lead poisoning
  - Sore throat, neck swelling – diphtheria
  - Canned food/honey – botulism
  - Drugs – vincristine, steroids (steroid myopathy)
  - Severe abdominal pain – porphyria
  - Fatiguable & diurnal variation - myasthenia
  - History of tick bite (tick paralysis)
- History on complications:
  - Respiratory distress, dysphagia, syncope (autonomic)
- Activities of daily living (p 255).

Past History

Similar episodes (multiple sclerosis/periodic paralysis).

Immunization

- OPV/IPV plus pulse polio doses, ask when the last dose of polio was given in children less than 5 years (many examiners are keen that the candidate knows pulse polio dates).
- Vaccines that may precipitate demyelination (e.g., rabies vaccine).
- Development & dietary history as routine.

Family History

Similar illness in family, surrounding areas: Polio, diphtheria, botulism.

Socioeconomic History

Water source, toilet facilities, etc are important in polio (faeco-oral transmission).

General Examination

General comment on sensorium and any typical posture adopted by the child.

Vitals

- Pulse and BP: May be unstable in GBS (autonomic manifestations).
- RR: Note the rate, pattern and whether the respiratory efforts are weak and shallow (respiratory distress will not be explicit as in a case of pneumonia because this can be central abnormality leading to hypopnoea and respiratory arrest or peripheral nerve involvement

leading on to respiratory muscle paralysis).

- Measure the temperature.
- Growth assessment (anthropometry) is usually normal and wasting is not expected in acute case even if the lesion is LMN.

Head to Foot Examination

- Face: Note if facial nerve is involved (GBS).
- Oral cavity: Blue line at gums (lead poisoning), tonsils (recent tonsillectomy – provocative polio during epidemics).
- BCG scar.
- Rash: May indicate dermatomyositis (heliotrope rash, Gottron's papules).
- Neurocutaneous markers.
- Bladder: Mention specifically whether retention is present; whether bladder fullness sensation can be appreciated; whether voluntary voiding is possible; or whether already catheterized.
- Spine: Any evidence of trauma/abscess/spinal dysraphism (scars/sinuses/lipoma/tuft of hair).

CNS Examination

- Higher mental functions are expected to be normal.
- Cranial nerves:
    - 2nd nerve: Pupillary response (autonomic manifestation); look for visual acuity, field of vision and colour vision.
    Fundus: Papilledema, optic atrophy (optic neuritis with myelitis suggests Devic's disease).
    - 3, 4, 6 nerves: Opthalmoplegia may be seen in Miller Fischer syndrome, a variant of GBS.
    - 7 nerve: Look for facial palsy (GBS).
    - 9, 10: Pooling of secretions, gag reflex.
- Motor system: Mention if there is tenderness on palpation (dermatomyositis, polymyositis).
- Tone: Hypotonia.
- Power: Grade individual groups of muscles (e.g., hip abductors grade 2).
- Specially mention the involvement of deltoid (difficulty in shoulder abduction beyond 15°); it is ominous as it indicates impending respiratory failure.
- Examine for neck flop and trunk muscle weakness.
- Respiratory muscles: Single breath count; individually examine diaphragm and then intercostal muscles. One can splint abdomen (with the examiner's hands) and ask the child to breathe to assess intercostals; or splint chest and ask the child to breathe to assess diaphragm.
- Examine co-ordination of movements and gait if possible (can be done only if power is more than grade 3).
- Tripod sign, kiss the knee test in polio.
- DTR: Usually not elicitable in GBS and polio, but may be reduced but still preserved till late in the course of illness in muscle diseases.
- Note if Beevor's sign is positive (p 213, indicates weakness of the lower part of trunk).
- Sensory system: In GBS, no objective sensory changes are expected though subjective sensory symptoms may be experienced by the patient in the early stages of illness.
- Carefully examine for a sensory level (transverse myelitis).
- Cerebellar signs: Any abnormality found is likely to be due to weakness rather than cerebellar involvement.
- Look for signs of meningeal irritation.
- Look for peripheral nerve thickening.
- Straight leg rising test may be positive in radiculopathy.
- Respiratory system: Assess respiratory efforts and look for aspiration pneumonia, if any.

Diagnosis

——year old male/female, with history of acute, progressive/non-progressive, symmetrical/asymmetrical flaccid weakness, with/without respiratory involvement, likely aetiology being GBS/—.

11

Approach

- Based on the nervous system examination findings, you will realize that AFP will be a lower motor neuron type of weakness and anatomical localization should be done as below.
- The lesion can be anywhere from:
  - Spinal cord (corticospinal tract) – Spinal shock stage of transverse myelitis, spinal cord infarction, spinal cord compression.
  - Anterior horn cell – Poliomyelitis, other enteroviruses.
  - Nerve roots – GBS, Lyme disease.
  - Nerve – Diptheria, porphyria, drug induced (vincristine, arsenic, lead).
  - Neuromuscular junction – Myasthenia gravis, botulism, tick paralysis.
  - Muscle – Inflammatory myopathy, periodic paralysis.
- Rarely, it can be associated with a lesion in the brain like ADEM, brainstem encephalitis, etc. So carefully look for any UMN signs despite flaccidity that may be found in the initial stages (e.g., extensor plantar response in a flaccid child).

Investigations in GBS

- CSF:
  - Albuminocytological dissociation *by the end of 1st week* (elevation of protein is much more compared to cells).
  - Protein: Elevated, > 40 mg/dL.
  - Cells: Not more than 10/mm^3.
- Nerve conduction velocity of motor nerves are decreased and F wave latency is increased.
- EMG (shows neuropathic pattern).
- ECG & BP monitoring in case of autonomic instability.
- Electrolytes and CPK are normal in GBS.

Treatment of GBS

- Majority are self limiting and hence if there is no progression one may wait for spontaneous improvement.
- In case of progression or respiratory muscle involvement, start treatment: the options are:
  - Intravenous immunoglobulin (IVIg)
  - Plasma exchange (plasmapheresis)

  Plasma exchange and IVIg provide similar degrees of benefits, but immunoglobulin is easier to administer. The dose of IVIg is 0.4 g immune globulin per kg per day for 5 days.
- Steroid is less preferred.
- Ventilatory support is needed in case of diaphragmatic paralysis or tiring respiration. Antihypertensive medications are better avoided because of chance of fluctuations of BP due to autonomic disturbances.

General

- Fluids and nutritional support
- Cardiac/BP monitoring
- Laxatives for constipation
- Deep vein thrombosis (DVT) prophylaxis in case of prolonged immobility

Prognosis

About 1/3rd of GBS patient may have some residual weakness.

Questions

1. What are the antibodies associated with GBS and Miller Fischer syndrome?
2. What is Asbury's diagnostic criteria for GBS?

NEURAL TUBE DEFECTS (SPINAL BIFIDA)

History

- The present hospitalization may be for urinary infection or for headache, vomiting and drowsiness (increased intracranial tension due to hydrocephalus).
- Ask for chocking while drinking, nasal regurgitation, stridor, etc.
- Must inquire about activities of daily living, EDTA, how eating, dressing, toileting and ambulation are managed.

- How incontinence is managed (pad, intermittent catheterization).
- Bowel care (is the child on periodic enemas, laxatives, etc).
- Antenatal, natal, postnatal: Periconceptional folic acid (must have started before getting pregnant); antenatal screening.
- Immunization: Additional pneumococcal vaccine is desirable in view of increased chance of meningitis.
- Development: Must be assessed in all domains. Apart from the disability due to paralysis or hydrocephalus, other delays are not expected.
- Dietary history.
- Family history of neural tube defects.
- Socioeconomic history: Burden on the family and siblings; child's schooling, play, availability of peers for play, effect of incontinence on schooling, etc. Any financial support or special schemes to care the child. How is the child adapting to the disability.
- General examination
- General comment
- Mention obvious findings like stridor, high pitched cry or hoarse voice (increased ICT due to hydrocephalus in Arnold Chiari malformation), nasogastric feeding tube, etc. Comment on the posture of baby like flexed at hip, extended at knee and dorsiflexion at ankle (p 529). Any obvious respiratory distress (aspiration is very common). Sensorium is normal unless altered by increased ICT.
- Vitals.
- Anthropometry.
  Height is usually less due to kyphoscoliosis and poor growth of the paralysed lower limbs. If you are calculating weight for height, the value will be skewed, as the height may not reflect the actual. A better assessment of age appropriate height is obtained from arm span with the usual age related allowance on span-height relations.
- Head to foot and neurological examination.
- Head: Large head; look for eye signs of hydrocephalus; mention prominence of scalp veins, shiny stretched skin, etc if seen; if any surgical shunt is visible, mention that. The candidate must know how to check for functioning of shunt. Any peculiar shape, e.g., in Arnold Chiari (ACM), there is significant frontal prominence but no occipital prominence. Palpate AF, PF, sutures, etc.
- Eyes: Look for nystagmus, squint, papilledema or optic atrophy (see under hydrocephalus, p 245).
- Cranial nerves: Special emphasis is on optic nerve, 6th nerve and lower cranial nerves (9–12); get history on suck/swallow; gag reflex may be tested; look for atrophy of tongue.
- Upper limbs: Carefully look for any spasticity: occasionally in ACM, herniating cerebellar tonsils or downward displacement may cause pressure effect.
- Chest: In long standing cases with chest deformity, look for cor pulmonale.
- Truncal ataxia or titubation in rare case of ACM.
- Hip: May be dislocated! Try to abduct and see.
- Back: Kyphosis, scoliosis, scars of any surgery. If meningomyelocele is there, describe its location.
- Skin: Dermatitis is very common due to soiling and constant wetness. Pressure sores.
- Abdomen:
  Mention if there is any scar of VP shunt or any procedures for urinary diversion.
- May have hydronephrotic kidneys.
- Bladder is palpable. Retention with overflow incontinence.
- Abdominal reflexes may not be elicitable in the involved quadrants.
- Comment on analsphincter tone.
- Lower limbs.
- Usually very much wasted.
- Measure the lower limb length. It will be short due to poor growth and contractures.

- In an infant with no spontaneous movements, a pin prick may initiate a flexion withdrawal due to spinal arc (not cerebrally mediated action). The child may not have appreciated the pain as evidenced by lack of any emotional response to pain. Please read paraplegia in flexion to understand this (see p 262).
- Look for tone, power, reflexes, sensations and contractures. Hypotonia, hyporeflexia and loss of sensations are expected. Regarding power, you may infer based on spontaneous movements or stimulus induced movements. Demonstrate the sensory level. Draw the blunt end of pin from leg upwards to quickly find the level at which sensation is appreciated.
- Counseling: There is an increased risk of neural tube defects in subsequent pregnancies. Antenatal α-fetoprotein will be elevated if carrying a fetus with open neural tube defect. Antenatal ultrasonogram also can detect. Folic acid 4 mg daily must be started a month before the next planned pregnancy.

TUBERCULAR MENINGITIS

Chief Complaints

- Fever (high/low grade, evening rise, long duration)
- Seizures (focal/generalized)
- Altered sensorium/lethargy (sudden/insidious)
- Focal neurological deficit

History of Presenting Illness

- *ODP* of presenting complaints (points to be elicited for each complaint, see Ch. 8).
- *Other CNS symptoms:*
  - Higher functions: Sensorium, seizures, memory, speech, comprehension.
  - Increased intracranial pressure: Vomiting, headache (especially early morning), irritability, drowsiness, seizures.
  - Cranial nerve palsy: Deviation of angle of mouth, problems with vision, hearing, swallowing, drooling of saliva and pooling of saliva in the throat.
  - Motor system: Focal neurological deficits, weakness, involuntary movements.
  - Sensory: Numbness or tingling.
  - Meningeal signs: Neck stiffness (photophobia is a usual complaint in meningitis and must be asked for).
  - Cerebellar signs (ask about gait, intention tremor, truncal ataxia and titubation).
  - Bowel and bladder complaints.
- *Aetiology:*
  - Fall (in yesteryears, it was common for tubercular meningitis to get noticed following a fall: often the fall was because the child had already become drowsy due to the ongoing meningitis!).
  - Otorrhoea (pyogenic meningitis).
  - Weight loss, evening rise of temperature, decreased appetite (TB).
  - Rash, viral illness/vaccination followed by altered sensorium (encephalitis/ADEM).
  - Contact with TB.
  - Recurrent diarrhoea, weight loss, recurrent infection (immunodeficiency, HIV encephalopathy).
  - Any treatment taken (partially treated meningitis).
- *Complications:*
  - Bed sore, contracture, tongue bite, increase in head size, skin changes, bowel/bladder disturbance, hearing/vision.
- *Treatment history and course in hospital:*
  - Any drugs: DOTS/IM injections, surgery (VP shunt), procedures done (lumbar puncture).
- *Activities of daily living:* EDTA, eating, dressing, toilet, ambulation.

Seizures in TBM could be due to:

- Early seizure due to febrile seizures, increased intra cranial tension, electrolyte imbalance, syndrome of inappropriate ADH, secretin etc.

- Later seizures are predominantly due to vasculitis/strangulating vessels due to thick exudates causing ischaemia and infarction to the brain.

Immunization History

- BCG, *H. influenza* vaccine, Pneumococcus, Meningococcal vaccine.
- Influenza, Japanese encephalitis, rabies vaccine (rarely rabies vaccine can precipitate demyelination).

Developmental History

- Were milestones attained normally/not till the present episode.
- Was there loss of attained milestones after present insult (sequelae).

Nutrition

Malnutrition, weight loss.

Family and Socioeconomic History

- History of seizures in the family.
- Overcrowding, hygiene and sanitation. Elicit history regarding overcrowding and ventilation at home.

Examination

1. General comment:
   - Child could be drowsy/comatose, may be lying with extended head or in decerebrate posture, could be emaciated.
2. Vital signs (compare with normal values for age):
   - Pulse rate, respiratory rate, blood pressure and temperature.
3. Assessment of growth (Anthropometry or Measurements): Must take measurements, as the child is likely to be malnourished.
4. Head to foot:
   Size of head, fontanel, crackpot sign (McEwan's sign), bruit over skull (AV malformations).
   - Eye: Phlycten, papilledema, choroid tubercles, vitamin A deficiency.
   - Lymph nodes
   - VP shunt tube
   - BCG scar
   - Mantoux reaction
   - Skull, spine, scars
   - Skin: Erythema nodosum, bedsores, callosity, neurocutaneous markers, bleeding (leukaemia can present with CNS manifestations).
   - Malnutrition and vitamin deficiency.

11

Examination of CNS

- Follow the CNS exam format (see p 2).
- Look for signs of increased intracranial pressure (symptoms already described p 263): bradycardia, elevated blood pressure, VI nerve palsy ("false localizing sign"), irregularity in respiration (a late event), etc.
- In a case of sequelae of CNS TB, look for them.
  - Hydrocephalus
  - Seizures
  - Mental retardation
  - Behaviour abnormalities
  - Paralysis, motor or cranial nerve (especially VII and II)
- Drug-induced hepatitis
- Look for shunt displacement

Also see p 529.

Diagnosis

Acute/subacute/chronic encephalopathy, meningo-encephalitis of infective aetiology with/without paresis, with/without cranial nerve palsy with/without vision or hearing involvement with/without evidence of increased intracranial tension, involuntary movements, malnutrition grade and vaccination status, probable aetiology being TBM.

Investigations

- The diagnosis of TB in general is by the combination of contact history, suggestive symptoms, Mantoux, X-ray chest and demonstration of AFB/histopathology. For TBM, specific additional investigations are LP and brain imaging.
- Lumbar puncture:
  - CSF is straw coloured, may form cob web on standing (smear from cob web is likely to yield AFB). PCR also may yield positive result.
  - CSF cell count is increased, shows >50% lymphocytes.
  - CSF sugar is less than 2/3rd of corresponding blood sugar value, but not very low (not <20 mg/dL).
  - CSF protein is elevated. Very high protein indicates TB meningitis with block to CSF circulation.
- CT with contrast/MRI: Basal exudates, hydrocephalus, focal areas of infarcts, tuberculomas, etc.
- Mantoux
- Chest X-ray
- Early morning gastric aspirate for AFB staining. If any lymph node is enlarged, FNAC or excision for histopathology to detect granuloma.
- Students may refer to Manual of Pediatric Practice by the same author for newer methods of diagnosis.

Treatment

Daily dose regimen: 2 months HRZE/S (Streptomycin given when visual defect is present or presumed)followed by 7–10 months of HRE. Total duration can extend to 12–24 monthsAdjunctive corticosteroids for 6–8 weeks.

Complications

- Cranial nerve palsies, including visual loss and hearing loss
- Focal neurological deficits
- Hydrocephalus
- Seizure disorder
- Behavioural abnormalities and learning disabilities

Table 11.1 Drugs used in the treatment of tuberculosis

Drug	Daily dose mg/kg/day	Adverse events
Isoniazid	10 (7–15)	Peripheral neuropathy, Hepatitis
Rifampicin	15 (10–20)	Hepatitis, flu-like illness
Pyrazinamide	35 (30–40)	Hepatitis
Ethambutol	20 (15–25)	Optic neuritis
Streptomycin	15–20	Tinnitus

Commonly Asked Questions

1. Discussion of differential diagnosis
2. Stages of coma
3. Stages of TBM & prognosis in each stage
4. Signs of meningeal irritation
5. Signs of increased intracranial pressure
6. Types of herniation
7. Management of TBM - supportive + definitive
8. Types of shunt & complications of shunt
9. Complication of TBM
10. Pathology in TBM & lesion localization
11. CT correlates in TBM
12. Precipitating factors in TBM
13. Poor prognostic factors in TBM
14. Role of steroids
15. Newer modalities of diagnosis of TBM

DEVELOPMENTAL REGRESSION

The examiners do not expect the candidate to have comprehensive knowledge of individual neurodegenerative disorders. The candidate must be able to narrow down the possibilities to a reasonable extent and then know names of a few conditions in that group. E.g., white matter degenerative disease with peripheral neuropathy. Possibilities are Krabbe, metachromatic leukodystrophy, adrenoleukodystrophy, etc to further narrow down, onset in early infancy favour Krabbe, and pigmentation favour adrenoleukodystrophy, etc.

Please read case sheet format of development delay. The same format is useful here.

Age and Sex

The candidate must have a working knowledge of sex-appropriate conditions and age-of-onset appropriate conditions. For example, Lesch Nyhan syndrome is X linked, so manifests in males only. Tay Sach syndrome manifests from very early infancy. SSPE, Wilson, Batten disease, etc manifest in older children.

Chief Complaints

- Loss of previously attained milestones, convulsions
- Personality changes/dementia
- Visual problems

HOPI

- ODP: Acute or chronic
  - Progressive
  - Onset and progression
  - Grey matter vs White matter
    - Grey – Dementia, personality change, seizure, speech, cognition, retinal changes.
      Clue – "RDS" is grey, i.e., retina, dementia, seizure.
    - White – Gait incoordination, optic atrophy, spasticity (tracts affected).
  - Gait – Adrenoleukodystrophy, metachromatic leukodystrophy
  - Focal deficit – Mitochondrial disease
  - Vision – Tay-Sach, Wilson's, neuronal ceroid lipofucinosis (NCL)
  - Hearing – ALD, mucopolysaccharidosis
- CNS history:
  - Higher functions
  - Cranial nerves
  - Motor
  - Sensory
  - Cerebellar
  - Autonomic, bowel/bladder
- Aetiology:
  - Rule out encephalitis: History of acute onset fever, altered sensorium
  - Behavioural syndrome (autism)
  - ICSOL
  - History of increased startle response – Tay Sachs (gray matter disease)
  - History of increased head size – Alexander, Canavan (both white matter disease)
  - History of repeated vomiting, failure to thrive from very early infancy: Krabbe
  - History of typical body odour – IEM
  - History of jaundice plus neurodegeneration – Wilson

11

- History of measles many years ago – SSPE
- History of self mutilation – Lesch Nyhan

- Complications:
  - Feeding difficulty
  - Respiratory infections
  - Contracture
  - Bed sores
  - Bowel/bladder
- Activities of daily living (ADL)
- Treatment history & advice

General Examination

- General comment (any dysmorphism)
- Vitals
- Anthropometry
- Head circumference
- Increased head size – typically in Alexander, Canavan. Large head may be seen in Tay Sach, MPS, hydrocephalus, etc
- Head size may be small in a lot of syndromes
- Short stature may be part of many syndromes

Development assessment by the candidate is important in cases of development regression. In case it is not practically feasible (uncooperative child), the candidate can bank on history and calculate DQ in various domains. For small infants, it is of advantage to do 180° flip manoeuvre (see p 256).

Head to Foot Examination

- Hair – Menke's kinky hair disease (feel the hair).
- Eye – Optic atrophy, KF ring, telengectesia (ataxia telengiectasia), cataract, retinitis pigmentosa, cherry red spot (Tay Sach).
- Ear: Hearing has to be evaluated (hearing defect in MPS).
- Dysmorphism of face Mucopolysaccharoidosis, Zellweger. ***Note***: Dysmorphism does not mean face only; morphological deviations from normal in hands, chest or anywhere is dysmorphism.
- Chest: CVS examination. Many syndromes are associated with heart diseases.
- Abdomen – Hepatosplenomegaly (Gaucher, GM1 gangliosidosis, Niemann Pick, Hurler).
- Genitalia: Large testes (post pubertal) in fragile X.
- Skin – Biotinidase deficiency; angiokeratoma in Fabry's disease.
- Cutaneous finding of tuberous sclerosis (p 521), ataxia telengiectasis (p 523), incontinentia pigmenti (p 519), thick coarse skin in MPS, eczema in phenyl ketonuria.
- Neurocutaneous markers.
- Subcutaneous nodules: Farber's disease.
- Trophic ulcers – sensory involvement.
- Peripheral nerve involvement – Krabbe's, MLD.
- Back: Scoliosis (Friedreich ataxia).

NERVOUS SYSTEM

Higher Functions

- Tone: Hypotonia in a variety of conditions like Leigh, Pompe, Zellweger, etc.
- Spasticity in white matter degenerative disease; rigidity in Wilson, Hallervorden Spatz.
- Power: Look for any weakness.
- Reflexes: Hyporeflexia of ankle in MLD, Krabbe. Generalized hypotonia and hyporeflexia in Leigh, Pompe.
- Primitive reflexes (see p 233).
- Involuntary movements: Extrapyramidal movements like dystonia and tremor in Wilson, Hallervorden Spatz, Huntington; myoclonus in SSPE, Batten (neuronal ceroid lipofucinosis); frank seizures in many conditions. The progression of symptoms of SSPE may be understood if we visualize it as progressing from cortex downwards: starts as intellectual regression (cortex), then myoclonus (sub cortical), and later involvement of vital structures of brainstem.

Diagnosis

—year old boy/girl, with insidious loss of previously attained milestones, with/without visual, hearing impairment, spasticity/hypotonia, macrocephaly, with/without seizures/involuntary movements, suggestive of grey/white matter involvement, with/without organomegaly, most probable diagnosis being —.

Investigations

- Urine metabolic screen.
- Thyroid function study for all.
- Karyotype in all dysmorphic babies.
- CSF study (measles antibody in SSPE, HIV antibody in AIDS; non specific findings in neurodegenerative diseases).
- CT/MRI wherever indicated.
- EEG if seizure. EEG in SSPE shows characteristic periodic complexes.
- Nerve conduction velocity in peripheral neuropathy (MLD, Krabbe).
- Other tests in specific situations:
  - Vitamin B_{12} assay as it may present with new neurological signs.
  - HIV serology (HIV encephalopathy).
  - Blood levels of ceruloplasmin (Wilson), measles antibody (SSPE), organic acids (organic aciduria), lactate and pyruvate (Leigh), ammonia (urea cycle disorders), uric acid (Lesch Nyhan).
  - BERA for hearing evaluation.
  - Visual evoked potentials (optic nerve is affected in white matter disease); electro retino graphy (retina is affected in gray matter disease).
- Specific white cell enzyme studies only if the diagnosis is narrowed down to a specific group of conditions (to be sent to specialized centres).

Questions

1. Approach to a case of neuroregression.
2. Various presentations of inborn errors of metabolism.
3. Causes of cherry red spot.
4. Treatable causes.

DUCHENNE MUSCULAR DYSTROPHY

- Baseline information.
- Think of a musclar dystrophy if the following points are present.
- Primary muscle involvement (as evidenced by proximal weakness more than distal; reflexes depressed in proportion to weakness).
- Progressive course (dystrophy has progressive course; myopathy has static course).
- Genetic basis (family history).
- Degeneration and death of muscle is seen at some stage of the disease (demonstrable histopathology; not useful as a clinical pointer).
- Age of first clinical presentation is usually 2–5 years in DMD. Congenital muscular dystrophy may be clinically evident from early infancy itself.
- Also read p 535–536.

Important differential diagnoses to be considered are

- Becker's muscular dystrophy (similar to DMD, but a more slow progression. Gene mutation and inheritance are same as DMD, i.e., Xp21; X-linked recessive inheritance).
- Myopathy: three groups
  - Congenital myopathy: In congenital myopathy, muscle is structurally abnormal to start with but there is no ongoing destruction of muscle (e.g., central core disease, nemaline rod, myotubular, etc). Thus, there is no progressive clinical deterioration. Creatine kinase (CPK) will remain normal as there is no destruction.

11

- Metabolic myopathy (glycogen storage disease, mitochondrial myopathy, etc).
- Inflammatory myopathy (dermatomyositis, polymyositis).

- Juvenile SMA (slowly progressive SMA).
- Kocher-Debre-Semelaigne syndrome (hypertrophied weak muscles in hypothyroidism).
- Rare differentials:
  - Emery Dreifuss muscular dystrophy
  - Limb-Girdle muscular dystrophy
  - Fukuyama congenital muscular dystrophy (has associated mental retardation): Described in Japan, possibly not common in our country, a fact that must be considered before offering this diagnosis.

Age

DMD generally will have some symptoms before 5 years of age, usually first noticed by 2 years of age.

Chief Complaints

- Weakness (lower limb > upper limb).
- Difficulty in getting up from squatting/sitting position; difficulty to climb stairs
  - Abnormal gait
  - Frequent falls, tripping
  - Prominent calf muscles

HOPI

- Weakness
  - Acute – Inflammatory, infective, traumatic, etc. DMD cannot present acutely.
  - Subacute – Hypothyroid, myasthenia.
  - Chronic – Congenital, metabolic.
  - Progressive (muscular dystrophy)/Static/Improving (GBS, inflammatory like polymyositis).
- More involvement of upper limb or lower limb. Lower limb is more involved in DMD.
- Calf muscle hypertrophy may have been noted by the parents.
- Predominant involvement of muscle groups: Distal (neuropathies except juvenile SMA) or proximal (myopathies except myotonic muscular dystrophy).
- Diurnal variation of weakness in myaesthenia.
- Associated with pain: E.g., polymyositis.
- Cranial nerve involvement (bulbar).
- Autonomic (dizziness on standing up, flushing, sweating).
- Bowel and bladder disturbances.

Aetiology

- History of family member with similar complaints.
- History of rash over face (dermatomyositis).
- History of joint pain, photophobia (collagen vascular disease).
- History of encephalopathy, seizures (mitochondrial diseases).
- History of drug intake (steroid).
- History of malabsorption (vit E deficiency).
- History of hypothyroidism (constipation, intolerance to cold, excessive sleepiness).
- History of repeated exacerbations (hypokalaemic periodic paralysis).
- History of ptosis, diurnal variation (myesthenia).

Complications

- History of respiratory infections.
- History of feeding difficulty.
- History of cardiac complaints: Breathlessness, chest pain, palpitations. Cardiomyopathy is a complication in the later stages of DMD.
- History of toe walking, bedsores, contractures.

Past History

Drugs; History of rash in dermatomyositis; Any recent IM injections (pseudo weakness due to pain or weakness due to traumatic nerve palsy); Is child already on physiotherapy.

Birth and Neonatal History

Decreased fetal movements (SMA), polyhydramnios. DMD babies appear normal at birth. Arthrogryposis may be seen even at birth in congenital muscular dystrophy.

Immunization

Development

Motor development is delayed. In DMD, milestones during infancy are somewhat normally achieved, and delay in motor milestones start beyond infancy.

Nutrition History

Will need good nutritional history to comment whether overweight, if any, is due to excess eating or immobility.

Family History

- Positive family history is likely in DMD, Becker, facioscapulohumeral dystrophy, etc.
- Weakness/wheel chair use by other members.
- Look for myopathic face, muscle hypertrophy, pes cavus, peroneal atrophy, etc in parents.
- Premature deaths.

General Examination

Vitals

- Pulse rate may be slow in hypothyroidism.
- Respiratory rate may be increased late in DMD when vital capacity is reduced due to muscle weakness.

Anthropometry

- Overweight is likely late in disease as the child is less mobile.
- Severe PEM may be associated with muscle weakness (nutritional myopathy).
- Short stature in hypothyroidism, steroid use.

Head to Foot Examination

- Facies: Myopathic, dysmorphic
- Cataract
- Ptosis: Ask the child to look up to the ceiling for 30 sec (myaesthnia): curtain sign
- Rash: Face, knuckles (dermatomyositis)
- Neck: Thyroid swelling: both hyper- and hypo thyroidism causes myopathy
- Joint: Joint swelling
- Limbs: Muscle hypertrophy or atrophy. Valley sign in DMD (p 535). Proximal muscle wasting in most myopathies. Distal muscle wasting in myotonic dystrophy and neuropathies. Fasciculation, if visible, point towards SMA. Pes cavus in lower limbs. 11
- Contracture:
  - Ask the child to walk normally, on toes, on heels (to do these need full power of muscles), heel to toe walking, climb stairs, jump, squat and get up (tests proximal muscle weakness), sit on floor and get up (Gower sign), etc.
  - Ask the child to keep both arms above the head for a few seconds (tests proximal muscle weakness). Ask the child to make a tight fist and release immediately a few times (brings out myotonia; this test is more sensitive than simple handshake). Percuss the thenar eminence for myotonia.
- Back: Scoliosis, kyphosis, lordosis.
- Testes

Examination of CNS

- Higher functions (intellectual retardation in hypothyroidism).
- Cranial nerves:
  Usually normal. Specifically look for bulbar weakness and any fibrillation on tongue.
- Motor system: Bulk: Weak hypertrophied muscles (calf, gluteus, deltoid, infraspinatus).

Specifically mention which all muscles are hypertrophied (e.g., in DMD, calf muscles, deltoid, infra spinatus, brachioradialis, etc).

- Tone is less. Palpate the hypertrophied muscle and describe the feel of it.
- Power: reduced. Dorsiflexion at ankle may be weak (hence tip toeing); deltoid, pelvic, calf muscles, etc may be weak.
- Mention if there is any contracture.
- Reflexes: Weak to absent. Distal reflexes (ankle) are preserved!
- Gait
- Waddling gait due to weak abductors.
- Gower's sign (weakness of extensors and abductors of hip).
- Sensory system: If involved, consider neuropathy rather than muscle disease.
- Skull and spine: Exaggerated lumbar lordosis (secondary to weakness of pelvic muscles).
- Features of hypothyroidism, if any.
- Features of Cushing syndrome, if any (steroid myopathy).
- Features of cardiac failure, if any (cardiomyopathy in DMD, Pompe; conduction disturbances in myotonic dystrophy).
- Features of respiratory failure, if any (may attempt single breath count).

Diagnosis

—year old, male child with/without family history, slowly progressive proximal muscle weakness, calf muscle hypertrophy, normal sensory system, likely cause is DMD with/without cardiac involvement, functional grade—.

Investigations in DMD

- CPK level are very high (indicates ongoing muscle destruction).
- Muscle biopsy shows muscle destruction.
- EMG will show myopathic pattern (brief small amplitude polyphasic potentials, BSA PP).
- Nerve conduction velocity is normal (this is a muscle disease not nerve disease!).
- Cardiac evaluation (ECG, X-ray, Echo).
- Pulmonary function studies.
- Genetic studies and chorionic villus sampling of next pregnancy for prenatal diagnosis.

Treatment of DMD

- Avoid overweight (obesity makes walking more difficult).
- Physiotherapy: Passive stretching to avoid contractures.
- Prompt treatment of all respiratory infections.
- Occupational therapy: Wheel chair, braces, etc.
- Additional vaccines like pneumococcal, influenza virus, etc must be considered.
- Emotional support.

Prognosis

- Invariably develop scoliosis in late childhood, which can interfere with respiration.
- Usually becomes wheel chair bound by 10 years and die before 20 years due to respiratory failure or cardiac failure.

Questions

1. What are the major tools for diagnosis?
2. Differentiating points from our main differential diagnosis.
3. Other causes of calf hypertrophy.

FEBRILE SEIZURES

Febrile seizures are seizures that occur between the age of 6 and 60 months with a temperature of 38°C (100.4°F) or higher, that are not the result of central nervous system infection or any metabolic imbalance, and that occur in the absence of a history of prior afebrile seizures.

History

- Age of the child (6m to 60 months, most common in 12-18 months)
- Duration of fever to seizures (fever 1-2 days prior to the event)
- Condition at the time of seizures (high/ low grade fever)
- Seizure generalized or focal
- Tonic clonic seizures or posturing or absent seizures (i.e. semiology of seizure)
- Duration of the seizure activity (<5 min usually, >30 min status)
- Mode of termination of the seizure (self-terminated or upon administration of drugs)
- Post termination sensorium (usually very short post ictal state)
- Anything to suggest atypicality (prolonged, focal, recurring within the same febrile illness)
- Complications noted - cyanosis, apnoea, aspiration any neurological abnormality.
- History of fall, vomiting, headache, irritability prior to the seizures (raised ICP)
- History of vaccination (consider vaccine encephalopathy)
- History of pica (iron deficiency)
- History related to the etiology of fever- HHV, Roseola (rashes), otitis media, shilgella (diarrhea), UTI, pneumonia
- History of any aura
- Drug intake history- past history of antibiotic intake in particular, and drugs lowering seizure threshold (aminophylline, isoniazid, metronidazole, penicillin, TCA, lidocaine, fentanyl, antihistamines, anticholinergics, baclofen, mefenamic acid, lithium)
- Poisonings- camphor
- Recurrent episodes of regurgitation of feeds with abnormal posturingà sandifer syndrome (not seizure)
- Past history of febrile seizures or seizure disorder
- Family history of seizure disorder or febrile seizures
- Assess the risk for recurrence of febrile seizure in the child- Major are: - first episode at age <1year, temperature 38-39 °C or duration of fever <24 hours, Minor risks are Parental history of febrile seizure, family history of epilepsy, day care attendance, males, any atypical features, low serum sodium at the time of occurrence (no risk factor 12 %, 1 risk factor- 25 – 50 %, 2 risk factors 50-59%, 3 or more 73-100%)
- Assess risk for subsequent epilepsy- status epilepticus, seizure recurring within 24 hours, developmental delay, family history of epilepsy, focal neurological deficit following a seizure, fever to seizure duration <1hour, focal seizure

Examination

- Vitals are to be monitored
- Temperature recording is a must
- Look for any dysmorphisms or coarse facies
- See for pallor
- See for tonsillar enlargement, ear discharge, rashes over the body, abscesses over the body
- Nail changes of iron deficiency
- See for any neurocutaneous markers, spinal dysraphisms
- See for any phimosis or synechia
- Skin hyperpigmentation, abnormality of genitalia
- Growth assessment
- Complete neurological assessment- see for any neurological defects.
- Respiratory system assessment- high chance for aspiration pneumonia
- GIT assessment - organomegaly

Diagnosis

- ______ year old male/ female child with normal development, immunized for age, with no malnutrition, with first episode of typical febrile seizure, family history +, no neurocutaneous markers secondary to______ (UTI, Pneumonia, Tonsillitis, Viral fever)

Investigations after first episode of Febrile seizure

- Blood glucose estimation
- Blood counts, sepsis screen, blood cultures
- RBC indices, peripheral smear
- Serum electrolytes including Sodium, Potassium, Calcium, Phosphorous, Magnesium
- Baseline RFT and LFT
- Iron studies
- Complete CSF analysis
- Routine lumbar puncture is strongly recommended in children of age < 6 months. 6months to 1 year lumbar puncture is desirable if the child has not been immunized for H. Influenza type B or S. pneumoniae. > 1 year LP need not be done provided it is a typical febrile seizure. Child on antibiotic therapy developing seizure needs to undergo a CSF analysis
- EEG done only after 2 weeks, Imaging (CT or MRI) not recommended if the child is neurologically normal

Treatment

- Protect from injury
- Semiprone position to prevent aspiration
- Oxygen inhalation
- Control seizures with diazepam 0.2–0.3 mg/kg iv or 0.5 mg/kg rectally. 0.2mg/kg midazolam iv or intranasal.
- Tepid sponging and antipyretics
- Reassure the parents, explain the risk for recurrence
- Iron supplementation in iron deficiency as it is a known trigger.

Prophylaxis

At the beginning of fever intermittent prophylaxis is adviced

- Tepid sponging
- Paracetamol round the clock x 3 days
- Diazcpam 0.33 mg/kg/dose tds x 3 days or Clobazam 0.25 – 1mg/kg/day x 3 days (clobazam has longer duration of action
- If fever persisting after 3 days then the child needs to be evaluated for the cause of fever.
- Continuous prophylaxis with phenobarbitone or valproate is not justified owing due to the adverse effects to these drugs

For extra reading (for PGs)

1. What is GEFS+, Dravet syndrome
2. What is FIRES
3. What is NORSE

CHAPTER 12

Cardiovascular System : Part–I

12

HISTORY

Symptoms Related to CVS

Chest Pain

Angina is a common symptom in adults but not in a child and in 25-45% is due to unknown reasons. In a child, pericarditis can produce chest pain. It is central chest pain, increased by deep inspiration, cough and even postural changes (hence easily confused with pleural pain, except for its location). Apart from pericarditis, other CVS conditions causing chest pain in children are mitral valve prolapse, severe aortic stenosis, moderate to severe aortic regurgitation, hypertrophic cardiomyopathy, anomalous left coronary from pulmonary artery (ALCAPA), Kawasaki disease, SLE, etc. Cardiac arrhythmias produce a perceivable uneasiness in chest, which is often complained of as chest pain. In addition, very rarely angina may occur in very fast tachyarrhythmias due to reduced diastolic interval. Angina equivalents in infants are episodes of irritable cry particularly in ALCAPA.

Aetiology of Chest Pain in Children

- **Respiratory**: Pleurisy (pain aggravated by pressing on the affected side, cough, deep breathing, etc), and rarely other diseases of respiratory system.
- **Cardiac (1-3% only)**: Pericarditis (which may be part of rheumatic pancarditis), rarely mitral valve prolapse. Other causes are discussed above.
- **Oesophagus**: Hiatus hernia, oesophagitis.
- **Chest wall**: Local cellulitis, trauma, costochondritis, herpes zoster, transverse myelitis (band of hyperaesthesia). Also see p 170.

Note: Mnemonic to describe chest pain: "SOCRATES"; **S**ite, **O**nset, **C**haracter, **R**adiation, **A**ssociated symptoms, **T**iming, **E**xacerbating and relieving factors, **S**everity.

Dyspnoea

This is an uncomfortable awareness of one's own breathing. Breathlessness is felt when the demand on the lungs is more than its capacity to respond. Enquire if it is on exertion or at rest, and what extent of exertion brings on dyspnoea (may be needed to know the severity of dyspnoea). Describe about the onset, progress, severity and diurnal variation of the breathlessness. Breathlessness in cardiac disease may be due to pulmonary congestion, which in turn may indicate left heart failure. When blood accumulates in the lung it becomes stiff and difficult to expand. In addition, the hydrostatic pressure in the pulmonary circulation may go above the oncotic pressure so that fluid that escapes the vascular compartment is not drawn back into venous end of the capillaries making it stiffer (pulmonary oedema). Dyspnoea on lying down may be a symptom of cardiac disease (like orthopnoea, paroxysmal nocturnal dyspnoea, etc), but one must remember that orthopnoea is much more common to be a presenting symptom of asthma (also see p 154).

Tachypnoea is an increase in respiratory rate. Dyspnoea is commonly associated with tachypnoea, but modest tachypnoea need not be associated with dyspnoea. Cyanotic heart diseases and lesions causing low cardiac output often have tachypnoea, especially during exertion, to compensate for poor peripheral oxygenation. In infants it is associated with suck- rest- suck cycle, head sweating, failure to thrive.

Orthopnoea

It is the dyspnoea occurring within minutes after lying down, and relief when put on to shoulders or sitting up. It is because of the redistribution of blood to the pulmonary circulation from the periphery when the patient is recumbent and also because of the abdominal contents pushing up the diaphragm compromising the space available for lung expansion. Orthopnoea gets relieved soon after getting up.

Paroxysmal Nocturnal Dyspnoea

This occurs only some 2–5 hrs after retiring to bed and is hence different from orthopnoea. The child wakes up from sleep fighting for breath. At times, one may find pink frothy sputum, characteristic of acute pulmonary oedema. It takes some 15–30 min for the patient to recover after assuming upright position, again differentiating it from orthopnoea. PND develops during rapid eye movement (REM) sleep. It is presumed that the venospasm occurring during REM sleep pushes blood from areas of pooling to pulmonary circulation. It is the classical symptom of left-sided heart failure.

New York Heart Association grading (NYHA): This is basically designed for adults and grades the cardinal cardiovascular symptoms (dyspnoea, palpitation, fatigue or angina in adults).

Class I	No symptoms with *ordinary* physical activity.
Class II	Has symptoms with ordinary physical activity like walking to school.
Class III	Has symptoms with activities of daily living like bathing, going to toilet, etc.
Class IV	Symptoms at rest.

Modified Ross Classification for Heart Failure in Children: The original Ross Classification was developed in 1987 by R.D. Ross which was later modified to incorporate children of all ages.

Class I	Asymptomatic.
Class II	Mild tachypnoea or diaphoresis with feeding in infants, no growth failure. Dyspnoea on exertion in older children.
Class III	Marked tachypnoea or diaphoresis with feeding in infants. Marked dyspnoea on exertion. Prolonged feeding times with growth failure.
Class IV	Symptoms such as tachypnoea, retractions, grunting or diaphoresis at rest.

Cyanosis

Cyanosis is difficult to detect in severe anaemia; it is said that a minimum of 5 g% of reduced Hb is needed for cyanosis to become easily appreciable.

Peripheral cyanosis becomes apparent in all conditions of circulatory stasis like shock, cold extremities, CCF, etc. Because of stasis there is increased extraction of oxygen from the blood and hence the cyanosis. The lip can very rarely become blue as part of peripheral cyanosis due to cold. But when tongue and mucous membrane of mouth and inside of lips are blue, it is central cyanosis.

Cyanosis of congenital cyanotic heart diseases may appear at birth (TGA, Pulmonary or Tricuspid Atresia, Severe PS with ASD), or within 3–5 days when the ductus closes. Tetralogy of Fallot is an exception, where the cyanosis occurs after only by 2–6 months (when infundibular stenosis has progressed in severity). In fact, in some TOF newborns, the infundibular stenosis is not tight to start with, so the murmur may sound like VSD in the newborn period (and there is no cyanosis), only to decrease in intensity in a couple of months and becomes a less loud ejection murmur and cyanosis makes its appearance.

Fatigue

It is a symptom of diuretic treatment or low cardiac output situations like AS, MS, MR, cardiac failure, etc. Feeding difficulty (suck-rest-suck cycles), head sweating during feeding, etc, may convey the message of fatigue in infants.

Note: Any young infant tiring rapidly with feeding and is sweating profusely with feeding may have cardiac failure. Subcostal retraction is a common accompaniment after feeding or exertion.

Palpitation

Most often, palpitation is the heartbeat perceived by an anxious child child or as increased precordial activity noted by the mother. Anaemia, anxiety and fever are the most common causes of palpitation. Sudden onset and cessation of palpitation may mean arrhythmia like supraventricular tachycardia. Always comment about any thyroid swelling in cases of palpitation. Also ask about any precipitating factors, e.g., salbutamol may cause palpitation in some children.

Syncope

This may be due to drugs that cause postural hypotension (like nifedipine), aortic outflow obstruction (AS, coarctation of aorta), severe PS, MVP, long QT syndrome, sick sinus syndrome, heart block, tachyarrhythmia, etc, but the most common cause is vasovagal syncope. One must enquire about preceding warning symptoms like feeling of weakness (light-headedness or dizziness), blurred vision, sweating, headache, yawning, etc, in vasovagal syncope. Also one must try to elicit history suggestive of fear, emotion, exhaustion, postural hypotension, hypoglycaemia, etc, before the episode. Cyanotic heart disease may be associated with syncope (also see p 154).

Oedema

12

It may indicate cardiac failure. The principle is that oedema accumulates behind the heart that fails. Thus, one expects oedema in legs and liver congestion in right heart failure. In left heart failure, the fluid accumulates in the lung (pulmonary oedema), the immediate area behind the left heart.

In small infants, rapid weight gain may indicate oedema. In young infants, pre-tibial oedema is less likely; more often oedema is peri-orbital and is usually preceded by tachypnoea, dyspnoea and hepatomegaly.

Mechanism of Oedema

The failing heart results in pump failure; the fluid accumulates in the veins, increases the hydrostatic pressure within the capillaries, which goes above the oncotic pressure exerted by the plasma proteins. Hence at the venous end of capillaries the fluid is not drawn back into the vasculature, but instead collects in the interstitial compartment. Effect of gravity makes it most likely to happen in dependant areas.

To examine for oedema, press against a bony part for about 30 sec and release; a pit will remain in this area if oedema is present ('pitting oedema'), also see p 169.

Squatting

This must be specifically asked for in cyanotic heart diseases. Similarly, history suggestive of cyanotic spell may be inquired into.

Arthritis

Arthritis and arthralgia are likely in rheumatic fever and infective endocarditis.

Note: Fatigue, reduced urine output, head sweating,oedema, failure to thrive, increased irritability, suck rest suck cycle, increased CFT are suggestive of Congestive Cardiac Failure.

Other Points in History

- Maternal history: Ask for history of irradiation, drugs, alcohol, etc, during pregnancy. Maternal diabetes has a higher risk of congenital heart disease. Preterm birth has higher chance of PDA. Maternal and antenatal history may include history of consanguinity, maternal age, history suggestive of intrauterine infections, etc. Cardiotoxic drugs in child (e.g., anthracycline used for leukaemia); Drugs like propranolol may explain bradycardia.
- History of sudden death (which may be forthcoming in hypertrophic cardiomyopathy) or Congenital Heart Disease in family.
- Fever, rash (KD, Acute Rheumatic Fever), subcutaneous nodules, abnormal movements, recurrent lower respiratory infections, etc. Other histories worth asking for include feeding history, conjunctivitis, peeling, lymph node enlargement, etc in relevant cases (e.g., Kawasaki disease, SLE).
- Treatment history.
- Activities of daily living affected by disease.

GENERAL EXAMINATION

- Look for Dysmorphic facies, Coarse facies (Hurler syndrome- Regurgitant lesions, coronary stenosis)
- Cyanotic heart disease:Polycythaemia, clubbing, cyanosis,conjunctival congestion, periorbital puffiness, prominent veins, congenital malformations.
- Marfan syndrome: Pectus excavatum, carinatum, Marfanoid features. Tall stature with arachnodactyly and arm span more than the height are seen in Marfan's syndrome. Here, mitral regurgitation may be seen.
- Rheumatic fever: Subcutaneous nodules, joint swelling, chorea, rash, etc.
- Infective endocarditis: Discussed elsewhere (p 303).
- Caries tooth.
- Any signs of orthopnoea.
- Skin laxity (Ehler Danlos syndrome, Marfan syndrome).
- Peripheral signs of AR (Pg. 282) X 303
- Malar flush: Mitral stenosis.
- Butterfly rash: SLE.
- Hyper- or hypotelorism in a variety of syndromes. Down syndrome has endocardial cushion defect as the typical cardiac lesion, but VSD, ASD and rarely TOF can occur.
- Cataract may be associated with congenital rubella syndrome.
- Webbing of neck is seen in Turner (CoA) and Noonan syndromes (PS). Shield chest is also characteristic of Turner.
- Elfin facies is described in Williams syndrome with supravalvular aortic stenosis (p 350).
- Supernumerary fingers of hands and feet in Ellis-van Creveld syndrome (p 509). Usually ASD or single atrium may be associated.
- In coarctation of aorta, the upper part of the body may be better developed compared to the lower part.
- Distal radial anomalies may be seen in Holt-Oram syndrome. Usually secondum ASD is associated (see p 412, 570).
- Cleft palate has a 20% chance of having a heart disease.
- Other abnormalities to look for are thumb anomalies and dermatoglyphics.
- Absence of Depressor AnguliOris muscle is associated with VDS, TOF, ASD.

Note: The student must be flexible in scheme of examination of the child. Auscultation should have been done before any procedure likely to make the child cry, like examining femoral or taking BP. In the end, the student can organize the whole examination findings in a systematic manner (see p 4 for scheme of CVS examination).

Pulse

One must look for the rate, rhythm, volume, character, peripheral pulses and radiofemoral delay. It is recommended that the student make it a habit to palpate all the peripheral pulses routinely. Conventionally, the right radial pulse is palpated first. For palpating the femoral artery, keep the thigh slightly abducted. For palpating the popliteal, the child must be supine with both hands of examiner encircling the knee from either side. The knee must be in slight flexion. Examination of pulse is discussed in more detail in the next chapter (p 306).

In selected cases, palpation of carotids may be needed (e.g., hemiplegia in a heart disease patient). Carotid is palpated with the child supine, using the thumb, only one side at a time (palpation of both carotids together may compromise blood flow to the brain and patient may become unconscious).

Blood Pressure

Blood pressure is discussed in detail in the next chapter (p 308).

Jugular Venous Pressure (JVP)

Comment on jugular venous pulsations (normal wave pattern or not), jugular venous pressure (measured height), and hepatojugular reflux.

Pulsations must be looked for in right internal jugular vein. Look carefully at the lower neck, just lateral to the clavicular end of sternomastoid muscle. Higher up, it moves beneath and then medial to sternomastoid muscle. The waves can be timed with simultaneous gentle palpation of *the opposite* carotid. JVP appears as a flickering double wave: the first or "a" wave comes just before the carotid pulse; the second or "v" wave along with the carotid pulse. Pressure over the vein at the root of the neck will obliterate the JVP (see p 310).

"x" descent is due to descent of tricuspid valve ring. "c" is when the tricuspid closes with the beginning of ventricular systole. "v" is due to passive atrial filling from vena cava. "y" descent is when the tricuspid valve opens allowing the atrial blood to go into ventricle. Towards the end of diastole, the atria contracts, thus producing "a" wave again (see p 311 & Figs. 13.6, 13.7).

Large fused "cv" waves are seen in tricuspid regurgitation.

Engorged non-pulsatile JVP indicates superior vena cava obstruction. 12

JVP is discussed in detail in the next chapter, p 310.

INSPECTION

In actual practice, one does inspection and palpation together, but when presenting a case to the examiner, they are presented as per format. The various areas where inspection/palpation are to be done are apex, left sternal border, pulmonary area, aortic area, right sternal border, epigastrium and suprasternal areas. The back should also be looked for especially in patients with COA to look for collaterals. Precordium is the area on the anterior chest wall overlying the heart.

Shape of Precordium

One may look for sulcus, precordial prominence, pulsations, bony deformities indrawings, etc.

Harrison's sulcus may be seen with outward flaring of inferior rib cage. Constant tachypnoea of cardiac failure may cause this sulcus to develop due to the pull of diaphragm.

Apical impulse and other Visible Pulsations

Apical impulse if visible should be described in relation to the nipple and may not always correspond to the apex palpated.

Special attention must be directed to the neck, second space on left side, parasternal area, epigastrium, neck, etc. Subtle precordial pulsations are common in ASD.

Dilated cardiomyopathy is probably the only one condition where there is huge cardiomegaly but no significant precordial pulsations.

Causes of Visible Pulsations

- Suprasternal pulsations: Hyperdynamic states, aortic regurgitation, coarctation of aorta.
- 2nd left space pulsations: Pulmonary hypertension, idiopathic dilatation of pulmonary artery, etc. May be seen in a thin child without any cardiac disease.
- Epigastric pulsations: Right ventricular hypertrophy, hepatic pulsations or aortic pulsations.
- Hepatic pulsations: Tricuspid regurgitation/ stenosis.

Dilated Vessels

In coarctation of aorta, dilated vessels may be seen in the interscapular and infrascapular areas in the back, with the child bending forwards. These vessels may at times show thrills and murmurs. In SVC obstruction dilated veins may be seen over the lateral chest wall (flow directed downwards), prominent neck veins with non-pulsatile raised JVP.

Surgical Scars

Median sternotomy scars indicate open heart surgeries. Lateral thoracotomy scars may be because of shunt surgeries, PDA ligation or coarctation repair.

PALPATION

Apex

Apex beat is the *lowermost and outermost* point in the precordium where a *definite* cardiac impulse is felt. Determine the site, character and presence or absence of thrill over the apex. First, the whole palm is placed over the precordium and then the exact point of apex beat is located using a single finger.

Note the space at which the apex is located and its position in relation to the midclavicular line, nature of apex beat, thrill, etc. The spaces are counted from the angle of Louis or sternal angle (the prominent ridge at the junction of manubrium and body of sternum). The midclavicular line is drawn midway between the medial end of clavicle and the tip of acromion. Anterior axillary line, midaxillary line and posterior axillary line are drawn from anterior axillary fold, apex of axilla and posterior axillary fold, respectively.

The apex is normally located ½–1 cm inside the left midclavicular line in the fifth space, on the left side (up to 2 years of age, the normal apex may be in the 4th space in midclavicular line). After 4–5 years, apex assumes the adult location. The apex is examined in the supine position. If it is difficult to locate, it may be under a rib. Subtle or impalpable apex may also be because of pericardial effusion, myocarditis, emphysema, obesity, etc. If the apex is not palpable in the conventional position, try the left lateral position or sitting up position to see if the apex can be palpable (if apex is located in such non-conventional positions, that fact must be mentioned when presenting the case to the examiner; e.g., apex in the 5th space in the left lateral position). In left lateral decubitus position, apex may be shifted about 1 cm laterally. If the apex is not palpable even in left lateral position, do not forget the possibility of dextrocardia.

During isovolumic systole, when the LV contracts the apex moves counterclock-wise and makes contact with chest wall. As the aortic valve opens (rapid ejection), the LV begins to move away from chest wall. Thus, the apex is normally felt during isovolumic systole and first half of ejection; the peak impulse felt at or just after aortic valve opening and start of ejection. During the latter half of systole, the apex retracts as LV size rapidly decreases. The normal apical impulse is:

- Gentle, non-sustained (lasts less than 1/3rd of systole).
- Felt only during the first 1/3rd of systole.
- Palpable in only one intercostal space and is <2.5 cm^2 in area.
- The adult position of the apex is reached only by mid childhood (4–5 years of age).

LV Apex vs RV Apex

Normally, the apex is occupied by the left ventricle (LV) and abnormal palpable impulse at apex is usually caused by pathology of LV. In some cases, the right ventricle (RV) occupies the apical area and produces what is known as RV apex. This occurs in RV volume overloaded (e.g., ASD) or pressure-overloaded (e.g., pulmonary arterial hypertension, severe PS) states.

Normally, RV impulse is not felt because of its low pressure. In systole as LV moves counterclockwise, RV moves away and hence normal RV movement is retraction during systole. Even when it is palpable in abnormal conditions the retraction pattern persists. The amplitude of left parasternal pulsations increases in both RV volume and pressure-overloaded states but in pressure-overloaded states the impulse is more sustained.

Both the RV impulse and the LV impulse can be palpable in situations like ASD with MR, VSD with hyperkinetic PAH, etc; here, the apex and left sternal border should be simultaneously palpated. The two pulsations are felt separately with a "normal area" in between the two.

Types of LV Apex

Sustained

Here, the amplitude and duration of the impulse is increased; i.e., outward movement persists through second half of systole. It is seen in:

- Pressure-overloaded states like aortic stenosis.
- Volume-overloaded states with LV dysfunction like late stages of severe MR (where LV ejection takes longer time).

In the former, the apex is not displaced (no cardiac enlargement only concentric hypertrophy), whereas in the latter it is displaced (cardiac enlargement is present).

In AS, the examining finger is elevated and the elevation is sustained for a short period of time (hence called ***heaving*** apex). When the LV is contracting against an obstruction as in AS or severe systemic hypertension, it takes longer time to expel its contents and hence the examining finger at apex experiences sustained elevation. Pumping against obstruction generally leads on to concentric hypertrophy without much dilatation.

12

Hyperkinetic

The amplitude of pulsations is increased but normal contour is maintained (i.e., early systolic outward and late systolic inward motion is preserved). Thus, this apical impulse is forceful but without any increase in duration (hence also called ***forceful*** apex). This type of apex is seen in volume-overloaded states. Examples are left-to-right shunts (VSD, PDA) and regurgitant lesions (AR, MR). Hyperdynamic apical impulse is more diffuse than the heaving apex, and may occupy more than one intercostal space (normal and the heaving apical impulses occupy only one intercostal space).

Double apex may be seen in hypertrophic cardiomyopathy. The doubleness is due to the impulse of atrial systole contributing to the LV filling during diastole.

Non-cardiac causes for shift of apex: Pectus excavatum, scoliosis, etc, can displace a normal cardiac apex. Pulmonary pathologies like collapse or pleural effusion will also shift the apex.

Left Parasternal Heave

Place the ulnar border of hand over the sternum at 4–5th ribs and watch the extended fingers of that hand, which act as a lever to magnify any subtle movement. Pulsations here may also be because of systolic expansion of a large left atrium (as in MR) causing anterior displacement of RV; however, only a pulsation rather than a lift (heave) is expected in this situation (it's felt but no lift!). In addition, it is late systolic in timing and is out of synchrony with LV apex when they are palpated together. Parasternal pulsations are obliterable with the examining hand, whereas in case of parasternal heave, the examining hand gets lifted up. There is no standard grading of left parasternal activity. But if one is to grade the parasternal activity, one may divide it into three. (i) Pulsations are felt but no lift; (ii) Pulsations are felt and there is a lift, but the lift is easily obliterated by slight pressure of hand; (iii) Even with such a pressure applied by the hand, the hand is still seen to be moving up and down (this is true parasternal heave).

Parasternal lift along with epigastric pulsations are invariably due to right ventricular hypertrophy.

Suprasternal pulsations may be normally seen in a few normal children; also may be seen in fever, exercise, anaemia, etc.

Pulsations without a lift along the right sternal edge is characteristic of a large right Atrium as in Ebstein Anomaly.

Epigastric Pulsations

- These are usually due to right ventricular hypertrophy, especially when associated with parasternal lift. Palpate with thumb (or with middle and index finger) just left of xiphoid process to feel the pulsations (normally no more than a faint impulse will be there).
- Hepatic pulsations of TR or TS may be appreciated in the epigastrium. Hepatic pulsations are easier to differentiate from others as the pulsations usually are continuous with that in the hypochondrium.
- In a thin nervous child, the pulsations of the abdominal aorta may be visible in the epigastrium and a little down. Placing a hand flat against the epigastrium with fingers insinuated upward into the subxiphoid region helps to differentiate it from RV impulse. If the pulsations are felt on the fingertips (i.e., from above), it is RV and if it is felt on the palmar side of fingers (i.e., from below) it is aortic.

Thrills

Thrills are palpable vibrations of murmurs. Palpate for thrills with the hypothenar eminence over all the conventional areas and also over the carotids, below the clavicle and the back. The timing and site of maximum palpability of the thrill must be mentioned (students may note that it is always less time consuming and more accurate to time the corresponding murmur and extrapolate that timing to the thrill!). Thrill of AS is best felt in sitting-up, leaning forward position; many a time in carotids as well. Thrill of MS is best appreciated in the left lateral position. VSD, MR and PDA are the other lesions likely to be associated with a thrill.

Other Palpable Sounds

Loud first sound of MS may become palpable as a tapping apex. P_2 may be palpable in pulmonary hypertension. Still rarely opening snap, S_3, S_4, ejection clicks, pericardial rub, etc, may become palpable. Palpate b/l carotids, b/l supraclavicular areas.

Palpation of Base of Heart

This is done with the child sitting up and preferably leaning forward. Place the whole palm transversely covering both aortic and pulmonary areas. Pulsation, thrill and palpable sounds may be looked for. Pulsations in aortic area may be due to aneurysm in adults, or thrill due to aortic stenosis. Palpable pulsations and palpable second sound may be seen in pulmonary area in pulmonary hypertension.

The pulsations felt in the pulmonary area can be due to dilated pulmonary artery or palpable P_2. In children without underlying cardiac diseases, PA pulsations are often felt because of thin chest wall. Abnormal pulsations are seen in:

- Enlarged PA:
  - Idiopathic dilatation of pulmonary artery (IDPA)
  - PS with post-stenotic dilatation
- Increased pulmonary blood flow:
  - ASD
  - VSD
- PAH:
  - MS
  - Eisenmenger

Pulsations due to PAH are more sustained and forceful, whereas pulsations in other conditions are quick and less sustained.

Mention must be made as to whether the second sound is palpable.

Palpation of Suprasternal Notch

One finger may be hooked into the suprasternal notch to look for pulsations. Pulsations may be felt if the aorta is dilated (in adults aortic aneurysm).

In children, coarctation with post stenotic dilatation and dilated aorta of PDA are the causes for pulsations in the suprasternal notch.

PERCUSSION

Cardiac percussion is actually a waste of time, except on rare occasions like pericardial effusion and dilated cardiomyopathy. However, it is important that it forms part of case presentation in examination.

Locate the upper border of liver dullness by percussion.

Cardiac borders (use light percussion only, e.g., flicking percussion): Locate the left followed by the right border. Percussion is done usually with pleximeter fingers parallel to the expected cardiac borders, starting from the resonant areas and moving towards the cardiac borders.

Percuss the pulmonary area and determine whether it is resonant or dull. Area of dullness in normal adult is 2.5 cm from the midline or less. There are no paediatric standards. A dilated pulmonary artery, mediastinal mass, pericardial effusion, etc, can produce dull second space.

Quick CVS examination before proceeding to auscultation: The following guide to quick assessment may help the student when time is short.

- Quick history: Dyspnoea, cyanosis, oedema, squatting episodes, joint symptoms
- Look for clubbing and cyanosis
- Look at the JVP
- Palpate the radial and femoral pulse
- Palpate the liver
- Palpate the apex, parasternal area and pulmonary area

AUSCULTATION

The diaphragm of stethoscope is used for auscultation most of the time. Bell may be useful in case of mitral stenosis. However, opening snap of MS is better heard with the diaphragm. Sometimes, S_3 and low-pitched murmurs are better made out with bell.

Usual Areas Auscultated

- **Mitral area**: Auscultate over the apex. Auscultate just inside the apex also because opening snap, etc, are better picked up here. Look for conduction of murmur; MR murmur is well conducted to the axilla (see p 300).
- **Tricuspid area**: Lower left sternal border.
- **Pulmonary area**: Second left space close to the sternum.
- **Aortic area**: Second right space close to the sternum. Murmur of AR is best heard with the patient sitting up, leaning forward and breath held in expiration. AS murmur being very loud will be picked up even otherwise. AS murmur may transmit along the carotids and to the apex.

- **Second aortic area**: Third left interspace close to the sternum.
- **Third and fourth space** close to the sternum: VSD murmurs are loudest here. A point of practical importance is that VSD murmur appears to be radiating to the right of sternum. PDA murmur, PR and AR murmurs may transmit down parasternally.
- **Below the clavicle** (left first intercostal space): PDA, venous hum, etc, are better made out here. Venous hum is well heard when the head is turned to left.
- **Carotids**: Here, the auscultation is mainly for bruits as in AS. AS is quite rare in a child, but AR, because of increased flow across the aortic valve produces a "functional or relative" stenosis of aortic valve and hence bruits may be heard.
- **Interscapular and infrascapular** areas may be auscultated for the murmurs of coarctation and collateral murmurs, respectively.
- **Axilla** may be auscultated, especially in MR to look for conduction of murmur.

Auscultation may be done as follows not to miss cardiac events of non conventional areas as well. Start with apex → midway between apex and lower left sternal border (Still's murmur is best heard here) → lower left sternal border → up the left sternal border, space by space (VSD murmur best heard in 3rd & 4th space) → 2nd left space → left infraclavicular area (PDA murmur is best heard here) → neck → move right to upper sternum and right infraclavicular area (venous hum is best heard here) → down to right second space → down to right sternal border (VSD murmurs are well heard here, as they are L to R shunts towards the right of border of sternum). Then auscultate the axilla and the back.

Dynamic Auscultation

Some of the methods of dynamic auscultations are listed below.

- Recumbent and standing; squatting and standing (in MVP)
- Inspiration and expiration
- Left lateral supine and sitting plus leaning forward
- At rest and after exercise
- Valsalva manoeuvre (forced expiration against closed glottis)
- Isometric handgrip

Right-sided cardiac events are better heard in inspiration and the left-sided ones are better heard in expiration (rare exception to this rule does exist, refer to ejection clicks in next chapter, p 319). Venous hum disappears if the patient is made to lie supine. MS murmur, which is not obvious, can be made out if examined after mild exertion. HOCM murmur is decreased with squat and hence this manoeuvre is used to differentiate between murmurs of AS and HOCM. Rheumatic MR and VSD murmurs are increased with isometric handgrip. MR murmur increases with squatting. It is because squatting increases the peripheral resistance so that it is more difficult to negotiate blood into the aorta, resulting in more blood being leaked into the left atrium.

The click and murmur of MVP becomes more obvious when the patient is standing up. It is easy to understand if we consider the mitral valve as a bit oversized for its opening: when supine the venous return is more, so the heart is relatively dilated to accommodate this blood and the valve perfectly fits in with the mitral opening. When standing up, there is some peripheral pooling so that the venous return is a bit less, and the heart is slightly smaller. So as the valve (which is now relatively larger for the orifice) closes the mitral orifice, it prolapses into the left atrium to produce the click and murmur. The sudden snatch of the slack chordae when the valve is prolapsed possibly produces the click. Other measures that decreases the end-diastolic volume of LV also produces the same effect (e.g., amyl nitrite, deep inspiration, etc).

Auscultation after exertion will bring out faint murmurs of MS. Exertion will also increase the intensity of innocent murmur heard at upper sternal border, due to increased flow across the aortic and pulmonary valves.

Drugs: Phenylephrine increases the systemic vascular resistance & BP and hence murmurs of MR, VSD, etc, increase. Amyl nitrite inhalation produces peripheral vasodilatation and hence a fall in BP, and decrease in venous return.

HEART SOUNDS

First Heart Sound (low pitched lubb)

Assess the first sound at apex. It can be normal, loud or soft. With experience, finding out which sound is the first comes naturally to the student; S_1–S_2 duration is shorter (systole) compared to S_2–S_1 duration (diastole) and getting used to this rhythm helps. But the beginner may better time it with the carotid. S_1 is produced by the closure of mitral and tricuspid valves (**Note**: Opening of valves are quiet events, producing no sounds). Conditions producing split first sound are so rare that if S_1 appears split, it is likely to be due to an additional sound like a click (or S_4 which is still rarer). Since the first heart sound is due to the closure of mitral and tricuspid valves, it is best assessed at the apex and tricuspid areas. It is best to ignore the second sound in these areas; it has to be assessed in the pulmonary and aortic areas only.

Loud S_1

Loud first sound is seen in fever, exercise, thyrotoxicosis and mitral stenosis. In mitral stenosis, because of the stenosed valve ventricular filling from the atria takes longer, keeps the mitral valve cusps open wide apart till the very end of diastole, thus resulting in a very forceful closure of the valve as the contraction of the left ventricle starts.

If there is associated mitral regurgitation along with MS, the S_1 becomes softer as the leaking valve does not support forceful approximation. MS with atrial fibrillation may have the loudness of S_1 preserved because despite the absence of effective atrial contraction, the retained blood in left atrium in case of mitral stenosis is quite large to produce sufficient gradient to keep on flowing to the left ventricle and hence to keep valve open till the very end of diastole.

Once you get the typical finding of mitral stenosis, expect to find the opening snap and evidence of pulmonary hypertension (so look for them carefully).

Loud S_1 is also expected in situations of shortened PR interval, Atrial myxoma, mechanical prosthetic valve. In tachycardia, diastole is shortened so that the flow of blood from the atria to ventricle proceeds till the very end of diastole and the valve remains open till the very end, causing forceful closure of the mitral valve and hence the loud first sound.

Soft S_1

In rheumatic fever where the PR interval is prolonged, the first sound is soft. Other types of AV blocks are also associated with soft S_1. Soft first sound is also expected in MR, myocarditis, dilated cardiomyopathy, calcified Mitral valve, shock, etc. Pericardial effusion and emphysematous lungs may impair conduction of heart sounds and hence S1 may appear soft.

Varying intensity of S_1 is expected in complete heart block. This is because the timing of the atrial and ventricular contractions are not inter related here. So, sometimes the atrial and ventricular contractions occur in close succession to produce loud first sound as the mitral valve starts closing even before the inflow from atria is completed. Varying intensity of S_1 is also likely in extrasystoles, MS with atrial fibrillation.

Split S1

Split S1 is seen in Ebstein anomaly, RBBB, large ASD, premature ventricular ectopics, severe PAH.

Second Heart Sound

The second sound must be assessed in the pulmonary area because it is the pulmonary component of S_2 that is most important clinically. P_2 is not to be assessed at apex. The second sound heard at the apex is more likely to represent A_2 because apex is part of LV, from which aorta originates. S_2 can be loud, attenuated or normal. It has two components, aortic and pulmonary, A_2 preceding P_2. If it appears widely split, it is vital to determine whether the split has the normal respiratory variations or is fixed. Normally, if we breathe out fully and stop breathing, the second sound appears single for 2–3 beats before the split becomes apparent again. This does not happen in wide fixed split of ASD. Conversely, if we breathe in fully, the venous return to heart increases, right ventricle takes longer to eject the extra blood, P_2 gets delayed so that A_2–P_2 distance increases, hence widening of second sound.

A_2 is louder than P_2 in adults (because the aortic valve closes under greater pressure) but in a child both can be of equal intensity normally, because of the proximity of the pulmonary artery to the thinner chest wall. S_2 will be loud in exercise and systemic hypertension because the valves closing under higher pressures produce louder sound. In TGA, the aorta is anterior to the pulmonary artery so that the aortic sound is conducted better to the chest wall, hence A_2 will be loud.

- Soft A_2 may be seen in valvar aortic stenosis.
- Loud A_2 may be seen in systemic hypertension.
- P_2 is soft in PS and TOF. It is nearly absent in pulmonary atresia.
- P_2 will be loud in pulmonary hypertension (likewise, A_2 will be loud in systemic hypertension). In lung diseases especially long-standing ones, pulmonary hypertension develops and hence P_2 can be loud. In children, P_2 may appear loud because of a thin chest wall (pulmonary artery is normally placed anterior to aorta).
- Fixed wide split of second sound: It is seen in ASD. The mechanism involved is discussed in the next chapter (see p 317).
- **Wide variable split of S_2**
  - In moderate VSDs, since part of the blood from the LV gets shunted to the RV, the LV systole gets shortened, aortic valve closes early and hence A_2 comes early. Since the RV gets extra blood shunted from the LV, it takes longer for the RV to complete its ejection, so that P_2 gets delayed. Thus, S_2 is widely split. Obviously, the split narrows with the development of PAH.
  - In MR also, S_2 can be widely split. The LV ejects part of the blood to the low pressure LA because of regurgitation, so that LV systole ends early to make A_2 come earlier. So S_2 is wide split.
  - In RBBB, the right ventricular systole is delayed due to delayed impulse transmission so that P_2 gets delayed, hence the S_2 is wide.
  - In PS, the RV takes longer to eject so that P_2 gets delayed and can produce wide split S_2. However, since the murmur of PS is rough and extends up to P_2, it masks the A_2 that comes before P_2. Hence, this predicted split of second sound is usually not useful clinically. In TOF, P_2 is hardly audible (pulmonary stenosis), the murmur is soft and short so that A_2 is clearly heard as a single S_2.
- **Single S_2 may be seen in**
  - Tetralogy of Fallot
  - Tricuspid atresia
  - TGA
  - Truncus arteriosus, etc (mnemonic: note that all are "T"s). In truncus arteriosus, there is only one semilunar valve and hence only one sound.

- Single S_2 may be because of subtle A_2 component (aortic stenosis) or subtle P_2 component (pulmonic stenosis in TOF).
- **Paradoxical splitting**: Normally, A_2 comes before P_2. If A_2 gets too delayed, it can come after P_2, the reversed split. It may occur in aortic stenosis. However, the P_2 that occurs earlier in such cases gets drowned in AS murmur, which extends to A_2. Systemic hypertension is another situation where one may get a reversed split. In LBBB, the A_2 gets delayed due to a delay in impulse transmission to LV. When it is delayed a bit, the sounds gets closer, but when it is very delayed A_2 gets delayed even beyond P_2 so that the split gets reversed, as P_2A_2. During inspiration P_2 gets delayed, thus moves closer to A_2 and hence S_2 appear single. During expiration, P_2 occurs earlier, hence S_2 appears split. Since this is opposite to what is expected normally, and hence it is called a paradoxical split. See hang out interval, p 315.

Important: Paradoxical split is usually not detectable by auscultation and hence the student should not commit to paradoxical splitting in a clinical examination.

S_3 and S_4

After assessing the first and second sounds, one must look for additional sounds like S_3, S_4, opening snap, clicks, pericardial rub, etc. S_3 is a ventricular distension sound and S_4 is an atrial contraction sound. They are discussed in detail in the next chapter (p 318). S_3 is best appreciated at apex.

For the beginner, if the second sound appears split at the apex, strongly suspect a third sound rather than a true split of second sound (split S_2 is expected to be heard at base of the heart, not at apex).

S_4 is very uncommon in a child. S_4 is due to atrial contraction against a non-compliant ventricle causing vibration of the ventricle and hence S4 is better felt (S4 is also called as Atrial sound as its production requires effective atrial contraction). Standing moves S_4 closer to S_1 (or it disappears). S_4 is seen in diastolic dysfunction (which forces atria to contract stronger), significant AS, etc. In practical sense, S_4 appears like a split S_1. It is clearly heard only at the apex in contrast to split first sound, which may be heard in other areas as well. In fact, a split S_1 is better appreciated at tricuspid area where a variation with respiration of the components of split S_1 may also be appreciable. It may appear ridiculous to think of picking up respiratory variation of split of S_1, but one who is good enough to pick up S_4 will pick up this as well! 12

Clicks

Normal valve openings are silent but abnormal valves may open with a click. Click in early systole is seen in valvular AS, PS, etc. Click of AS and PS are respectively heard in their corresponding areas and apex/left sternal border, respectively. Aortic ejection click may be heard at apex in addition to the upper sternal border (because aorta arises from the left ventricle and hence the sound is conducted well to the apex).

Ejection click of PS is better heard in expiration (yes, expiration) (see p 319). Absence of click in a pulmonary stenosis could mean that the stenosis is not at the valve, e.g., infundibular stenosis. Dilatation of aorta or pulmonary artery in systemic or pulmonary hypertension, respectively will also result in a click. Mid-systolic click (non-ejection click) is characteristic of MVP. Severe tetralogy of Fallot also may have a click from dilated aorta. Multiple clicks are seen (clustered around the second sound) in PDA.

Rule of thumb: Normally, S_1 is louder at the apex than the base. If S_1 appears to be louder at base then that sound is more likely to have been augmented by an ejection click. Also click is a sharper sound than S_1.

Pericardial Rub

This is a to and fro friction rub. It can have one, two or three components. Typically, it is triple phased, with mid-systole and mid and late diastole components. It is a scratchy/leathery sound produced by apposition of abnormal visceral and parietal pericardial surfaces. It can be augmented with firm stethoscope pressure and breath held in exhalation and the child leaning forward. Rub is better heard with the child sitting up and leaning forward (as it brings the anterior pericardial coverings in close proximity to the chest wall) with the stethoscope held over the left 2nd and 3rd intercostal spaces immediately to the left of the sternum. It is very often heard for only a short duration of time, disappears, and reappears—something that a student should keep in mind. Pericardial rub synchronizes with cardiac cycle (but may be systolic, diastolic or systolodiastolic) and continues to be audible after holding the breath (pleural rub is abolished by holding the breath). Pericardial rub is usually localized to a small area. It changes in site or character as time progresses.

When there is pleurisy of the anterior portion of pleura in contact with the heart, pleural rub may synchronize with cardiac cycle, as it is a pleuropericardial rub in reality. However, even this will be abolished by holding breath, thus helping to differentiate it from true pericardial rub.

Pericardial Knock

It is a common finding in constrictive pericarditis and is heard all over the precordium. It occurs in early diastole, just before S3. It is caused by sudden cessation of ventricular filling and may be augmented with inspiration.

Opening Snap

It is a high-pitched sharp sound in diastole, falling between S_2 and S_3 (only in timing; not that S_3 and opening snap will occur together, which is exceptionally rare). In a combined MS–MR lesion if the dominant lesion is MR, S_3 is heard but not the opening snap. Opening snap is best heard inside the apex rather than at the apex, using the diaphragm of the stethoscope.

Both the murmur of MS and the opening snap in MS are accentuated with exercise. Opening snap may not disappear even when there is atrial fibrillation. Do not diagnose opening snap if the first sound appears soft, you will almost invariably be wrong. Closer the opening snap to S_2, the tighter the MS.

Murmurs

If a murmur is detected, comment on its timing, intensity, character, area where it is best heard, its conduction, any associated thrill and changes with manoeuvres like exercise, posture, Valsalva's manoeuvre, etc. Auscultate for conduction of the murmur in axilla and carotids. Frankly, the conduction is not really true, most often it is only radiation even in MR. It is termed as conduction when it is heard with the same intensity at a different location and called radiation when it is heard with a slightly reduced intensity. Nowadays, the term conduction is not used; radiation is the current standard term.

Levine Grading scale of Intensity of Murmurs

- Grade I: Very faint, can be made out only on careful auscultation in a quiet room. It may take several beats to recognize this. Only picked up by the experienced.
- Grade II: Faint, but easily identified on examination.
- Grade III: Loud murmur without a thrill (when the murmur is more obvious than the heart sound, it may be taken as loud).
- Grade IV: Loud murmur with a thrill.
- Grade V: Very loud murmur heard even with one edge of stethoscope off the chest.
- Grade VI: So loud that the murmur can be heard even with the stethoscope fully taken off the chest wall.

This grading is primarily for systolic murmurs but the same can be used for diastolic murmurs also, but most authorities grade diastolic murmurs up to grade IV only. It makes no difference, because in that grading, the only difference is that grades V and VI of the above grading are taken off. Thus, diastolic murmurs can be graded as follows.

- Grade I: Very faint
- Grade II: Easily identified on examination
- Grade III: Loud murmur without a thrill
- Grade IV: Loud murmur with a thrill

For evaluation of a murmur, see p 321.

Character of Murmurs

- Rough and rumbling in MS
- Machinery or train-in-tunnel murmur in PDA
- Soft blowing in AR
- Sea gull murmur of rheumatic carditis
- Harsh grating murmur in AS
- Changing character of the murmur from day to day in infective endocarditis, and atrial myxoma.
- Higher pitched murmurs originate where the velocity of flow is high and lower pitched murmurs originate where the velocity of flow is less (e.g., MS).

Timing of Murmurs

- **Early systolic murmur**: It may be seen in very small muscular VSD where the defect practically closes as the contraction of ventricle proceeds. It may also be seen in VSD with pulmonary hypertension. Early ejection murmurs are likely with increased cardiac output situations like exercise, fever, thyrotoxicosis, etc. Here, rapid rate along with the high contractile force generated so rapidly by the ventricles leaves practically no time gap in between closure of atrioventricular valves and the opening of semilunar valves. Functional carotid murmurs also may be heard in situations of high output. *Carotid murmurs need not always indicate AS.* In VSD with pulmonary hypertension, the pansystolic murmur may start as expected but stops much earlier than S_2 because the pressure difference between the two ventricles becomes negligible soon after the onset of systole. Hence, there may be just an early systolic murmur. When the pulmonary hypertension further progresses, the murmur of VSD becomes still shorter and ultimately gets replaced by the ejection murmur of pulmonary hypertension.
- **Mid-systolic murmur** (crescendo-decrescendo or diamond shaped): This is otherwise called ejection systolic murmur. The murmur begins a little after S_1 and proceeds for a variable period of time through systole but never reaches the semilunar valve closure sound (A_2 or P_2). It is seen in AS, PS, etc. In AS, PS, etc, the pressure difference between the aorta and the left ventricle or pulmonary artery and the right ventricle progressively decreases as the systole progresses and hence the murmur stops short of S_2 to produce ejection systolic murmurs. At the start of systole, the mitral/tricuspid valves close to produce S_1. However, the murmur starts a bit later, when the pressure generated by the ventricular contraction exceeds that of the aorta or pulmonary artery. Hence the murmur starts after S_1 and not along with it. The murmur stops just before the semilunar valve closure and hence the murmur does not extend to S_2. Obviously, the valve can close only after the ventricular ejection is over. The murmur is diamond shaped in accordance with the pressure generation by the ventricles.
- **Late systolic murmur**: This is seen in mitral valve prolapse, because the valve prolapses late in systole. Late systolic murmur may *occasionally* be heard between the scapula in the back in coarctation of aorta. It is due to coarctation itself, and one may assume that the murmur is later in the systole because the murmur originates in the aorta in a region away from the heart. Please note that the most common murmur in CoA in this location is due to

12

collaterals and not a late systolic murmur. Murmur is late in peripheral pulmonary stenosis also because the blood reaches here late. Hypertrophic cardiomyopathy is the other condition where a late systolic murmur may be heard.

- **Holosystolic or pansystolic murmur**: Occupies the whole of systole (MR, TR, VSD).

  The pansystolic nature is most classical in VSD. In VSD, there is no valve and there is a pressure difference between the chambers throughout systole and hence the pressure difference between the chambers is free to be communicated throughout the systole. Hence, the murmur is pansystolic.

  In MR, throughout systole, there is a big pressure difference between the LV and LA and hence the murmur is pansystolic (the pressure difference between the LV and aorta is less and hence the LV finds it easier to eject longer into LA). MR murmur appears true pansystolic at apex as it drowns S_2 at the apex because the A_2 component of S_2 is the one heard at apex. Ventricular systole is over with the aortic valve closure and hence the murmur also stops. At the pulmonary area, the second sound may be heard in MR as the pulmonary valve closes later than the aortic valve normally and the murmur of MR stops with A_2. Thus, please note that even though the murmur of MR is pansystolic, P_2 may be well heard at pulmonary area.

  The students always have a confusion as to whether S_1 can be appreciated when there is a holosystolic murmur (as murmur covers the whole of systole, how can S_1 be differentiated). However, it is not true. The pitch of S_1 and murmur are different and hence although S_1 is drowned in the murmur, it may still be heard. Its like appreciating your friend's conversation in a background of big noises; it's difficult but possible.

  TR is usually part of pulmonary hypertension in children (hence one may look for it in conditions where pulmonary hypertension is expected, like MS). The systolic murmur is best heard at the lower sternal border and is louder with inspiration (these differentiate it from MR).

- **Early diastolic murmurs**: AR, PR. Clinical differentiation of the two is discussed in the next chapter (see p 322).
- **Mid-diastolic murmurs**: It is seen in MS. Flow murmurs of VSD, PDA, MR, etc, are mid-diastolic at apex. Carey Coombs murmur and Austin Flint murmur are also mid-diastolic. Carey Coombs murmur is thought to be due to oedematous unevenness of valve cusps. Carcy Coombs murmur of acute rheumatic fever is mid-diastolic, soft, low-pitched, apical murmur, which is transient. It is never associated with a thrill. In ASD, one may find a mid-diastolic rumble at tricuspid area indicating increased flow across that valve. It increases with inspiration and also by raising the leg of supine patient; both procedures increasing the venous return (also see p 322).
- **Late diastolic murmur**: Also called presystolic murmur. Example is MS (it is usually mid-diastolic murmur peaking at late diastole).

  Note: The term pan diastolic murmur is never used.

- **Continuous murmur**: It is seen in PDA, AV fistula, venous hum, etc. It is discussed in detail in the next chapter (see p 323).
- **Multiple murmurs**: When two different murmurs are heard, it is important to decide whether they are the same murmur or different ones. Here, one may look at the character of the murmur auscultating inch by inch from one area to the other other (inching technique) determining whether the intensity changes gradually to that of the next area or a different murmur picks up in intensity. Also one may note the character, which if different strongly argues for two different murmurs rather than a single one. Also keep in mind the fact that some murmurs are well heard in more than one area; e.g., AS murmur at upper sternal

THE CARDIAC CYCLE: EVENTS

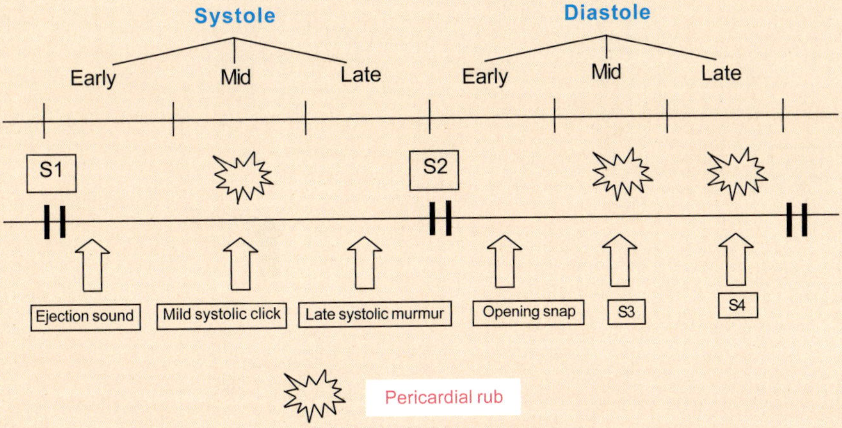

Aortic Stenosis

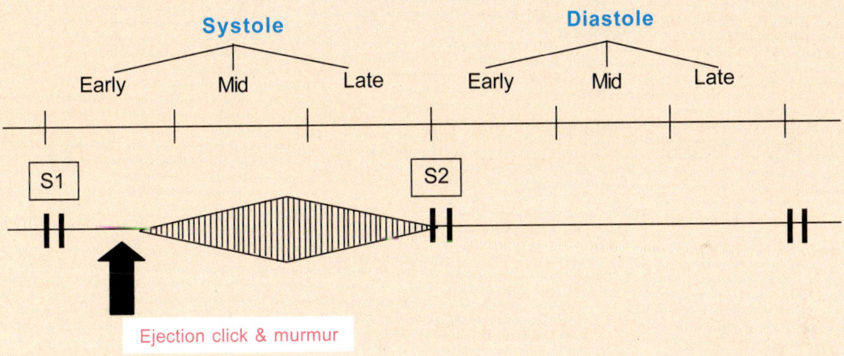

Aortic Regurgitation

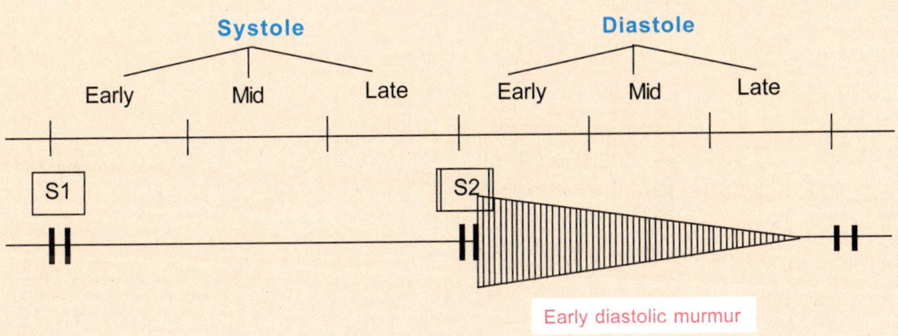

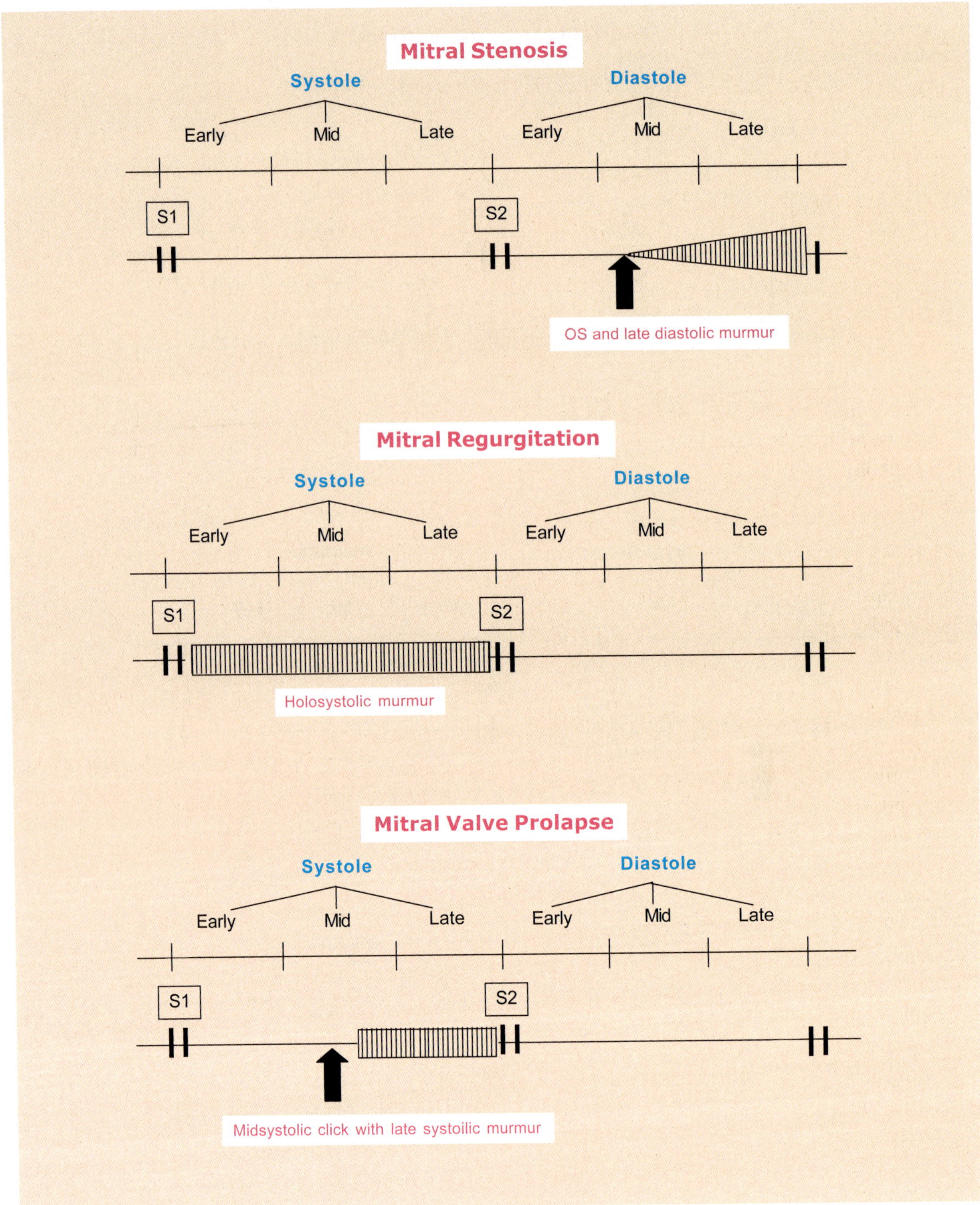
Mitral Stenosis
Systole
Diastole
Early
Mid
Late
Early
Mid
Late
S1
S2
OS and late diastolic murmur
Mitral Regurgitation
Systole
Diastole
Early
Mid
Late
Early
Mid
Late
S1
S2
Holosystolic murmur
Mitral Valve Prolapse
Systole
Diastole
Early
Mid
Late
Early
Mid
Late
S1
S2
Midsystolic click with late systoilic murmur

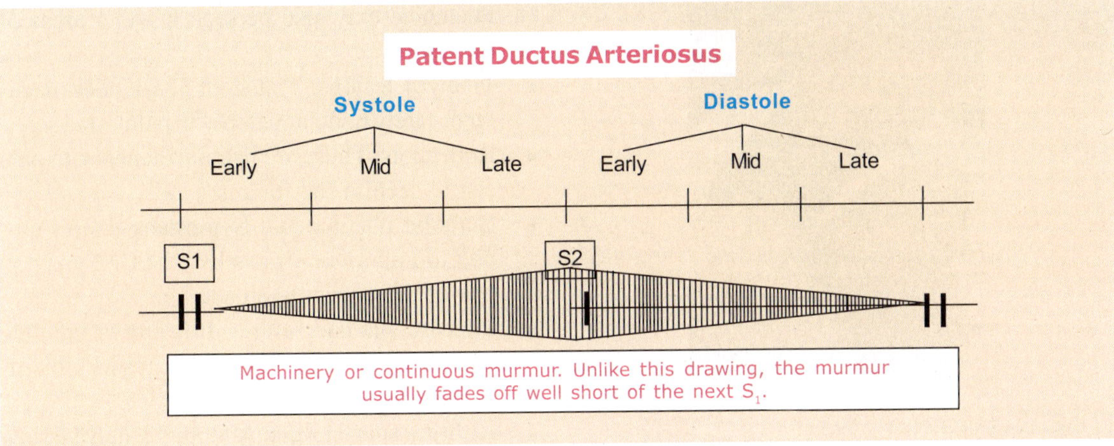

border and apex. Also note that AS murmur can be of slightly different quality at apex, less rough compared to that at upper sternal border.

PERIPHERAL SIGNS IN AR

- Collapsing pulse: Method of elicitation is discussed in the next chapter (p 306).
- Dancing brachials: Visible pulsations of brachials.
- Lighthouse sign: Flushing of forehead with each cardiac cycle.
- Capillary pulsation on tongue (demonstrated by pressing with a glass slide).
- Muller's sign: Uvular pulsation.
- Becker's sign: Retinal arterial pulsations on fundus examination.
- Landolffe's sign: Dilatation and contraction of pupils.
- Corrigan's sign: Prominent carotid pulsations seen in the neck, dancing carotids. It may become severe enough to cause head nodding with each systole (Alfred de Musset's sign).
- Hill's sign: The blood pressure difference between the upper and lower limbs is more than 20 mmHg (see p 348).
- Duroziez murmur: This is the diastolic murmur heard on distal compression of the artery (tested in femoral usually). It is usually a sign of very florid AR and rarely, if ever, found in children with rheumatic heart disease. A systolic murmur may be heard on proximal compression but it is non-specific.
- Pistol shot sounds: It is heard with the stethoscope over the arteries like the brachial and femoral in cases of significant AR. It is due to the sudden distention of the vessel. Sometimes referred to as Traube's sign.
- Quincke sign: Capillary pulsations of the nail bed. Gentle pressure at the tip of nail to blanch it partially will show pulsations of the edge of blood column seen through the nail. Gentle compression of mucous membrane of lip with a glass slide also will help to elicit the pulsations.
- Hepatic pulsations (Rosenbach's sign); splenic pulsation (Gerhardt's sign).

SIGNS IN INFECTIVE ENDOCARDITIS

- Prolonged fever
- New cardiac murmurs
- Cardiac failure: It is possibly due to the valvular lesion but may also be due to the toxic effects of persistent infection.
- Clubbing: It used to be common in the preantibiotic era. Since it takes time for clubbing to develop (average about 6 weeks), it is not seen if the endocarditis is detected and treated early.

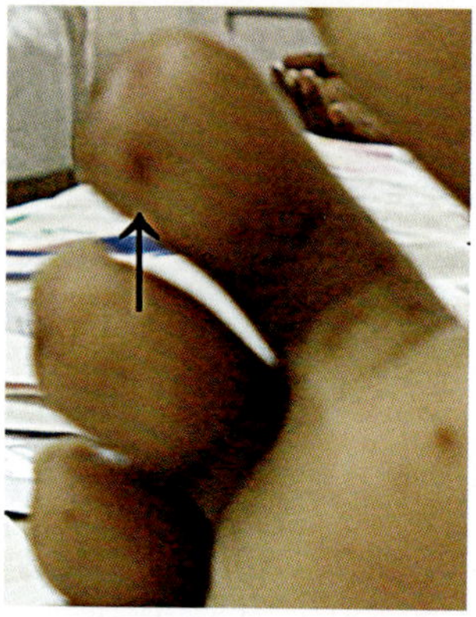

Fig.12.1 Osler's nodes

- Splenomegaly
- Osler's nodes: Tender nodules in the pulp of fingers and toes.
- Splinter haemorrhages: It is seen in fingernails (Fig. 6.114, p 124). It may be seen in arteritis of various aetiologies. Frankly the most common reason for this lesion is local trauma! Petechiae may also be seen in other areas of the body.
- Janeway lesions: Transient non-tender macular or rarely nodular patches in palms and soles.
- Roth spots: These are haemorrhages with pale centre seen in the fundus.
- Embolic phenomena: Symptoms due to emboli to important organs like the CNS may be one of the presentations.
- Microscopic haematuria: It is due to immune complex-mediated focal or diffuse glomerulonephritis.
- Arthritis or arthralgia: Although it may be seen in endocarditis its presence is more characteristic of rheumatic fever rather than endocarditis.
- Weight loss, fatigue, etc, are due to the prolonged nature of the illness and are not specific for endocarditis.

CHAPTER 13

Cardiovascular System : Part–II

PULSE

Look for the Pulse Rate, Rhythm, Volume, Character, Radio-Femoral delay, distal pulsations, pulse deficit, vessel wall thickness (familial hyperlipidemia, progeria syndrome).

Pulse Rate

Pulse rate is counted for 1 min by palpating the radial artery.

Bradycardia

Bradycardia (sinus bradycardia) may be normal in sleep and in highly trained athletes (high vagal tone in athletes).

Pathological bradycardia may be seen in:

- Hypothyroidism
- Hypothermia
- Obstructive jaundice
- Raised intracranial tension
- Heart blocks
- Drug toxicity (propranolol, digoxin, etc)

Tachycardia

Physiologically, tachycardia is expected during exertion, emotion, etc.

Pathological tachycardia may be seen in:

- Shock
- High-output states like fever, anaemia, hyperthyroidism, beriberi, etc.
- Tachyarrhythmias like supraventricular tachycardia (SVT).
- Drugs (thyroxine, nifedipine, atropine, catecholamines like adrenaline, etc).

Pulse deficit: When the pulse rate does not match the heart rate, there is a pulse deficit. Ideally, the pulse and heart rate are to be counted simultaneously for 1 min; obviously it needs an assistant for help. Pulse deficit may be seen in atrial fibrillation and in certain ectopic beats, usually ventricular prema-ture beats. Presence of "a" wave in JVP helps to differentiate ventricular premature beats from atrial fibrillation. In atrial fibrillation, a pulse deficit of >10 is expected.

Rhythm of Pulse

Rhythm (regularity of the pulse) is assessed by palpating the radial artery.

Irregularity of Pulse

The most common cause in a child is ***sinus arrhythmia***. It is the irregularity timed with phases of respiration, accelerating during inspiration and decelerating during expiration.

Regularly irregular pulse may be seen in certain ectopic focus of impulse generation. Ventricular bigemini is an example.

Irregularly irregular pulse is seen in atrial fibrillation. Look for a pulse deficit in such a situation.

Volume and Character of Pulse

Volume of pulse depends on the pulse pressure (i.e., the difference between the systolic and diastolic BP). Normal pulse pressure is about 30–40 mmHg. Higher the pulse pressure, higher the "volume" of pulse.

High-volume pulse (bounding pulse) may be seen in anxiety, after exercise, fever, anaemia, hyperthyroidism, AV fistula, etc (due to increased stroke volume and hence a higher systolic pressure plus or minus decreased peripheral vascular resistance, which brings down the diastolic pressure). Among structural heart diseases, high volume pulse is seen in PDA and AR. The pulse may appear bounding in early septic shock (warm shock), due to peripheral vasodilatation (here there is a fall in diastolic BP and hence a wider pulse pressure). This is not a happy sign at all in sepsis and hence must be detected and treated promptly; otherwise, systolic BP will also fall with catastrophic consequences.

Note: One should not have the impression that the pulse pressure will be wide in all shocks. It depends. For example, in hypovolaemic shock the peripheral vessels constrict to preserve BP, so that the pulse pressure will be narrow due to the elevated peripheral vascular resistance.

In advanced status asthmaticus, the pulse may appear bounding with warm extremities, due to the vasodilator properties of retained CO_2.

Difference in pulse volume between the upper and lower limbs may be seen in coarctation of aorta. Difference in pulse volume between the left and right upper limbs may also be seen rarely in coarctation of aorta (diminished left upper limb pulse is seen when coarctation is at or proximal to left subclavian artery).

Water hammer pulse (Collapsing or Corrigan's pulse): This can occur in conditions producing a bounding pulse, and is classically seen in AR and PDA. Also seen in A-P Window, AV Fistula, RSOV. Water hammer is a toy of sealed glass tube containing water and vacuum. On inversion, the water drops through the vacuum to give a thud. The patient's forearm is gripped using the examiner's left palm with sufficient pressure so that the pulse is just palpable. While this pressure is kept exactly the same, the patient's arm is lifted using the examiner's right hand when a thud will be felt if the pulse is "water hammer."

Low volume pulse (or low amplitude pulse or **pulsus parvus**) is seen when the pulse pressure is narrow, like CCF, shock, severe AS or coarctation of aorta, severe mitral stenosis, etc. In mitral stenosis, the volume of blood that reaches left ventricle is less due to the stenosed mitral valve and hence the output from left ventricle decreases and hence the low pulse volume. Small volume pulse with tachycardia is termed as thready pulse (seen in shock).

Character of pulse describes the pulse waveform. Some information on the waveform of pulse may be obtainable by palpation of carotids, as it is closest to the heart and the waveform is not dampened by multiple branching (Fig. 13.1). Frankly no clinically useful information on the waveform can be made out by palpation.

Arterial Pulse Wave

The palpable arterial pulse is the pressure pulse transmitted along the arterial system when the blood is ejected by the LV into the proximal aorta. The pulse wave is faster (5 m/sec) than the actual movement of blood (50 cm/sec) along the arterial tree.

The normal arterial pulse consists of two positive waves in systole.

- Percussion wave, due to the rapid upstroke.
- Tidal wave due to reflected waves from aortic bifurcation.

The end of systole is indicated by a sharp notch, the dicrotic notch, which is then followed by a small positive wave, the dicrotic wave. The dicrotic notch corresponds to closure of aortic valve. Figure 13.1 shows a normal arterial pulse.

- **Pulsus tardus**: A slow rising low volume pulse characterized by late peaking, close to S2 is seen in AS (pulsus tardus), because the left ventricle takes a much longer time to push the blood through the stenosed valve.

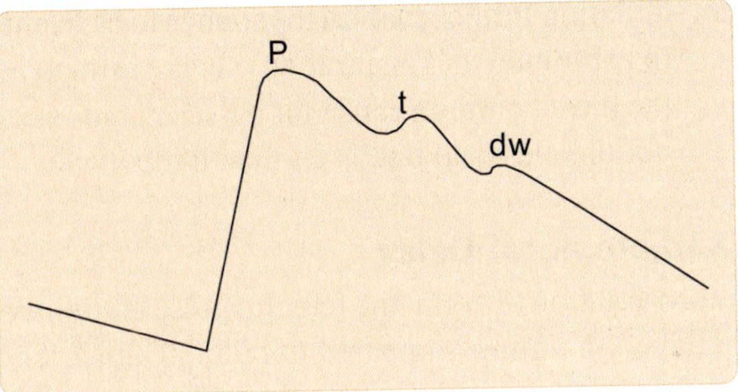

Fig.13.1 Normal arterial pulse

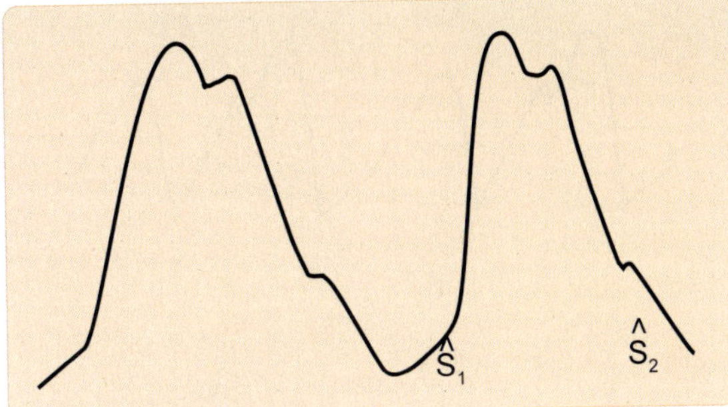

Fig.13.2 Pulsus bisferiens

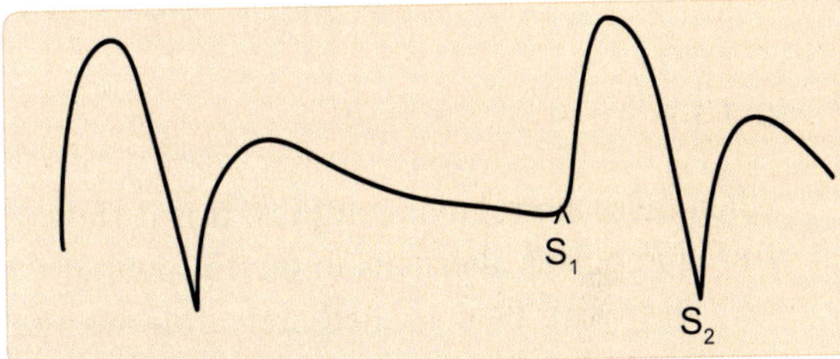

Fig.13.3 Dicrotic pulse

- **Pulsus bisferiens** or double-peak pulse may be seen in hypertrophic cardiomyopathy. It has two peaks, *both in systole* (percussion and tidal waves). In HOCM, initially there is no obstruction to left ventricular outflow, then there is obstruction as the hypertrophied septum comes in the way of the outflow and later it is somewhat overcome. Severe AR, combined AR/AS with predominant AR are other situations where a similar pulse may be seen as in Fig. 13.2.
- **Dicrotic pulse**: Here also two peaks are present, but one is in systole and the other is in diastole. It occurs in conditions with high peripheral vascular resistance and low cardiac output as in severe cardiac failure (cardiomyopathy, myocarditis, etc) or cardiac tamponade (Fig. 13.3). The dicrotic wave in diastole is the result of reflected waves from aorta and its branches.
- **Anacrotic pulse**: It is a low volume pulse with slow systolic upstroke. So here the second impulse occurs in the anacrotic upstroke much before the start of tidal wave.
- **Jerky pulse** may be seen in severe MR. There is LV overload, which the LV ejects at the beginning of systole. After sometime as the aortic pressure builds up, it becomes easier for the blood to go to the low pressure area of the left atrium through the regurgitant jet. Hence, the flow to the aorta is rapidly reduced. The initial high volume giving way to sudden cessation gives the feel of jerkiness. Jerky pulse may also be seen in hypertrophic cardiomyopathy, because of the sudden cut-off of forward flow by the hypertrophied septum. *Important*: Jerky pulse is a terminology of yesteryears. Most standard textbooks of today do not discuss the entity "jerky pulse" and hence the student should not commit "jerky pulse" as a clinical finding in the clinical examination scenario, unless specifically asked for.
- **Pulsus alternans**: This denotes alternating large and small volume beats in *regular rhythm*. It may be seen in severe LV dysfunction where there are alternating strong and weak beats, which are regularly spaced. In case it is doubted, during measurement of BP, deflate the cuff very slowly to look for sudden doubling of Korotkoff's sounds when deflated a few mm below systolic BP (Fig. 13.4a).
- **Pulsus bigeminus**: Here also weaker and stronger beats alternate (Fig. 13.4b). It is seen

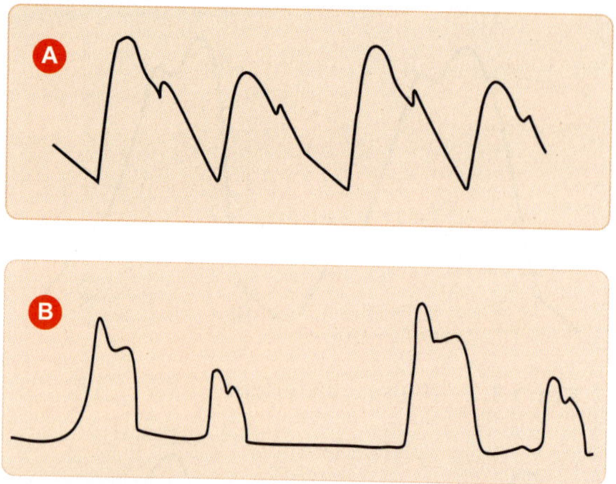

Fig.13.4 Pulsus alternans

when there are regular ectopics. It is different from the pulsus alternans in the following:

- The weak beat immediately follows the strong beat.
- There is a gap between the weak beat and next strong beat (this compensatory pause is absent in pulsus alternans).

- **Pulsus Trigeminus**: Coupling of 3 beats because of ectopic ventricular premature beats occurring regularly after 2 normal beats.
- **Pulsus paradoxus**: Normally systolic BP (and hence the pulse volume) falls during inspiration, but never more than 10 mmHg (usual fall is 5 mmHg or less). This is because during inspiration the lung capacity increases, pooling very large quantities of blood in the lung, thus reducing venous return to the left side of heart and hence less blood is pumped out to the systemic circulation and hence the fall in BP. When the fall exceeds 10 mmHg, it is termed pulsus paradoxus. Thus, it is an exaggeration of normal fall. This can be documented using BP apparatus, but to a trained hand excessive fall in pulse volume can be appreciated by examining the pulse itself. BP cuff is inflated well above the expected systolic BP and then slowly deflated. First, the Korotkoff's sounds are heard only during expiration. Slow deflation further enables the sounds to be heard in expiration and inspiration. Severe asthma is the most common cause for pulsus paradoxus, but the classical one is cardiac tamponade.

Radiofemoral Delay

In coarctation of aorta, the femoral pulse is slightly delayed in timing compared to radial. Both arteries are to be palpated simultaneously keeping radial and femoral artery side by side to appreciate this. Some authorities look for brachiofemoral delay.

Notes

- In combined lesions, the pulse differs according to the severity of individual lesions.
- Always correlate the pulse with clinical condition, e.g., CHF is associated with tachycardia most of the time; if slow heart rate is associated with features of CHF suspect a bradyarrhythmia like congenital heart block as the cause of CHF.
- Always evaluate all the peripheral pulses if relevant, especially the femoral, even if it requires sedation in a younger child. Missing an absent femoral may prove fatal for an examination candidate!

BLOOD PRESSURE

If there is difficulty to record BP by auscultation (e.g., shock), palpatory method may be used. Earlier the muffling of sounds (phase IV of Korotkoff) used to be taken as the diastolic BP but presently the disappearance of sounds (phase V) is recommended to be accepted as the diastolic pressure at all ages. However, in certain situations like AR, the Korotkoff sounds may be heard right up to the zero mark. In such situations, muffling of Korotkoff sounds may be taken as the diastolic BP. If Korotkoff sounds are difficult to make out, tie the BP cuff and then keep the limb elevated for a few seconds; then inflate the BP cuff with hand elevated, then bring it down and proceed with BP recording.

This procedure may also help in avoiding "auscultatory gap." As one deflates the BP cuff, Korotkoff sounds appear, then they disappears only to reappear again – this gap being termed as auscultatory gap. May be when BP cuff is deflated a little, Korotkoff sounds appear as blood is allowed to flow through artery, but soon the pressure difference gets reduced due to retained venous blood, which is not yet draining (increased distal resistance due to inflated BP cuff). When BP cuff is deflated further, venous flow starts, distal vascular resistance decreases and the Korotkoff sounds reappear. When we elevate the limb before inflating the cuff, it allows venous blood to drain before cuff is inflated. Thus, when cuff is deflated progressively, there is a good pressure difference and hence Korotkoff sounds are well heard without a gap. In palpatory method, prior elevation of limb is not essential as diastolic pressure is not measured.

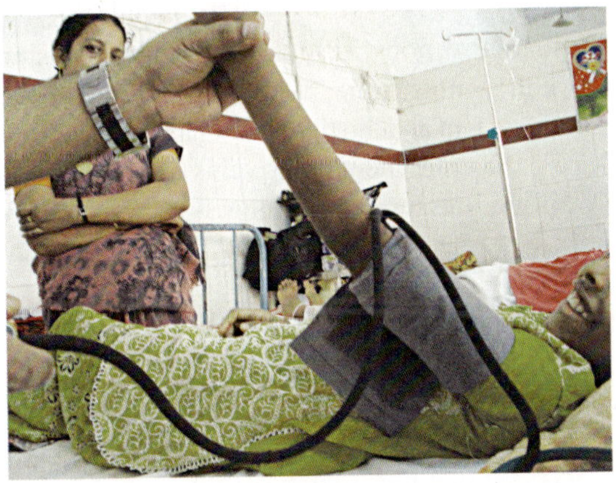

Fig.13.5 Arm is best raised while inflating BP cuff

Korotkoff's Sounds

1. Sounds begin to appear (low intensity sounds). This is systolic BP.
2. Louder sounds, sometimes with a murmur-like tail.
3. Higher intensity tapping sounds.
4. Muffling.
5. Total disappearance of sounds.

When Korotkoff's sounds are not audible in attempting to record BP, ask the patient to raise the cuffed upper limb and open and close the fist a few times before trying BP recording again. This may help in some cases, but not in a patient in shock in whom actually the BP is too low to be recorded.

Lower limb BP is taken with the patient prone, and stethoscope applied in the popliteal fossa. Systolic pressure in the lower limb is normally 10 mmHg, or more, higher than in the upper limb, but the diastolic pressure is the same. It is not because of the effect of gravity because it is demonstrable with the child lying down. Femoral is a larger artery and is more in direct line with aorta to receive larger quantities of blood. Supine and standing BP may have to be taken if postural hypotension is suspected (e.g., history of syncope, patient on nifedipine, etc).

There may be subtle difference of blood pressure between the right and left arm in normal adults, being slightly higher on the right side. Hence, the measurement of BP must be on right arm so that it becomes comparable to published normal values. A difference of more than 10 mmHg between the two limbs must make one suspicious of coarctation of aorta. Supravalvular aortic stenosis, because of the directional peculiarity of the jet, may produce a similar difference of BP between the arms.

Apart from palpatory and auscultatory methods, the other methods of BP recording are flush method and Doppler method.

Flush Method

Flush method is rarely used, sometimes it is useful in newborn. This is useful in infants and in pulseless limbs (as for legs in COA). An uninflated cuff is applied to the patient's forearm and is elevated. The limb distal to the cuff is massaged with both hands of one examiner to induce blanching. With the limb still elevated, the cuff is fully inflated by a second examiner and the limb is then brought down. Now the cuff is gradually deflated and the point of appearance of flushing of the limb distal to the BP cuff will be verbally notified by the second examiner; this corresponds to the mean arterial pressure. The obvious limitation of this method is the inability to measure the systolic and diastolic pressure separately. Some use crape bandage or similar things to drive off the blood from the limb before inflating the BP cuff.

Doppler and oscillometric methods are the other methods available for recording BP in ICU set up, but are not useful in the scenario of clinical examination.

BP Cuff Size for Different Ages

- The *length* of inflatable bladder should encircle the arm without overlapping, or must cover at least 80% of the circumference.
- The *width* of the bladder should cover at least 2/3rd of the length of arm from axilla to antecubital fossa (Ref. 5).
- In children, it is better to use a larger cuff than smaller one if the ideal size is not available because errors are more with the use of smaller cuffs (small cuff tends to produce falsely high BP).
- Recommended bladder width in the paediatric age group is 6 cm for infants, 8 cm for a child and 10 cm for adolescent. (The inflatable bag of the cuff is to be 20% wider than the diameter of the limb on which it is used.) Adult cuff size is 12.5 cm.

Upper Limit of Normal BP in Children

BP above the 95th centile for the age is called hypertension and between the 90th and 95th centile is called high normal (pre-hypertension). An easy way to remember the 90th centile of systolic BP in children is as follows (note that it is the 90th centile and not the average BP of different ages. This mnemonic is used to say whether the child has got hypertension or not). Hypertension should be diagnosed when there are 3 readings>95th centile at 3 different settings.

Newborn	90 mm (**n**ewborn-**n**inety)
Infants	100 mm (1 month to 1 year–100). One year, one hundred!
Preschool	110 mm
School age	110 + 2 mm for each year above 6 years till adult value of 120 mm is reached (e.g., for 7 year old–112 mm, 8 year old–114 mm and so on)

For all age groups, 50th centile SBP is 90+2x and diastolic BP is 55 +2x.
Hypotension is <5th centile (70+2x).

JUGULAR VENOUS PRESSURE (JVP)

The jugular venous pulse reflects the relationship between venous tone, volume of blood in the venous system and the right heart haemodynamics. During diastole, the jugular veins directly reflect RV filling pressure and during systole it mirrors the RA pressure.

Waveforms (Fig. 13.7, p 313)

'a' Wave (a = Atrial Contraction)

- It occurs during right atrial contraction.
- It follows the P of ECG.
- Occurs just before the carotid upstroke.
- It is almost synchronous with or just before S_1 in clinical examination.

Following 'a' wave, blood from the RA empties to the RV and thus RA pressure decreases and forms the 'x' descent. This is interrupted by the 'c' wave, which is a reflection of slight RA pressure elevation during the closure of the tricuspid valve and this corresponds to the carotid upstroke (c = tri**C**uspid). The portion of 'x' descent after 'c' wave is called x' descent and is due to the continued fall in RA pressure. Thus, x and x' occur during ventricular systole and are between S_1 and S_2.

'v' Wave (v = Ventricular Contraction, Venous Filling)

This occurs during ventricular systole when the atrium begins to fill. Thus, it is synchronous with carotid pulsation and peaks just after S_2.

'y' Descent (emptYing of atrium)

This occurs with the onset of ventricular diastole when the atrial blood flows to ventricle with a consequent decrease in atrial pressure. The end of atrial filling is characterized by atrial contraction ('a' wave) and the cycle continues.

Normally in the right atrium, 'a' is more than 'v' and the same is reflected in the JVP.

Clinical Significance of JVP

- Jugular veins represent a direct pipeline to RA and are hence useful in assessing RA and venous pressure.
- Changes in the pulse wave amplitude indicates dysfunction of right heart.
- Using the relation of 'a' to 'v' waves, some arrhythmias can be recognized at the bedside.

Position to Measure JVP

The patient lies supine, propped up by 45°, head is turned slightly away to the opposite side and neck relaxed (a tense sternomastoid will mask JVP) and shine a torch over the root of neck tangentially. The right atrium is lower than the jugular vein and hence the venous pressure is slightly more positive so as to facilitate proper drainage. So in the supine position, the jugular veins can be distended normally and abnormalities cannot be discerned. In the upright position, because the right atrium is much lower, even if the jugulars are congested it may not be seen above the clavicle unless the pressure is very high. At an angle of 45°, the jugular veins and RA are related in such a way that the veins normally are filled up to the level of clavicle. So any increase in venous pressure is immediately manifested above the clavicle and hence easily measured.

Whatever the position is used, the head and neck should be in straight line.

Sternal angle is always used to measure the JVP because the distance between the sternal angle and right atrium is constant at all positions and is around 4–5 cm in adults. So the right atrial pressure will be then measured as JVP + 5 cm of water (to convert to mm of Hg divide by 1.3 because 1.3 cm of water or blood corresponds to 1 mm of Hg). 13

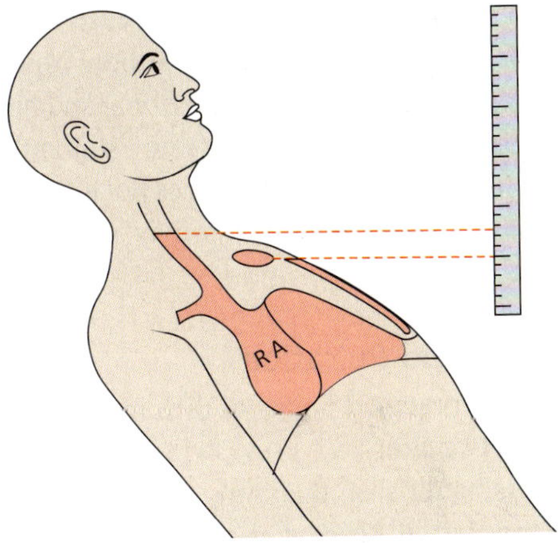

Fig.13.6 JVP examination

ABDOMINOJUGULAR REFLUX

This is a better term than hepatojugular reflux because abdominal compression anywhere elicits similar response. Here, the patient is made upright or elevated to an angle and the abdomen is compressed for 30–60 sec. Normally, the venous return gets increased and the jugulars become congested. But the increased return of blood to the right side of heart elicits Frank-Starling mechanism, the cardiac output increases and the JVP falls on continued compression. Thus, the normal hepatojugular reflux response is a transient increase in JVP followed by fall. In abnormal situations, the heart cannot accommodate the increased venous return and this causes the JVP to *remain elevated* for the period of compression. This occurs in CHF, restrictive diseases (e.g., endomyo-cardial fibrosis), etc.

Kussmaul's Sign

Normally with inspiration, the JVP falls as venous return to the right heart increases. If JVP does not fall or increases on inspiration, it denotes a positive Kussmaul's sign (denotes impaired filling of right ventricle). Inspiratory increase in blood flow to the veins is the normal response, and it normally empties into the heart. In case of constrictive pericarditis, restrictive cardiomyopathy, etc, there is obstruction to cardiac filling and hence the Kussmaul's sign. In very severe asthma there is marked air trapping and this does not allow cardiac filling and the neck veins may remain distended.

JVP vs Carotid Pulsation

Some of the practical points of differentiation between the two are:

- JVP is better seen than felt.
- JVP is better seen at the root of the neck, whereas carotids are best seen halfway up the neck where it is more superficial.
- JVP is associated with 2 positive waves per cardiac cycle (if there is no atrial fibrillation). Thus, it looks wavy.
- JVP increases with abdominal compression.
- Compression at the root of neck obliterates JVP but not the carotids.
- Respiratory variations are seen with JVP and not with the carotids.
- JVP upstrokes are gradual, with dramatic collapse and 2 pulsations per systole but in carotids are dramatic with gradual collapse and one pulsation per systole.

Prominent 'a' Waves vs Cannon Waves

Prominent 'a' waves are seen with PS, PAH (Eisenmenger), TS, etc. These are late diastolic waves (occur before S_1) corresponding with atrial contraction. In congenital heart block, off and on the atrial contraction gets so timed that the tricuspid valve has not yet opened; the atria contracts against the closed AV valves to produce large 'a' waves called cannon waves, but these occur during ventricular systole (i.e., between S_1 and S_2).

JVP in Congenital Heart Diseases

- *In large ASD,* the JVP shows equal 'a' and 'v' waves; this is because of free communication between the RA and LA (normally in RA a > v and in LA a < v).
- If JVP is prominent in a cyanotic CHD it can be:
  - Severe PS with intact ventricular septum.
  - Cyanotic congenital heart disease with increased pulmonary blood flow.
  - Tricuspid atresia (one may find large 'a' waves).
- *In CCHD* of TOF physiology JVP is not prominent. *TOF* is almost never associated with prominent JVP; if it is associated with a prominent JVP, it can be due to:
  - Restrictive VSD due to prolapse of septal leaflet of tricuspid valve.
  - In adults especially with hypertension.
- *In Eisenmenger,* 'a' wave will be prominent. JVP is elevated only with the onset of right heart failure and in such cases cyanosis is usually inevitable.
- Large 'v' or 'cv' waves in TR, ASD with MR.
- Decreased or absent 'x' descend seen in constrictive pericarditis.
- Absent 'y' descend seen in cardiac tamponade.
- Rapid and deep 'y' descend (Friedrich sign) seen in constrictive pericarditis.

As the 'a' wave is because of atrial contraction, 'a' wave will be absent in atrial fibrillation. Large 'a' waves are expected when the atria contracts against obstruction, as in tricuspid stenosis/atresia. Indirect obstruction to atrial contraction may be expected (and hence large 'a' waves) in pulmonary stenosis or pulmonary hypertension.

Elevated JVP indicates cardiac failure; but not invariably so. Any acute increase in circulating volume amounting to circulatory congestion will raise the JVP. Examples are IV fluid overload and acute glomerulonephritis. Steroid therapy at times results in sufficient retention of salt and water to raise JVP (observant students may be able to recall a few patients who while on steroids for rheumatic fever developed elevated JVP and liver enlargement). In these situations, it is not frank cardiac failure but just circulatory congestion. Raised intrathoracic (e.g., acute severe asthma) or intra-abdominal pressure can also elevate JVP marginally (a tight trouser may also do the same!).

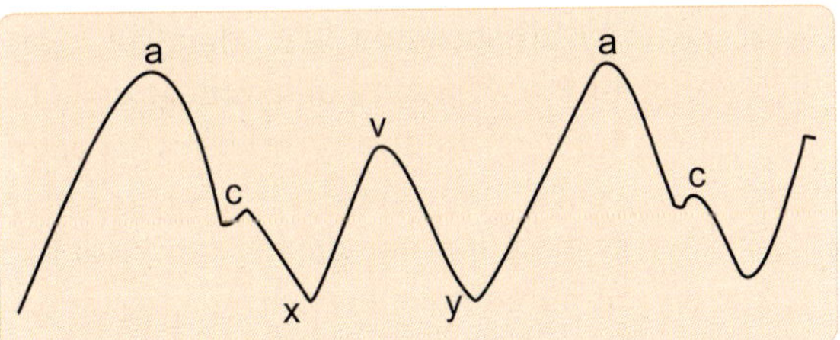

Fig.13.7 Normal jugular wave pattern

Non-pulsatile JVP is due to superior vena caval obstruction and hence very uncommon in a child. SVC obstruction may cause the face to be swollen; dilated veins may be seen in SVC drainage areas.

FIRST HEART SOUND

S_1 is a combination of tricuspid and mitral closure. Thus, it is composed of two components, mitral and tricuspid (M_1 and T_1). M_1 occurs first followed by T_1. Hence, it is possible to have split S_1 when there is delay in closure of these two valves. However, it is extremely uncommon in children.

It is proposed that S_1 is produced by all of the following and not merely due to a single event.

- Valvar components, during valve closure.
- Vibrations of cardiohaemic system during AV valve closure.
- Contributions of myocardial and vascular components.

The intensity is determined by several factors. Important ones are listed below.

1. **Position of AV valve at the time of ventricular contraction** 13

   Normally at the end of diastole, the mitral valve is in a semi-closed position as the leaflets float up in ventricle, which has already filled. With the onset of ventricular contraction the LV pressure exceeds LA pressure and the mitral valve is closed completely. If at the onset of ventricular contraction, the MV is in a widely open position than normal, then it has to move a larger distance before closing and this produces a loud first heart sound. This occurs in several situations:

   - *Prolonged diastolic ventricular filling*: E.g., left-to-right shunts like ASD; atrioventricular valve stenosis like mitral and tricuspid stenosis
   - *Early rapid diastolic filling of ventricles*: E.g., tachycardia shortens the diastole; hence ventricular contraction occurs sooner after diastole and finds the valves relatively farther apart.
   - *Recent atrial contraction*: E.g., short PR interval: Atrial contraction (occurring with P of ECG) keeps the AV valves open and because the PR interval is short, ventricular systole (R of ECG) starts soon and finds the AV valves widely separated and causes a loud S_1. The opposite conditions result in soft S_1, e.g., long PR interval

[where valves have time to float to a semi-closed position during the gap between P (atrial contraction) and R (ventricular contraction)] of ECG.

2. **Structural integrity of AV valves**
Normal AV valves are thin and pliable. Thickened valves tend to produce a loud S_1 provided they remain mobile. A calcified immobile valve as in advanced severe MS tends to produce a soft S_1 (in adults). Similarly, infective endocarditis with damage to AV valves produces a soft S_1.
3. **Integrity of isovolumic systole**
Isovolumic systole occurs after closure of the AV valves (at which time the semilunar valves also remain closed). The LV pressure rapidly increases to a peak. The onset of LV isovolumic systole is responsible for the AV valve closure and production of normal S_1.
Isovolumic systole can be interrupted in the following conditions:
   - Mitral regurgitation
   - VSD
   - Ventricular aneurysm
   - Aortic regurgitation

   With the above conditions, the LV pressure cannot increase to its peak rapidly and this affects closure of the AV valves and hence S_1 becomes soft.
4. **Myocardial contractility**
It directly affects the intensity of S_1. Hence, hyperkinetic states like exercise cause a loud S_1, whereas LV dysfunction as in myocarditis produces a soft S_1.
5. **The pressure at LV-LA pressure crossover**
During diastole, the LA pressure decreases and LV pressure increases. When the LV pressure exceeds LA pressure the AV valves close.
Normally, the pressure at which it occurs is low. In MS, the LA pressure is high and so the LV pressure has to increase more to become higher than the LA pressure. This high pressure at the crossover point also results in a loud S_1.

Two parameters are important in the assessment of S_1; they are the intensity and the split.

1. **Intensity of S_1**
Intensity may be classified as normal, accentuated, diminished or varying:
   - Loud S_1 in mitral stenosis is due to:
     - Wide open mitral valve at end diastole.
     - Higher LV pressure at mitral valve closure.
     - Thickened but mobile mitral leaflets.
   - Soft S_1 in mitral regurgitation is due to:
     - Loss of isovolumic systole (as blood leaks back to LA).
     - Failure of the leaflets to close perfectly.
     - Fibrous shortening and diminished mobility of the valve.
   - Varying intensity of S_1 occurs mainly in two situations:
     - AV dissociation like complete heart block: The atria and ventricles contract without any relation to each other. In some cycles, ventricular contraction immediately follows the atrial contraction, whereas in others it is delayed. Hence, the position of the AV valves at time of onset of ventricular contraction varies (recent atrial contraction tends to produce loud S_1).
     - Atrial fibrillation: In AF not all atrial impulses conduct to ventricles. Ventricular response is irregular too, hence the duration of ventricular diastole is different. Short R-R interval implies that the next ventricular contraction occurs earlier and finds the AV valves in its rapid filling phase and hence a loud S_1, whereas with a long

R-R interval, the ventricular contraction occurs after the AV valves have moved up to a semi-closed position and hence a soft S_1.

But in the case of AF with complete heart block as with digitalis intoxication, S_1 remains constant because the ventricular response is regular (rhythm is ventricular) and atrial contraction is ineffective in altering the position of AV valves.

PR interval and S_1

When PR interval is very prolonged, the ventricles have almost filled up and hence the valves are floating almost to the position of closure when the ventricles start contracting. So S_1 will be faint. When the patient stands up the heart rate tends to increase and hence PR shortens and so S_1 becomes louder. In complete heart block, there is beat to beat variation of PR interval and hence beat to beat variation of intensity of S_1. This differentiate heart block from sinus bradycardia.

2. **Splitting of S_1**

   Wide splitting of S_1 is difficult to appreciate. Hence, it is best not mentioned in clinical examination (also see p 296). It tends to occur in:
   - RBBB (RV component of S_1 gets delayed)
   - ASD
   - Ebstein's anomaly of tricuspid valve

SECOND HEART SOUND

S_2 is called the 'key to auscultation of the heart.'

Components

S_2 has two components: aortic (A_2) and pulmonary (P_2). They occur just after the actual closure of valve cusps and the sounds represent the abrupt tensing of the closed leaflets, which sets the cardiohaemic system (the valves, outflow tracts, great arteries and blood) into vibration.

Hangout Interval

During the process of closure of the semilunar valves, the pressure in the corresponding ventricles decrease and that of the corresponding great arteries increase. But valves do not close at the time of this pressure crossover; rather it is delayed a little (i.e., A_2 does not occur at the point when the LV pressure falls below the aortic pressure and the same is true with pulmonary system). The time interval between the time of pressure crossover and the actual valve closure is called the hangout interval.

Since the pulmonary vascular resistance is lower than the systemic vascular resistance the pulmonary arteries are more distensible than the aorta. The hangout interval is thus more in PA and hence P_2 occurs after A_2.

13

Evaluation of S_2

Intensity

Normally, the intensity of P_2 is less than that of A_2 because PA pressure is less than the aortic pressure. P_2 is usually heard only in the pulmonary area, whereas A_2 is heard widely and even here the intensity of the P_2 is less than of A_2. Thus, P_2 is considered loud if P_2 is equal to or more than A_2 (in fact, P_2 should be expressed as $P_2 = A_2$ or $P_2 > A_2$ in such cases). The grading of P_2 intensity correlates with severity of PAH (the louder the P_2 the more the pulmonary artery pressure). But in children, P_2 may appear loud due to the thinness of chest and so associated findings of PAH like left parasternal heave, epigastric pulsations, etc, should always be looked for before commenting on PAH.

Intensity of A_2 or P_2 is affected by:
- Pressure beyond the valve: PAH has loud P_2 and systemic hypertension has loud A_2.
- Flow across the valve: In left-to-right shunts with increased pulmonary blood flow P_2 may be accentuated. Similarly in hyperkinetic states

with increased flow across the aortic valves A_2 is increased in intensity.

- Size of vessel beyond the valve: In PAH, left-to-right shunts, idiopathic dilatation of the pulmonary artery, etc, pulmonary arteries are dilated contributing to the increased intensity of P_2. Likewise ascending aorta aneurysm has an associated loud A_2.
- Valve stenosis: Generally, stenotic valve produces softening of sounds (e.g., PS is associated with soft P_2). But in congenital bicuspid aortic valve, the A_2 may be normal even with stenosis.
- Valve regurgitation: This also softens the intensity of sounds. In AR, the intensity of A_2 plays an important role in identifying its aetiology; soft A_2 denotes valvular AR as in rheumatic, whereas normal or loud A_2 denotes AR secondary to dilated aortic root where the valves are essentially normal.

Masking

Loudness of one sound can mask the other. In PAH, a loud P_2 can mask A_2 and in TOF a loud A_2 masks a soft P_2.

Splitting

As mentioned earlier, the hangout interval in the PA is more than in the aorta and hence P_2 occurs after A_2 producing the A_2–P_2 sequence.

Normal Split of S_2

With inspiration, A_2–P_2 widens and are heard separately, whereas in expiration it narrows and so only a single sound is heard (only sounds that are more than 30 ms apart can be heard by our ears as separate).

Mechanism of Normal Split

During inspiration:

- The venous return to the right side of the heart increases and pulmonary distensibility increases. This results in:
  - increase in PA hangout interval and
  - increase in RV ejection time causing a *delayed P_2*.
- The venous return to the left side of heart decreases and causes a *early A_2*.

The opposite occurs during expiration. Thus, S_2 is split in inspiration and nearly single in expiration. Although all the above mechanisms are probably responsible, the major reason for the normal split is the increase in PA hangout interval occurring with inspiration.

Wide Split

If the split is heard in expiration also, it is a wide split. In children, the expiratory split may be normally heard in the supine position; so always *auscultate in the upright posture* before commenting on split in a child.

Wide split can be fixed (where the split is same in inspiration and expiration) or mobile (where the expiratory split is audible but the split further increases in inspiration).

Causes of Wide Split

1. Usually it is due to a *delayed P_2*, which occurs:
   - When electrical activation of RV is delayed—as in RBBB, LV ectopic beats, etc.
   - When RV ejection time is prolonged—as in PS, PAH, etc.
   - Hangout interval (p 315) in pulmonary artery is increased—as in ASD, IDPA (idiopathic dilatation of pulmonary artery), etc.
2. An *early A_2* is also responsible for wide split S_2 in some cases as in MR and VSD.
   Among the above, the *split is fixed* in:
   - ASD
   - In other causes if there is associated RV failure; this is because the increased venous return during inspiration does not affect the RV, which has already failed and

cannot increase its stroke volume. Severe PS has wide mobile split S_2 but when RV fails in late stages the split becomes fixed.

Mechanism of Wide and Fixed Split in ASD

In ASD, there is free communication between LA and RA, which means the pressure change in one chamber, affects the other. During expiration, although the systemic venous return to the right side of heart is reduced, the venous return to the left side of heart is increased. In ASD, therefore the decreased venous return to the right heart is compensated by the increase in the left-to-right shunt across the free communication between the atria. Hence, S_2 is split in expiration. During *ins*piration, the venous return to the right heart is increased, but the flow across the ASD is correspondingly reduced because the flow to the left heart is reduced, so the net effect on right heart is unchanged and the split does not widen further resulting in a fixed split.

Partial anomalous pulmonary venous connection with intact atrial septum has a similar physiology as that of ASD because it also has a pre tricuspid left-to-right shunt. But since the atrial septum is intact, the split is only wide and mobile and not fixed.

Single S_2: Only one sound is heard in both phases of respiration. The single sound heard can be:

- P_2—In severe PAH where the loud P_2 masks A_2 and in severe AS where A_2 is very soft.
- A_2—In TOF like situations where the loud A_2 masks the soft P_2.

Reverse split (paradoxic split), i.e., the split sequence is P_2–A_2 and not the normal A_2–P_2.

It occurs where A_2 gets unduly delayed or P_2 occurs very early.

Delayed A_2 occurs in

- Delayed electrical activation of LV—as in LBBB, RV paced (pace maker) beats.
- Prolonged LV ejection time—as in severe left ventricular outflow tract obstruction (AS).
- Increased hangout interval in aorta—as in PDA (dilated ascending aorta) and ascending aorta dilatation (in AS or AR).

Early P_2 occurs with early electrical activation of right ventricle as in right-sided WPW syndrome.

Reverse split (P_2-A_2) can be of 3 types

- In inspiration, P_2 is very much delayed and A_2 occurs very early so that only one sound is heard. So S_2 will be split in expiration and single in inspiration—the exact reverse of normal. This is the one which can be easily recognized in the bedside in an older child. In AS, the presence of paradoxic split suggests severity.
- In inspiration, P_2 is delayed but remains separate from A_2. So S_2 will be split both in inspiration and expiration but a careful observer can make out that the split widens in expiration.
- In both inspiration and expiration, the components cannot be separated and S_2 is single but phonocardiography will show that the sequence is reversed, i.e., P_2–A_2. It is not recognizable at the bedside.

13

Split of S_2 in Various Types of Heart Diseases When they Progress to Eisenmenger

- ASD Eisenmenger: The split remains wide and fixed in the majority.
- VSD Eisenmenger: S_2 is single because the RV and LV act as a common chamber with equal pressures. If S_2 is split in patients with clinical picture suggestive of VSD-Eisenmenger, always rule out associated ASD or AV canal defect or the occurrence of right heart failure.
- PDA Eisenmenger: In the majority, the split is normal.

Congenital cyanotic heart disease (CCHD) with wide split S_2 occurs in:

- Common atrium
- ASD-Eisenmenger
- Ebstein's anomaly

CCHD with single S_2 occurs in:

- TOF
- TGA
- Double outlet right ventricle (DORV)
- Truncus arteriosus
- Tricuspid atresia

Thus, normal S_2 in a cyanotic child is extremely rare and if it is actually so, think of other causes of cyanosis like methaemoglobinaemia, pulmonary AV fistula, etc.

THIRD HEART SOUND (S_3)

This a low frequency sound 0.14–0.22 sec after S_2 (mid diastole). It is generated during the rapid ventricular filling phase in diastole (before the atrial contraction). S_3 occurs during the stage of rapid ventricular filling and when active ventricular relaxation ends and passive distension occurs. Various theories are proposed on its genesis like valvar theory, ventricular theory and the impact theory. It may be normally heard in children and pregnancy. It may be is best heard with the bell of stethoscope. LV S_3 is best heard at the apex, whereas RV S_3 best heard at the LLSB or subxiphoid area (RV S_3 is louder with inspiration and can be augmented by passive leg raise).

S_3 occurs in conditions like VSD, PDA and in MR where there is increased flow across the AV valve.

Pathological S_3 is of early onset (i.e., more close to S_2) and louder compared to physiological S_3. S_3 is louder with greater volume of blood flowing across the AV valves, greater velocity of inflow and less complete myocardial relaxation. It occurs in:

- Left-to-right shunts: The presence of S_3 denotes significant shunt of at least 1.5:1; presence of mid-diastolic murmur indicates a shunt-of at least 2:1.
- In cyanotic congenital heart diseases with *increased* pulmonary blood flow.
- Hyperkinetic states like anaemia, beri-beri, thyrotoxicosis.
- Valvular regurgitation:
    - Mitral regurgitation where its presence usually indicates severity.
    - Aortic regurgitation where it occurs in acute AR (e.g., following infective endocarditis) or with left ventricular dysfunction (e.g., chronic AR producing LV dysfunction over a period of time).
- Ventricular failure: E.g., dilated cardiomyopathy or myocarditis where presence of S_3 denotes low ejection fraction of <40%.

Note: In patients with ASD, even with a large shunt, right ventricular S_3 may not be heard because the tricuspid valve is more capacious. If RVS_3 is well heard in patients with features of ASD, always think of the following: Ebstein's anomaly, large shunt in ASD due to associated mitral valve disease (i.e., Lutembacher syndrome), or an endocardial cushion defect with associated tricuspid regurgitation.

FOURTH HEART SOUND

This is a low frequency sound 0.08–0.20 sec before S_1 (presystolic). It is generated due to atrial assistance to presystolic ventricular filling. It occurs during atrial contraction at the end of diastole just before the first heart sound.

Unlike S_3, the presence of S_4 in paediatric population is always pathological. It is heard in patients with LV outflow tract obstruction (LV S_4 in severe aortic stenosis or coarctation) or RV outflow tract obstruction (RV S_4 in severe pulmonary stenosis or pulmonary arterial hypertension).

The presence of S_4 in such conditions is an indicator of severity of the lesion.

Triple rhythm (S_1,S_2,S_3)may be normal in children if unassociated with any other evidence of heart disease. Quadruple rhythm is S_1, S_2, S_3, S_4. Gallop rhythm is tachycardia with three or more heart sounds, e.g., S_3 gallop, S_4 gallop, etc.

CLICKS (SYSTOLIC SOUNDS)

There are two types of systolic sounds, the ejection sounds and non-ejection sounds.

Ejection Sounds

There are two mechanisms for an ejection sound (ejection click):

- Valvular, due to snapping open or doming of a stenotic, thickened or malformed semilunar valve.
- Vascular, due to sudden tensing or reverberation of a dilated great artery (proximal aorta or main pulmonary artery).

Valvular Clicks

They occur with either PS or AS. Their recognition is important in that the presence of a click localizes the level of stenosis to the valve (in other words, supravalvar or subvalvar AS or PS do not produce clicks).

With bicuspid aortic valve, the click may be heard well even in non-stenotic valves; the loudness of click is thus related to the mobility of the abnormal valve than to the degree of obstruction.

Pulmonary ejection click (PEC) differs from aortic ejection click (AEC) in that it is phasic; i.e., changes with respiration. Unlike other right-sided cardiac events, PEC decreases in intensity with inspiration, whereas AEC does not show any variation ("constant ejection click").

Mechanism of phasic pulmonary ejection click (PEC) is as follows.

Intensity of PEC depends on the position of the pulmonary valve leaflet at the time of its opening (isovolumic contraction). With inspiration there is increased blood flow to the right side of heart. In normal individuals, the RV end-diastolic pressure (RVED) is low, whereas in patients with PS the RVED is high due to RV hypertrophy and decreased compliance. During inspiration, the increased venous return to RA causes forceful RA contraction, which elevates the RVED, and this is transmitted to the base of the PV valve leaflets. Since the PA diastolic pressure in PS is low, this transmitted pressure tends to partly open the PV and thus the resultant PEC occurring with ventricular contraction is low in intensity. The reverse happens in expiration. 13

As PS becomes more severe, the RVED pressure increases further and PEC occurs earlier. With severe PS, the RVED may be so high so as to cause opening of PV in diastole itself and in such situations PEC is absent.

Similar changes happen in the aorta and LV but AEC remains constant with respiration (i.e., do not decrease with expiration). This is because the aortic diastolic pressure can never fall less than LV end diastolic pressure (LVED) even in severe AS (normal LVED = 8, aortic diastolic pressure = 80, RVED = 4, PA diastolic pressure = 4 mm).

Valvular clicks are not heard with calcified and immobile valves (but calcification is expected only in the elderly).

Vascular Clicks

This occurs in condition with a dilated proximal aorta (as in systemic hypertension, aortic aneurysm) or dilated, tense pulmonary artery (as in pulmonary arterial hypertension and idiopathic dilatation of pulmonary artery).

It may be difficult to differentiate valvular and vascular clicks; the accompanying clinical features help. The vascular clicks with PAH may not show respiratory variation. Unlike in PS where clicks occur *earlier* with increasing severity, the clicks in pulmonary hypertension occur *later* with increasing severity. This is because in PAH the PA diastolic pressures are also elevated causing delayed opening of the valve (PA diastolic pressure is low in PS).

Mid to Late Systolic Clicks (Non-ejection clicks, NEC)

These are due to systolic sounds occurring at the AV valves due to prolapse of the mitral valve or tricuspid valve secondary to myxomatous degeneration of the valve.

The clicks may be single or multiple, although multiple clicks do not imply an adverse situation. The NEC as the name implies is not related to ejection. It occurs at the precise moment when the MV or TV prolapses (whole leaflet or part of it) to atria. The prolapse occurs only when the LV volume has decreased a little and hence they are usually mid-to-late systolic in timing. However, in severe conditions prolapse can be holosystolic and the clicks can occur earlier and can even 'fuse' with S_1 producing a 'loud S_1' (see p 297).

Any condition producing a decrease in LV volume makes the NEC click to occur earlier. Thus inspiration, sudden standing and Valsalva manoeuvre tend to bring the click earlier.

In many ways the murmur of hypertrophic cardiomyopathy and click murmur of MVP behave similarly. A difference between the two may be noticeable with the change seen after an ectopic beat. Post ectopic beat is characterized by more blood in the ventricle with resultant increased contractility. In HCM, the increased contractility is responsible for a louder murmur, whereas in MVP the more blood volume decreases prolapse and the click murmur occurs late.

OPENING SNAPS

Opening snaps can be of mitral or tricuspid origin. The following discussion is on mitral OS. Among the diastolic events, opening snaps occur first (OS, tumour plop, pericardial knock, S_3, S_4 in that order). The OS does not represent the onset of MV opening; rather it occurs at the maximal opening movement of AML; even before OS, the LV has begun to fill from LA. It is a sharp sound heard best just medial to apex and if loud, can be conducted widely.

Note: Tumour plop is a diastolic sound heard in cases of atrial myxomas, which are quite mobile. Pericardial knock is a diastolic sound heard in constrictive pericarditis due to the abrupt halt of diastolic filling.

Intensity of OS

OS is a medium- to high-frequency sound; sharp and distinct. A pliable valve with a maintained cardiac output can produce a loud opening snap. Patients with severe MS can have diminished or indistinct opening snaps due to: (i) a calcified valve with calcium extending on to the valve tips, (ii) low cardiac output situations such as CHF, severe PAH, (iii) thick chest wall, (iv) associated lesions like AS/AR, etc. However, a calcified valve with tips remaining free of calcium can still produce OS. This is not of much significance in children as calcified valves are rare in children.

A_2-OS interval

This is one of the most important parameters to assess the severity of MS. The timing of OS depends on the pressure in LA. With severe MS, high LA pressure opens the MV earlier and results in a short A_2-OS interval. Shorter the A_2-OS interval, higher the left atrial pressure and higher the pressure gradient across the mitral valve. But other factors also affect this interval. They are:

- **Aortic systolic pressure**: Systolic hypertension increases the interval.
- **Rate of decline of LV pressure during the isovolumic relaxation**: If LV relaxation is rapid, then LV pressure falls below LA pressure sooner and OS occurs earlier. In conditions like cardiomyopathy or adults with diastolic dysfunction due to hypertension or coronary artery disease, the LV relaxation is affected and the OS is delayed and increases the A_2-OS interval.

- **Heart rate**: Bradycardia increases the available diastolic time and thus helps in more complete LA emptying. So LA pressure falls to a lower value and hence OS is delayed and the A_2-OS interval is widened. Tachycardia shortens the A_2-OS interval by opposite mechanism.
- **Aortic valve disease**: Aortic regurgitation causes early aortic valve closure and early A_2 and increased A_2-OS interval. Aortic stenosis causes the opposite.
- **Mitral valve disease**: Mitral regurgitation causes earlier closure of aortic valve (A_2) and hence widens the interval.
- **Atrial fibrillation**: A_2-OS interval is directly related to cycle length, i.e., with long R-R interval the LA pressure falls to a lower value (as with bradycardia) and hence long A_2-OS interval and vice versa.

A_2-OS vs A_2–P_2

- P_2 is best heard in the left upper sternal border (pulmonary area), whereas OS is best heard medial to the apex.
- Inspiration widens the A_2–P_2 interval but no change is likely with A_2-OS interval.
- In an older child, auscultation in the upright posture may help. The venous return decreases in the upright posture. In the right heart, this causes an early P_2 and therefore a narrow A_2–P_2 interval. In the left heart LA pressure falls, hence the OS gets delayed and the A_2-OS interval widens.

A_2-OS vs S_2-LVS_3

- S_3 is lower pitched, occurs later and is best heard at apex and is usually localized.

MURMURS

Types of Murmurs

Marriot has described murmurs as:

- *Organic*—Due to intrinsic cardiovascular disease.
- *Functional*—Cardiovascular murmurs but are produced by disturbances of circulation other than due to cardiovascular cause (like anaemia, thyrotoxicosis, etc).
- *Innocent*—May be cardiovascular or extra cardiac, but not due to any pathology of these. Their precise origin may not be clear in some cases.

Evaluation of Murmurs

Murmurs should be evaluated for following features:

- **Timing**: Systolic/diastolic/continuous.
- **Site**: Of maximal intensity and of propagation.
- **Loudness**: Grade 1 to 6. Samuel Levine has graded murmurs as has been discussed in the previous chapter.
- **Pitch or frequency**: Classified as
  - Low pitched—25–125 cycles/sec, e.g., mitral stenosis.
  - Medium pitched—125–300 cycles/sec, e.g., innocent murmurs.
  - High pitched—>300 cycles/sec, e.g., AR/MR.
- **Shape**: Crescendo, decrescendo, plateau, diamond shaped etc.
- **Changes with manoeuvres**: E.g., manoeuvres like Valsalva, inspiration, etc (right-sided murmurs generally increase with inspiration—Caravallo's sign).
- Radiation

Pathologic Significance of Murmurs

All murmurs may not be pathological or necessarily associated with cardiac disease.

Generally pansystolic murmurs, louder systolic murmurs (> grade 3) and diastolic murmurs are associated with underlying cardiac disease. **Nadas** has proposed a criteria, which help in assessing a child for the presence of heart disease.

13

Major

- Systolic murmur of > grade 3
- Diastolic murmur
- Cyanosis
- CHF

Minor

- Systolic murmur of < grade 3
- Abnormal S_2
- Abnormal ECG
- Abnormal CXR
- Abnormal BP

Presence of 1 major or 2 minor criteria suggests the presence of heart disease.

Systolic Murmurs

(Please refer to the discussion of murmurs in previous chapter p 298).

- Pansystolic or holosystolic murmurs result when the blood is regurgitated from a high-pressure chamber to a low pressure system and pressure difference is maintained throughout the cardiac cycle, e.g., MR (LV to LA), VSD (LV to RV).
- Ejection murmurs are generated during the ejection phase from one chamber to a great artery, which has nearly the same pressures, e.g., PS (RV to PA), AS (LV to aorta). Ejection murmurs are greatly affected by flow. Even with severe aortic stenosis, the murmur may not be prominent if flow is reduced as is the case when associated with CHF.
- Early systolic murmurs begins with S_1 and end in mid-systole. Early systolic murmurs are seen in small muscular VSD and large VSD with PAH (discussed in the previous chapter p 299). They may also be seen in low pressure tricuspid regurgitation as in Ebstein's anomaly and in rare cases of mitral regurgitation, e.g., acute MR due to infective endocarditis.
- Late systolic murmurs begin in mid systole or later and usually reach S_2. They are seen in MVP, HCM, etc. In coarctation of aorta and peripheral PS also the murmur originating in the vessels is late systolic because the blood reaches the site of obstruction only later in systole.

Table 13.1 Sites of maximal intensity

Aortic area	AS, aortic flow murmurs
Pulmonary area	PS, pulmonary flow murmurs, PDA (left infraclavicular)
Tricuspid area	TR, VSD (3rd & 4th space close to sternum)
Apex	MR, AS
Back	COA, peripheral PS, pulmonary AV fistula

Diastolic Murmurs

Mechanisms—there are three mechanisms:

- Semilunar valve regurgitation (pumonary/aortic)
- AV valve stenosis (mitral/tricuspid)
- Increased blood flow across AV valves

Semilunar Valve Regurgitation

An EDM is heard in AR and PR. Among causes of PR, only those seen with PAH (high-pressure PR—Graham Steell murmur) is heard prominently. An EDM due to AR may be missed if not carefully sought; auscultate with the diaphragm of the stethoscope with the patient sitting and leaning forward and breath held in expiration.

PR murmur can be differentiated from AR murmur by the following:

- Associated features of PAH.
- Increases with inspiration.
- An appreciable gap between the S_2 and the onset of PR murmur (A_2-murmur interval).
- AR murmurs may be associated with peripheral signs, whereas PR murmurs are not.

AV Valve Stenosis

In MS and TS and conditions simulating these (like cor triatriatum, atrial myxoma, etc), the murmur is mid-diastolic with presystolic accentuation.

MS murmur should be carefully looked for—light exercise like sitting ups 10–12 times and then auscultating in the left lateral position with the bell of stethoscope will help in difficult cases.

Other Mid-Diastolic Murmurs vs MDM of MS

- Flow murmurs of MR and left-to-right shunts like VSD: The murmur is softer and shorter. If S_3 is heard along with MDM it can never be MS, because S_3 is a rapid ventricular filling sound; ventricular filling is not rapid in MS. But S_3 at times may be difficult to differentiate from OS. Presence of cardiac enlargement, LV apex, etc, also suggests that the murmur may be flow related.
- Carey Coombs murmur is seen in acute rheumatic fever. It is softer and relatively higher pitched than MS murmur. No presystolic accentuation.
- Austin Flint murmur occurs when AR is at least moderate. Helpful features of differentiation are:
  - Presence of peripheral signs of AR.
  - If the presystolic component is not heard it is more likely to be Austin Flint because in severe AR the mitral valve tends to close prematurely and this prevents the atrial contribution to the murmur. But one must remember that in MS with atrial fibrillation the pre-systolic murmur may not be heard.
  - Isometric handgrip is a useful bedside method.
    It increases the systemic vascular resistance and increases the regurgitation across the aortic valve and therefore the Austin Flint murmur.

Table 13.2 Sites of maximal intensity

Sites	Possible murmurs
Mitral area	MDM of MS, Austin Flint and flow murmurs
Tricuspid area	MDM of TS, EDM of PR
Second aortic area (3rd LICS)	EDM of AR
Pulmonary area	EDM of PR

Note: If EDM of AR murmur is best heard along the right sternal border always rule out aortic root dilatation (like in Marfan's syndrome) as the cause of AR.

13

Continuous Murmurs

They begin in systole and continue uninterrupted into diastole but do not necessarily occupy the whole length of systole and diastole. The to and fro murmurs mimic a continuous murmur but they do not extend beyond S_2 or peak at S_2. Recognition of a to and fro murmur is important because they represent two different murmurs and hence two different lesions like AS/AR, VSD/AR, etc, whereas continuous murmurs are due to a single lesion like PDA, RSOV (rupture of sinus of Valsalva), etc.

Mechanism of Continuous Murmur

Continuous murmurs are seen with following conditions:

- Blood flows from a relatively high pressure area to a low pressure area throughout the cardiac cycle.
  - From aorta to pulmonary artery in PDA, APW (aortopulmonary window).
    Note: The aortopulmonary window is more likely to produce systolic murmurs mimicking VSD than a continuous murmur. Aortopulmonary window is also a connection between the aorta and pulmonary

artery like PDA, but the communication is very wide to equalize the pressure to some extent, so that the murmur is most often systolic rather than continuous.
- From aorta to elsewhere: RSOV, ALCAPA later in life.
- From systemic artery to venous system: Coronary AV fistula, bronchopulmonary collaterals.
- From PA to pulmonary vein: Pulmonary AV fistula.
- From left to right atria: In Lutembacher's (MS +ASD) syndrome, the murmur may be continuous if the ASD is restrictive. *Note*: However, it is an exception because restrictive ASD is rare in Lutembacher's.

- Blood flows across a severely constricted region or artery:
  - Peripheral pulmonary stenosis
  - Coarctation of aorta (COA)
- Blood flows through dilated tortuous anastomotic channels:
  - Collaterals in COA/Pulmonary atresia
  - Mammary souffle in pregnancy

4. Turbulent venous flow:
   - Venous hum
   - TAPVC

In CCHD, continuous murmurs should be always looked for all over the chest and back.

They are seen in:
- Severe TOF/Pulmonary atresia where murmur arises from PDA or collaterals.
- Post BT shunt cases.
- Truncus Arteriosus

Continuous murmurs over back are also seen in:
- COA
- Peripheral PS
- Pulmonary AV fistula

Continous murmurs over pulmonary artery are seen in:
- PDA
- Rupture of sinus of valsalva (RSOV) to PA
- Coronary arteriovenous fistula (CAVF) to PA

Pseudo continuous murmur are seen in:
- VSD (PSM) + AR (EDM)
- AS (ESM) + AR (EDM)
- MR + AR
- TR + MS

Innocent Murmurs

General features of innocent murmurs are that they are systolic, not very loud, short (never pan-systolic) with otherwise normal cardiac examination.

Various types are:
- Venous hum (discussed below)
- Vibratory (Still's) murmur (discussed below)
- Pulmonary systolic murmur (from pulmonary trunk).

  Pulmonary systolic murmur is heard to the left of sternal border in the second space and never associated with a thrill. This is a flow related murmur and is audible because PA is anterior to the aorta and because children have thin chest walls. Make sure that the second sound is moving normally before stamping this murmur as innocent.
- Peripheral pulmonic murmur (from pulmonary branches). It is commonly heard over the lung fields in newborn.
- Supraclavicular systolic murmur (from brachiocephalic arteries).
- Aortic systolic murmur (in adults with sclerotic AV; in children due to very high flow). Heard to the right of sternal border at the second space. This may be associated with a low-pitched bruit sound over the carotid.

Of the above murmurs, Still's murmur is a vibratory murmur (vibration of tissue); all others are "flow murmurs" (produced by the turbulence of high flow). Flow murmurs usually are associated with other evidences of high stroke volume. Systolic flow murmurs greatly diminish in intensity or even disappear on standing up as the flow reduces under the effect of gravity.

For all practical purposes, there is no diastolic murmur that is innocent (non-organic). Two very rare situations where one may find innocent diastolic murmurs are extreme bradycardia and high blood pressure; these will disappear with the correction of bradycardia or hypertension.

Venous Hum

This is very common in children. It is due to the turbulence in the jugulars and brachiocephalic veins. It is common in children because of the increased cardiac output. It is also seen in hyperkinetic states like anaemia, thyrotoxicosis, etc, which cause venous turbulence. If widely conducted it may be mistaken for a PDA murmur.

Differentiating features include:

- Venous hum is best heard at the root of the neck on the right side (supraclavicular and infraclavicular areas).
- It increases on sitting/standing up.
- It disappears on lying down (because there is no venous turbulence in that position).
- Turning the head to left increases the hum because of increased stretch.
- Flexing the neck or compressing the jugulars decreases the hum.
- Disappears with Valsalva maneuver or head turning to right.

Still's Murmur

This is heard in children between 3 years of age and adolescence. It is usually less than grade 3 in intensity. It is vibratory in nature with medium frequency. High stroke volume ejected forcefully (which is the usual scenario in healthy children) causes tissue of left ventricle to vibrate and hence the murmur. Vibratory murmurs are due to vibration of tissues; vibration has harmonics and hence can be musical (like vibration of string producing musical sound). But unfortunately not all examiners can appreciate the musical quality. A medium-pitched "musical" murmur may sound only like a hum to some students. However, high-pitched notes will be appreciable to many students, and it will sound like seagull's cry. Still's murmur is confined to the first half of systole with a long gap between the end of murmur and S_2 S2and is diamond shaped. It is best heard in the supine position (unlike venous hum).

Fever, exercise, etc, increase the intensity (as stroke volume and force of ejection increases). It is best heard in the area between 3rd/4th left intercostal space and the apex.

Rule of thumb: A murmur that sounds musical or hums in an asymptomatic child is likely to be innocent.

13

1. Syndromes associated with cardiovascular disease

Name of syndrome/disease	Predominant heart lesions
Heritable diseases	
Holt-Oram	ASD
TAR	ASD
Ellis-van Creveld	ASD
Noonan	Dysplastic pulmonary valve (PS), HCM
Tuberous sclerosis	Rhabdomyoma
Leopard	PS
Apert	VSD

contd.

Crouzon	PDA/COA
Williams	Supravalvar AS/PS (peripheral)
Connective tissue diseases	
Marfan	Aortic dilatation, MR
Ehlers-Danlos	Aortic dilatation, MR
Metabolic disorders	
Mucopolysaccharidosis	Mutivalvar disease
Pompe's	Cardiomyopathy
Homocystinuria	Early CAD, venous thrombosis, medial necrosis of aorta
Chromosomal abnormalities	
Down	ECD, VSD, ASD, TOF
Trisomy 18	VSD, PDA
Trisomy 13	VSD, DORV
Turner	COA, BAV
DiGeorge	Conotruncal anomalies (interrupted aortic arch)
Sporadic	
VATER	VSD
CHARGE	TOF
Cornelia de Lange	VSD
Teratogenic	
Rubella	PDA, PS (valvar, peripheral), ASD
Dilantin	PS, AS, COA, PDA
Nearly 20% mothers with PKU may have babies with TOF.	

2. **Eyes**

Lesions	Pathology/Syndromes
Blue sclera	Osteog. imperfecta, Marfan, Ehlers-Danlos
Iridodonesis	Marfan, homocystinuria
Brushfield spots	Down
Cataract	Congenital rubella
Ocular protrusion	Severe tricuspid regurgitation
Petechiae	Infective endocarditis
Jaundice	Congestive hepatitis secondary to PAH, TR, CHF

3. **Skin**

Lesions	Pathology/Syndromes
Lentigines	Leopard (HCM, PS)
Erythema marginatum, subcutaneous nodules	Acute rheumatic fever
Petechiae	Infective endocarditis
Telangiectasia	Osler-Rendu-Weber (pulmonary AV fistula)
Angiokeratoma	Fabry's (valve regurgitation, arrhythmias)
Livedo reticularis	SLE (endocarditis)

4. **Extremities**

Broad thumb	Rubinstein-Taybi (PS, PDA)
Absent thumb	Holt-Oram (ASD)
Simple polydactyly	VSD, Primum ASD
Cutaneous syndatyly of 2/3rd toes	Smith-Lemli-Opitz (VSD)

Other syndromes associated with abnormal extremities and cardiac manifestations are Down, Marfan, Turner, trisomy 16 and 18.

5. **Face**

Syndrome with abnormal facies	Cardiac lesions
William	Supravalvar AS, PS
Noonan	PS (dysplastic PV), ASD, HCM
Klippel-Feil	VSD
Cornelia de Lange	VSD
Hurler	Valve regurgitation
Kearns-Sayre	CHB, CHF
Pierre Robin	VSD, ASD

Other syndromes with abnormal facies and cardiac manifestations are Down, Rubinstein-Taybi, Leopard, etc.

13

CHAPTER 14

Cardiovascular System: Case Sheet Formats

History

1. **Age**

   Congenital heart diseases (except secondum ASD) usually manifests clinically from birth to few years of life according to severity. Rheumatic fever typically presents in the age group of 5–15 years. Infective endocarditis is rare before the age of 1–2 years. Myocarditis is usually in infancy and arrhythmias at any age.

2. **Presenting complaints**
   - Presenting complaints:
     - *Acyanotic CHD*: The usual presenting complaints in L to R shunt lesions (VSD or PDA; ASD is rarely symptomatic in childhood) are:

       Breathing difficulty, cough, effort intolerance (all because of cardiac failure; manifest as feeding difficulty in infants: forehead sweating during feeding and suck-rest cycles; equivalent symptoms in older children are breathlessness and exertional dyspnoea), recurrent lower respiratory infections, and FTT.
     - *Cyanotic heart disease:* In congenital cyanotic heart disease cyanosis, squatting, breathlessness (spells), etc may be the complaints. Headache or seizure in a cyanotic heart disease could be due to cerebral thrombosis (<2 years age, especially following dehydration) or cerebral abscess (>2 years age). Plethora and mild bleeding may be a there in cyanotic CHD.
     - *Rheumatic fever:* In rheumatic fever, fever, sorethroat, joint pains (arthritis and heart disease in rheumatic fever, endocarditis, Kawasaki, SLE, etc), palpitation, chest pain, oliguria, nocturia (cardiac failure), chorea, etc.

       Huge left atrium of rheumatic mitral valve disease may press on the recurrent laryngeal nerve to produce hoarseness (very rare).

       Syncope, palpitation, "funny feeling in chest," etc could mean arrhythmia. Causes of palpitation need not always be cardiac (tachycardia or arrhythmia): other causes could be hyperthyroidism, hypoglycaemia, anxiety, anaemia, fever, sympathomimetics, vasodilators or atropine. Chest pain due to myocardial ischaemia is unlikely in childhood; rarely pericarditis may be the reason for chest pain (practical point: most often chest pain in children is musculoskeletal).

3. **History of the present illness**: Each presenting symptom may be probed in detail as discussed in Ch. 8.
   - Cardiac features:
     - Cyanosis, spell, squatting in cyanotic heart diseases (in TOF).
     - Congestive cardiac failure in L to R shunt lesions:
       - Infant – Suck-rest-suck, head sweating, irritability.

- Child – Dyspnoea, orthopnoea, paroxysmal nocturnal dyspnoea, easy fatigability, abdominal pain (could be due to congestive gastropathy, hepatomegaly, mesenteric emboli), vomiting, anorexia. Fatigue cough and effort intolerance without fever is likely to be cardiac failure; with fever could be respiratory infection with or without cardiac failure.

- Focus/aetiology that has led to the present admission:
  - Find focus of infection (usually respiratory).
- Complications due to the acute problem or the pre-existing cardiac problem:
  - The reason for acute problem is usually respiratory infection and hence look for the danger signs of ARI and look for wheeze: because pneumonia or exacerbation of wheeze could be severe; inquire about acute life-threatening episodes in the past (which means the present episode also could progress to life-threatening episode).
  - FTT, poor weight gain, feeding problems, and development delay may be there in L to R shunt lesions.
- Course in hospital:
  - Whether started on any drugs/injections.
  - Advice that has been given regarding fluid, salt intake.
  - Any counselling given as to the need for surgery or antibiotic prophylaxis for endocarditis.
- Activities of daily living: Whether compromised or not. Was the child advised any exercise limitations.
- Treatment history: E.g., endocarditis prophylaxis, heart failure medications, rheumatic prophylaxis, etc.

Focused history on chronological evolution of symptoms also is important: e.g., child with L-R shunt lesion who was having recurrent respiratory infections and symptoms suggestive of cardiac failure is now improved without any more respiratory infection could mean either the child is getting better or child is developing obstructive pulmonary hyperten-sion.

4. **Antenatal, natal & postnatal history**
   - Antenatal:
     - Relevant antenatal histories include maternal rubella (fever with rash during the first trimester), smoking, alcohol, irradiation (maximum permissible radiation exposure during the whole of pregnancy period is 500 rads), etc.
     - Antenatal drugs: Lithium, warfarin, phenytoin, etc. NSAIDs (fetal demise due to intrauterine closure of ductus arteriosus), vit D (supravalvular aortic stenosis). Fetal hydantoin and fetal alcohol syndromes have CHD as part of it (VSD, ASD, PDA, etc).
     - Maternal SLE: Congenital heart block; maternal diabetes: transient asymmetric septal hypertrophy (hypertrophic cardiomyopathy), TGA.
     - Consanguinity; history of sibling with CHD.
     - Maternal age at conception has implications in the form of higher risk of Down's syndrome babies. Age of father is less important: a higher chance of connective tissue diseases such as Marfan's may be found in advanced paternal age.
     - Whether the mother has had her quota of iron, folic acid tablets.
     - Any anomalies detected by antenatal ultra sonography.
   - Natal history:
     - Term or preterm; birth weight.

- Pre-term babies have a higher predisposition for PDA. Also CHDs may be found in association with intra-uterine infections, which may manifest as small for gestational (SGA); infants of diabetic mother who usually have LGA babies, occasionally associated with CHDs such as TGA.
- Respiratory distress or cyanosis.
- Sucking and feeding normal or interrupted.
- Poor weight gain in neonatal period.

5. **Immunization history**: Ask about the adequacy and timing of vaccine shots. There could have been delays or missed shots due to unwell child. Was any additional vaccines advised.
6. **Development history**: Development delay is common in L-to-R shunt lesions, especially motor delay due to the poor exercise tolerance.
7. **Dietary history**: The nutritional intake is likely to be inadequate. The paradox is that in cardiac failure the child requires more calories than normal, but can take only less than normal due to feeding difficulty. Inquire if the child is on salt or fluid restriction.
8. **Family and socioeconomic history**: Impact of disease on the child (missed school days/ academic performance, restrictions on recreational activities, self-esteem, etc). Impact of disease on family expenses; impact of this child's illness on care of sibling (like less parental attention to normal sibling).
   Overcrowding must be inquired into in rheumatic fever as streptococcal infections are more common in that scenario.
   Any cardiovascular-related diagnosis in the family (e.g., Marfan syndrome) or cardiac deaths at young age (hypertrophic cardiomyopathy, long QT syndrome, arrhythmia as in WPW syndrome).
   Its also important to know about any CHD in the family. Recurrence risk of CHD is 2–6% when there is one affected sibling.

Note: It is best to start examination after a very brief history; rest of the relevant history can be elicited while you are examining the child or after finishing the examination.

In small infants, its rewarding to do auscultation first before the baby becomes uncooperative.

Blood pressure, JVP and femoral pulse may be examined last because they may be time consuming in small babies. If neck is very short as in small infants, it may not be possible to examine JVP meaningfully and most examiners will accept this fact if stated so. Although examined last, while presenting the case to the examiner, you should place BP and JVP as per the standard examination scheme.

General Examination

1. **General comment**
   - Is the child sick looking, tachypnoeic/dyspnoeic? Comment on syndromic feature if any.
   - Elfin facies - Williams (supravalvular aortic stenosis).
   - Mongoloid facies - Down (VSD, endocardial cushion defect).
   - Webbed neck, cubitus valgus - Turner (coarctation of aorta).
   - Tall stature, arachnodactyly - Marfan (AR).
   - Hypertelorism, short philtrum, downslanting eyes - Di George.
   - Noonan (PS, ASD); Kartagener syndrome (dextrocardia, situs inversus); radial deformity in Holt-Oram syndrome (ASD); Ellis-van Creveld (ASD, common atrium); congential rubella (PDA).
2. **Vital signs** (compare with normal values for the age):
   - Pulse rate, respiratory rate, blood pressure and temperature.

     If radial pulse is not obvious go on to brachial pulse before coming back to search radial.

3. **Anthropometry**
   - Usually growth will be retarded in CHD. Both poor nutritional intake (feeding difficulty due to cardiac failure and increased energy expenditure due to cardiac failure) and marked hypoxia (in cyanotic heart disease) can cause growth retardation. Failure to thrive may be part of syndromic heart diseases and intrauterine infections associated with heart disease.
   - Short stature (Down, Turner, etc) and tall stature (Marfan) can be associated with heart disease.
   - Head circumference may be low in syndromes and intrauterine infections.
4. **Assessment of Development**
   In cases of developmental retardation (e.g., syndromic child), the student is required to assess development by examination rather than depending totally on history. However, in a CVS case, development assessment from history is all that is needed.
5. **Head to Foot Examination**
   - Eyes: Look for pallor; congested conjunctiva in cyanotic heart disease.
   - Mouth: Must mention if there is carious teeth.
   - Nails: Look for clubbing and cyanosis; look for differential clubbing and differential cyanosis.
   - Osler nodes, Janeway lesions, splinter haemorrhages in endocarditis.

   Chest: Any surgical scars
   - Median sternostomy scars in all surgeries needing cardiac bypass (i.e., all intracardiac repairs).
   - Left lateral thoracostomy scars are seen in BT shunt, PDA ligation, coarctation repair, pulmonary artery banding, etc. Modified BT may be via right thoracostomy, but otherwise right thoracostomy scars are more likely to be due to pulmonary surgeries. Absent right brachial, right thoracostomy scar and continuous murmur on the right side of chest: most probably child has cyanotic heart disease and has undergone a palliative shunt procedure.

     Median thoracostomy scar in a child who is still cyanotic may indicate a palliative shunt procedure where a definitive correction is not feasible.
   - Harrison sulcus, precordial bulge, precordial pulsations or quiet precordium (precordium is quiet in pericardial effusion).
   - If you find dextrocardia on exam, its important to palpate liver and auscultate lungs for bronchiectasis. 14
   - Kyphosis, scoliosis if present must be mentioned, because these may shift the apex position.
   - Look for oedema at ankle (sacral oedema in bed ridden patient).
   - Fundus: Roth spots in endocarditis.
   - Any abnormal movement (chorea).
   - Skin: Subcutaneous nodules, erythema marginaturm (rheumatic fever).
   - In cases of aortic regurgitation and endocarditis, look for related peripheral signs.

CARDIOVASCULAR SYSTEM

1. General

- **Pulse** (rate, rhythm, volume, character, radio-femoral delay): If radial pulse is not obvious go directly to brachial pulse before coming back to search radial. Palpate all peripheral pulses. Mention pulse deficit, if any. It is more convenient to look for brachiofemoral delay rather than radiofemoral delay.

  Large volume and collapsing pulse may be appreciable in AR and PDA.

  Beware of weak/absent right radial/brachial pulse; e.g., absent right brachial, right thoracostomy scar and continuous murmur right side of chest could mean that most probably child had cyanotic heart disease and undergone a palliative shunt procedure.

- **Blood pressure** (all four limbs when indicated). Wide pulse pressure may be seen in PDA and AR.
- **JVP** (mention the waves seen, the height of JVP and hepatojugular reflux). If the neck is very short as in small infants, it may not be possible to examine JVP meaningfully and most examiners will accept this fact if stated so.

  JVP is elevated in case of cardiac failure; if there is large 'v' wave it could mean associated TR due to PAH (rare).

VENTRICULAR SEPTAL DEFECT

Inspection of Precordium

- Shape of precordium: Large VSD may show precordial prominence; small defects may not have precordial prominence.
- Apex beat: In large VSDs. the apex is shifted down and out (unlikely in small defects).
- Precordial pulsations: Large VSD may show hyperdynamic precordium; small size defects may not have pulsations.
- Dilated veins or any surgical scars may be looked for.

Palpation

- Apex beat: Apex is shifted down and out and is forceful (hyperdynamic) in character.
- Systolic thrill, maximal at 3rd and 4th intercostal spaces at the left sternal edge.
- Left parasternal heave (indicates right ventricular hypertrophy) is often seen in large VSD (unlikely in small defects).
- Palpable P2 in the second space is expected if there is pulmonary hypertension.

Table 14.1 Diagnostic importance of second sound in VSD

Magnitude of shunt	PAH	Second sound
Small L to R shunt	No PAH	S2 wide split with respiratory variations. P2 is of normal intensity.
Large L to R shunt	PAH (hyperkinetic)	S2 wide split with respiratory variations. P2 is loud. All haemodynamically significant shunts will have loud P2 (usually equal to A2) due to hyperkinetic PAH.
Small L to R shunt	PAH present, possibly progressing to obliterative PAH. This means that although shunt is small, the VSD is not small. The shunt is small because of PAH.	S2 closely split with respiratory variations (split appreciable in inspiration; nearly single during expiration). P2 is loud.
R to L shunt (reversal of shunt; Eisenmenger)	Severe irreversible PAH (obliterative PAH). Inoperable	Loud S2. A2 and P2 close together, hence heard as single. Loudness is due to loud P2.
L to R shunt with acquired pulmonary stenosis	No PAH. PS	S2 wide split with respiratory variations. P2 is of diminished intensity.

Additional sounds: S_3 may be there; may be difficult to appreciate if the primary murmur is loud.

Percussion

- Locate the upper border of liver dullness.
- Cardiac borders (use light percussion only).
- Determine whether the pulmonary area is resonant or dull.

Auscultation

Heart Sounds

VSD: S1 may get immersed in murmur, or could be heard with normal intensity. S2 is widely split and movable. P2 may be loud if there is pulmonary hypertension.

Since part of the blood destined to go to the aorta is now going in to the right ventricle, the left ventricular systole is shortened and hence A_2 occurs earlier. Since there is extra blood for the right ventricle to pump into the pulmonary artery, the P_2 gets delayed. Thus, the second sound is widely split but with normal respiratory variations.

Murmurs

VSD murmur is pansystolic of good loudness (usually 3 to 4/6 in intensity), best heard in left sternal border, transmitted very well to the right sternal border and lower sternal border. A practical point is that the VSD murmur may appear to radiate well to the right of sternum. Loudness of murmur need not correlate with the size of VSD. Small VSDs usually produce loud murmur.

A mid-diastolic low intensity (2/6) flow murmur may be heard at the apex due to increased flow across normal mitral valve in moderate and large VSDs (indicates a shunt of > 2:1). Also look for diastolic murmur of AR, as it may develop as a complication of VSD. TR murmur is rarely audible (as in PAH of any aetiology, not just VSD).

Palpation of abdomen: Hepatomegaly is likely. Determine liver span; liver could be pulsatile in tricuspid regurgitation. Look for spleen (Infective endocarditis).

The diagnosis must be given as congenital acyanotic heart disease, L to R shunt lesion, small/medium/large VSD; the child is in sinus rhythm, with/without CCF, with/without PAH, with/without evidence of infective endocarditis, with/without PEM, with/without development delay and immunization status being adequate/not.

Differential Diagnosis

Consider other causes of systolic murmurs (see p 298, 322).

Investigations

1. In small asymptomatic VSDs, ECG and X ray are likely to be normal.
2. In symptomatic medium sized and large VSDs:
   - X ray: Cardiomegaly; pulmonary vascular markings are increased; prominent pulmary artery segment may be seen; left atrial enlargement may be seen (shadow-in-shadow on the right side of cardiac shadow).
   - ECG: Left ventricle enlargement of volume overload type is seen. There may be evidence of right ventricle hypertrophy and enlargement of left atrium.
   - Abnormal QRS axis that may be present occasionally may help in inlet VSD has right upper quadrant axis; equiphasic RS pattern in V2–V5 (Katz Wachtel phenomenon) suggests significant L to R shunt.

14

Treatment

Small Defects (Asymptomatic; no cardiomegaly, no cardiac failure)

- Small defects without haemodynamic changes require no medical or surgical treatment.
- They require infective endocarditis prophylaxis before minor surgical procedures (p 337).
- Correction of anaemia (if any) by iron therapy is warranted.

Medium-sized Defect (with cardiac enlargement)

- May benefit from digoxin.
- They require treatment of respiratory infections, prophylaxis for endocarditis, attention to nutrition and additional vaccines (like influenza virus vaccine).

- Surgical closure at an elective date.

Large Defects (cardiomegaly and cardiac failure)

- Early surgical closure before pulmonary hypertension is established is a must.
- Till then, medical management with digoxin, frusemide, etc (see p 337).
- Treatment of respiratory infections, prophylaxis for endocarditis, attention to nutrition and additional vaccines (like influenza virus vaccine).
- High calorie low volume feeds at more frequent intervals when there is cardiac failure.

Follow-up

Periodic evaluation (yearly for small defects, more frequently for larger defects) is planned for assessing growth, immunization, frequency of respiratory infections, cardiac failure, pulmonary hypertension, pulmonary stenosis or aortic regurgitation.

Prognosis

Natural history of VSD: Up to 80% of small defects close spontaneously (mostly perimembraneous ones). If it closes, most often it does so within the first 2 years of life. Medium and large VSDs are less likely to close, but still the size of the defect may come down.

Medium and large defects produce recurrent respiratory infections and cardiac failure.

Medium and large defects will have hyperkinetic pulmonary hypertension, which may progress to obliterative pulmonary artery hypertension and Eisenmenger syndrome in later life. VSDs in syndromic children are more likely to progress to Eisenmenger (e.g., Down).

Some may develop aortic regurgitation due to prolapse of the valve cusp (due to the drag by the VSD jet). It is common in sub pulmonic VSD ("outlet VSD").

An occasional one may develop pulmonary stenosis due to hypertrophy of right ventricular infundibulum. It may then start behaving somewhat like TOF. Even small defects are predisposed to develop infective endocarditis.

Notes

- VSD is the most common congenital heart lesion accounting for approximately one-third of CHDs.
- Usually 'multifactorial inheritance'; recurrence risk if there is one affected child or parent is 1–4%.
- Symptoms may not be present at birth, but manifest by 4–6 weeks of life (when the pulmonary vascular resistance falls). Large VSDs and VSD in preterm babies may clinically present earlier, 2–4 weeks of life. There is increased incidence of recurrent lower respiratory infections. History of suck-rest-suck cycle and excessive perspiration during feeding are useful points in infants to detect cardiac failure.
- General examination: Look for any dysmorphic features as VSD could be part of many syndromes.
- Anthropometry: Evidence of PEM (if the child is well grown, the defect is likely to be small).
- No cyanosis, no clubbing.
- Normal pulses.
- JVP may be elevated, depending on whether there is cardiac failure. No cardiac failure in small defects.
- Breathlessness with signs of increased work of breathing (unlikely in small defects) may be present. Look for signs of increased work of breathing; e.g., intercostal recession or chest wall deformity (e.g., Harrison's sulci).
- Outcome depends on the size of defect and position of defect in the septum. Small defects are more likely to close than large defects; defects in the perimembraneous area are more likely to close.

Locations of VSD are:

Perimembranous VSD (membranous defect but often with slight extension to muscular part of septum; location is subaortic); this is the commonest and most likely to close spontaneously.

- Inlet VSD.
- Outlet VSD (infundibular VSD, as it is related to the infundibulum of right ventricle; also called sub pulmonic).
- Muscular VSD (trabecular) has some chance of spontaneous closure. However, multiple muscular VSDs (swiss cheese) do not close.

Clinical Assessment of Size of Defects

- Small size VSD/PDA: Normal growth of the child; no cardiomegaly; no cardiac failure.
- Medium size VSD/PDA: There will be *cardiomegaly* and may develop cardiac failure, when there is associated respiratory infection. MDM at apex implies significant shunt (>2:1 shunt) in VSD and PDA.
- Large size VSD/PDA: There will be heart failure, growth failure and frequent respiratory tract infections.

PATENT DUCTUS ARTERIOSUS

See case sheet format for CVS, p 328. In general examination, specifically look for features of congenital rubella syndrome and any other dysmorphism.

Inspection of Precordium

- Shape of precordium: May or may not show precordial prominence depending on the shunt.
- Apex beat: In large PDA, the apex is shifted to left.
- Precordial pulsations over the 2nd left intercostal space may be seen with PDA.

Palpation

- Apex beat will be displaced to left if shunt is significant; usually the apex is forceful (hyperdynamic) in character.
- Thrill is felt in first and second left intercostal spaces and/or infraclavicular area (thrill in PDA could be continuous or just systolic as the murmur tapers off during diastole to an intensity not loud enough to produce the thrill). Palpable impulse of ascending aorta may be felt in the suprasternal notch (finger pushed into the suprasternal notch may feel aortic pulsations in PDA; this finding is not likely in any other L to R shunt lesions).

Auscultation

- S1 and S2 could be normal or loud (depending on tachycardia and pulmonary hyper-tension, respectively) but usually gets immersed in murmur. Theoretically reversed splitting of S2 is possible in PDA, but almost never clinically appreciable to a student (S2 itself is difficult to evaluate as the murmur peaks at S2). Reverse splitting is because A2 gets delayed due to prolonged left ventricular emptying time.
- Continuous 'machinery' murmur β loudest at second left intercostal space radiating to below the left clavicle (Gibson murmir); reaches maximal intensity towards the end of systole, may have multiple clicks near S_2 and then fades away in diastole. The murmur is crescendo during systole, peaks at S2 and then is decrescendo during diastole. Multiple clicks may be heard near S2 where the intensity of murmur peaks.
- Intensity of murmur does not indicate the severity of shunt. Severity of the shunt is indicated by wide pulse pressure, apical diastolic flow murmur and left ventricular hypertrophy. PDA murmur most often is of grade 3 to 4/6. Only systolic murmur may be heard in a PDA in the following situations:
  - < 6 weeks of age due to slower resolution of fetal pulmonary hypertension.
  - Decreased flow due to cardiac failure.
  - Severe pulmonary arterial hypertension (as the gradient between aorta and the pulmonary artery becomes less).
  - Small PDA.

- A mid-diastolic murmur may be heard at the apex due to increased flow across normal mitral valve (indicates a shunt of > 2:1).

  This may be difficult to appreciate if PDA murmur is loud.
- Examine the abdomen for liver (cardiac failure) and spleen (infective endarteritis).
- A small ductus arteriosus is likely to be asymptomatic; with increasing size of shunt there may be poor weight gain, reduced exercise tolerance or heart failure.
- Clinical assessment of size of PDA:
  - Small PDA: High volume pulse, continuous murmur, normal growth, no cardiomegaly, no cardiac failure.
  - Moderate or medium sized PDA: Cardiomegaly, S3 at apex, mid diastolic murmur at apex.
  - Large PDA: Cardiac failure in addition to features of moderate PDA.

Differential Diagnosis

Consider other causes of continuous murmurs:

- Venous hum: see p 325.
- AR with ventricular septal defect: Usually, the second sound is audible, unlike PDA. The murmur will have a systolo diastolic nature rather than "continuous" nature.
- Aorto pulmonary window (APW): The location of the murmur is a little medial to and lower down compared to PDA and only 10% of APW will have a continuous murmur; 90% will have only systolic murmur.
- Rupture of sinus of valsalva: The right/non coronary sinus ruptures into the right atrium, right ventricle or pulmonary artery. The murmur is lower down than in PDA.
- Coronary AV fistula: Here, the murmur is more audible during diastole, because the major part of coronary flow is during diastole. In PDA, murmur is more audible during systole
- Pulmonary AV fistula: There is cyanosis.
- Systemic AV fistula: Originates in the internal mammary artery and thus the maximum intensity of murmur is located there.
- Tetralogy of Fallot with absent pulmonary valve syndrome: Due to the absence of valve, there is diastolic murmur also. Obviously, it is a cyanotic heart disease.
- Truncus arteriosus: Cyanosis is present in this condition.

Investigations

- **X-ray**: Cardiomegaly with left ventricular contour. The main pulmonary artery is prominent. A prominent aortic knuckle is present, which differentiates it from a ventricular septal defect.
- **ECG**: Left ventricular hypertrophy of volume overload type. If right ventricular hypertrophy is present, it indicates pulmonary arterial hypertension (uncomplicated PDA will not have right ventricular hypertrophy). This is in contrast to VSD, where biventricular hypertrophy is the rule.

Treatment

Pharmacological closure with indomethacin may be successful in the newborn period in preterm babies with PDA. Beyond newborn period, there is no drugs that can obliterate the PDA.

There is no spontaneous closure of even small PDA beyond newborn period. So even small PDA need to be closed at an elective time.

PDA is nowadays closed with coil (Gianturco coils) or device (Amplatzer) or surgery (triple ligation), surgery is used only in a small percentage of cases where the former is not feasible (e.g., calcified ductus with aneurysm).

- Treatment of recurrent respiratory infections.
- Treatment of cardiac failure (p 337).
- High calorie low volume feeds at more frequent intervals when there is cardiac failure.
- Infective endarteritis prophylaxis is needed before minor surgical procedures (p 337).

Notes

- In PDA, symptoms may not be present at birth, but manifest beyond 4–6 weeks of life (when the pulmonary vascular resistance falls). There is increased incidence of recurrent lower respiratory infections.
- There is a strong association with prematurity. Also, increased incidence of PDA is likely if the baby is born at high altitude.
- Look for any dysmorphic features.
- Assess the growth and development.
- May have been a low birth weight baby with maternal history suggestive of antenatal exanthem (congenital rubella).
- A persistent ductus arteriosus is common in extremely premature babies, unlike in mature infants; it is often managed successfully with fluid restriction and indomethacin in the newborn period. PDA that is patent beyond 3 months of age is unlikely to close naturally.
- No cyanosis, no clubbing.
- Pulse is high volume and collapsing in character (wide pulse pressure).

Notes on L to R Shunt Lesions

Usual age of first clinical presentation is at 6–10 weeks (except secondum ASD, which generally is not symptomatic during childhood).

MDM at apex, poor weight gain (always assess if contributed by syndromic status or nutrition), and feeding difficulty suggest significant L to R shunt. In all congenital heart diseases (except secondum ASD, which anyway will not be an exam case), make sure you look for signs of infective endocarditis.

In all L–R shunts, make sure that you search for signs of development of Eisen-menger syndrome. Progression to Eisenmenger should be suspected when patient with large shunt shows disappearance of MDM, shortening of lengthy pan systolic VSD murmur or continuous murmur of PDA (which indicates the shunt becoming smaller) and persistence of loud P2 (> A2) with symptomatic improvement.

Cyanosis, clubbing, polycythemia, etc will not be obvious till shunt reversal (which happens much later).

Infective Endocarditis Prophylaxis

Low risk procedures (e.g., dental procedures, upper respiratory procedures, etc) in low risk patients: Oral amoxycillin 50 mg/kg (max. 3 g) 1 hr before the procedure. In case of penicillin allergy, clindamycin, cephalexin or azithromycin.

For high-risk patients (e.g., pre existing rheumatic valvular lesion, history of previous endocarditis, complex cyanotic heart disease like transposition of great vessels, prosthetic valve, etc) or high-risk procedures (e.g., genitourinary or gastrointestinal procedures): IV Ampicillin 50 mg/kg plus gentamicin 1.5 mg/kg ½ hr before the procedure. The drugs may be repeated once 6 hrs later.

Management of Cardiac Failure

Mnemonic: **ROAD**: **R**est in propped up position, **O**xygen, management of **A**ssociated conditions (e.g., anaemia, rheumatic fever, endocarditis, etc) and **D**iuretics, **D**igoxin, **D**iet (salt/fluid restriction), vaso **D**ilators (ACE inhibitors), **D**opamine/ **D**obutamine (dopamine and dobutamine are only for cardiac failure with circulatory shock).

ATRIAL SEPTAL DEFECT (Secundum)

Note: ASD is hardly ever kept for examination. Hence in case of L to R shunt lesions the differential diagnosis is essentially VSD/PDA.

- Accounts for about 8% of congenital defects.
- Look for any features suggestive of syndromes (e.g., Holt-Oram, Noonan's syndrome, trisomy, etc).
- Growth and development are usually normal.
- No cyanosis, no clubbing.
- Normal pulse.
- Right ventricular heave in left parasternal area is less likely. However, pulsations in left

14

parasternal area is common due to large right atrium.

Pulsations of precordium and epigastric areas are common in ASD.

S1 is normal and S2 wide split and fixed in ASD. P2 usually is not loud (pulmonary hypertension is unlikely during childhood in ASD).

- Fixed splitting of the second heart sound (if not convincing, re-examine with the child standing).

  During inspiration, the negative intrathoracic pressure attracts more venous return to the right side of the heart so that the right ventricle takes longer time to eject. Thus, P_2 gets delayed and the split of the second sound widens in a normal child. Negative intrathoracic pressure increases the capacity of pulmonary vasculature and hence less blood returns to the left side of the heart. In ASD, there is a non restrictive communication between the two atria so that these two effects gets mutually cancelled during inspiration and expiration and hence there is no respiratory variation of split of second sound (also see p 317).

  The fixed split of S2 narrows down (but still persists) with the development of PAH in later life, with loud P2.
- Soft ejection systolic murmur (usually 2-3/6) loudest at the second left intercostal space. May have a click.
- With a large shunt there may also be a diastolic murmur in the tricuspid area due to increased flow across the tricuspid valve (right atrium receives additional blood from left atrium due to L to R shunt across ASD). This murmur is better heard if legs of the supine patient are elevated by the examiner to increase the venous return.

  Once PAH develops in adult life, diastolic tricuspid murmur is no longer audible, and instead tricuspid regurgitation murmur (systolic murmur) appears. This TR may be audible in PAH of any aetiology, not just ASD or VSD.
- Rarely causes symptoms in childhood, but untreated, it may present with pulmonary hypertension, heart failure or arrhythmias in early *adult life*. One must always remember that symptomatic secundum ASD is rare in childhood; one must think twice if it really is ASD if the child is symptomatic. If so, whether it can be primum ASD rather than secondum one.
- ***Ostium primum ASD***: This may present with failure to thrive and heart failure in infancy or childhood. May be associated with Down syndrome as part of endocardial cushion defect. The defect occurs in the lowest part of the atrial septum, with a cleft in the anterior leaflet of the mitral valve. Thus, the presence of additional MR murmur strongly favours a diagnosis of primum defect. ECG findings are left axis deviation, biventricular hypertrophy (if MR is also significant) and incomplete right bundle branch block (rSR pattern in the right precordial leads like V_1, V_2).

Investigations

- X-ray: There is right atrial and right ventricular enlargement, prominent main pulmonary artery segment and increased pulmonary vascularity.
- ECG: Demonstrates normal or right axis deviation, right bundle branch block (rSR pattern in V_1) and usually right ventricular hypertrophy (compare with primum atrial septal defect).
- In *ostium primum type of ASD,* there is left axis deviation.

Treatment

Treatment is surgical, using cardiopulmonary bypass with either direct suturing or a patch. Device closure is another option. Usually, the closure is done at around 5 years of age.

Infective endocarditis prophylaxis is generally not required for ASD as there is no high pressure gradient flow. After correction (device/patch), IE prophylaxis is given for 6 months.

TETRALOGY OF FALLOT

The four abnormalities are RVOT obstruction at infundibuluar/valvar/supravalvar level, ventricular septal defect, hypertrophy of the right ventricle, overriding of aorta. In 25% of cases, there may be a right aortic arch.

When there is an additional atrial septal defect also it is described as ***pentalogy***. When the pulmonary obstruction is not severe enough to cause right to left shunt, it allows bidirectional shunt across the VSD and frank cyanosis is absent. Then the condition is called ***pink Fallot***. A combination of right ventricular hypertrophy, pulmonary stenosis and atrial septal defect is sometimes referred to as ***trilogy of Fallot***.

The clustering of the above four defects is because of a specific abnormality occurring during fetal life. This abnormality is an *anterior and cephaloid deviation of the infundibular septum*. Thus, the infundibular septum fails to fuse with the muscular part of the septum producing VSD. The anterior deviation of the infundibular septum encroaches on to the outflow tract of the anteriorly placed right ventricle, which is the reason for the obstruction at infundibulum. Right ventricle pumping against this obstruction invariably results in right ventricular hypertrophy. The anterior displacement of the infundibular septum drags the aortic root along with it so that it overrides the ventricular septal defect.

TOF may be associated with chromosomal anomalies - deletion 10q, syndromes such as Goldenhaar, VATER, DiGeorge, maternal PKU, etc.

Check for complications of paradoxical embolism such as thrombosis causing neurological deficits (which may also occur secondary to brain abscess).

Note: In the scenario of examination, the student must keep in mind that a cyanotic heart disease kept for examination is most likely to be TOF. Without corrective surgery, more than 90% all other congenital cyanotic heart diseases will die. And the acquired cyanotic heart disease namely Eisenmenger syndrome is rare in paediatric age group (generally in second decade and beyond). So in a case of cyanotic heart disease not fitting in with the classic features of TOF, always consider whether it can fit into some uncommon presentations of TOF before offering some alternate diagnoses.

Symptoms and Signs

1. Cyanosis and Clubbing: Cyanosis in TOF is generally not present at birth, but is delayed for a few weeks to months (2–6 months) possibly due to:
   - Closure of the PDA that may have been persisting (and hence preventing cyanosis) for some weeks after birth.
   - Progressive infundibular stenosis due to infundibular hypertrophy.
   - Increased oxygen demand due to the activity of the growing infant.
2. Dyspnoea:
   - Dyspnoea occurs on exertion and it is relieved by squatting for a few minutes. Squatting blocks venous return and prevents highly unsaturated venous blood from lower limbs from reaching the heart. This also exerts pressure on arteries increasing the peripheral resistance so that more blood is diverted to the pulmonary circulation (which has much less pressure).

History of Present Illness

Ask for history of spells, squatting, history suggestive of any neurological event, haemoptysis, etc. Headache, if complained of, may be because of polycythaemia or early evidence of more serious CNS problems like cerebral abscess. If there is a history of diarrhoea, always think of dehydration and associated cerebral thrombosis, especially if the child is less than 2 years. It is not a bad idea to ask about any recent procedures like dental work.

1. **Pulse** - Normal volume pulse. High volume pulse is rare, e.g., when there are plenty of collaterals. Beware of bradycardia as many patients are on propranolol for prevention of spells. Compare pulse between two upper limbs, if post-BT shunt there could be a difference in volume.
2. **BP** - Normal; anisosphygmia (BP difference between two upper limbs) if post-BT shunt.
3. **JVP** - Normal.

General Examination

- Always comment on oral hygiene.
- Growth and development: Some delay in the development may be there, especially motor, due to the restriction of activity due to the heart disease. Growth retardation because of cyanotic heart disease is unlikely unless hypoxia is so severe. Hence, must think of alternate reasons for growth delay in case it is present.

Inspection

Normal precordium. Pulsations if visible at right upper sternal border, may be explained as due to right aortic arch.

Palpation

Normal apex beat (neither forceful, nor heaving); generally no cardiac enlargement on clinical examination; subxiphoid pulsations suggestive of right ventricular hypertrophy; parasternal heave is less likely. Since the RV directly empties into the aorta through the VSD (thus there is no expansile impulse on to the anterior chest wall) and because of the narrow infundibular chamber situated beneath the sternum, the left parasternal heave, so characteristic of RVH, is not seen in TOF. However, RV pulsation may be felt over the epigastrium. A thrill is unlikely as the pulmonary flow is restricted.

Auscultation

S1 - Normal

S2 - Usually, soft, P2 delayed (but often cannot be appreciated), S2 may be heard as single in pulmonary area; loud S2 if heard, is A2 and is due to the dextroposed anteriorly placed dilated aortic root.

Click: In TOF, the stenosis is commonly infundibular and not valvular. Hence, a click when heard is unlikely to be of pulmonary origin. It is more likely to be originating from the dilated aorta. Dilatation of aorta is expected as aorta receives additional quantities of blood shunted through VSD, due to pulmonary stenosis not allowing normal blood flow to pulmonary circulation. Note that the murmur in TOF is never due to the VSD as the R–L shunt across the large VSD does not have a large pressure gradient to generate a murmur.

Murmurs

The murmur of tetralogy of Fallot is the *ejection systolic murmur* of pulmonary stenosis best heard at 2nd or sometimes 3rd left ICS close to the sternum; since the pulmonary stenosis is often infundibular, the murmur is often heard lower down, like third or even fourth left space in addition to second space. Intensity of murmur is about 2-3/6. In tight stenosis, the murmur may hardly be audible (intensity and duration of murmur is lesser if the stenosis is tighter). Always look for collateral murmurs elsewhere in the chest and back, in severe TOF.

Important: Significant cardiomegaly and cardiac failure *do not* occur in TOF. Because the aorta overrides the septal defect, right ventricle is able to decompress directly into the aorta. Thus, supra-systemic pressures do not develop in RV and hence is protected from developing heart failure.

The presence of cardiac failure in TOF is exceptionally rare. Examples are:

- Severe anaemia
- Infective endocarditis
- Systemic hypertension
- Coincidental myocardial disease (e.g., myocarditis)
- TOF with absent pulmonary valve syndrome

Differential Diagnosis

Congenital cyanotic heart diseases can be remembered as 5 "T": TOF, TGA, TAPVR, truncus arteriosus and tricuspid valve anomalies (tricuspid atresia, tricuspid valve downward displacement in Ebstein anomaly).

The term 'admixture lesions' are used to describe conditions where the cyanosis results from obligatory mixing of desaturated and oxygenated blood. The mixing can occur at venous level (total anomalous pulmonary venous return), atrial level (common atrium), ventricular level (single ventricle) or great artery level (truncus arteriosus). The cyanosis is usually mild.

Investigations

- Blood: PCV (to detect hemoconcentration), MCHC and red cell distribution width (because of polycythemia, anaemia cannot be reliably detected by haemoglobin estimation), platelet count and peripheral smear.
- ECG may show evidence of RVH, early transition of predominant r wave in chest lead V_1 changing to predominant S wave in V_{2-3}. X-ray may show an upturned apex, no shadow of main pulmonary artery, right aortic arch if present, and oligemic lung fields (clear lung fields and hilum). The X-ray appearance is often called "boot shaped."

Management

- Correction of anaemia with iron.
- Proper attention to dental hygiene to prevent infective endocarditis.
- Prophylaxis against infective endocarditis (p 337).
- Reduction of PCV when it is high (PCV above 65% is an indication for partial exchange transfusion).
- Treatment of complications.
- Definitive surgery: Closure of VSD and relief of pulmonary obstruction. Timing and type of surgical treatment depend on the clinical severity of the lesion though in most centres all TOF are now operated as early as possible, irrespective of symptoms.
- Palliative shunt procedure (e.g., Blalock-Taussig operation) may be required before definitive surgery if the right ventricular outflow tract is poorly developed. The surgery consists of anastamosing subclavian artery with pulmonary artery to increase the pulmonary blood flow.

14

Complications

1. **Cyanotic (hypoxic) spells**: Cyanotic (hypoxic) spell is due to decreased pulmonary blood flow; it can occur following crying and exertion like straining at stool; 'squatting' may increase systemic vascular resistance, reduce venous return from the legs and improve pulmonary blood flow and help relieve the spell.
   - *Treatment of Hypoxic Spell*
     Mnemonic: **POMP**. **P**osition, **O**xygen, **M**orphine and **P**ropranolol.
     - *Knee chest position*: This acts like squatting by increasing peripheral resistance.
     - *100% oxygen inhalation.*
     - *Morphine*: This calms the child thus decreases respiratory rate, and hence reduces oxygen requirement. It may relieve infundibular spasm.
     - *IV propranolol*: Reduces infundibular spasm; also β block allows unopposed α action in peripheral vessels allowing increase in peripheral vascular resistance.

- Others: Sodium bicarbonate, IV fluids. To increase peripheral vascular resistance one may use methoxamine or phenyl ephrine.
- *Prevention of further episodes* can be done by oral propranolol & correction of anaemia with iron.
- Frequent spells is an indication for early surgery.

2. **Cerebral thrombosis** (<2 years age, usually following diarrhoea and dehydration); rapid correction of dehydration with IV fluids is the treatment.
3. **Cerebral abscess** (>2 years age): Paradoxical embolism (peripheral embolus bypassing the pulmonary vascular bed because of right to left shunt) may bring the infection to the brain. Fever, signs of increased intracranial tension, and localizing neurological signs. Bacteria by-pass the filtering mechanism of lung (by R–L shunt) and localizes in the hypoxic brain (the organisms are anaerobic or micro aerophilic; hence the initial antibiotics are penicillin and metronidazole).
4. **Bacterial endocarditis**
5. **Haemorrhagic tendency** (hemoptysis): Platelet dysfunction due to hypoxia.

RHEUMATIC FEVER WITH CARDITIS

Arthritis: Large joints are affected in rheumatic fever; one joint may get relieved when the next joint gets affected; or multiple joints are affected simultaneously. Small joint involvement, temporomandibular joint involvement and morning stiffness are pointers to rheumatoid rather than rheumatic arthritis. Signs of active carditis may be resting tachycardia, S_3 gallop, soft S_1, cardiomegaly/failure, pericardial rub or murmurs due to valvulitis. CCF may not improve in spite of treatment in the following situations: anaemia, co-existing infections, infective endocarditis, poor compliance of drugs (usually due to gastritis), etc.

Always look for rash (erythema marginatum), subcutaneous nodules (better seen than felt) and abnormal movements (chorea).

Rheumatic Carditis

- **Pulse** - Tachycardia if there is active carditis; usually pulse is of normal character, except in aortic regurgitation where we may get high volume pulse. Be careful to look for arrhythmias, especially atrial fibrillation.
- **BP** - Wide pulse pressure in cases of AR.
- **JVP** - Elevated if associated with CCF.

Inspection

Bulging precordium in long standing valvular lesions; no bulge likely in acute carditis of initial rheumatic episode.

Palpation

Shifting of apex beat; associated thrills (depending on the lesion).

Percussion

Cardiomegaly may be demonstrable.

Table 14.2 Revised Jones criteria 2015 for the diagnosis of rheumatic fever

Low risk	Moderate/High risk
Major Criteria: 1) Carditis clinical/subclinical; 2) Polyarthritis; 3) Chorea; 4) Erythema marginatum 5) Subcutaneous nodules	**Major Criteria**: 1) Carditis clinical/subclinical; 2) Mono arthritis/Polyarthritis/polyarthralgia; 3) Chorea; 4) Erythema marginatum; 5) Subcutaneous nodules
Minor Criteria: 1) Polyarthralgia; 2) Fever > 38.5°C; 3) ESR > 60 mm/hr, CRP > 3 mg%; 4) Prolonged PR interval (unless carditis is a major criteria)	**Minor Criteria**: 1) Mono arthralgia; 2) Fever > 38.5°C; 3) ESR > 30 mm/hr, CRP > 3 mg%; 4) Prolonged PR interval (unless carditis is a major criteria)

Note: Low risk-RF incidence in school aged children <2/100,000 or RHD prevalence <1/1000 population/year.

Auscultation

- **S1** - Muffled or soft
- **S2** - Normal
- **S3** gallop if in CCF

Murmurs

Pan systolic murmur at apex generally 3/6, may or may not be radiating to the axilla and back (MR murmur is almost universal in rheumatic carditis) Apical mid diastolic murmur (Carey Coomb's murmur) due to funtional mitral stenosis (valve oedema).

Rarely, early diastolic murmur of aortic regurgitation, and pericardial friction rub may be audible.

Investigations

- Blood counts (total count is elevated), ESR (high), CRP (high). Unlike ESR, CRP is not affected by cardiac failure or co-existing anaemia.
- ECG (prolonged PR interval, >0.16 sec)
- X-ray chest (cardiomegaly)
- ASO titre (elevated titre)
- Throat culture (optional; may be positive for streptococcus)
- Echocardiography

Treatment

- Bed rest (till the ESR normalizes). Usual minimum is 2 weeks.
- Injection procaine penicillin IM once daily for 10 days. Oral penicillin (penicillin V 250 mg 3–4 times daily for 10 days) is the alternative.
- Rheumatic arthritis with or without carditis but without cardiomegaly or cardiac failure: Aspirin 75–100 mg/kg/day for minimum 6 weeks (8 weeks if mild carditis).
- Rheumatic carditis with cardiomegaly or heart failure: Prednisolone 2 mg/kg/day for 2 weeks. If the ESR has come down, start tapering the dose, taking off one tablet (5 mg) every third day till the steroid is totally taken off. While tapering of steroid is started, aspirin is added (75 mg/kg/day) and continued to complete a total of 12 weeks of anti-inflammatory therapy.
- Cardiac failure: Usually responds to steroids itself. Consider the standard management of cardiac failure (however, digoxin is avoided or used in reduced dose).
- Rheumatic chorea: Haloperidol 0.1 mg/kg/day.
- Prophylaxis: This is needed for all children who already had rheumatic fever. Injection benzathene penicillin 12 lakh units once in 3 weeks after test dose each time, or oral penicillin V 250 mg twice daily: till 21 years for rheumatic arthritis (as per American Heart Association, 1997) and at least until 40 years or lifelong for rheumatic heart disease.

Prognosis

Majority of mitral regurgitation following the initial episode of rheumatic fever disappear by the end of first year. AR if present on initial presentation, is likely to persist.

MITRAL REGURGITATION

Symptoms

- Dyspnoea (stiff lungs due to pulmonary venous congestion).
- Palpitation (tachycardia to compensate for the reduced cardiac output; palpitation due to atrial fibrillation is quite rare in paediatrics).
- Fatigue (since part of the blood leaks into the left atrium during systole, the forward output through the aorta is insufficient to meet the demands of exertion and hence the fatigue).
- **Pulse** may be normal volume ("pseudo collapsing" low volume pulse described in yesteryear literature is difficult to appreciate in children).
- **BP** normal. Pulse pressure may normal or slightly wider than normal.
- **JVP** not elevated but can be elevated if associated with cardiac failure.

Inspection

Apex: Shifted downwards and outwards, with hyperkinetic precordium in severe MR.

Palpation

- In moderate to severe MR, apex is shifted downwards and outwards, and precordium may be hyperkinetic.
- Left parasternal pulsation (rather than heave) is more common, which may be due to the huge left atrial enlargement and less likely to be due to right ventricular hypertrophy. Although the blood regurgitates to the dilated left atrium during systole, as there is no stenosis to mitral valve, all this blood is free to come down to left ventricle during diastole, and hence there is no back pressure to pulmonary venous side. Hence, pulmonary hypertension is less common compared to MS.
- Systolic thrill in the mitral area may be present.
- Mild MR can have normal precordium to palpation and normal apex.

Auscultation

- **S1** - Soft.
- **S2** - Normal split in mild MR and widely split and movable with respiration in moderate or severe MR (as part of the blood is pushed to left atrium during systole, left ventricular systolic phase ends earlier causing early A2, and hence widened split of S2).
- **S3** may be audible at apex (rapid filling of excess blood from left atrium to left ventricle).

Murmurs

High pitched, soft blowing pan systolic murmur (sounds like "shhh") conducted to the axilla (or to the back when anterior leaflet is involved and to the precordium when the posterior leaflet is involved). The pansystolic murmur of MR decreases on standing (the peripheral resistance is decreased, so more blood is pumped into the systemic circulation and the MR decreases); MR murmur increases on squatting and hand grip (these procedures that increase the peripheral resistance will make pumping to systemic circulation more difficult and hence more blood leaks to the low pressure chamber, namely left atrium).

Functional mid diastolic murmur due to increased flow across the mitral valve.

Investigations

- ***CXR***: Cardiomegaly; left atrial enlargement may be seen as shadow in shadow on the right heart border.
- ***ECG***: Evidence of left atrial enlargement and left ventricle volume overload (deep q and tall T in V5, V6) may be seen in ECG.
- ***Echocardiography***: It will assess the severity of MR; can detect other causes of MR like mitral valve prolapse. It will also help in assessing the left ventricular function.

Differential Diagnosis

Tricuspid regurgitation (murmur increases on inspiration), VSD, hypertrophic obstructive cardiomyopathy, etc.

Other causes of MR: Mitral valve prolapse, infective endocarditis, dilated cardiomyopathy, collagen vascular disease like SLE or rheumatoid arthritis, congenital conditions like parachute mitral valve.

Complications

Left ventricular failure, infective endocarditis, atrial fibrillation, etc.

Management

Mild MR does not require any cardiac medication. They only require prophylaxis against infective endocarditis and rheumatic fever.

Treatment of Severe MR

- Digoxin and Diuretics:
  Reduction of afterload using angiotensin converting enzyme inhibitors. Vasodilators reduces

the peripheral vascular resistance and thus the resistance against which the left ventricle has to pump is reduced. Thus, more blood reaches systemic circulation rather than left atrium.

- *Infective endocarditis prophylaxis*
- *Rheumatic prophylaxis*
- Warfarin if left atrial clot is present or in case of atrial fibrillation (both are likely in adults, not childen).
- Surgery is considered in severe MR that is symptomatic despite medical management.

Useful Points on MR

- Most common cardiac lesion seen in patients with acute rheumatic carditis and established rheumatic heart disease is MR.
- MR murmur may disappear in a significant percentage of patients (within 1 year or so), especially if the initial MR is mild, there is no CHF and there is no recurrence of rheumatic fever.
- MR murmur is less likely to disappear if the patient has severe MR, CHF or clinical pericarditis at presentation.
- In some cases, the MR gradually disappears or decreases and then presents with features of MS later.
- Although mortality in acute rheumatic fever is low now, the main cause of mortality is acute severe MR; valve replacement in this setting has been shown to improve survival.
- Brisk pulse may be seen with severe MR (may appear high volume at start due to high volume output from left ventricle but suddenly the pulse volume drops as the blood gushes to the lower pressure left atrium).
- Presence of cardiac enlargement, presence of LV apex, loudness of murmur and presence of S_3 and mid-diastolic flow murmur are indicators of severity.
- In combined MS/MR if S_3 is present, significant MS is unlikely; but first make sure 'S_3 is S_3' and not opening snap.
- Mitral valve repair or replacement is the treatment in severe MR with symptoms of left ventricular dysfunction.

MITRAL STENOSIS

Usual presenting symptoms are fatigue and exercise intolerance (because of mitral stenosis, less blood reaches left ventricle during exertion and hence these symptoms); dyspnoea on exertion; paroxysmal nocturnal dyspnoea (because of stenosis at mitral valve, blood in pulmonary circulation stagnates and seeps out to produce pulmonary oedema); chest pain; hemoptysis (rupture of vessels due to back pressure on pulmonary circulation). 14

Facies: Malar flush that was described in MS in yesteryears is hardly seen nowadays possibly because of earlier detection and correction of MS.

Oatner's syndrome: It is hoarseness of voice due to compression of left recurrent laryngeal nerve by the enlarged left atrium. Hardly seen nowadays.

- **Pulse** - Low volume pulse, pulse volume decreases with the severity of stenosis (because of mitral stenosis, less blood reaches left ventricle, and hence less blood pumped to peripheral circulation). The pulse may be irregularly irregular in the presence of atrial fibrillation.
- Respiratory rate may be increased as there is invariably pulmonary venous congestion.
- **BP** - Normal or low.
- **JVP** - Prominent 'a' waves.

Inspection

Apex beat may be visible.

Palpation

- Apex beat: Tapping apex, may be displaced outwards due to RVH. There may be palpable P2 (associated PAH is almost universal). A diastolic thrill may be elicited in the mitral area.

Auscultation

- **S1** - Loud
- **S2** - May be loud with loud P2 component (PAH)
  Opening snap if present is heard after the second sound (best heard at or just inside the apex), with diaphragm pressed firmly on chest wall.

Murmurs

Low-pitched mid-diastolic rough and rumbling murmur with pre-systolic accentuation, best heard with bell of stethoscope with patient in left lateral position (sounds like urrrrrrub with loudness increasing towards the end). Murmur will start with opening snap, if snap is audible. If murmur is not audible, try auscultating in left lateral position with breath held in expiration. Still inaudible murmurs may be made out after exertion (like going up and down the stairs: but get permission from examiners before doing so, because MS patients tolerate exertion poorly).

Rarely, ejection systolic murmur is heard in pulmonary area in case of associated pulmonary hypertension.

Differential Diagnosis

Tricuspid stenosis (murmur increases with inspiration), congenital MS (extremely rare), Carey coomb's murmur (in the acute phase of rheumatic carditis), Austin Flint murmur, etc. They are discussed elsewhere.

Combination of MR and MS is very common in rheumatic heart disease. Clinically, MS can be considered the prominant lesion when there is loud S1, opening snap or presystolic accentuation of diastolic murmur. MR may be the dominant lesion when these are absent, apex is forceful & S_3 is audible.

Complications

Infective endocarditis, right ventricular failure, atrial fibrillation.

Investigations

- ***X ray***: The enlargement of the left atrium is shown in the X-ray chest as a double outline of the *right* cardiac border. The left atrial appendage will show up as a bulge in the *left* cardiac border just below the pulmonary artery. The pulmonary artery, the left atrial appendage and the ventricular border together gives the appearance of straightening of left cardiac border. The lung fields appear congested and Kerley B lines *may* be seen (fine horizontal lines of engorged lymphatics at the costophrenic angles). Upper lobe veins may be prominent (the X-ray picture is likened to "stag's horn"). Since there is obstruction to venous return from pulmonary circulation, the blood, flowing under gravity stagnates in upper lobe veins in upright position.
- **ECG**: If the patient is in sinus rhythm, the P wave will be wide (best seen in lead L2) or bifid (in V1 lead) due to the electrical conduction through the large left atrium taking a longer duration. There will be evidence of right ventricular hypertrophy.

Management

Medical

- Rheumatic prophylaxis.
- Infective endocarditis prophylaxis.
- Diuretic if there is dyspnoea (to reduce pulmonary venous load).
- Beta blocker to reduce the heart rate (prolongs the diastolic time, so more time for blood to flow via stenotic valve).
- Digoxin is not indicated in normal sinus rhythm (may be considered in atrial fibrillation).
- Anticoagulation must be considered in atrial fibrillation to prevent formation of atrial clot.

Surgical

- Balloon mitral valvuloplasty: It is the procedure of choice in severe MS in children.
- Closed mitral valvotomy
- Open mitral valvotomy
- If there is associated significant mitral regurgitation, valve replacement is preferred.

Additional Points on Mitral Stenosis

- History of rheumatic fever may be *absent* in up to 50% of cases of mitral stenosis.
- Juvenile rheumatic MS is defined as that occurring in those less than 20 years of age.
- Juvenile rheumatic MS is more common in Indian population, i.e., the latent period from acute rheumatic fever to the development of MS is shorter in Indians. Increased virulence of organism, more frequent rheumatic recurrences, etc, are some of the proposed explanations for this phenomenon.
- Exertional dyspnoea and fatigue (rather than palpitations) are more common in isolated MS. Ask for history suggestive of paroxysmal nocturnal dyspnoea.
- Chance of acute pulmonary oedema is less in patients with severe PAH as the pulmonary bed is partly protected from over circulation and hence the interstitial leak.
- Compared to adults, frequency of atrial fibrillation is less in juvenile MS.
- Note that the murmur of MS may be sharply localized to a small area and may be missed unless specifically looked for. Look for opening snap.
- Presystolic accentuation will be absent in case of atrial fibrillation.
- The murmur of MS may be difficult to hear in the following situations: severe pulmonary arterial hypertension and right ventricular hypertrophy with right ventricle forming the apex; associated significant aortic valve lesions; low cardiac output states; patients with thick chest wall.
- In difficult cases, mild exercise like few sit ups or walking a few times across the room may bring out the murmur of MS.
- A_2-opening snap interval is inversely related to severity of MS.
- Length and loudness of murmur is related to severity.

AORTIC REGURGITATION

Symptoms

- Palpitation (to compensate for the reduced forward flow due to the leaking back of blood into the left ventricle during diastole, the heart rate is maintained high)
- Chest pain
- Exertional dyspnoea
- **Pulse**: The pulse is high volume, collapsing
- **BP**: The pulse pressure is wide. At times, the Korotkoff sound never disappears, remains audible till the cuff is deflated to zero. In such instances, the diastolic pressure must be taken as the muffling of Korotkoff, not its disappear-ance.
- **JVP**- Not elevated.

Inspection

Apex - Shifted downwards and outwards, in severe AR.

Palpation

In moderate to severe AR, apex is shifted downwards and outwards; precordium is hyperkinetic. Thrill due to AR is unlikely. Carotid thrill due to increased flow through the carotids (unlikely to be due to associated AS).

Auscultation

- **S1** - Soft
- **S2** - Normal
- **S3** is not usual, when audible, indicates left ventricular diastolic dysfunction.

Murmurs

High-pitched early diastolic decrescendo murmur, blowing in quality, best heard in the third space in the left sternal boarder and also in the second space in the right upper sternal boarder. Faint murmurs can be picked up if the patient is made to sit up, lean forward and hold the breath in expiration.

Other murmurs that can occur in AR are

- *Austin Flint murmur*: It is a mid diastolic murmur. It is possibly due to the fluttering of the mitral valve interposed between the two diastolic flows - one from the aorta and the other from the left atrium (see p 322).
- Aortic ejection systolic murmur due to high flow across the left ventricular outflow tract (it is due to increased flow and not due to AS). If this is due to organic aortic stenosis, one cannot have a high volume pulse.

The following indicates severity of AR

- High volume collapsing pulse and wide pulse pressure.
- Cardiomegaly with left ventricular apex.
- Hill sign (the difference between the lower limb and upper limb BP, 20-39 = mild AR; 40-59 = moderate AR; >60 = severe AR).
- *Long* early diastolic murmur.
- Austin Flint murmur.
- Peripheral signs (seen only in severe AR, mostly in adults).

The peripheral signs in AR

See p 303.

Investigations

- ***X-ray***: Cardiomegaly.
- ***ECG***: Usually, the rhythm is sinus. Left ventricular hypertrophy of volume overload type (deep Q and tall T in left chest leads) and left axis deviation.
- ***Echo***: It can assess the severity of AR and can also assess the left ventricular contractile function. Also can recognize whether the AR is due to congenital bicuspid aortic valve.

Aortic Regurgitation vs. Pulmonary Regurgitation Murmur

Inspiratory increase is seen in PR murmur (venous return to the right side of heart increases on inspiration, see p 322).

If second sound is well audible, one can make out that AR murmur begins after A2 while PR murmur begins after P2.

Handgrip increases the murmur in AR while PR murmur is unaffected (increase in peripheral systemic vascular resistance will make it difficult to pump to systemic circulation and hence increase AR murmur).

Complications

Left ventricular failure, infective endocarditis, atrial fibrillation.

Management

Medical

- Mild AR:
  - Infective endocarditis prophylaxis
  - Rheumatic prophylaxis
  - Normal activity at school except competitive sports
- Moderate to severe AR:
  Generally have subtle or frank cardiac failure. Depending on the risk of cardiac failure, one can start digoxin before clinically detectable cardiac failure (this helps by aug-menting contractility).
- Digoxin
- Diuretics
- Vasodilators: Angiotensin converting enzyme inhibitors (ACEI); it brings down the peripheral resistance so that more blood reaches the systemic circulation.

- Rheumatic and endocarditis prophylaxis.
- Surgery is advised if the left ventricle function is decreasing while on optimum medical management.

Additional Points on Aortic Regurgitation

- Look for marfanoid features in addition to history of rheumatic fever.
- *Isolated* AR in acute rheumatic fever is unusual; however, AR occurs in up to 25% of cases of rheumatic heart disease along with mitral regurgitation.
- Peripheral signs are seen only with severe AR.
- Length of murmur is an indicator of severity.
- Early diastolic murmur at left upper sternal border may be well heard at lower sternal border as well. Because of the big pressure gradient, the leak starts immediately after the A_2. It must be looked for very carefully not to miss the faint murmur (best auscultated with diaphragm of stethoscope firmly pressed). It is a high-pitched, blowing "Shhh" murmur. It is usually best heard in the third left space close to the sternum rather than the classical aortic area. Murmur may be best heard in sitting up, leaning forward and breath held in expiration. Elevation of arms also helps in making the murmur clearer as this manoeuvre increases diastolic leak by gravity. Manoeuvres that raise the peripheral resistance increase diastolic leak so that squatting and isometric hand grip may increase the murmur. So in doubtful cases auscultation may be repeated in the squatting position, which by increasing peripheral resistance, increases the regurgitation.
- Mid-diastolic murmur seen with AR (Austin Flint) is a sign of severity of AR, but should not be confused with the mid-diastolic murmur of MS. Austin Flint murmur is because of the anterior mitral cusp vibration between the diastolic stream of blood from LA to LV and regurgitant stream of AR.
- Acute development of AR (as in infective endocarditis) even if severe, may not have the classical features of chronic severe AR like peripheral signs, long EDM or Austin Flint murmur.
- If you are hearing a click also, meticulously look for evidence of AS. Click plus systolic and diastolic murmur may point towards a congenital bicuspid aortic valve. However, it is worth remembering that even when there is no organic AS, there may be a systolic murmur because of increased volume output from the LV. This flow murmur will be early peaking and shorter than the mid-to-late peaking and longer murmur seen with organic AS.
- PR murmur of pulmonary hypertension was originally described in cases of MS (Graham Steell's murmur), where pulmonary hypertension is almost universal. It is practically impossible to differentiate AR murmur from PR murmur. Hence, one may have to look for associated features. If the child is having pulmonary hypertension, it is a PR murmur. Also PR murmur is not associated with peripheral signs of AR (see p 303). Surgical correction of PS usually results in some PR where the murmur sounds very different, i.e., it is of rougher quality (lower pitch).

The following lesions are not typical examination cases. However, these lesions may form part of the syndromes of cases kept for examination and hence some knowledge of these lesions becomes necessary for the candidate.

Hence the following are discussed.

PULMONARY ARTERIAL HYPERTENSION

- Central cyanosis may be there (Eisenmenger)
- Finger clubbing (Eisenmenger)
- Normal pulse
- Right ventricular heave*

14

- No significant cardiac enlargement
- Palpable second sound in pulmonary area*
- Pulmonary area may be dull to percussion*
- Loud second heart sound in the pulmonary area*. Tip: If second sound is louder than the first at apex, consider pulmonary hypertension.
- Short ejection systolic murmur in pulmonary area* often preceded by an ejection click.*
- With established pulmonary hypertension, there is gradually increasing cyanosis and heart failure.
- ***Eisenmenger***: Eisenmenger syndrome describes pulmonary hypertension at systemic level due to pulmonary vascular resistance with reversed or bidirectional shunting. The term 'Eisenmenger complex' was used when the same was detected in ventricular septal defects. This was the original case reported and thus of historical importance only. Cyanosis and clubbing are likely.
- Eisenmenger syndrome secondary to PDA may have differential cyanosis and clubbing, the lower limbs being cyanotic and not the upper limbs. It is because the unsaturated blood is shunted to aorta from pulmonary artery distal to the area of origin of subclavian artery.
- Pulmonary hypertension may be primary (idiopathic); it may be secondary to congenital heart defects with increased pulmonary blood flow or raised pulmonary venous pressure.

  Treatment modalities in established pulmonary vascular disease include vasodilators like calcium channel blockers and prostaglandins, oral anticoagulation.

  Heart–lung transplantation is a possible treatment option.
- Sildenafil also is a useful drug.

AORTIC STENOSIS

- Look for dysmorphic features (e.g., Williams syndrome, Turner's syndrome). Elfin facies is described in case of congenital supravalvular AS. Note that here the stenosis is supravalvular. Since valves are not involved, ejection clicks will not be heard. May ask for history of vitamin D during pregnancy. Facies of Williams syndrome is shown in the photo (Fig. 14.1); prominent thick lips with open mouth, smooth long philtrum, anteverted nares, etc.

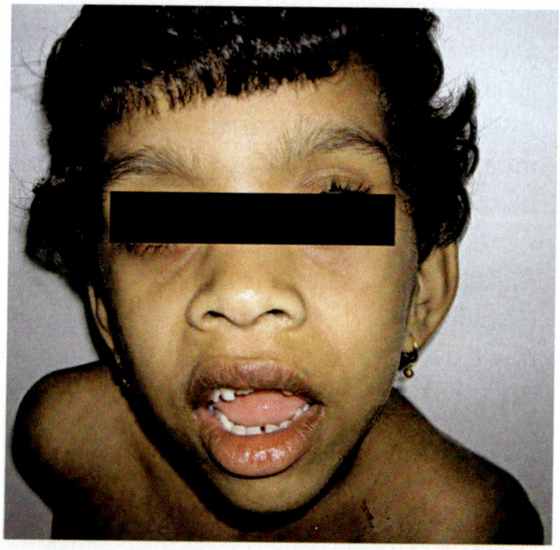

Fig.14.1 Williams syndrome

- Growth and development are not usually affected.
- No cyanosis, no clubbing, usually no oedema, no hepatic enlargement, JVP is normal.
- Usually asymptomatic; syncope and exertional dyspnoea are rarely the presentations.
- Pulse: Small volume and slow rising pulse.
- Heaving apex (examining fingers are raised and the lift is sustained).
- Clinically detectable cardiac enlargement is minimal, as it is concentric hypertrophy without dilatation.
- Systolic thrill in suprasternal notch.
- Ejection systolic murmur loudest over second right intercostal space and at cardiac apex; radiates to the neck and over the carotid arteries. It stands to common sense to believe that the later the maximum peak of murmur is reached, the greater is the stenosis because it

indicates that it took longer time to negotiate the obstruction. The murmur when heard at apex may appear softer and higher pitched than what is heard at the upper sternal border. When this is heard at apex one may suspect additional MR, but note that AS murmur is ejection and MR murmur is pansystolic. If A_2 is clearly audible at apex, it is unlikely that it is a pansystolic murmur.

- Often an ejection click precedes the murmur and is well heard at the apex also (best during expiration); the difference from pulmonary click in that it is 'constant ejection click.'
- Aortic second heart sound is soft and delayed; in congenital AS the A_2 may be normal.
- Paradoxical splitting of second heart sound may occur in severe stenosis (**Important**: Cannot be made out by auscultation).
- Accounts for about 5% of congenital heart lesions and is more common in boys; in fact, all congenital left ventricle outflow tract obstructive lesions (another example is COA) are more common in boys.
- Aortic valve in AS is commonly bicuspid with partial fusion of commissures, but it may be unicuspid or non-cusped.
- Obstruction may occur above the valve (supravalvular stenosis; see William syndrome discussed above) or below the valve (due to fibrous diaphragm).
- Valvotomy is required for severe stenosis, but if possible valve replacement should be postponed until adult life.
- Look for evidence of coarctation of aorta because bicuspid aortic valve is a common association in coarctation of aorta.
- Look carefully for AR murmur. Many of the congenital bicuspid aortic valves may have both AS and AR.

Note: **Coanda effect** is seen in supravalvar AS which is the preferential streaming of the jet into the innominate artery so that the right arm BP may be 10-15 mm more than the left arm BP.

PULMONARY STENOSIS

- Look for dysmorphic features (e.g., Noonan's syndrome, congenital rubella, etc).
- Growth and development are not usually affected because of the heart lesion per se.
- Normal pulse.
- Left parasternal heave (right ventricular hypertrophy).
- Systolic thrill in the second left intercostal space.
- Ejection click may be heard if valvular in origin; it is 'phasic' (p 319).
- Pulmonary component of second heart sound is soft.
- Harsh ejection systolic murmur loudest over the second left intercostal space; increasing severity of stenosis prolongs the duration of murmur.
- Splitting of the second heart sound widens with increasing severity of stenosis.
- In mild stenosis, the right ventricular to pulmonary artery pressure gradient is <25–30 mmHg and no treatment is required apart from antibiotic prophylaxis for infective endocarditis.
- The pressure gradient is >75–80 mmHg in severe stenosis.
- Balloon dilation valvuloplasty is now the preferred treatment.
- Severe stenosis can present in infancy with cyanosis (due to right-to-left shunt at the atrial level through the foramen ovale) and heart failure.

COARCTATION OF THE AORTA (COA)

- Look for features suggestive of Turner syndrome.
- Normal radial and brachial pulses; weak or absent femoral pulses and there may be radiofemoral delay.
- Elevated blood pressure in the right arm; reduced systolic and pulse pressure in the legs.

14

- Look for features suggestive of valvular aortic stenosis (see above).
- A late systolic murmur is often heard best at the back between the scapulae; in fact, the site of maximum intensity of the murmur helps to localize the site of COA.
- Collateral vessels may be palpable in the intercostals space and on the medial borders of the scapulae.
- The constriction usually occurs just distal to the origin of the left subclavian artery.
- Occasionally, the narrowing is above the origin of the left subclavian artery, giving rise to weak pulses in lower limbs plus reduced left upper limb pulses.
- In COA, pulse difference will not be seen in the *unusual situation* of COA with involvement of ostium of left subclavian artery and the right subclavian artery originating aberrantly from descending aorta distal to co arctation.
- Surgery is often used as the primary mode of treatment and balloon dilation if re-stenosis occurs, although recently the latter is increasingly being used as the first-line treatment in selected cases.

CHAPTER 15

Respiratory System

In a respiratory case, special stress is to be given to the following in history/general examination:

- History of measles, pertussis, history suggestive of foreign body aspiration, history of contact with tuberculosis, history of asthma, parental smoking, smoky kitchen, polluting factories, etc. In case of asthma, obtain history of pets at home, any known allergies, medications (e.g., relief with nebulization), smoking members in the family, exercise induced cough, school absenteeism, etc.
- Warm hands are seen in CO_2 retention, as in *severe* asthma. Altered sensorium, bounding pulse and warm extremities could mean impending respiratory failure.
- If the differential diagnosis includes tuberculosis as a strong possibility, look for phlyctenular conjunctivitis (p 527), erythema nodosum (p 543), scar/sinuses (indicating old lymph nodes), lymphadenopathy, etc.
- Severe hyperinflation (e.g., asthma) and tension pneumothorax may cause rise in JVP because of increased intrathoracic pressure not allowing free emptying of veins into the right atrium. Non-pulsatile raised JVP is seen in superior vena cava obstruction, usually the obstruction is by lymph nodes of mediastinum. SVC obstruction also causes swelling or reddening/cyanosis of the face and distended veins over the chest (sometimes Horner's syndrome as well).
- In long-standing pulmonary problems, mention if there is any evidence of PAH or cardiac failure.
- Mention if there is halitosis or not (bronchiectasis, lung abcess, sinusitis, poor oral hygiene, etc.
- Preference to lie on one side may mean a painful lesion on that side. 15
- Some of the facial chubbiness of infants with asthma may be due to steroids. So ask the mother if she feels there is puffy face or not.
- Recurrent respiratory infection: This is considered significant if more than 6 episodes in urban and more than 4 episodes in rural areas.

History suggestive of obstructive sleep apnoea: Decreased or no breath sounds during periods of apnoea but chest and abdomen move in an attempt to breath against an obstructed upper airway (e.g., Pierre Robin, adenoids, etc). The apnoeic episodes culminate in body disturbances, snoring and ultimately the child may wake up. This is in sharp contrast to central apnoea in preterm newborns where there is no breathing efforts at all during periods of apnoea.

ANATOMICAL CONSIDERATIONS

For describing the findings on clinical examination, the anterior chest is divided into supraclavicular (above clavicle), infraclavicular (up to the level of 2nd rib), mammary (up to the level of 5th rib) and inframammary areas (this terminology is not accepted by all authorities). Laterally, up to the 4th rib between the lines from anterior and poste-rior axillary fold is called axillary area and below it is infra-axillary area (Ref. 26). In the back, there is suprascapular, interscapular and infrascapular areas.

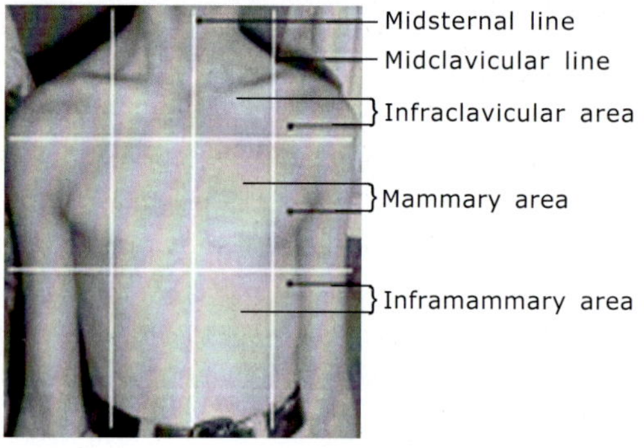

Fig.15.1 Anatomical areas in front

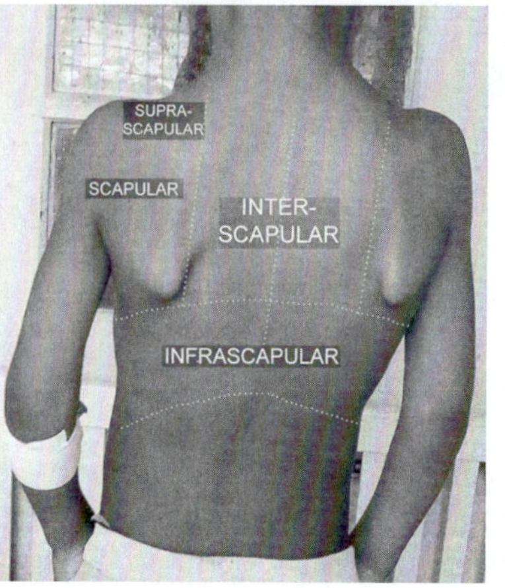

Fig.15.2 Anatomical areas of back

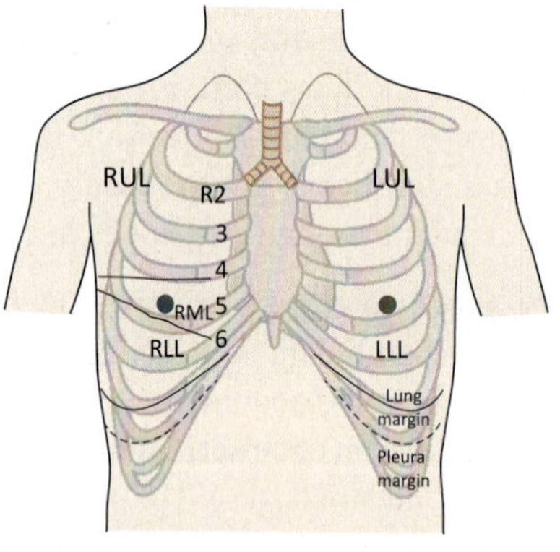

Fig.15.3 Front of chest

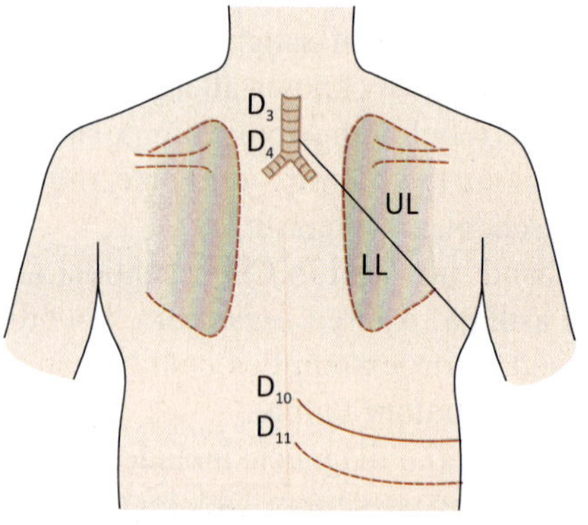

Fig.15.4 Back of chest

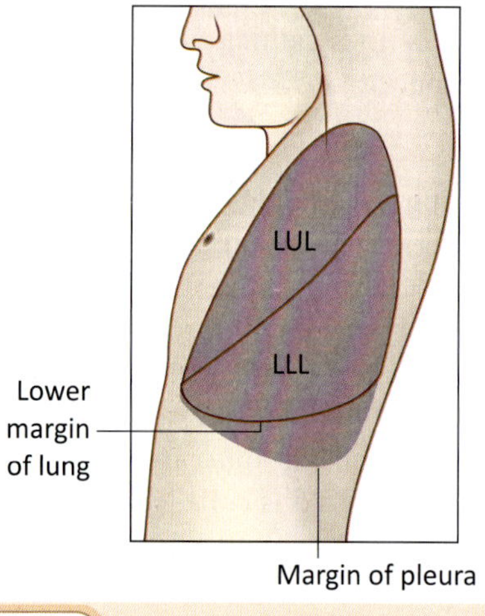

Fig.15.5 Left side of chest

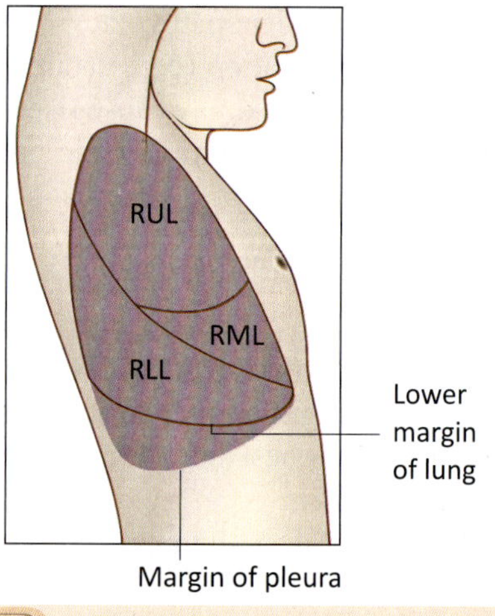

Fig.15.6 Right side of chest

Major Fissure

A curved line from the second thoracic spine in the back to the 6th costochondral junction (i.e., 6th rib in mammary line) in front represents the major fissure. A line from sternum at the level of fourth costal cartilage, joining the oblique or major fissure at midaxillary line represents the ***minor fissure*** on the right side. When one's hands are lifted up over the head, the vertebral border of the tilted scapula will approximately correspond to the major fissure posteriorly.

Ribs can be counted anteriorly from the ***angle of Louis*** (correspond to the 2nd rib joining the sternum) and posteriorly counted from C7 spine (the most prominent cervical spine).

At the lower border, the pleura extends beyond the lower lung border. The lower lung borders are 6th costal cartilage in the midclavicular line, 8th rib at midaxillary line, and 10th rib at midscapular line. The corresponding levels for the pleura are 6th, 10th and 12th ribs.

Bronchopulmonary segments are relatively independent units with their own airways and blood supply with minimal communication with the adjacent ones.

UPPER RESPIRATORY TRACT (see p 5)

Upper respiratory tract extends from nostrils to the laryngeal inlet. If the child has a nasal voice, it could be due to blocked nose, submucous cleft of the palate, etc. Submucous cleft of the palate is not visible, but can be palpated. Obstructed nostrils can be detected by placing a piece of cotton below each nostril and observing for its movement with respiration. Also one may look for mist in a glass slide placed beneath each nostril.

Comment if there is any nasal discharge, deviated nasal septum, etc. Nasal speculum examination is resented by most children and hence need not be attempted as a routine. The nasal septum is most pain sensitive and hence take care to see that the speculum (if used) is not directed medially.

15

Right upper lobe	Left upper lobe
Apical Anterior Posterior	Apical Anterior Posterior (on the left side, apical and posterior are sometimes together called apicoposterior)
Right middle lobe	**Left upper lobe, lingular segment**
Medial Lateral	Superior Inferior On the left side, there is no middle lobe, but instead has lingular lobe (which is part of upper lobe, thus it corresponds to the middle lobe on right side)
Right lower lobe	**Left lower lobe**
Apical (superior) Medial basal Anterior basal Lateral basal Posterior basal	Apical (superior) Anterior basal Lateral basal Posterior basal On the left side, because of the presence of heart there is hardly any medial basal segment

One may even use the otoscope and its speculum for nasal examination. The inside of the nose is more horizontal than is apparent by the external appearance and hence speculum examination with the child sitting (with the nose slightly upturned by the examiner's thumb) is preferable to the child lying down. The inferior turbinate is quite swollen in allergic children and this must not be confused with a polyp. One can note any bleeding or pus in the nasal cavity (in epistaxis, the bleeding points are usually seen at the lower end of the septum). Watery or mucoid discharge indicates viral rhinitis or allergic rhinitis. Purulent discharge may point towards sinusitis or nasopharyngitis. Look for frontal and maxillary sinus tenderness (note that frontal sinus is not fully pneumatized until 6–7 years of age). Ethmoid and maxillary sinuses are present at birth but quite small. Thus, sinusitis is unlikely in infancy and toddlerhood. Pushing the medial corner of the orbit, against the side of the nasal bridge, can elicit tenderness in the ethmoid sinus. Frontal sinus tenderness is elicited by percussion over the frontal area and maxillary sinus tenderness may be elicited by pressing over the maxilla. Sinusitis may present itself with indirect symptoms like headache (frontal sinus), peri-orbital oedema (ethmoid sinusitis), toothache (maxillary sinus), etc. Note that one of the important causes of *unilateral* persistent bloody/purulent nasal discharge is foreign body (rarely polyp).

Nasal obstruction (blocked nose): This is very common in allergic rhinitis, common cold, etc. Persistent unilateral nasal obstruction could be due to foreign body or polyp.

Allergic shiners: Bluish discolouration of lower lids. This is basically due to venous stasis resulting from inflammatory oedema.

Allergic salute: Line between the cartilaginous and bony portion of nasal septum. This is because of the constant rubbing of the nose upwards due to allergic irritation.

Dennie-Morgan line: Fold of skin just below the lower eyelid, bilaterally.

Allergic shiners, allergic salute and Dennie line indicate that the child is atopic. Allergic conjunctivitis may be part of the spectrum of allergic diseases in an asthmatic child.

Presence of conjunctivitis or history of conjunctivitis in the mother of a child 4–16 weeks age with pneumonia may point towards chlamydia pneumonia.

Inspection of pharynx, tonsils and ear is also part of examination of the upper respiratory tract. Sometimes, postnasal drip may be visible on examination of pharynx. A few round swellings in the pharynx are normal. In pharyngitis, their number increases and appears very red (the child may be requested to say ahh or one may use spatula to visualize the pharynx). Look for any torticollis, which could be related to upper respiratory problems like parapharyngeal abscess. Look for tragus tenderness, mastoid tenderness and have a look at tympanic membrane using otoscope. The Fig. 15.7 shows the normal appearance of landmarks of tympanic membrane. The pars flaccida is the region where redness is noted earliest in case of middle ear infection. Later there will be generalized redness of tympanic membrane, disappearance of cone of light, etc. Pneumatic otoscopy need not be attempted by the paediatrician.

A small child can be restrained by keeping him in mother's lap facing the examiner, one hand of mother pressing the child's head to her chest and

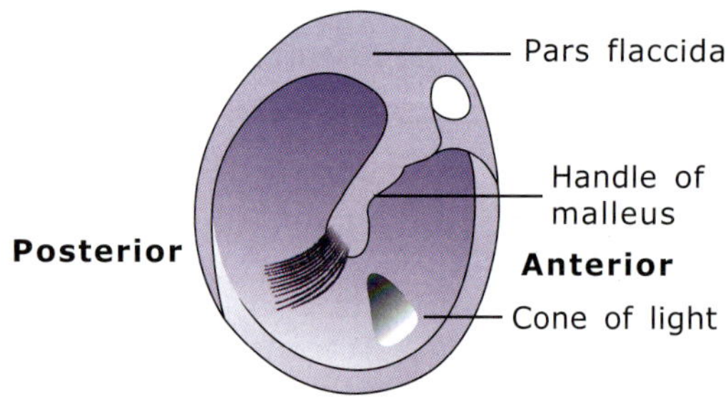

Fig.15.7 Right tympanic membrane

the other hand encircling the child's belly with both his hands restrained underneath it. Hold the otoscope in right hand; with left thumb and forefinger grasp pinna and pull it away and posteriorly to straighten the normally curved auditory canal. One may look for wax, foreign body, tympanic membrane, etc.

EXAMINATION OF THE CHEST (see p 5)

Inspection

Fully expose the chest and abdomen of the child. Comment on whether the child is dyspnoeic/tachypnoeic/accessory muscles of respiration are acting or not. Look for visible contractions of the sternomastoid, indrawing of supracalvicular fossa, flaring of alae nasi, etc. In severe dyspnoea, there may even be head bobbing.

It is best to inspect in the supine and sitting/standing positions. Examine from the front, back and also by looking over the shoulder from the back (flattening of infraclavicular areas are best made out looking down from the back with the child standing). Tangential views yield more information and hence in a supine patient one may squat and look from the foot end of bed, head end of bed, side of bed, etc.

Make a note of scars, aspiration site, etc, if present. Any localized bulge or swelling or dilated veins, if present, must be mentioned.

Respiratory rate and rhythm: Comment on the respiratory rate, rhythm (example of an abnormal rhythm is Cheyne-Stokes breathing) and character (predominantly abdominal or thoracic). Some irregularity of respiration may be voluntary or emotional (e.g., about to cry). In children, the respiration is most often abdominothoracic. Predominantly, thoracic breathing points towards some abnormality in the abdomen like massive hepatosplenomegaly, ascites, peritonitis, etc.

Normal resting respiratory rates in children:

- Newborn: 40–60/min
- Infants: 30–40/min
- Toddler: 20–30/min
- School age: 15–20/min

Normal ratio of respiration to pulse rate is 1:4. It may become 1:3 or 1:2 in pneumonia.

Abnormal rate is defined as that which is beyond 2 SD of mean respiratory rate for that age.

Decreased rate of respiration may be seen in narcotic poisoning, increased intracranial pressure, metabolic alkalosis, hypothyroidism, etc. In narcotic overdose, the respiration will be shallow with low rate, but rhythm may be regular.

Tachypnoea may be due to excitement, fever, diseases of lung or heart, acidosis, etc. There is no accepted standard on degree C rise in temperature and the respiratory rate. Very rapid and deep breathing (Kussmaul breathing) is seen in acidosis (mnemonic: ketoacidosis, uremia, sepsis, salicylates, methanol, aldehyde, lactic acidosis). Rapid but shallow breathing is seen in pulmonary oedema and pneumonias. This is basically because when the lung is stiff as in pulmonary oedema, it is economical for the body to spend less energy by shallow but rapid breathing. 15

Prolonged inspiration is characteristic of upper airway obstruction like obstruction of glottis, whereas prolonged expiration is characteristic of lower airway obstruction like asthma. Upper airway obstruction produces stridor, whereas lower airway obstruction produces wheeze.

Various abnormal rhythms of respiration are discussed in Ch. 10 ["breathing patterns and CNS localization" (p 239)].

Respiratory effort: See for use of accessory muscles of respiration.

Trachea: If one sternomastoid appears to stand out, it could mean a tracheal shift to that side (trail sign). Trachea is normally central or minimally shifted to the right.

Apex: See if the apex can be visually located.

Shape & Symmetry of Chest

Normal shape with bilateral symmetry is expected in normal child.

Antero posterior distance can be measured using two cardboards, one placed anteriorly & one posteriorly. Thoracic index is the ratio of A-P diameter to transverse diameter. Normally it is <1.

Points to look for in shape of chest are:

- Barrel-shaped chest. (Thoracic index >1)
- Pigeon chest (pectus carinatum)
- Funnel-shaped chest (pectus excavatum)
  Inspect to see if the chest is bilaterally symmetrical. Shape of chest is best inspected from the front and then from the side. Barrel chest is found in emphysema of adults and possibly some cases of asthma in children. Normally, the chest is elliptical in cross section. In infancy, the cylindrical chest may be normal and may not indicate any disease.

Points to look for in symmetry of chest wall are bulging or flattening:

Bulging of chest or part of chest may be seen in:

- Pleural effusion/hydropneumothorax/ empyema.
- Pneumothorax.
- Precordial bulge due to heart diseases.
- Local chest wall bulges due to abscess, traumatic contusion, etc.

Localized flattening may be seen in:

- Collapse (atelectasis)
- Fibrosis (pulmonary fibrosis is uncommon in children)

Examine the back to ensure that the asymmetry is not due to spinal curvature (kyphosis/scoliosis).

Comment on any swelling. Swelling may be there in advanced empyema pointing outwards through the chest wall (empyema necessitans), air leak producing subcutaneou emphysema etc. One side of the chest may appear bulging in tension pneumothorax, pleural effusion, etc. However, one must not fail to see if the bulging is just an apparent one due to scoliosis.

Look for any flattening or drooping of shoulder (Figs. 15.8 & 15.9). Flattening may be seen in collapse of lung. Also look for crowding of ribs, scoliosis and kyphosis.

Slightly better developed pectorals on the right side may be normally seen in right-handed adults but uncommon in children. So look again, it could be a congenitally absent pectoralis major on the flat side!

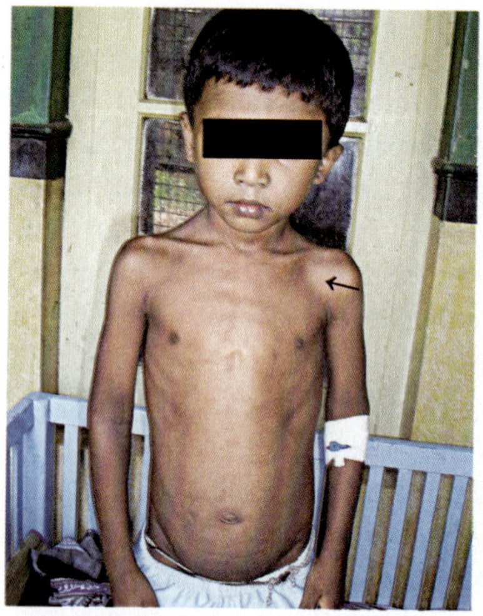

Fig.15.8 Flattening of infraclavicular area

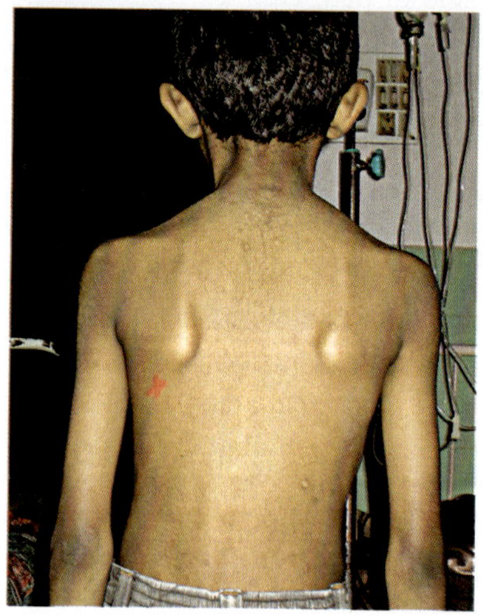

Fig.15.9 Drooping of left shoulder. Note the level of scapula.

Pigeon Chest or Pectus Carinatum

Marked forward protrution of sternum. Historically linked to rickets, the association now appears quite weak (Fig. 15.10a & b).

Pectus Excavatum (Funnel Chest)

This is the depression of the lower part of sternum. Historically, it is related to rickets; however, it is usually an exaggeration of normal depression of lower sternum (may run in family). It is also seen in Marfan syndrome. Significant pectus excavatum may shift the apex to left and may mechanically compromise the ventilatory capacity of the lung (Fig. 15.11).

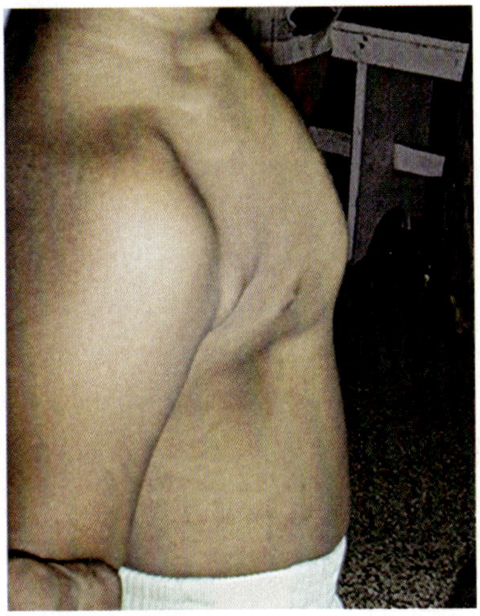

Fig.15.10a Pigeon chest (lateral view)

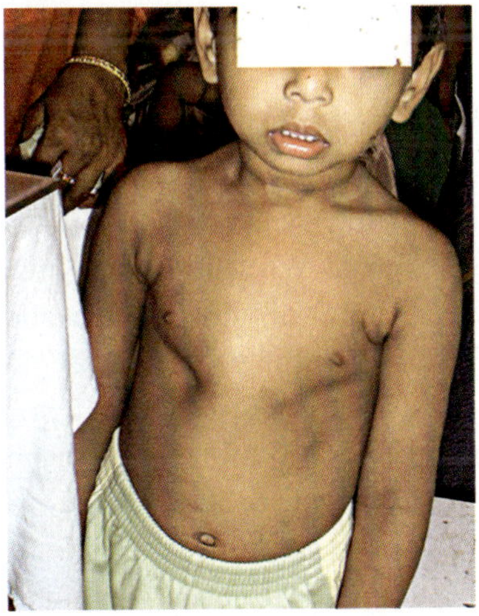

Fig.15.10b Pigeon chest (frontal view)

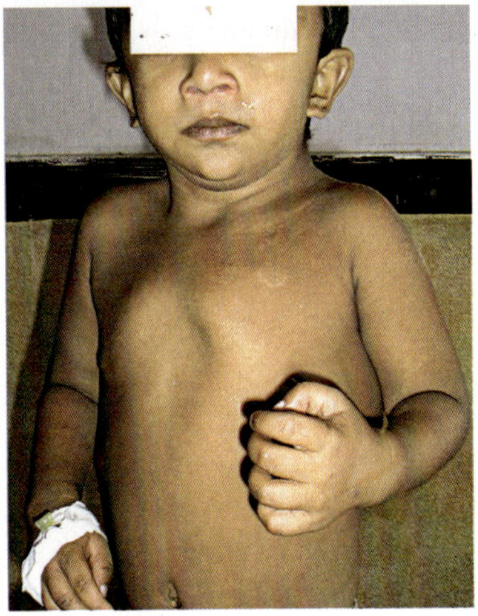

Fig.15.11 Pectus excavatum

Harrison's Sulcus

This is seen along the attachment of diaphragm and is produced by the pulling of diaphragm on a weak chest wall. Again historically linked to rickets, the association now appears to be more with recurrent respiratory problems in early infancy like L to R shunt lesions of the heart, asthma, upper airway block due to adenoids, etc (Fig. 15.12).

Rachitic Rosary

Knob-like swellings of the costochondral junctions (p 490). This may be related to accumulation of uncalcified osteoid in rickets. Rosary of scurvy (scorbutic rosary) is the protrusion of rib ends because of displacement from the joint. So the sternum appears depressed rather than projecting out (pectus carinatum is expected more commonly in rickets). Children with rickets come with recurrent respiratory infections and hence a mention of rachitic rosary is made here.

15

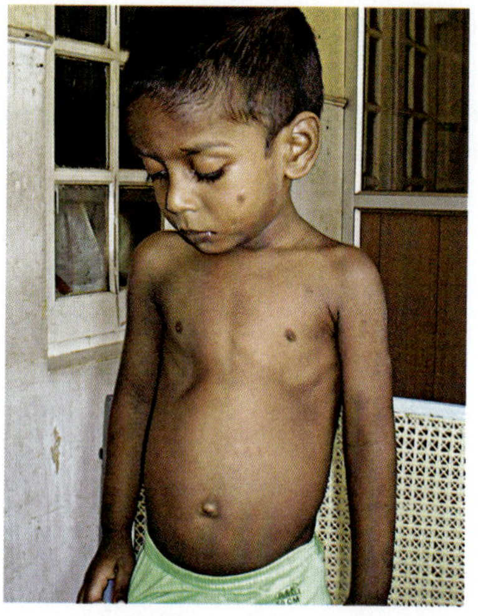

Fig.15.12 Harrison's sulcus

Broad chest with widely spaced nipples may be seen in Turner's syndrome [shield-like chest (p 518)].

Small thoracic cage as seen in the Ellis-van Creveld syndrome (p 509).

Absence of the clavicle is seen in cleidocranial dysostosis. Here, both shoulders can be almost approximated in front (p 501).

Movement of Chest

Both sides of normal chest must be symmetrical in mobility. Comment whether all areas of both sides are symmetrical in movements. Also comment on any pulsations (apical, parasternal, epigastric). The side or part that is less mobile is the diseased one (there is no pathology that makes the affected part move more than normal!).

Unilateral reduction in chest wall movements may be seen in:

- Pleural effusion/Empyema
- Pneumothorax
- Consolidation
- Collapse (atelectasis)
- Fibrosis
- Pleural adhesions (result of improperly treated empyema)
- Bilateral reduction in chest wall movements may be seen in:
    - Bronchiolitis
    - Bronchial asthma
    - Emphysema

Movement of the chest is upwards in both thorax and abdomen during normal inspiration. One may be tempted to think that the lower costal margins must go inwards during inspiration due to the pull of descending diaphragm. But actually this effect is mostly overpowered by the outward pull of intercostal muscles in health (although diaphragm is much stronger than the intercostals, there is only mild diaphragmatic activity during quiet breathing. However, during stronger breathing efforts, the diaphragm acts stronger and easily overpowers the intercostal action). In case of weak chest wall like rickets or increased diaph-ragmatic work like in asthma, the inward costal movement becomes obvious. If long standing, it leads on to Harrison's sulcus.

Comment on any retractions or pulsations. Retractions may indicate respiratory distress. Lower chest indrawing points towards severe pneumonia as per WHO ARI criteria.

Hoover's Sign

The subcostal angle is the angle between the xiphoid process and the costal margin. Normally, during inspiration the chest expands laterally, increasing this angle. When the diaphragms are flattened (as in COPD of old age), inhalation paradoxically causes the angle to decrease due to the change in angle of diaphragmatic pull. In children, a similar situation is possible when diaphragm is maximally flattened by obstructed airway; and further inspiration may cause a similar narrowing of subcostal angle. However, it is important to note that in clinical medicine, Hoover's sign generally refers to that connected with neurological examination (see p 213 and not the inspiratory indrawing. Hence, it is advised that the students should not mention this sign in examination, unless specifically asked for.

Flail Chest

Secondary to multiple rib fractures, depression of diaphragm causes injured area to cave inward producing a "paradoxical inward thoracic movement" in inspiration.

Palpation

1. **Trachea**: The trachea must be palpated to find if there is any shift. Palpate using middle finger with index and ring finger on the sternal attach-ment of sternomastoids. Look for the space between trachea and sternomasoid muscle; the space will be narrow to the side to which trachea is shifted. The trachea is shifted to the same side of lesion in collapse and to the opposite side in pleural effusion and tension pneumothorax.
2. **Apex**: Apex beat may be palpated to see if there is any shift (indicating shift of mediastinum). Apex may be obscured in obesity, emphysema, pericardial effusion and rarely when the apex comes under a rib. Apex may be shifted in cases of funnel chest and scoliosis.
3. **Movement with respiration**: Expansion of chest may be measured in deep inspiration. If it is not symmetrical bilaterally, try to document the differential expansion. Chest expansion of adolescent children is on the average 5 cm (5–8 cm, may be slightly less for girls).

   Placing the two hands of the examiner on either side of the patient's chest, the thumbs are stretched towards the midline; then look for separation of thumbs with respiratory movements. The emphasis is on encircling the lateral chest and not on approximating the thumbs on midline. Maximum expansion is on lateral chest & hence the importance of encircling the lateral chest. For palpating the apical region, the examiner places two hands over supraclavicular fossa from behind in a sitting patient, approximating the thumbs in the midline at the back; look for the upward movement of thumbs. See p 368-369 for illustrations.

   Place one hand over the abdomen and one over the chest. Both should move up during inspiration. Paradoxical inward movement of abdomen during inspiration occurs in diaphragmatic paralysis, in severe respiratory distress signifying impending respiratory failure. When only one diaphragm is paralyzed, during inspiration one side of abdomen bulges out while the other side is drawn in and vice versa in expiration. This see-saw movement is demonstrable by placing two hands over the left and right side of abdomen. Localized tenderness may be due to trauma, empyema, pleurisy, etc. Presternal oedema is rarely seen in association with mumps. Sternal tenderness may be noticed in leukaemia. Crepitus on palpation is the sensation of air over the chest wall. It is found in air leak producing "surgical emphysema." Surgical emphysema or sub-cutaneous emphysema is felt as crackling under the palpating fingers.
4. **Palpable sounds**: Wheeze (rhonchi), crackles and pleural rub may all become palpable at times. Of these, rhonchi (wheeze) is the most common one to become palpable.

   Vocal fremitus is looked for indifferent areas comparing with the corresponding areas of the other side of the chest using the ulnar border of palm. The significance is the same as vocal resonance and hence one may even avoid wasting time examining vocal fremitus!

Percussion

The middle finger of the left hand is placed firmly over the chest wall. The other fingers of this hand are slightly lifted off to avoid dampening of vibrations. Percussion is made with the index or middle finger of the right hand (depending on personal preference). The percussion stroke is a smooth sudden stroke on to the pleximeter finger placed on the chest wall and the percussing finger springs off immediately after making the stroke to avoid dampening of the sound generated. The movement of stroke originates at the wrist and not at the elbow. The pleximeter finger is generally placed parallel to the ribs but for percussing the right border of the heart, the pleximeter finger may be placed vertically on the right border of the sternum (the pleximeter finger is placed parallel to the area of expected dullness). The clavicle is percussed directly over the bone without the intervening pleximeter finger. For percussing the axillary areas, the patient may keep his hands above on to the back of the head. For percussing the interscapular area, the child can place the hands over his opposite shoulders, crossing the arms in front of chest; this keeps the scapulae spread apart to make the percussion easier. Percussing the interscapular area keeping pleximeter finger parallel to the vertebral column is advocated by some, but is not a desirable method. Percussion must proceed from a resonant area to a dull area. Corresponding areas of both sides are to be percussed and compared.

It should be mentioned whether one is getting normal resonance, impaired resonance, dull note or stony dull note. If any abnormality is detected, it is to be described by areas. In case a dullness is obtained, look for a higher level in axilla and shifting dullness (explained further).

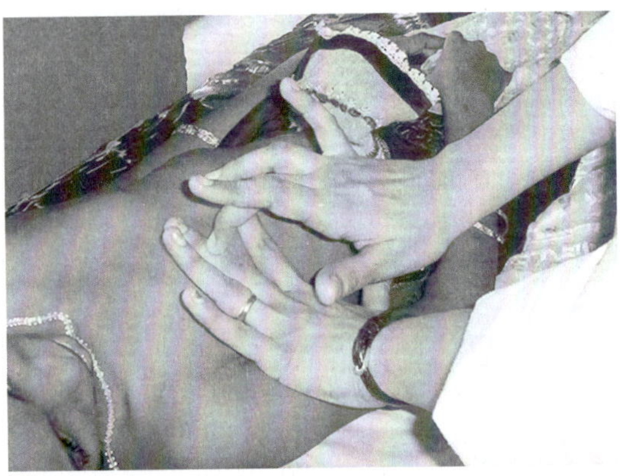

Fig.15.13 Method of percussion

Cardiac dullness: For percussing out the borders of heart, the pleximeter finger is kept parallel to the various expected borders of the heart.

Light percussion must be used (flicking percussion is preferred).

Note: Flicking percussion is easier and more rewarding for an experienced person and the author himself is a proponent of it. However, the examiners are unlikely to accept this method and hence the students should adhere to the classical method of percussion during their examination.

Various Percussion Notes

Tympanitic resonance is expected over the stomach; hyperresonant in pneumothorax; impaired note in consolidation or collapse (especially if the consolidated or collapsed segment is away from the chest wall); dull note in consolidation; stony dull note (flat note) in pleural effusion.

Traube's space: Traube's space is bounded by the pulmonary resonance (= level of 6th rib) above, left costal margin below, and mid-axillary line to the left. Normally, tympanic resonance is obtained here due to the underlying stomach, but will be dull in case of left-sided pleural effusion. Rarely, Traube's space may be dull due to splenic enlargement or marked enlargement of left lobe of liver.

Tidal percussion: The upper border of liver dullness must be percussed out. Following this, percussion on deep inspiration is done. The dullness due to liver moves down, whereas the dullness due to pleural effusion tends to remain stationary; this is because of restricted expansion of the lung due to parenchymal or pleural pathology (during inspiration air is preferentially directed to other areas offering lesser resistance to expansion).

Shifting dullness: This is found in hydropneumothorax. A horizontal upper level of dullness above which there is a hyperresonant area is classical of hydropneumothorax. In contrast to popular belief, the dullness does shift in large pleural effusions and hence demonstration of horizontal upper level of dullness is the most important clinical finding in the diagnosis of hydropneumothorax.

In pleural effusion, the upper level of dullness is higher at axilla. It is attributed to capillary suction effect. It is also possible that because of the fluid, the lung tends to collapse towards the hilum (hilum is at a more superior location than the mid-portion of the lung) so that the higher level can only be in the axilla (Fig. 15.14).

In case of pleural effusion, maximum dullness is observed at the lung bases where thickness of fluid is greatest. Clinically, the upper limit of dullness is at least one space higher in the axilla compared to the limits of dullness anteriorly and posteriorly. Shift in the dull note with posture indicates free pleural fluid, (as against loculated effusion, where the dullness does not shift). To demonstrate shifting dullness, the child may be percussed in sitting position first, followed by percussion of the same area in the lateral decubitus position. Care must be taken to differentiate the shifting dullness of a pleural effusion with that of hydropneumothorax where the upper level of dullness is horizontal. In emphysema, the area of cardiac and liver dullness may be reduced. Splenic dullness, if located, is most likely to be found around the 9th space in midaxillary line, in a normal child.

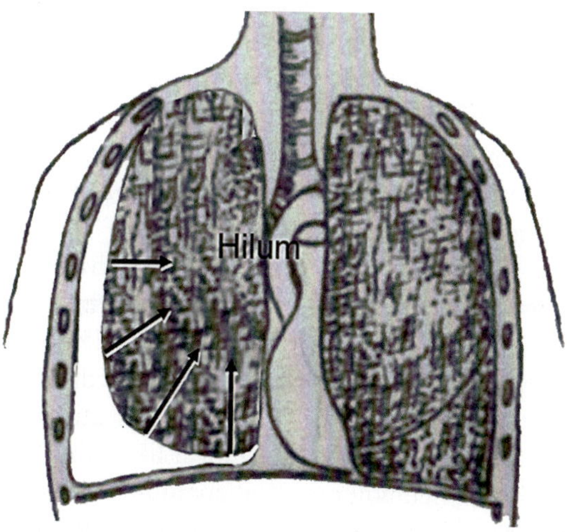

Fig.15.14 Lung collapsing towards the hilum

Auscultation

With the patient relaxed and breathing normally, auscultate the upper, middle and lower lung fields posteriorly, laterally and anteriorly, each time comparing the corresponding areas of both sides. 15

During auscultation, one looks for breath sounds (intensity), adventitious sounds (location, timing) and VR. Normal breath sounds are vesicular. If the breath sounds are vesicular, one must see if they are of normal intensity or reduced intensity and if they are equal in corresponding areas on either side. ***Note***: A trained ear must know that breath sounds are not exactly equal in corresponding areas of either side in health. Examples would be louder breath sounds over the right apex, lower intensity breath sounds over the left precordium, etc.

If there is a bronchial breathing, it is to be described by areas and whenever possible by type—tubular, amphoric or cavernous.

One must look for any adventitious sounds like crackles, wheeze or pleural rub. Vocal resonance is tested by asking the child to repeat words like 99. However, in small children even their cry may be used as a tool to assess resonance. One must assess if the vocal resonance is normal, decreased or increased. If it is increased, look for any whispering pectoriloquy or aegophony.

Vesicular breathing: This is rustling in character; the expiration is shorter than inspiration (about a third) and there is no pause between inspiration and expiration as the elastic recoil of lung initiates expiration immediately at the end of inspiration. Actually, the duration of expiration is equal to inspiration; however, only the early portion of expiration is audible as the elastic recoil is maximum early in expiration.

Airflow in small airways is slow without turbulence and hence not much sound is expected to be produced there. The breath sounds that we hear by auscultation originate from bronchi where there is lot of turbulence. But it does not sound "bronchial" in the normal child, as these are transmitted to the chest wall after getting filtered and muted by the intervening lung tissue and thus the vesicular character is obtained. When the intervening lung between the patent bronchus and the chest wall gets consolidated, the bronchial sounds get transmitted as such without intervening modification and hence we hear bronchial breathing.

Vesicular breath sounds of increased intensity: The characters are the same as vesicular breathing but appear louder or harsher than usual. It may be seen with excitation, exertion, etc. When one side of the chest is grossly affected by a pathology (e.g., pleural effusion, pneumothorax, etc), the normal lung will allow preferentially more air entry to produce this type of breathing.

Vesicular breath sounds of diminished intensity: This is a better descriptive term than saying that the air entry at a particular area is diminished. It may be because of blocked airway (lymph node obstruction, foreign body obstruction, severe asthma, etc) or barrier to transmission of breath sounds to the chest wall (pleural effusion, pneumothorax, pleural thickening, etc) or weakness of respiratory muscles (e.g., paralysis of respiratory muscles in polio).

Vesicular breath sounds with prolonged expiration: These are seen in asthma. Expiration is a passive process normally. But when it is through the narrowed airways of asthma, it takes longer, as it requires the patient to exhale actively.

Bronchial breathing: Bronchial breathing is heard normally when the stethoscope is placed over the trachea and this fact may be used by the beginners to get to know how it sounds. It sounds harsher, expiration is at least equal to inspiration in duration and there is a definite pause between inspiration and expiration. Expiration is louder and of higher pitch (aspirate in quality; sounds like haa) than inspiration. This is heard in consolidation and less commonly in atelectasis. Rarely, it may be heard just above the level of pleural effusion. It is possible that the lung tissue that is compressed by the accumulated pleural fluid acts like a consolidated area to produce bronchial breathing.

Why there is a pause in bronchial breathing? Imagine that one whole lobe is consolidated. The air entering the bronchi supplying this consolidated lobe cannot go beyond the bronchus to alveoli and hence stops there. However, air flow goes on beyond the bronchi into the alveoli in other parts of the normal lung; after this only the expiration starts. So in the consolidated part, there is a silent phase between the time the air gets blocked from further flow into the alveoli and start of expiration. Hence, there is a pause between inspiration and expiration in bronchial breathing.

Low-pitched bronchial breathing is called cavernous, the medium-pitched one simply called bronchial breathing and the high-pitched bronchial breathing is called tubular breathing. ***Cavernous*** breathing is heard over a cavity with a large communicating bronchus. ***Tubular*** breathing is heard in consolidation (sounds from the "tubes" directly conveyed to the chest wall without modification by the aerated lung). When it echoes like blowing into a bottle with narrow neck, it is called ***amphoric*** breathing, characteristic of large cavity (A large cavity with smooth margins and a narrow bronchus opening into it is almost like a bottle!). At times, pneumothorax that communicates with a bronchus may also produce similar amphoric breathing. The student may blow into a big bottle with narrow opening to know how it sounds like. It has a high-pitched whistling quality.

Bronchovesicular breathing has some (but not all) characteristics of both bronchial and vesicular breathing; e.g., expiration may be prolonged or has a hollow quality to it. This is not synonymous with harsh vesicular breathing, which is only a loud vesicular breathing, which retains all the characteristics of vesicular breathing.

Bronchovesicular breathing may be heard over the right interscapular area and at the right apical area. The tracheobronchial tree is close to the chest wall without much surrounding lung tissue in the regions close to right sternoclavicular joint and right interscapular area.

Rhonchi vs wheeze: Rhonchi (wheeze) are dry continuous sounds that are produced by the oscillation of opposing narrowed airways when there is high velocity airflow through them; continuous means at least 250 msec in duration (American Thoracic Society). That is, "continuous" still may have interruptions. Wheeze and rhonchi are the same, *but one tends to use the term wheeze when it is high-pitched musical in quality and rhonchi when it is low-pitched snoring or gurgling in quality.* Some authors describe the former as sibilant rhonchi and the latter as sonorous rhonchi. Sibilant rhonchi (high-pitched rhonchi) is produced by the high velocity air movement through the narrowed small "smooth inside" airways. The sonorous rhonchi is due to the vibra-tion of constricted inflamed bigger airways "irregular inside" as the air goes through it. Although continuous, sonorous rhonchi (low-pitched rhonchi) has a vibratory character; this is probably because of the air negotiating the airway lumen irregularities produced by inflammatory oedema and/or adherent mucus secretions. Rhonchi (wheeze) can occur during inspiration and expiration, but more commonly during expiration because the airway calibre is smaller during expiration. Sometimes, asthmatic patient in very severe distress may not wheeze at all ("silent chest with severe respiratory distress"), either because the airways are closed down or narrowed so much that the flow through them is too slow to produce any sound. Sibilant rhonchi (wheeze) originating from smaller airways are mostly heard during expiration and are more musical (e.g., wheeze in asthma). Musical rhonchi is possible when small airways are constricted to give a narrow smooth passage for the air to go out. Rhonchi originating from larger airways may be heard during expiration and inspiration and are lower pitched and sonorous (e.g., rhonchi in bronchitis). ***Note***: Having said this, the practical point that a student must keep in mind is that both inspiratory and expiratory wheezes are heard in the majority of asthmatic children (as inflamation is part of asthma).

15

Fixed monophonic rhonchi (rhonchi of constant character, timing and site) indicate foreign body obstruction, lymph node obstruction, etc. In asthma, rhonchi may be polyphonic because the obstruction in various places are not equal in magnitude; even if monophonic, it may be varying in timing and site.

Note: Wheeze that is missed on auscultation over the lung fields may be picked up by auscultation over the trachea. This is because wheeze produced anywhere will be conducted to trachea, because all airways are peripheral branches of trachea only!

Rhonchi (wheeze) should not be confused with snoring, a continuous vibratory sound produced during sleep due to fluttering of soft tissues of oropharynx.

Stridor, another continuous sound of respiratory system, is much lower pitched than rhonchi and is heard usually in inspiration only (although it may occasionally be heard during expiration also, especially when trachea or main bronchus is involved). Stridor originates from large airways, which are not subjected to much variation in caliber during the respiratory cycle. Stridor is heard in laryngotracheobronchitis, foreign body in large airways, epiglottitis, diphtheria, etc.

Wheeze vs crackle: Continuous sound is wheeze (rhonchi). Crackles are may be of different qualities like popping, clicking, bubbling or rattling sounds. However, in clinical case presentation it will suffice to say whether the crackles are fine or coarse.

Crackles or rales or crepitations are interrupted (discontinuous), short, non-musical popping sounds. Crackle can best be simulated to the fire crackling in wooden stove or crackling sound heard when dry leaves are put to fire. They occur in bursts and not as a single sound. Crackles are usually heard during inspiration (it may be heard during expiration as well, but much less frequently). Crackle probably results when the sticky terminal airways or alveoli open up with inspiration (hence there may be a shower of crackles as the inspiration proceeds).

Conventionally, fine crackles are called by the name crepitations although currently this term is used interchangeably with crackles.

Note: Some use the term rales as a common name for all adventitious sounds, so that rhonchi are called dry rales! Majority prefers to use the term rales synonymous with crackles.

Early crackles are heard in disease associated with airway obstruction (sticky air ways open up with a crackle).

Late crackles: In pulmonary oedema, the leakage of fluid is likely in lung bases due to gravity and crackles are heard late in inspiration as the air reaches these areas late (thus they open up late in inspiration to produce late crackles).

In bronchiectasis, there may be bubbly **coarse crackles** or bubbly crackles, possibly due to air going through the stagnant secretions in the dilated airways. Naturally, one can expect to hear it both during inspiration and expiration. Many a time, coarse crackles are palpable as well. Crackles of bronchiectasis are sometimes described as "leathery" (not a standard textbook description). Because of the irregularity of the inside of airways and the stagnant secretions in the pockets formed within the dilated airways, rhonchi in bronchiectasis may be sonorous or gurgling.

Fine crackles are seen in early stage of pneumonia, possibly due to the sticky small airways and alveoli opening up (indux crepitations). Velcro crepitations are heard in ILD.

Fine crackles may be heard also in acute pulmonary oedema and interstitial lung disease. Crackles without sputum production may indicate interstitial lung disease, whereas crackles with sputum production may mean parenchymal lung disease (pneumonia). Coarse crepitations are heard in resolving pneumonia.

Crackle–wheeze combination in asthma: The student is often confused as to why he hears crackles in addition to wheeze in a case of pure asthma. Inspiration opens the sticky airway with a crackle. But the airway is small due to bronchospasm and hence they vibrate as the air goes in and out. Thus, crackles and rhonchi are possible in asthma without accompanying pneumonia.

Post-tussive crepitation: The child is asked to cough a few times followed by a deep inspiration, with the examiner listening to this inspiration for crackles that were not there initially. Possibly small amount of secretions from different areas are brought together to a common place to give this crepitation. In the same procedure, if a sucking sound is heard in inspiration (***post-tussive suction***), it may indicate a thin-walled cavity in communication with a bronchus. It collapses with expiration after a series of coughing and then suddenly the air gushes in to expand it on inspiration; this produces the suction sound.

Interestingly, the crackles produced by the airway secretions in COPD (adult patient) typically disappears after a cough, because the patient has coughed out those secretions.

Can crackles be heard in normal lung? Some crackles may occasionally be heard over the anterior chest in normal old age subjects breathing in low tidal volume for a long time. They can be made to disappear with a few deep breaths, because the alveoli get opened up by deep breathing so that the minimal fluid that was there inside gets absorbed and the stickiness of alveoli disappears. They are usually seen in old age and not in children or young adults.

Stertor: It is the sound produced by the air traversing the accumulated secretions of extrathoracic airways. It is best heard over the trachea, as discontinuous coarse bubbling sound both during inspiration and expiration.

Coarse bubbling originating at the throat are conducted sounds, due to secretions that stagnate in the throat or upper airway, due to inability to cough it out (e.g., paralysis, unconsciousness). It is usually termed ***rattle***, which in a seriously ill child often signifies a dying child.

Squawk: It is best described as a very short wheeze (cannot describe it as crackle varient, because it is generally a single sound and not a burst of sounds; and the duration is much longer than a crackle). Closed airways suddenly open during inspiration and the airway walls briefly remain in contact to produce the squawk as the air column negotiate that area. Then it opens up to allow quiet inspiration. It is described in adults with fibrotic disorders and rarely in hypersensitivity pneumonia.

Grunt is a sound that is produced at the beginning of expiration due to expiration against a partially closed glottis. It is the effort on the part of the patient to create a positive end expiratory pressure so that the alveoli can be kept open. It is usually seen in severe pneumonia. It is never expected in acute asthma, as there is already air trapping and end expiratory pressure is already high (hence no need for grunt) (see p 157).

Pleural rub: Its quality is described as leathery or rubbing or grating, but one has to hear it to know how it sounds. Suffice to say that it sounds like crackles, becoming louder as one presses the stethoscope firmly on to the chest (possibly firm pressure makes the pleural layers rub closely). It is usually heard at the lower part of the axilla where the excursions of pleura are maximum. It is repeatedly heard at the corresponding phases of inspiration and expiration (because at that stage of lung expansion the pleural layers rub together). There is no change on coughing (quality or location of crackles may change with cough). It is usually well localized to a small area where the pleural layers rub together. There may be pain at the site on inspiration, and at times can have local tenderness. Sometimes, pleural rub may become palpable. Pleuropericardial rub, an unusual cause of rub, may be differentiated from pleural rub by the fact that it synchronizes with heart beat (pleural rub comes on with respiration).

Succussion splash: When the patient is suddenly shaken with examiner's hands, a splash sound is heard, either with stethoscope or unaided ear. If using stethoscope, place it at the upper level of dullness. It is characteristic of a large hydropneumothorax. The sound is similar to the sound that is heard from the stomach when the patient is shaken after drinking water.

Coin sound: In large pneumothorax and large hydropneumothorax, it may be elicitable. On the side of pneumothorax, place a coin on the front of chest wall and strike it with another coin. Listening to the diagonally opposite surface of the same side of chest (i.e., back of chest wall in this case) will yield a high-pitched metallic echoing sound (like ringing bell). This test described in 1890s is seldom done these days.

Vocal Resonance (VR)

Spoken sound produced by the vibrations of vocal cord is transmitted through the air column of the airways to the lung parenchyma and then to the chest wall to produce the vocal resonance. Let the child say "ninety-nine" and auscultate to compare the corresponding areas on either side. Normally, it is heard as muffled sound with individual syllables indistinguishable. VR is increased over an area of consolidation by the same mechanism as bronchial breathing (consolidated lung is a better conductor). When VR is louder and clearer and heard as if originating close to the ears of the examiner, then it is called ***bronchophony*** (somewhat similar to the intensity of what is heard over the trachea). In bronchophony as well, individual syllables may remain indistinguishable. As in case of bronchial breathing, VR may occasionally be accentuated over an area just above pleural effusion (see the explanation under bronchial breathing, p 364). When spoken words are heard with clearly distinguishable individual syllables, it is referred to as ***pectoriloquy***. When pectoriloquy is elicited with whispered words, it is called whispering pectoriloquy (in normal person, the whispered words are heard only as faint sounds or nothing at all). The larynx does not play a part in whisper, so that unlike spoken words, *intense* vibrations of air column by the sound waves are not produced during whispering. Thus, whispered sounds are not heard in most of the lungs in health (but may be heard over the trachea). If the whispered voice is heard over the lung with distinguishable syllables, it indicates that even small vibrations in the air column are getting transmitted with sufficient clarity to the chest wall. As expected, it occurs in consolidation, the mechanism of better transmission of sound being the same as in bronchial breathing.

VR is decreased over areas of pleural effusion and pneumothorax. Also in conditions where voice production is weak, VR will be decreased (e.g., vocal cord paralysis, Guillain-Barre syndrome affecting respiratory muscles, etc).

Aegophony: Here, VR has a nasal quality, like the bleating of a goat. Ask the patient to say "ee" continuously. Auscultate the suspected abnormal area and compare with the symmetrical area of the other lung. Normally, one should hear a muffled "ee" sound. If one hears an "ay" sound this is referred to as egophony ("E > A"). It may be heard at the upper level of pleural effusion. When there is a thick layer of pleural fluid, all sound waves are blocked so that VR is greatly reduced.

But at the upper level of a pleural effusion, there is only a thin layer of fluid, so that only some frequencies are filtered out. It seems that high-pitched nasal sounds are allowed to be transmitted, but the other frequencies are filtered out to produce the aegophony.

Note: American Thoracic Society and American College of Chest Physicians do not agree with this definition of aegophony.

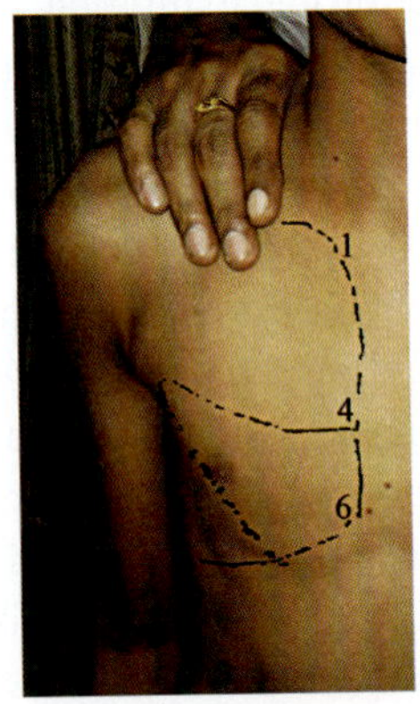

Fig.15.15 Surface marking of long lobes

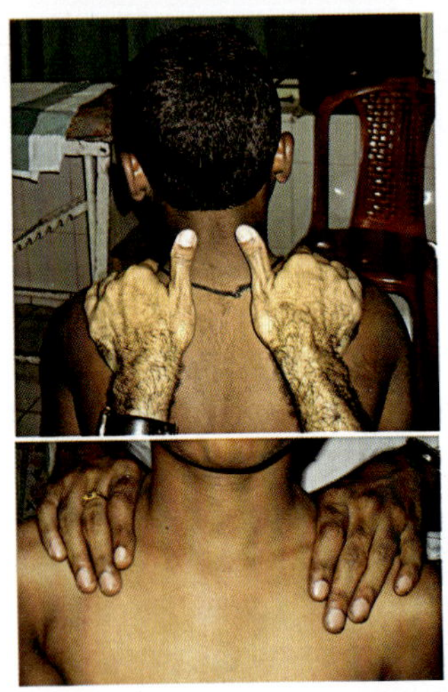

Fig.15.16 Supra scapular area is examined from the back as shown. The bottom picture is the same procedure when viewed from the front.

When the patient is unconscious, one may try to produce sounds by tapping over the trachea and then listening for transmission of this sound over the lung fields (obviously a very crude method). If there is gross difference between the intensity of transmitted sounds between identical areas of two sides, one may assume some abnormality of vocal resonance.

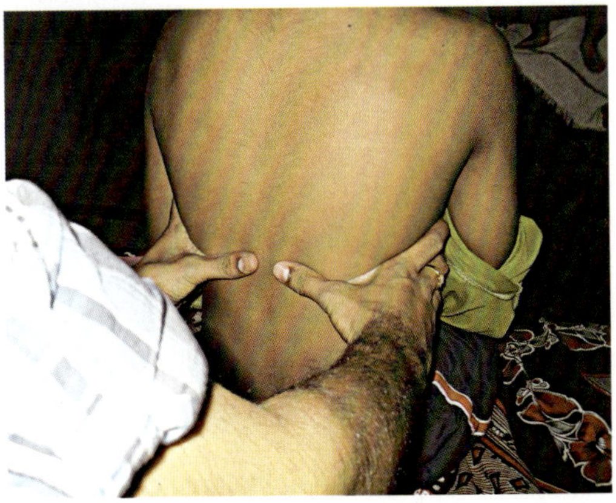

Fig.15.17 Infra scapular area

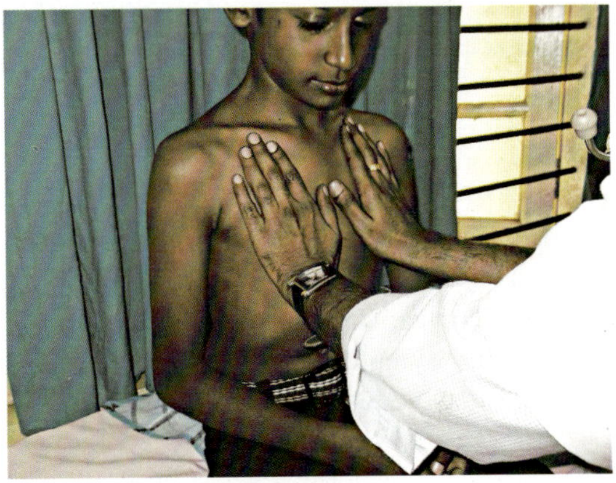

Fig.15.18 Infraclavicular region. Place the hands flat and observe movement on deep inspiration.

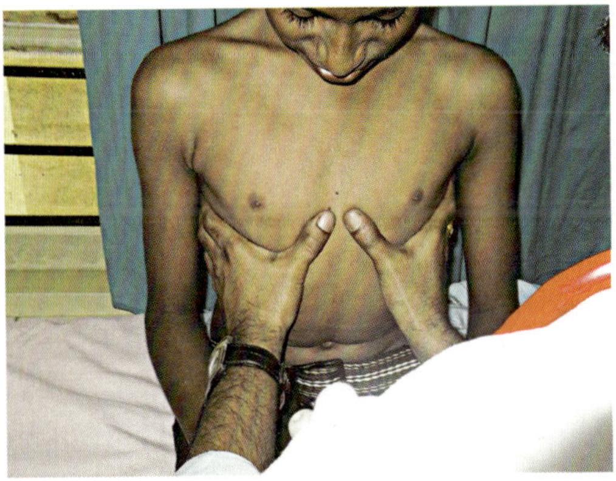

Fig.15.19 Mammary area

CHAPTER 16

Disorders of Respiratory System: Case Sheet Formats

Symptoms (Complaints)

The usual complaints pertaining to respiratory system are cough, fever, breathlessness, noisy breathing, coryza, chest pain, etc.

Other rare symptoms include hemoptysis and halitosis (lung abscess, bronchiectasis).

History of Present Illness

1. *Expand chief complaints*: Onset, duration, progress of complaints
2. *History of other respiratory symptoms*: Whether chief complaint associated with fever, cough with/without expectoration, hemoptysis, breathlessness, chest pain.
   a) Cough:
      - Sudden onset (choking); paroxysmal (whooping cough, asthma; in both these paroxysm may terminate with vomiting; in whooping cough, in between paroxysms, the child remains ok, including normal respiratory rate).
      - Productive or dry ("moist or dry"). Sputum if brought out, whether whitish (asthma), yellow (pneumonia, bronchitis, bronchiectasis, etc), frothy & blood stained in pulmonary oedema. Very foul smelling sputum in lung abscess (anaerobes).
      - Initiating or aggravating factors of cough.
      - Diurnal or positional variations of cough.
      - Dyspnoea

   b) Chest pain: Site of pain, intensity of pain aggravating or relieving factors (e.g., pleural pain is increased on deep breath).
   c) Noisy breathing: Stridor in acute laryngotracheo-bronchitis, epiglottitis, foreign body lodged in upper airway, etc; Wheeze in asthma.
   d) Drooling of saliva: In acute epiglottitis.
3. *History of Aetiology:*
   - History of sorethroat, nasal discharge, ear pain or discharge, skin pustules.
   - History of foreign body aspiration.
   - History of choking, regurgitation of feeds, vomiting - GERD.
   - History of halitosis, mouth breathing, snoring.
   - History of weight loss/evening rise of temperature/contact with TB.
   - History of congestive cardiac failure (suck -rest suck cycle, head sweating, dyspnoea on exertion).
   - History of trauma to chest.
   - Bone pains and bleeding manifestations (malignancy can cause pleural effusion).
   - History of rash illness: Bronchopneumonia follows measles.
   - Skin infections, history of rapid deterioration: Staphylococcus.
4. *History of complications*:
   - History of danger signs like poor feeding, drowsiness, severe chest indrawing, cyanosis, seizures.
   - History of splinting chest/lying down on one side pleurisy.

5. *Treatment history and course in hospital:*
   - Whether on oral or IV medicines, nebulizations, physiotherapy, sputum test done.
   - Since admission how has the child improved in terms of each symptom.
6. *Activities of daily living:*
   - How is the present illness affecting the patients. Activites of daily living: eating, dressing, toilet, ambulation, EDTA, school, emotions and behaviour.

Past History

- History of previous episodes of recurrent LRTI, allergy (wheeze, night cough, atopy, eczema, allergic rhinitis) or similar complaints.
- History of hospital admissions, pertusis or measles in recent past.
- History of aspiration (temporal relation to feeding; seizure may have lead to aspiration without getting noticed).
- History of allergies: nasal, skin, respiratory or others.
- Contact with tuberculosis.
- Day care centre attendance, passive smoking, overcrowded house, etc.
- Recurrent sino pulmonary infections (immunodeficiency).

Antenatal, Natal and Postnatal History

- Respiratory distress soon after birth.
- Delayed passage of meconium (cystic fibrosis).
- Premature baby (bronchiolitis more likely).

Immunization

BCG, pertusis, measles, pneumococcal, influenza are the vaccines that may modify respiratory infections. Mention if BCG scar is seen or not. BCG scar is expected to be seen within 90 days of vaccination.

Development History

Diet

- Breast feeding or on cows milk.
- Dietary allergies.

Family and Socioeconomic History

- TB, bronchial asthma, atopic dermatitis, lower respiratory tract infection, high risk behviour.
- Hygiene, overcrowding, smoking, firewood, coils, pets, dust, cockroach, pollen.

General Examination

- Any sensorial alterations; difficulty to speak; activity of accessory muscles of respiration; lower chest indrawing; depression of intercostals spaces.
- Any definite position the child prefers to lie.
- Vital & anthropometry as usual.
- Hand to head and head to foot examination.
- Clubbing: Bronchiectasis, congenital cyanotic heart disease, cystic fibrosis.
- Cyanosis indicates severe pneumonia or severe asthma (respiratory failure).
- Lymphadenopathy.
- Face: Allergic salute, Shiners, Dennie-Morgan folds.
- Nose: Mention if you have noticed any abnormality in nose (deviated septum, oedematous inferior turbinate in nasal allergy, nasal discharge, bleeding, flaring of ala nasi, etc). Pale mucosa is seen in chronic allergic rhinitis.
- Look for sinus tenderness in relevant cases.
- Ears must be examined with otoscope in relevant cases (e.g., ear discharge).
- Eyes: Conjunctival erythema, subconjunctival bleed, discharge, phlyctenular conjunctivitis.
- Sinus: Look for tenderness frontal and maxillary sinus.
- Oral thrush: Beyond newborn period, may suggest immunodeficiency.
- Throat: Tonsils, pharynx.
- Chest: Intercostal tenderness/fullness, flattening, harrisons sulcus, shoulder drooping.

- Skin: Sinus, pyoderma, erythema nodosum, large haemangioma (increased risk of intra thoracic lesion).

PNEUMONIC CONSOLIDATION

1. **Symptoms and signs**
   - Fever, cough, tachypnea, lower chest indrawing, etc; rarely blood tinged sputum.
   - Uncommon features of pneumonia:
     - Lower lobe pneumonia may cause referred pain to the abdomen due to its proximity to the diaphragm. However, a more common reason for abdominal pain is the repeated contractions of the abdominal muscles due to cough. Upper lobe pneumonia may cause meningismus. Subpleural location of pneumonia may produce pleurisy and hence pleuritic type of pain. Retro-sternal chest pain may be due to tracheitis.
     - Grunt is the sound produced due to expiration against a partially closed glottis. This is the body's attempt to increase end expiratory pressure to prevent the end expiratory collapse of the alveoli and it indicates severe pneumonia.
2. **Inspection**
   - Respiration: ***Respiratory rate*** is increased (the inflamed lung is stiff and less distensible so that the child will have to increase the rate of respiration to compensate for the poor distensibility). Look for any catch during respiratory movement on deep breath, e.g., in pleural rub the child may suddenly stop breathing movement when pleural rub producing pain. Ala nasi and other accessory muscles of respiration may be active during breathing.
   - Trachea: Position of trachea is central.
   - Apex: Normal position.
   - Shape of chest: Expected to be bilaterally symmetrical. If there is asymmetry, look for any scoliosis, usually due to bending to the side of pleural pain. No drooping of shoulder, hollowing, flattening/bulging.
   - Movement of chest: Movement will be restricted in the affected side or affected area. ***Indrawing of lower chest wall*** may be present. Other retractions to look for are intercostal supraclavicular and suprasternal retractions and tracheal tug.
   - There will be no dilated veins or pulsations because of consolidation.
   - Scars: Specifically look for scars of intercostal drains, because the case may have had effusion along with consolidation.
3. **Palpation**
   - Trachea and apex beat (mediastinum) are at normal position.
   - Expansion of chest with inspiration, may be restricted at the affected area (measure during full inspiration and expiration; compare with normal side). Try to document the differential expansion, although it is likely to be far from accurate. Place both palms on chest at the level of nipples with thumbs stretched towards each other in midline; during inspiration thumbs separate giving some idea on the difference in expansion (see p 369).
   - Vocal fremitus, in affected areas may be increased (feel with the ulnar aspect of palm).
   - Palpable crepitations or rub may or may not be present. Palpable rhonchi is likely in bronchopneumonia, unlikely in lobar consolidation (bronchus must be involved for rhonchi to be produced).
   - Tenderness may be elicitable if there is pleural pain.
4. **Percussion**
   - Dullness is expected in the area of consolidation. If dullness is detected, look for

a higher level in axilla as there may be associated pleural effusion as well.
- Cardiac dullness if feasible (to document any shift of mediastinum).
- Upper border of liver dullness (confirm by tidal percussion).
- Percuss Traube's space in left sided lesion (synpneumonic effusion is possible).

5. **Auscultation**
   - Intensity of breath sounds: Breath sounds, if normal in character (vesicular), it will be of grossly reduced intensity. Bronchial breath sounds may not be audible always because bronchi in the involved areas may be blocked by thick plugs. If there is a bronchial breathing, describe it.
   - Adventitious sounds: Crackle, pleural rub. Fine crackles early in pneumonia and coarse crackles during the phase of resolution. Crackles may be scanty or even absent when the bronchus feeding the area is completely blocked. Wheeze (rhonchi) may be abundant in bronchopneumonia, less likely in lobar consolidation (still may be present). Look for post-tussive crepitations if crepitations are not readily obvious even after deep breathing.
   - Vocal resonance: It is likely to be increased; but need not be always so, due to blocked airways (widespread block of airways may even cause decreased VR). Look for any whispering pectoriloquy.

Investigations in Pneumonia

- Pulse oximetry to document oxygen saturation. This will help decide which child is sick enough to be hospitalized.
- ABG if the child is sick.
- Complete blood cell (CBC) count, ESR, CRP.
- Sputum microscopy, gram stain, cultures (results may be confusing because of contamination with pharyngeal flora).
- Blood culture: Beyond newborn period most pneumonias are not bacteremic and hence as much as 2/3rd of all cultures could be negative.
- Cold agglutinin test in school age children (because significant percentage of infections are with mycoplasma).
- Mantoux test.
- Chest X-ray.
- Ultrasonography: Most useful when synpneumonic effusions are suspected, but can detect consolidation as well.
- Rapid antigen tests and serology when available.

16

Treatment of Pneumonia

- Oxygen inhalation if indicated.
- Oral fluids or IV fluids as is needed
- Antibiotics:
  - First-line antibiotic is amoxicillin. Second line is cefuroxime (covers usual organisms like pneumococci and *H. influenzae*).
  - For small infants and in those suspected to have staphylococcal pneumonia, add cloxacillin to the above antibiotic.

The clinical pointers towards possible staphylococcal pneumonia are
- Severe pneumonia in *infants*.
- Focus of infection like pyoderma.
- Hospital-acquired pneumonia.
- Rapid progression of symptoms and signs.
- Clinical evidence of empyema, subcutaneous emphysema, etc.

- Macrolides for well looking school age child (mycoplasma pneumonia).
- Infants less than 3 months of age may be treated with regimen for newborn (e.g., cefotaxime and aminoglycosides).
- Viral pneumonia (H1N1) may be treated with oseltamivir.
- Bronchodilators: Bronchopneumonia will invariably require bronchodilators.

- A thin layer of pleural effusion is common (synpneumonic effusion). This may resolve with antibiotic for pneumonia. Pleural tap for therapeutic purpose is not needed, but may be considered for diagnostic purpose.
- Continue normal feeding as per tolerance of the child.

BRONCHOPNEUMONIA

Bronchopneumonia generally follows an upper respiratory infection; the consequent denudation of airway epithelium facilitates the upper respiratory organisms to go down the bronchus and reach lung parenchyma to produce pneumonia. Thus, bronchopneumonia consists of inflamed bronchi (hence wheeze) plus numeruous small areas of parenchymal involvement (organisms reaching via the airway feeding the area), producing minute areas of consolidations. These areas may be so minute as to be inconspicuous even in X ray, leave alone clinical examination. Since these areas are quite small and are surrounded by normally aerated lungs, it is unlikely to be detected as consolidation by clinical examination.

Since the infection tracks down the airways, it obviously irritates the airways and cause cough and wheeze. In fact, there is no bronchopneumonia without wheeze. Hence, there is no need to put the diagnosis as bronchopneumonia with wheeze. However, some examiners want such a diagnosis and hence the student is advised to follow the scheme of his/her teacher.

The clinical diagnosis of bronchopneumonia revolves around the following three factors: (i) significant wheeze plus crackles in a (ii) sick or significantly febrile (iii) infant or toddler. Lower chest indrawing, when present helps a lot in differentiating bronchopneumonia from asthma. So also, grunt points towards pneumonia rather than asthma (grunt is the body's effort to open up the closed sticky alveoli; in asthma, these are already open with air trapping so that there is no need to grunt).

In older child (school age child), the inter alveolar connections have already developed, so much so a small area of consolidation will spread laterally to adjoining lung parenchyma to produce a lobar or lobular consolidation. Hence, consolidation is more likely in school age child and bronchopneumonia in small child. Hence, the diagnosis of bronchopneumonia is best entertained in small children.

1. **Symptoms and signs**
   Fever, cough, tachypnoea, chest indrawing, etc. Almost always it is a continuum from a upper respiratory infection.
2. **Inspection**
   - Respiration: Respiratory rate is increased. Ala nasi and other accessory muscles of respiration may be active during breathing.
   - Trachea: Position of trachea is central.
   - Apex: Normal position.
   - Shape of chest: Expected to be bilaterally symmetrical. No drooping of shoulder, hollowing, flattening/or bulging.
   - Movement of chest: Movement will be normal or slightly reduced. Indrawing of lower chest wall may be present. Other retractions to look for are intercostal, supra clavicular and suprasternal retractions.
   - There will be no dilated veins or pulsations because of bronchopneumonia.
3. **Palpation**
   - Trachea and apex beat (mediastinum) are at normal position.
   - Expansion of chest with inspiration, may be normal or restricted. Try to document the expansion, although it is likely to be far from accurate. Do the measurement at last, to avoid provoking the child's cry. Measurement of chest expansion is not an important step and many examiners would not mind even if the candidate skips this step.

- Vocal fremitus, usually remains normal, but may be increased in some areas.
- Palpable crepitations or rub may or may not be present. Palpable rhonchi is likely in bronchopneumonia (bronchus is involved and hence rhonchi).
- Tenderness may be looked for, but generally not seen, except in a rare case of pleural pain.

4. **Percussion**
   - Dullness is unlikely as there are no large areas of consolidation. Some areas may have even increased resonance if there is air trapping due to bronchospasm.
   - Look for cardiac dullness.
   - Percuss the upper border of liver dullness (confirm by tidal percussion).
   - Percuss Traube's space.
5. **Auscultation**
   - Intensity of breath sounds: Breath sounds, usually are normal or reduced intensity; vesicular in quality. Bronchial breath sounds are unlikely; if at all, it is more likely to be bronchovesicular rather than bronchial.
   - Adventitious sounds: Both crackle and wheeze (rhonchi) are abundant in bronchopneumonia.
   - Vocal resonance: It is likely to be normal or increased in some areas.

Investigations and Treatment

See under consolidation p 373.

COLLAPSE OR ATELECTASIS

1. **Symptoms and signs**
   This depends on the acuteness of collapse and extent of area involved. Acute collapse may have symptoms like that of pneumonia. Long standing collapse may have practically no symptoms.
2. **Inspection**
   - Respiration: Respiratory rate may or may not be increased depending on the acuteness of the collapse and extent of lung area involved. Ala nasi and other accessory muscles of respiration may or may not be active.
   - Trachea: Position of trachea is likely to be shifted to the side of collapse.
   - Apex: May be shifted towards the side of collapse, but only if collapse involves sufficient lung area.
   - Shape of chest: Drooping of shoulder, hollowing, flattening, etc may be present in large collapse.
   - Movement of chest: Movement will be restricted in the affected area.
   - There will be no dilated veins or pulsations because of collapse.
3. **Palpation**
   - Trachea and apex beat (mediastinum) may be shifted to the side of collapse.
   - Expansion of chest with inspiration may be restricted at the affected area (compare with normal side). Try to document the differential expansion, although it is likely to be far from accurate.
   - Vocal fremitus, in affected areas may be increased if bronchus is patent, but decreased if the bronchus is blocked.
   - No palpable events.
4. **Percussion**
   - Dullness or impaired resonance is expected in the area. Impaired resonance is more likely because the collapsed lung will be surrounded by normally aerated lung, which takes up the vacant space left by the collapse.
5. **Auscultation**
   - Intensity of breath sounds: Breath sounds will be of grossly reduced intensity or even totally absent when the bronchus is blocked. Rarely, bronchial breath sounds

may be audible when there is a patent bronchus (collapsed segment acts as a consolidated area conducting the bronchial sounds).

Caution: It is extremely unlikely that there is a patent bronchus; in fact, generally it is a blocked bronchus that lead on to the collapse (absorption collapse). In a very rare scenario, e.g., external compression to the lung can produce compression collapse where bronchus will be patent. The most common scenario of compression collapse is pleural effusion where findings suggestive of pleural effusion will predominate and in addition may have a bronchial breath sound at the top edge of pleural effusion. To make it clear: if there is mediastinal shift to same side and bronchial breathing one may diagnose collapse (some prefer to call this collapse consolidation, meaning consolidated collapsed segment). In the same scenario, if there is no mediastinal shift, offer the diagnosis of consolidation only, not collapse.

- Adventitious sounds: None likely.
- Vocal resonance: Classically, it is reduced; however, in a rare case of patent bronchus, it may be increased.

Notes:

1. Bulging intercostal spaces and tenderness indicate an ***empyema*** rather than a simple effusion.
2. The surrounding normal lung will expand and cover the collapsed lung so that the dullness may not be obvious.
3. There will be a higher level of dullness in the axilla in pleural effusion. This is partly due to the capillary action drawing the fluid up and partly due to the lung collapsing in a curvilinear manner towards the hilum as the fluid collects. Pain during percussion is indicative of a pleuritic pain or empyema.
4. In case of ***hydropneumothorax***, there will be a sharp horizontal level of dullness followed by hyper resonance above that. In addition, this level can be shown to change with the change of position of the patient. When we shake the patient, a splash sound can be heard indicating the free movement of the fluid in the pleural cavity because of the air fluid mixture inside.
5. In regions where the fluid collection is thin, some of the sound frequencies may be filtered off while some are conducted. This may lead on to a bleating quality of the vocal resonance (***aegophony***).
6. The presence of bronchial breathing depends on the presence of a patent bronchus and proximity of the consolidated lung tissue to the chest wall. Thus, bronchial breathing may not be heard always. In this situation, the breath sounds are likely to be vesicular but of diminished intensity due to the poor air entry to the consolidated lung.
7. As the pleural fluid collects, it compresses and collapses the overlying lung tissue so that this portion of lung tissue acts as a solidified segment. *Thus, at the upper border of a pleural effusion one may occasionally hear a bronchial breathing and increased VR.*
8. Crepitations (crackles) may be totally absent. If all the affected alveoli are solidified and are not opening up with inspiration, then one cannot have crepitations. However, the crepitations will appear at some stage of the disease, finer ones early and coarser ones later.

   Caution: When crepitations are absent as discussed above, many students have been misled to diagnosing pneumonia on the normal side. When there is a large area of consolidation on one side, the air entry on the normal side is enhanced so much to compensate for it that the breathing on the normal side may appear loud and harsh. Here, the harsh loud sound is more on inspiration; thus, bronchial

Table 16.1 Clinical comparison

	Consolidation	Collapse	Pleural effusion	Pneumothorax
Shape of chest	Unaffected	Maybe flattened	See note (1)	May be bulging if under tension
Movements of affected side	Maybe reduced	Maybe reduced	Maybe reduced	Maybe reduced
Trachea/mediastinum	Normally placed	Shifted to same side	Shifted to opposite side	Shifted to opposite side
Percussion	Impaired/dull	Impaired (2)	Stony dull (3)	Hyper resonance (4)
Vocal resonance	Increased	Diminished	Diminished (5)	Diminished
Breath sounds	Diminished or bronchial (6)	Diminished	Diminished (7)	Diminished
Adventitious sound	Crepitations (8)	None	None	None

breathing must be diagnosed only after carefully listening to expiration.

9. When the features of collapse and consolidation together are found, it is sometimes called collapse consolidation meaning that part of the area is collapsed and part is consolidated. For example, there are findings suggestive of consolidation but the mediastinum is shifted to the same side.

PLEURAL EFFUSION

1. **Symptoms and signs**
   Fever, cough, tachypnoea, etc.
2. **Inspection**
   - Respiration: Respiratory rate is increased. Look for any catch during respiratory movement on deep breath, e.g., in pleural rub the child may suddenly stop breathing movement when pleural rub producing pain. Ala nasi and other accessory muscles of respiration may be active during breathing.
   - Trachea: Position of trachea is shifted to opposite side.
   - Apex: Shifted to opposite side.
   - Shape of chest: The affected side may (or may not) show a generalized bulge (prominence) compared to the normal side. Look for any scoliosis, usually due to bending to the side of pleural pain. Drooping of shoulder, if present, may be part of scoliosis due to pain. Chest wall oedema is favour of empyema rather than simple effusion. Localized bulge in the intercostal space may be seen in empyema (empyema tracking into the subcutaneous space; this entity used to be called empyema necessitatis in yesteryear literatures).
   - Movement of chest: Movement will be diminished on the affected side, more so towards the lower part.
   - There will be no dilated veins or pulsations because of effusion.

16

- Scars: Specifically look for scars of intercostal drains, because the case may have had a diagnostic or therapeutic tap.

3. **Palpation**
   - Trachea and apex beat (mediastinum) are shifted to opposite side.
   - Expansion of chest with inspiration, may be restricted on the affected side (compare with normal side). Try to document the differential expansion, although it is likely to be far from accurate.
   - Vocal fremitus, on the affected side is decreased.
   - Palpable rub may be present on a rare occasion.
   - Tenderness may be elicitable in case of empyema. Rarely in pleural effusions there may be pain at the area of pleural rub.
4. **Percussion**
   - Stony dullness is expected in the area of pleural effusion. If dullness is detected, look for a higher level in axilla.

     Large pleural effusions do shift with change of position. This is best demonstrated anteriorly when the child is sitting and then in supine position.
   - Upper border of liver dullness must be confirmed by tidal percussion in all right sided small effusions to differentiate whether the dullness is due to liver or effusion.
   - Percuss Traube's space in all left sided effusions. Traube's space is normally hyper resonant due to the air in underlying fundus of stomach.
   - Occasionally in large effusions, the mediastinum pushed to the opposite side may produce a triangular area of dullness posteriorly on the opposite side of chest. This author has never been able to demonstrate this in a paediatric patient; remember to have demonstrated it in an adult with malignant effusion. Suffice to say that the student need not mention this sign at all.
5. **Auscultation**
   - Intensity of breath sounds: Breath sounds are normal in character (vesicular), but it will be of grossly reduced intensity (or even inaudible). Bronchial breath sounds may be audible rarely just above the effusion due to the compression collapse of the overlying lung acting as a consolidated segment.
   - Adventitious sounds: None, except for occasional pleural rub (carefully examine at the upper level of effusion; large effusion may not show the rub as the pleural surfaces are widely separated). If pleural rub is found, confirm it is rub by pressing the diaphragm of stethoscope firmly on to the chest wall, examination after coughing, etc (see p 367).
   - Vocal resonance: It is decreased; rarely there may be a small area of increased VR just above the upper border of effusion due to compression collapse of the over lying lung (refer to aegophony in text, p 368).
   - Look for succussion splash, when hydropneumothorax is suspected.

Investigations in Pleural Effusion and Empyema

- Total leukocyte count and differential
- Blood cultures (yield will be poor)
- X ray
- Ultrasonography
- Mantoux test
- Pleural fluid aspiration
- Most effusions are exudates. Transudate is unlikely in pulmonary pathology; it is seen in congestive heart failure, nephrotic syndrome, etc.
- Simple pleural effusion is clear, pale yellow fluid. Milky fluid suggest chylothorax (usually following injury in thoracic surgery). Blood stained fluid may be seen in trauma, malignancy, pancreatitis, etc.

- Tests to be done with pleural aspirate: Cells, protein, sugar, gram stain, culture, pH, LDH; AFB stain and AFB culture; pleural fluid adenosine deaminase.
- Exudates vs transudate (Light criteria).
- Pleural fluid lactate dehydrogenase to serum LDH ratio more than 0.6 or
  Pleural fluid protein to serum protein ratio more than 0.5.

Characteristics of Pleural Fluid in Empyema

- Protein more than 50% of serum proteins.
- LDH more than 1000 IU.
- pH often less than 7.1.
- Glucose less than 40 mg/dL.

Treatment

- Antibiotics: All pneumonia causing organisms can cause pleural effusion (examples are *pneumococci, H. influenzae, staphylococci,* etc).
- Anaerobes are possible in case of empyema (putrid odour suggests an anaerobic empyema). The usual starting antibiotics contains an anti-staphylococcal agent also (e.g., cefuroxime plus cloxacillin).
- Tube drainage (for simple pleural effusion, needle drainage may be enough).
- Intrapleural fibrinolytic therapy (controversial).
- Breathing exercises after drainage to help lung re-expand.
- Video-assisted thoracoscopic (VATS) surgery or conventional surgical decortication in organized empyema.

PNEUMOTHORAX

1. **Symptoms and signs**
   In acute onset tension pneumothorax, the complaints will be chest pain and severe respiratory distress and shock. There may be history of distressing cough (which may have precipitated air leak); history of tuberculosis; hemoptysis, etc.
2. **Inspection**
   - Respiration: Respiratory rate is increased. Ala nasi and other accessory muscles of respiration may be active during breathing.
   - Trachea: Position of trachea is shifted to the opposite side.
   - Apex: May be shifted to the opposite side.
   - Shape of chest: There may be bulging of the affected hemithorax.
   - Movement of chest: Movement will be restricted on the affected hemithorax. Look for respiratory accessory muscle activity.
   - Scars: Specifically look for scars of intercostal drains.
3. **Palpation**
   - Trachea and apex beat (mediastinum) are at shifted to opposite side.
   - Expansion of chest with inspiration, is very much reduced (sometimes nearly absent) on the affected hemithorax (compare with normal side). Try to document the differential expansion. Often crepitus of subcutaneous emphysema may be palpable (air escaping via mediastinum).
   - Vocal fremitus, on the affected areas is decreased (or absent).
4. **Percussion**
   - Hyper resonant note is expected in the affected side. It may even sound tympanic in very large pneumothorax.
5. **Auscultation**
   - Intensity of breath sounds: Breath sounds, if present is normal in character (vesicular), but of grossly reduced intensity. Breath sounds may even be absent. In non-tension pneumothorax that is "open" amphoric breath sounds at the site of pleural rent may be audible (because the pneumothorax acting as a big cavity and pleural rent acting as a narrow entry into the large cavity; this is exceedingly rare in paediatrics and hence the students are

unlikely to see one in their life time, leave alone during exam!).

- Adventitious sounds: None are expected.
- Vocal resonance: Decreased.
- Coin sound may be elicitable (rarely done these days) (see p 367).

Investigations and Treatment

- Pulse oximetry (tension pneumothorax may have life-threateningly poor oxygen saturation).
- ABG
- Transillumination in infants.
- X-ray chest.
- Ultrasonography.
- In an emergency, needle drainage in second space (in mid clavicular line) with IV set with the other end immersed in water will be diagnostic and also relieves some pressure effect.
- Oxygen inhalation (preferably by non-rebreathing bag).
- Chest tube drainage.
- Paracetamol for pain.
- Anti-staphylococcal antibiotics if pneumothorax is a complication of pneumonia.

HYDROPNEUMOTHORAX

This is a combination of pneumothorax and pleural effusion. The stony dullness of pleural effusion will have a horizontal upper level, above which it is hyper resonant. If examination is done in supine position, then make the child sit up and repeat the percussion. The area of dullness has shifted now (shifting dullness), but still there is stony dullness in the lower part, a horizontal upper level to this dullness, above which there is hyper resonance. Shifting dullness with horizontal upper level even after shifting clinches the diagnosis of hydropneumothorax. Succussion splash may be elicitable. There may be tinkling metallic sounds on auscultation, may be due fluid drop movements.

Investigations and Treatment

See under pleural effusion and pneumothorax.

CAVITY

Large cavities are unlikely in paediatric population. Cavity usually is not clinically detectable unless it is large and located superficially close to the chest wall. The clinical findings described below pertains to a large superficial cavity with patent bronchus.

1. **Inspection**: There may not be anything remarkable on inspection. There may or may not be a localized reduction in chest wall movement. Trachea and mediastinum are normally positioned.
2. **Palpation**: Vocal fremitus may be increased (assuming a patent bronchus).
3. **Percussion**: Percussion note may be dull (assuming significant fibrosis or cavity contains pus). Empty cavity located close to the chest wall will have hyper resonant note.
4. **Auscultation**: Large empty cavity with patent bronchus may have cavernous breath sounds. Pus-filled cavity will have diminished breath sounds.

   VR may be increased if feeding bronchus is patent. In pus-filled cavity, crackles may be audible.

PULMONARY FIBROISIS

1. **Symptoms and signs**

   Pulmonary fibrosis is not seen in children in modern era. Even in yesteryears, it was extremely uncommon in childhood (but common in adults with tuberculosis; TB in child heals by calcification, whereas TB in adults heals by fibrosis). However, rarely TB in children may lead on to fibrosis and bronchiectasis and occasionally bronchial stenosis, all of which are uncommon in the modern era. So if a student is making a diagnosis of fibrosis, he is more likely to be wrong than right.

Fibrosis is the end result of a healing process. Thus, if fibrosis is there at all, the child comes to medical attention because of associated problems like bronchiectasis or consolidation. So findings of these conditions will add on to the findings suggestive of fibrosis.

And lastly one needs extensive/dense fibrosis to get typical clinical findings suggestive of fibrosis. Extensive fibrosis is unlikely in children.

2. **Inspection**
   - Respiration: Respiratory rate depends on the associated problems (see above).
   - Trachea and apex beat: Shifted towards the affected side.
   - Shape of chest: Localized flattening of chest wall may be seen. Drooping of shoulder is likely when the upper lobe is involved.
   - Movement of chest: Movement will be diminished in the affected area. No indrawing or retractions with respiratory excursions.
3. **Palpation**
   - Trachea and apex beat (mediastinum) are shifted to the affected side.
   - Expansion of chest with inspiration, may be restricted at the affected area (compare with normal side). Try to document the differential expansion, although it is likely to be far from accurate.
   - Vocal fremitus, in affected areas may be decreased. But if it is increased, consider associated consolidation.
   - Palpable adventitious sounds are unlikely.
4. **Percussion**
   - Impaired resonance/dullness is expected in the area of fibrosis.
5. **Auscultation**
   - Intensity of breath sounds: Breath sounds are normal in character (vesicular), but will be of reduced intensity. Bronchial breath sounds if present, must be due to associated consolidation. Bronchial breath sounds from a patent bronchus getting conducted to chest wall by a dense extensive fibrosis is too much of an imagination than reality. So it is best not to commit bronchial breathing to be caused by fibrosis per se.
   - Adventitious sounds: Fibrosis per se does not have any adventitious sounds. Presence of adventitious sounds are due to associated issues like consolidation or bronchiectasis.
   - Vocal resonance: It is reduced; but may be increased if there is associated consolidation.

16

EMPHYSEMA

Emphysema as part of COPD is a disease of adults. In paediatrics, emphysema is found as bilateral hyperinfated lungs in asthma and bronchiolitis.

Unilateral or segmental obstructive emphysema is seen in foreign body obstruction, lymph node obstruction, etc. These are discussed further.

In the very rare cases of long standing emphysema in a child, always consider cystic fibrosis and α_1-anti trypsin deficiency. Thus, history of bulky sticky stools, failure to thrive, history suggestive of liver disease, etc becomes important (these precede pulmonary symptoms). Equally important is to look for bronchiectasis.

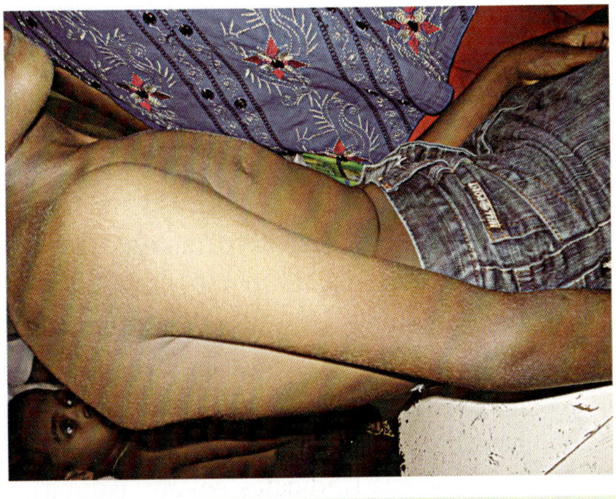

Fig.16.1 Emphysema of chest

BRONCHIAL ASTHMA

1. **Symptoms and signs**

   In case of an acute exacerbation, there may be a preceding history of viral upper respiratory infection or exposure to triggers (like dust, smoke, viral upper respiratory infection, etc). The main symptoms are breathlessness and cough (cough during the initial phase is dry, which later becomes wet). Fever is mild or totally absent. Fever if present initially, may be related to the initiating URI.

   Fever that appears days later in the course of illness could be due to secondary infection of stagnant secretions.

   History should focus on necessary information to diagnose asthma.

   - Three or more episodes of reversible airway obstruction (reversibility is assumed by the history prompt relief with nebulization).
   - Family history of asthma, allergic rhinitis, hay fever, etc.
   - Trigger factors for exacerbation (ask about URI, parental smoking, smoke from kitchen, in-house dusts, cockroaches, flowering plants, relation with exertion, pets, etc).
   - Relatively afebrile episodes.
   - In the child ask for history suggestive of allergic rhinitis also and look for evidence of allergic rhinitis (see p 356).

   General examination:

   - Anthropometry is important as growth may be impaired in poorly treated asthma.
   - General comment: Comment on sensorium (normal/drowsy/irritable).

   Hand to head and head to toe examination:

   - Nails: Clubbing is unlikely in asthma and hence its presence must indicate alternate diagnosis or additional diagnosis (e.g., bronchiectasis, cystic fibrosis, etc). Look for cyanosis (indicates severe asthma).
   - Pulse: Could be bounding in severe asthma with CO_2 retention. In severe exacerbation, one may find pulses paradoxus.
   - Look for cyanosis of lips/tongue.
   - Face: Look for evidences of allergy like allergic shiners, transverse crease on nose, etc.
   - Look for cushingoid features, likely in long-term steroid therapy.
   - Mention if the child has any intervention devices like prongs, oxygen masks or monitoring devices.
   - Chest: Look for chest wall deformities like pectus excavatum/carinatum, Harrison sulcus, etc.
   - Abdomen: Look for organomegaly (pushed down liver).

2. **Inspection of chest**

   - Respiration: Respiratory rate is increased.
   - Trachea and apex: Normal position.
   - Shape of chest: Bilaterally symmetrical bulging chest (antero-posterior diameter may be increased: "barrel-shaped chest"). Comment on any chest deformity like sulcus (likely in long standing cases).
   - Movement of chest: Chest wall expansile movement will be diminished bilaterally. There may be evidence of working of accessory muscles of respiration (flaring ala nasi, suprasternal indrawing, intercostals indrawing, etc); however, lower chest indrawing is not seen because the chest is already over expanded due to air trapping and hence there is no reason for lower chest to be drawn in during inspiration. All the other indrawings described above are efforts to augment the inspiratory effort by accessory muscles of respiration or intercostals muscles. Presence of lower chest indrawing must point towards pneumonia.

3. **Palpation**
   - Trachea and apex beat (mediastinum) are at normal position.
   - Expansion of chest with inspiration will be diminished bilaterally (this will be a subjective impression as there is no scope to compare with a normal side). Try to measure expansion.
   - Vocal fremitus, may be normal or diminished.
   - Palpable rhonchi is common in asthma.
4. **Percussion**
   - Hyper resonant percussion note (often percussion note may be normal or difficult to comment as it is bilaterally hyper resonant). Rarely, localized area of hyper resonance may be noticed due to localized air trapping secondary to mucous plug obstruction.
     Although asthma is a generalized disease, localized areas of air trapping could be there.
   - Cardiac dullness may be obliterated.
   - Upper border of liver dullness will be at a lower position (pushed down by the emphysematous lung).
5. **Auscultation**
   - Intensity of breath sounds: Breath sounds are vesicular with diminished intensity. Expiration may be prolonged in asthma.
   - Wheeze may be audible in asthma; crackles are also likely (secondary to inflammation) but as a rule, wheeze is much more pronounced than crackles.
   - Vocal resonance: Bilaterally normal or rarely decreased. Since there is no normal area to compare, this will have to be subjectively commented on.
6. **Other systems**: Examine CVS for evidence of pulmonary hypertension. Acute respiratory conditions can also cause temporary pulmonary hypertension.

Investigations

- Complete blood count, ESR (normal values are expected; may have eosinophila)
- Pulse oximetry and ABG during acute severe asthma exacerbations
- Mantoux
- X-ray chest
- Peak flow measurement
- Spirometry
- Skin prick test for allergen identification
- Total serum IgE (expected to be elevated; if extremely high values, consider allergic broncho-pulmonary aspergillosis)

16

Management of Acute Exacerbation of Asthma

Assess ABC:

- A: Alertness and good tone (drowsy child will be flaccid).
- B: Work of breathing as evidenced by activity of accessory muscles of respiration.
- C: Circulation as evidenced by capillary refill time.

1. Mild Exacerbation

ABC: A: Alert child. B: Work of breathing is not increased (respiratory rate may be increased). C: Capillary refill is normal. ABC is normal.

Nebulized salbutamol 150 mcg/kg/dose of salbutamol (but the minimum dose is 2.5 mg, i.e., 0.5 mL asthalin respirator solution) in 3 mL of saline once.

⇩

Assess for response.

⇩

Response is adequate and the child is comfortable (if the child is not improving adequately, shift to the management protocol of moderate exacerbation).

contd.

Discharge* on oral salbutamol (0.1–0.2 mg/kg/dose 6 hourly). If the child is already used to inhaler technique, salbutamol inhaler puffs, 2 puffs 4–6 hourly instead of oral salbutamol. Majority of children with mild exacerbation will require only oral salbutamol and no nebulizations.

⇩

*If the child has had a recent life threatening asthma episode, that child has to be kept under observation for at least 4 hours before discharge, to ensure that the initial relief is lasting.

2. Moderate Exacerbation

ABC: A: Alert child. B: Work of breathing is increased (clues include interrupted speech and interrupted feeding). C: Capillary refill is normal. Only B is abnormal.

Nebulized salbutamol (dose as above) every 20 min for three times in 1 hr. Use oxygen driven nebulizer if possible.

⇩

Assess for response.

⇩

(1) If the response is adequate, space out nebulization intervals to 2–4 hourly. Observe the child for 6–8 hrs. If the relief is sustained, discharge the child on oral salbutamol (0.1–0.2 mg/kg/dose 6 hourly) or salbutamol inhaler puffs, 2 puffs 4–6 hourly.

(2) If the response is only partial, start oral steroids (predinisolone 1–2 mg/kg/day); continue nebulizations. When improved (usually takes 1–2 days), discharge the child on oral salbutamol and steroids for 3–5 days. The child is fit for discharge if he feeds well and sleeps well.

(3) In case of deterioration manage as severe exacerbation.

If the nebulizer is not available, 2–4 puffs of salbutamol by metered dose inhaler using spacer (and mask for smaller children) every 20 min for three times or subcutaneous injection of terbutaline may be considered.

3. Severe Exacerbation (Acute Severe Asthma)

Assess ABC: A: Child may be drowsy; B: Work of breathing is increased (clues include interrupted speech and interrupted feeding); C: Capillary refill is abnormal; may have cyanosis. ABC abnormal.

Admit in the ICU.

⇩

Connect to pulse oximeter.

⇩

Oxygen inhalation.

⇩

Oxygen driven nebulization with salbutamol (dose as above) and ipratropium (125 mcg for infants and toddlers, 250 mcg for >5 years, 500 mcg for adolescents) every 20 min for three doses.

⇩

IV hydrocortisone 10 mg/kg initially followed by 4–5 mg/kg/dose every 6 hourly or IV methyl prednisolone 2 mg/kg/dose or if oral is tolerated, oral prednisolone 2 mg/kg/day.

⇩

IV Magnesium sulphate: 0.1 mL/kg 50% $MgSO_4$ in normal saline infusion over 30 min.

Injection aminophylline 5 mg/kg/dose diluted as IV infusion 6 hourly. Alternative is constant infusion at 0.7–0.9 mg/kg/hr.

⇩

If improvement is inadequate, consider continuous oxygen-driven nebulization with salbutamol*, 0.5 mg/kg or hourly nebulizations. Ipratropium can be spaced out to 4 hourly, mixed with the corresponding doses of salbutamol.

⇩

IV Terbutaline 10 mcg/kg bolus infusion over 30 min, followed by 0.4 mcg/kg/min increasing gradually, to maximum 4 mcg/kg/min.

⇩

Ketamine

⇩

Mechanical ventilation

Table 16.2 Long term Asthma Management in Children aged 6–11 years - Initial treatment

Presenting Symptoms	Preferred Initial Treatment	Step
Infrequent asthma symptoms < twice a month & no risk factors for exacerbation	As needed SABA ICS whenever SABA is taken	1
Asthma symptoms or need for reliever twice a month/more	Low dose ICS with as needed SABA Other options are daily LTRA or taking ICS whenever SABA is taken	2
Troublesome asthma symptoms on most days; Or waking due to asthma once a week/more, Especially if any risk factors exist	Low dose ICS - LABA with as needed SABA Medium dose ICS with as needed SABA Very low dose ICS - Formoterol maintenance and reliever Low dose ICS with daily LTRA, with as needed SABA	3
Initial asthma presentation is with severely uncontrolled asthma, or with an acute exacerbation	Medium dose ICS - LABA with as needed SABA or Low dose ICS-Formoterol maintenance & reliever Short course of oral steroids may be needed	4

Table 16.3 Long term Asthma Management in Adolescents & Adults - Initial treatment

Presenting symptoms	Preferred Initial Treatment	Alternative Initial treatment	Step
Infrequent asthma symptoms < twice a month& no risk factors for exacerbation	As needed low dose ICS - Formoterol	ICS taken whenever SABA is taken	1
Asthma symptoms or need for reliever twice a month/more	As needed low dose ICS - Formoterol	Low dose ICS with as needed SABA	2
Troublesome asthma symptoms on most days; Or waking due to asthma once a week/more, Especially if any risk factors exist	Low dose ICS - Formoterol maintenance & reliever therapy	Low dose ICS - LABA with as needed SABA Or Medium dose ICS with as needed SABA	3
Initial asthma presentation is with severely uncontrolled asthma, or with an acute exacerbation	Medium dose ICS - Formoterol maintenance & reliever therapy Short course of oral steroids may be needed	High dose ICS Or Medium dose ICS - LABA with as needed SABA Short course of oral steroids may be needed	4

Mild asthma	Moderate asthma	Severe asthma
Well controlled on step 1 or step 2	Well controlled on step 3 or step 4	Uncontrolled symptoms even on optimal step 3 or step 4

ACUTE BRONCHIOLITIS

1. **Symptoms and signs**
   - The whole episode may have started with a viral upper respiratory infection.
   - Main symptoms are breathlessness and cough. Fever is mild or totally absent. Fever if present initially, may be related to the initiating URI. Fever that appears days later in the course of illness could be due to secondary infection of stagnant secretions. Recurrent episodes of bronchiolitis is unlikely and hence bronchiolitis is a safe clinical diagnosis only for the first episode.

   General examination:
   - General comment: Comment on sensorium (normal/drowsy/irritable).

   Hand to head and head to toe examination:
   - Nails: Look for cyanosis (indicates severe disease).
   - Look for cyanosis of lips/tongue.
   - Mention if the child has any intervention devices like prongs, oxygen masks or monitoring devices.
   - Abdomen: Look for organomegaly (pushed down liver).
2. **Inspection**
   - Respiration: Respiratory rate is increased.
   - Trachea and apex: Normal position.
   - Shape of chest: Bilaterally symmetrical bulging chest ("barrel-shaped chest").
   - Movement of chest: Chest wall expansile movement will be diminished bilaterally. There may be evidence of working of accessory muscles of respiration (flaring ala nasi, suprasternal indrawing, intercostals indrawing, etc); however, lower chest indrawing is not seen because the chest is already over expanded due to air trapping and hence there is no reason for lower chest to be drawn in during inspiration. All the other indrawings described above are efforts to augment the inspiratory effort by accessory muscles of respiration or intercostals muscles. Presence of lower chest indrawing must point towards brancho pneumonia.
3. **Palpation**
   - Trachea and apex beat (mediastinum) are at normal position.
   - Expansion of chest with inspiration will be diminished bilaterally (this will be a subjective impression as there is no scope to compare with a normal side). Try to measure expansion, but this measurement must be reserved for last to avoid provoking the child to cry.
   - Vocal fremitus, may be normal or diminished.
   - Palpable rhonchi may be there.
4. **Percussion**
   - Hyper resonant percussion note.
   - Cardiac dullness may be obliterated.
   - Upper border of liver dullness will be at a lower position (pushed down by the emphysematous lung)
5. **Auscultation**
   - Intensity of breath sounds: Breath sounds are vesicular with diminished intensity. Expiration may be prolonged as in asthma but difficult to appreciate due to high rate. Wheeze may be audible but in severe cases the chest may be almost silent due to widespread bronchiolar obstruction and inability of baby to generate enough inspiratory effort to overcome this.
   - Vocal resonance: Bilaterally normal or rarely decreased. Since there is no normal area to compare, this will have to be subjectively commented on.

Investigations

- Blood counts are either normal or show lymphocyte predominance suggestive of viral infection.
- X ray show hyperinflation.
- Pulse oximetry and ABG.

- Nasal swab: Fluorescent antibody detection of RSV.

Treatment

- Adequate hydration. If oral intake is not sufficient, supplement with IV fluids.
- Humidified oxygen.
- Nebulized adrenaline 0.1–0.3 mL of 1:1000 solution of adrenaline per kg per dose diluted in saline. The dose may have to be repeated 4 hourly.
- Nebulization with hypertonic saline (3%) to thin down the tenacious mucous.
- Steroids are not indicated.
- Nebulized ribavirin may be beneficial if the fluorescent RSV antibody test is positive (presently this is reserved for high risk groups like congenital heart disease).
- RSV immunoglobulin may be used prophylactically during RSV season in high risk patients (e.g., premature babies with chronic lung disease).
- Anti-RSV monoclonal antibody is presently preferred to RSV immunoglobulin.

UNILATERAL HYPERINFLATED (EMPHYSEMATOUS) LUNG

This situation is generally due to partial obstruction of bronchus (foreign body, lymph node, etc):

1. **Symptoms and signs**
   These are related to the underlying conditions.
2. **Inspection**
   - Respiration: Respiratory rate may be normal or increased.
   - Trachea and apex: Shifted to opposite side.
   - Shape of chest: Unilateral bulging hemithorax.
   - Movement of chest: Movement will be diminished on the affected side.
3. **Palpation**
   - Trachea and apex beat (mediastinum) are shifted to the opposite side.
   - Expansion of chest with inspiration, will be diminished on the affected side.
   - Vocal fremitus, may be diminished.
4. **Percussion**
   - Hyper resonant percussion note.
   - Cardiac dullness may be obliterated if left side is affected.
   - Upper border of liver dullness will be at a lower position (pushed down by the emphysematous lung), if right side is affected.
5. **Auscultation**
   - Intensity of breath sounds: Breath sounds are vesicular with diminished intensity. Sometimes, localized wheeze may be audible at the site of obstruction.
   - Vocal resonance: Decreased on the affected side.

16

BRONCHIECTASIS

1. **Symptoms and signs**
   Fever, tachypnoea, chest indrawing, chronic cough, copious sputum, weight loss, loss of appetite, etc. One must ask in detail about the sputum (copious sputum for a long time, but presently it has turned yellow or foul smelling is the usual history).

   Must ask about suggestive history of chronic sinusitis (the association may be seen in Kartagener). Exercise tolerance, bronchodilator use, any recent worsening of symptoms, etc must be inquired into. The treatment the child is already on may be documented (exercise, physiotherapy, home nebulizers, etc).
2. **Past history**
   - Previous history of hemoptysis: As cystic fibrosis may be a cause for bronchiectasis, ask for weight loss, bulky offensive sticky stools, etc. Recurrent infections in various locations may point towards immunodeficiency as the cause of bronchiectasis.

- History of TB in the family.
- Past history of measles or whooping cough.

3. **General examination**
   - Vitals: Pulse may be normal or bounding due to hypercarbia.
   - Assessment of growth (anthropometry): Bronchiectasis being a chronic illness will have growth retardation.
   - Head to foot: Nails (clubbing, cyanosis); Ears: recurrent otitis in immunodeficiency or celiary dyskinesia; Chest: look for chest wall deformities and dextrocardia.
   - Tanner staging. Pubertal delay is common in chronic diseases.
4. **Inspection**
   - Respiration: Respiratory rate may be increased. Ala nasi and other accessory muscles of respiration may be active during breathing.
   - Trachea: Position of trachea is central; may be altered due to associated issues, like fibrosis or collapse.
   - Apex: Normal position.
   - Shape of chest: Hyperinflation is likely. So chest wall may appear prominent.
   - Movement of chest: Movement may or may not be restricted in the affected side.
3. **Palpation**
   - Trachea and apex beat (mediastinum) are at normal position (unless there are associated problems).
   - Expansion of chest with inspiration, may be restricted. Measure A-P diameter (using two boards or books). Try to document the differential expansion, although it is likely to be far from accurate.
   - Vocal fremitus, in affected areas may be normal or decreased depending on the patency of the bronchus (VF may be increased if there is associated consolidation).
   - Palpable crackles and wheeze are common.
4. **Percussion**
   - No diagnostic findings in uncomplicated bronchiectasis.
5. **Auscultation**
   - Intensity of breath sounds: Breath sounds, may be normal in character (vesicular). If there is a bronchial breathing, associated consolidation is likely.
   - Adventitious sounds: Coarse crackles are common. Wheeze is also common.
   - Vocal resonance: Depends on associated consolidation.

Do not forget to examine the heart. There may be dextrocardia (Kartagener), loud pulmonary second sound (pulmonary hypertension secondary to chronic lung problem) or right sided cardiac failure.

Investigations

- Imaging: X-ray chest and CT. High-resolution CT (HRCT) is the diagnostic standard. Railroad/tram track streaking, honey combing, signet ring, etc may be seen (Fig. 25.51, p 574).
- Pulmonary function test may show obstructive, restrictive or mixed pattern.
- Investigations to detect aetiology:
  - Investigations for tuberculosis.
  - Bronchoscopy: Obstruction – foreign body, tumour.
  - Sweat chloride test – increased sodium and chloride in cystic fibrosis.
  - Immunoglobulin profile.
  - HIV test.
  - Cilia function and structure – Kartagener syndrome.
  - Sputum culture or deep oropharyngeal swab in younger children.
  - α_1-antitrypsin levels.

Treatment

- Antibiotics for exacerbations.
- Postural drainage and chest physiotherapy.
- Surgical removal of the affected area if localized bronchiectasis.
- Nebulized gentamicin or tobramycin as continuous preventive antibiotics.
- Inhaled mucolytics: N-acetyl cysteine.
- Beta agonist only if there is bronchospasm.
- Additional vaccines: E.g., conjugate pneumococcal vaccine and yearly influenza vaccines.

CHAPTER 17

Gastrointestinal System

The usual complaints pertaining to disorders of gastrointestinal system are:
Diarrhoea, constipation, vomiting, abdominal pain, abdominal distension, hemetemesis, malena, hematochezia (fresh blood per rectum), jaundice, itching, oedema, etc. These individual complaints are discussed in ch. 8.

EXAMINATION OF UPPER GI TRACT

Please refer to scheme of examination, p 6.

Lips

- Look for angular stomatitis (angular cheilitis), dry fissured lips (cheilosis), wet inflamed lip (cheilitis; cheilosis with inflammation is cheilitis; most common cause is excess salivation), herpetic ulcers, perleche, rhagades. Classically, cheilosis is fissuring due to riboflavin deficiency. Fissuring of lips is also found in Kawasaki disease. Cracked lips are common in cold weather.
- Perleche: Fissuring, scaling, maceration and crusting of the angles of mouth (angular cheilitis/stomatitis). Cheilitis due to persistent licking or collection of moisture is called perleche.
- Rhagades: Radiating scars at the angle of mouth that extend into the mouth; seen in congenital syphilis. To convey how it will look like, the closest approximation that one can think of is the radiating lines from lips of very old characters in English films.
- Pigmented lips and buccal mucosa may be seen in Peutz-Jeghers syndrome, Addison's disease, etc.

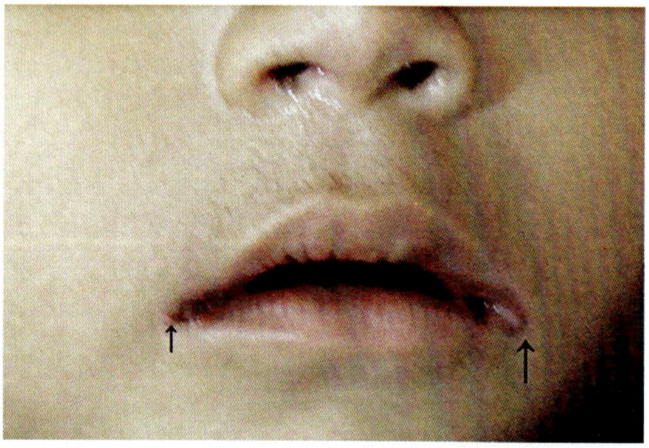

Fig.17.1 Angular stomatitis (angular cheilitis). Possible aetiology is riboflavin deficiency. Similar appearance may be seen in Candida infection as well (perleche).

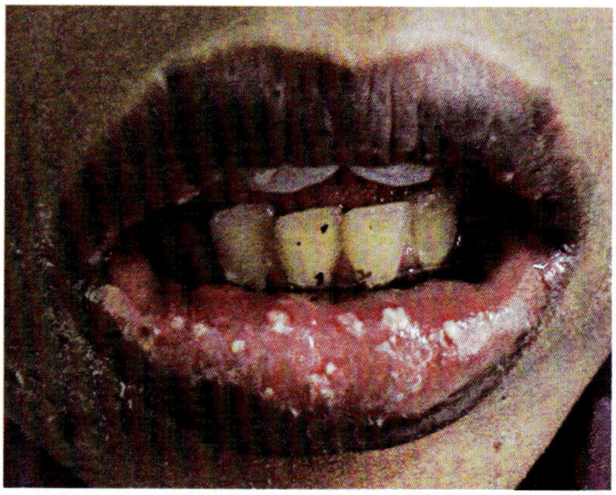

Fig.17.2 Herpes labialis

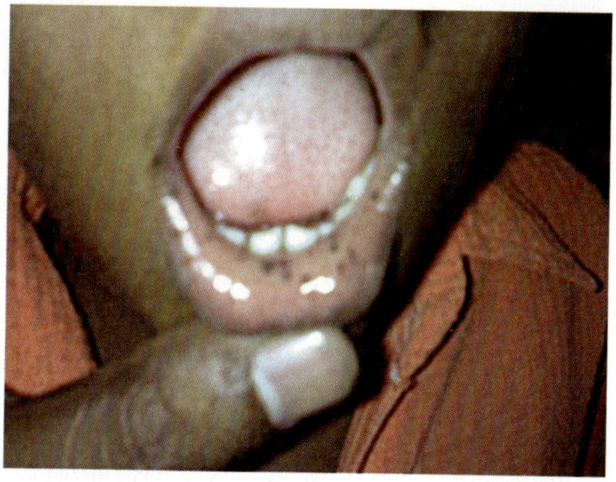

Fig.17.3 Peutz Jegher syndrome

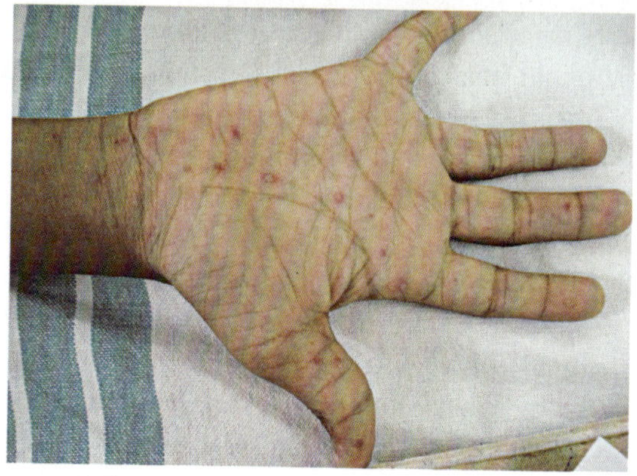

Fig.17.4 Lesions of hand-foot-mouth disease

Oral Cavity

Examine the lips, gums, teeth, tongue, palate, pharynx and tonsil.

- Aphthous ulcer: Small painful ulcer with a yellowish white base, on a hyperaemic surrounding area; aphthous ulcer may be recurrent. Traumatic ulcer also may look similar but history of trauma may be elicitable (e.g., trauma by tooth brush). Other causes of ulcers in oral cavity are herpes simplex, hand-foot-mouth disease, herpangina, agranulocytosis, etc.
- Strawberry tongue with prominent papillae is seen in scarlet fever. When red papillae are seen in the background of white coating of tongue, it is called white strawberry tongue, which is usual in early scarlet fever. Later this coating is shed so that the red papillae are seen in red background, hence the red strawberry tongue.
- Magenta tongue (purplish red) and angular stomatitis are seen in riboflavin deficiency.
- Raw beefy tongue with atrophic papillae is seen in long standing B_{12} deficiency.
- Bald tongue (atrophic glossitis) without papillae may be seen in riboflavin, niacin or iron deficiency. Atrophic glossitis is seen only in long standing deficiency.

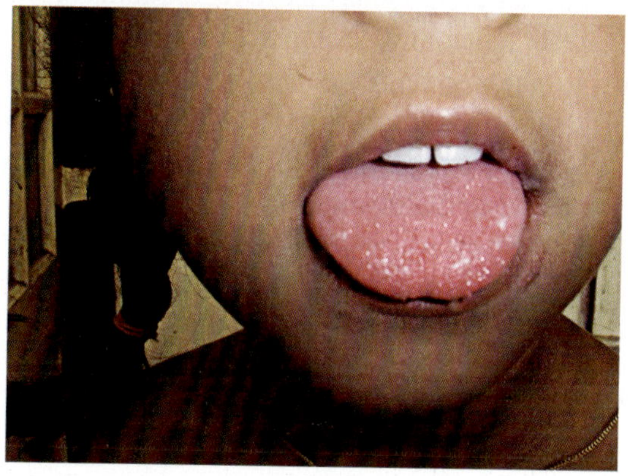

Fig.17.5 Red strawberry tongue. May be seen in scarlet fever, Kawasaki disease, etc. The appearance is due to the enlargement and reddening of paplllae of tongue.

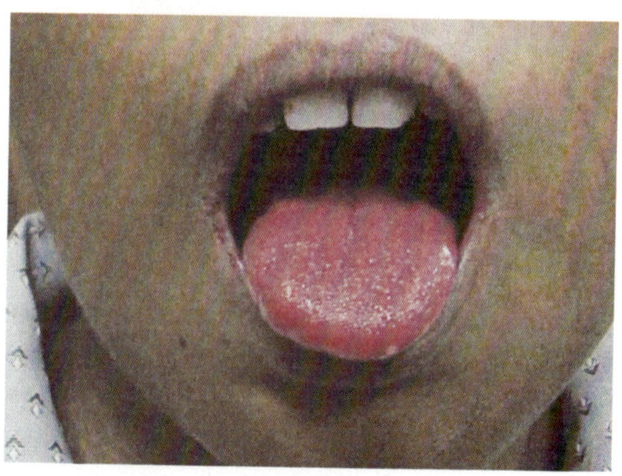

Fig.17.6 Magenta tongue

- Coated tongue is classically described in typhoid, which consists of central coating and retained redness in the periphery.
- Black pigmentation of tongue is seen in Peutz-Jeghers syndrome, Addison disease, dyskeratosis congenita, etc.
- Look for bleeding gums of scurvy. Gum hypertrophy may occur in poor oral hygiene (gingivitis), AML and phenytoin therapy. It can be detected by passing a paper between the gum and crown of teeth to demonstrate the space in between. This space is created by the projected out gum.
- Blue line (Burtonian line) over the gum at gum-teeth junction is seen in lead poisoning.
- Koplik's spots seen opposite lower 2nd molar tooth is pathognomonic of measles (white spots with reddish base). It appears before the appearance of rashes of measles, is very transient and is usually not found once the measles exanthem appears **(Fig. 17.7)**.
- Look for oral thrush. Oral thrush is difficult to remove and leaves bleeding points (hence it is easily differentiated from white patches left by milk feeding).
- Look for the presence/absence of tonsils and its inflammation. Absence of tonsils is often due to surgical removal; may also indicate T cell immunodeficiency.

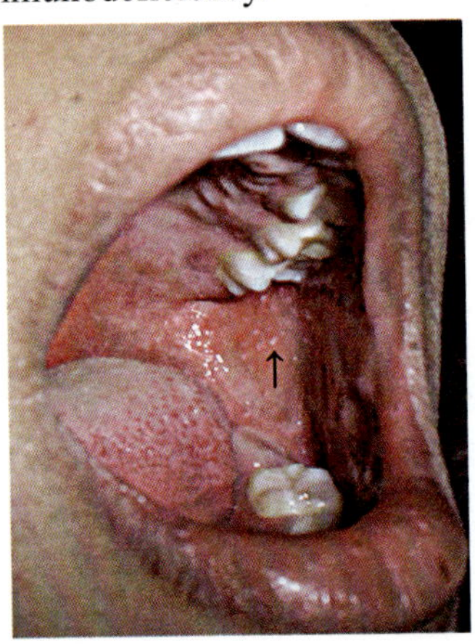

Fig.17.7 Koplik spot

Posterior to the last molar is two vertical webs of tissue (tonsillar pillars) between which is the tonsil. At birth, the tonsils are barely visible; it progressively enlarges, reaches maximum size by 6–8 years and then slowly involutes to adult size over the years. Thus in a school-aged child, the tonsils are bigger by adult standards. Past infections leave tonsils hypertrophied, pitted and even with white concretions for many months. It is like cervical lymph nodes persisting for months after an infection in the drainage area. Also if a child can say a good Ahh — with protrusion of tongue, the tonsils will project out giving a false impression of hypertrophy (hence better make the child say Ahh without protruding out the tongue). The message is that one must concentrate on the redness and exudates on the tonsils rather than its size. The student must be familiar with the normal appearance of tonsils because normally the tonsils are a shade redder than the buccal mucosa. Small nodules giving a bumpy appearance to posterior pharyngeal wall ("pharyngeal tonsil") indicates lymphoid hyperplasia there and thus indicates pharyngitis.

- Inflamed tonsils and pharynx often cause drooling from mouth. (***Note***: Drooling in those less than 2 years of age is most often physiological.)
- Look for grayish white membrane over the fauces and tonsils in diphtheria.

Differential diagnosis of white patch in tonsil are:

- Group A β-haemolytic streptococci: Exudates in follicles, easily removable without bleeding.
- Diphtheria: Difficult to remove dirty gray patch, bleeds on attempted removal.
- Thrush: The patch white, may extend to tongue and oral mucosa.
- IMN: Patch somewhat like streptococci.

- Painful ulcers over anterior pillar of fauces is seen in herpangina **(Fig. 17.8)**.
- Caries teeth involving inner side of upper central incisors indicates bottle baby syndrome (enquire about the baby sleeping with bottle or breast at night) **(Fig. 6.79, p 112)**.

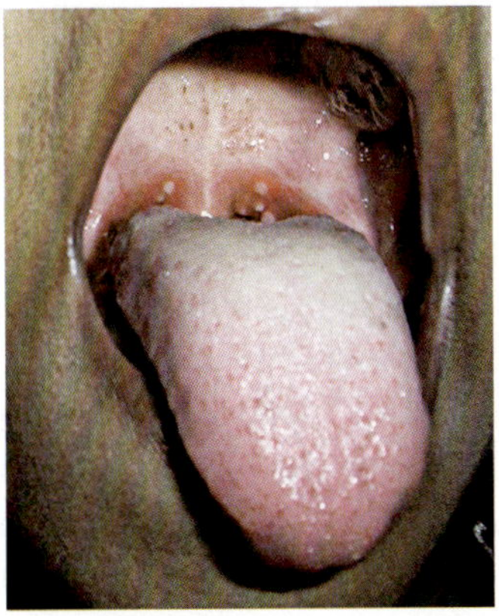

Fig.17.8 Herpangina

- Look for pigmentation of oral mucosa as in Peutz-Jeghers, dyskeratosis congenita and Addison's disease.

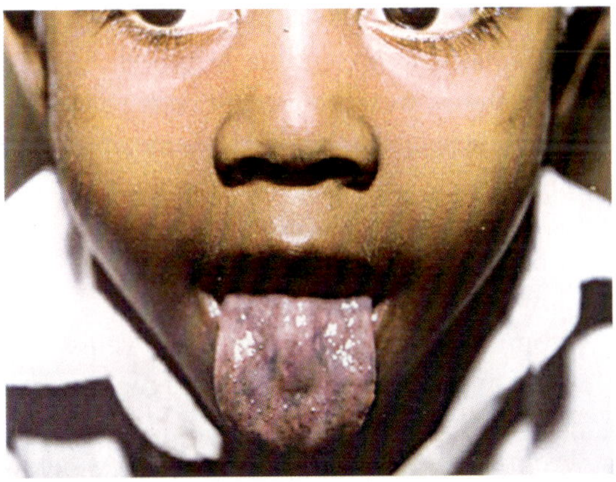

Fig.17.9 Pigmented tongue

- Listen to the speech. If nasal twang is present but no cleft palate seen, palpate for submucous cleft.
- Smell the breath. Halitosis is expected in poor oral hygiene, bronchiectasis and lung abscess. Fruity odour (similar to that of nail polish remover) suggests diabetic ketoacidosis, which may present with abdominal pain and vomiting.

EXAMINATION OF ABDOMEN

See p 6 for organized case sheet of GIT.
Examination should be done in supine position and in toddlers standing position is also acceptable. Abdomen can be divided into nine quadrants by two vertical and two horizontal lines **(see Fig. 17.10)**.

17

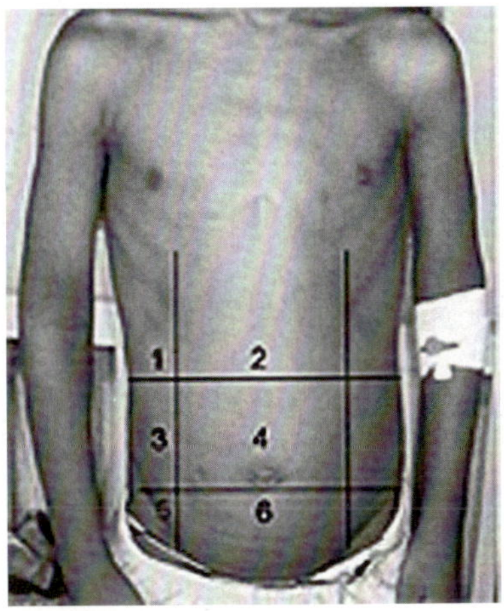

Fig.17.10 Abdomen markings

Two vertical lines pass through the mid-inguinal point (midway between the midline of abdomen and anterior superior iliac spine) upwards to mid clavicular point.

Horizontal lines: The upper horizontal line connects the two lowermost points of costal margins, and the lower horizontal line connects two iliac crests. The areas marked in **Fig. 17.10** are hypochondrium (1), epigastrium (2), lumbar area (3), umbilical area (4), iliac fossa (5), and hypogastrium (6).

Inspection

Inspection of the abdomen comprises of:

- Shape of the abdomen
- Skin (scars, sinuses, dilated veins)
- Movements with respiration
- Umbilicus
- Visible pulsations
- Visible peristalsis
- Hernial orifices
- External genitalia

For inspection of the abdomen, it is best for the examiner to sit beside the child as it brings his eyes at level with the anterior abdominal wall (minor variations in contour are picked up this way). Hernia and engorged veins are detected by inspection with the patient in standing position. Watch the position and attitude of the patient. Restlessness and irritability are suggestive of colicky pain. A child who is afraid to move may have peritonitis.

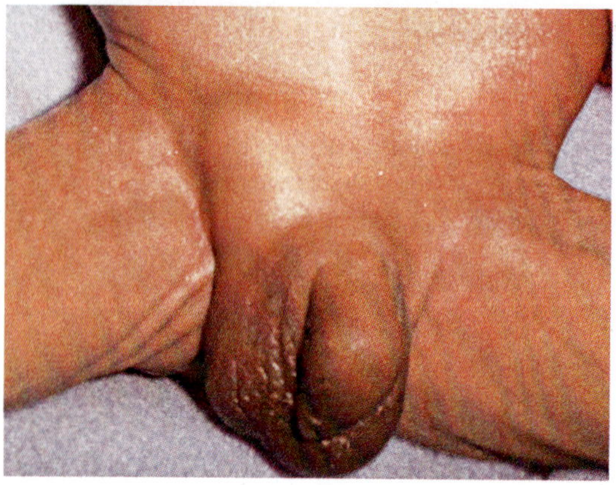

Fig.17.11 Inguinal hernia

Shape of Abdomen

Scaphoid abdomen is normal in adult males and not in a child. In small children under five, a protuberant abdomen is actually the normal one expected (partly due to exaggerated lumbar lordosis). Scaphoid abdomen is abnormal in newborn, it being pathognomonic of diaphragmatic hernia (abdomen is scaphoid as its contents have gone into the chest). Occasionally, scaphoid abdomen may be seen in marasmus. If there is distention, look for any asymmetry in distention. For example, a suprapubic bulge could be due to bladder. Localized fullness may also be seen in organ enlargements like hepatomegaly, splenomegaly or other masses. Mention if the flanks appear full or not. Symmetrical distention could be due to gas, obesity or ascites. Unilateral flank swelling could be kidney mass as well. Remember the old mnemonic of five Fs—Fat, Flatus, Faeces, Fluid and Fetus. With adolescent care slowly coming to paediatrics, fetus is also a possibility!

Abdominal distention due to lax abdominal wall is seen in rickets, hypothyroidism, celiac disease, etc. Remember the typical presentation of celiac disease: symptoms starting after weaning; severely wasted child with markedly protuberant abdomen. Divarication of recti muscle is noticed as a linear protrusion, as the child tries to raise his shoulder from bed (Fig. 6.136). It can be a normal variant or because of abdominal distention like ascites.

Skin Over the Abdomen

In tense ascites, the skin may look tense and glistening. In prune belly syndrome, the abdominal skin is totally wrinkled due to the absence of abdominal wall muscles (sort of floating abdomen with fullness in flanks and skin folds radiating from umbilicus; **(Fig. 24.52, p 513)**. Look for dilated veins, scars, etc.

- Prominent abdominal veins suggest venous flow obstruction.
- Prominent dilated peri umbilical veins with flow away from umbilicus suggest portal hypertension.
- Prominent veins in the flanks with flow below upwards inferior vena cava obstruction.

Striae, may be due to recent weight loss in the obese, steroid therapy or Cushing's syndrome. Striae of steroids initially may look pinkish, but ultimately becomes white and looks similar to the striae due to other causes. Striae are usually seen over the lower abdomen (laterally), thigh, axilla, etc.

Movement with Respiration

Abdominothoracic breathing is the normal pattern in children. Thoraco-abdominal breathing may be seen when abdominal distension/pain is present. Normal abdominal movement during respiration is bulging out during inspiration and collapsing during expiration. The reverse (paradoxic) abdominal movements are seen in diaphragmatic paralysis. Abdomen is held rigid without any movement in peritonitis. Asymmetry of movement of abdomen may indicate localized pathology.

Visible Lump, Pulsations and Peristalsis

Epigastric pulsations are normally seen in thin children. Epigastric pulsations may originate from aorta, liver or enlarged right ventricle.

Visible peristalsis is sometimes seen normally in thin individuals. Abnormal visible peristalsis: In pyloric stenosis, the peristalsis is from left to right in the left hypochondrium. In small intestinal obstruction, the peristalsis is around the umbilicus in various directions. In transverse colon obstruction, the peristalsis is from right to left, midway between xiphisternum and umbilicus. In obstruction of ascending and decending colons, one gets vertical, upward or downward peristaltic movements on the flanks. Frankly one never gets to see these typical peristalsis waves.

Umbilicus

It is normally inverted or flat. Everted umbilicus may be due to umbilical hernia, which in majority of infants will resolve by 4 years. Defects over 2 cm and the cosmetically unacceptable umbilical hernia may be surgically corrected after waiting for a minimum of 4 years. In contrast, paraumbilical hernias do not close spontaneously and need surgical correction. Umbilical hernia is also a pointer towards hypothyroidism, ascites, etc. Transversely stretched umbilicus (smiling umbilicus) is described in ascites. Umbilical granuloma is a reddish swelling without any pedicle seen in the post newborn period (in contrast, polyp will have a pedicle). Note any discharge from the umbilicus. If present, note if it is due to infection (foul smell, erythema, induration). If urine/faeces comes through the umbilicus, consider persistent urachus/omphalomesenteric duct (they are usually associated with umbilical polyps). In case of ascites, always measure the abdominal girth (at the level of umbilicus), as it is needed to follow-up for increasing ascites. Note that the examiner expects the student to do this measurement. Before finishing the inspection of abdomen, have a look at hernial orifices and external genitalia.

17

Related General Examinations to be Done

- Look for the evidence of fat malabsorption like stigmata of fat-soluble vitamin deficiencies, xanthomas (raised, yellowish, cholesterol rich deposits), trace element deficiencies like zinc (acrodermatitis), etc.
- Look for petechiae, ecchymosis, proptosis, bone tenderness, etc (especially in a patient with organomegaly).
- Bluish subcutaneous nodules are seen in neuroblastoma with metastatic skin involvement.
- Look for arthritis, uveitis, skin rash, and erythema nodosum in a patient with a chronic history of diarrhoea and abdominal pain (inflammatory bowel disease).
- Clubbing is not a sign limited to cardiac and pulmonary diseases alone. GIT causes of clubbing include ulcerative colitis, celiac disease, cirrhosis and cystic fibrosis.
- It is important to count the respiratory rate in ascites and in "acute" abdomen.
- Look for KF ring, cataract, spider naevi, palmar erythema, scratch marks, flapping tremor, testicular atrophy and gynaecomastia in a child with jaundice.

Palpation

Warm approach and warm hands are essential prerequisites for a successful abdominal palpation. Flexing the hips and taking deep breaths will help in relaxation of abdomen. In a crying child, the only chance is to palpate when the child pauses to take a breath. Dipping palpation may be attempted in an obese child.

Painful areas must be palpated last or else the cooperation of the child will be lost. There is no definite sequence of palpation, but one recommendation is to start palpating from left iliac fossa, proceeding anticlockwise to left kidney, spleen, liver, right kidney, right iliac fossa, urinary bladder, groins and genitals.

If the area, which is said to have pain, is painless on palpation, press firmly down and release suddenly to look for rebound tenderness (indicates peritoneal irritation, like appendicitis). Pain due to spastic bowel is relieved by pressure or squeeze, whereas the same manoeuvre aggravates the pain of inflammatory conditions like peritonitis. Loin tenderness is related to the kidney.

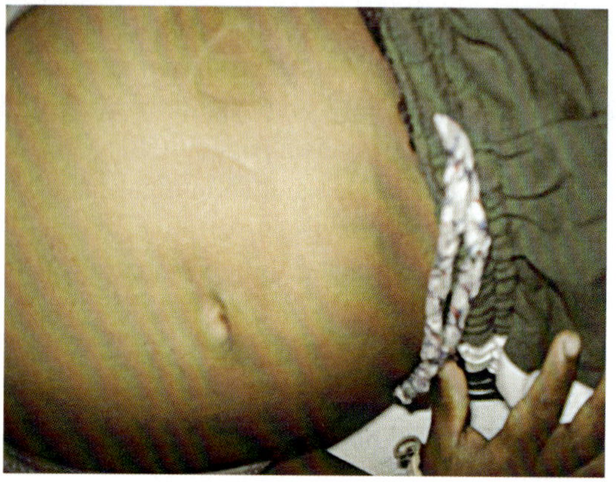

Fig.17.12 Abdominal wall oedema

Feel of Abdomen

Comment whether the abdomen feels soft, firm, tense, doughy, etc. Abdomen is normally soft. It is very soft in prune-belly syndrome; doughy in abdominal tuberculosis; localized firmness may be seen over swellings; rigid in peritonitis and tetanus. It is difficult to describe the doughy feel. The closest approximation would be the feel of the lax abdomen of an obese multiparous woman. Localized rigidity may be due to a localized cause like acute appendicitis. But the most common cause of "rigid" abdomen is the apprehensive child holding it tight. Palpable coils of intestine could mean spastic coils of intestine, worms or faeces. If it is due to spastic coils, there will be associated abdominal pain as well. If relevant to the case at hand, look for skin turgor or abdominal wall oedema.

Skin turgor: Skin turgor must be tested for by picking up a thick fold of skin with subcutaneous tissue over the abdominal wall; use thumb and four fingers to pinch, (not just thumb and one finger) vertically, midway between the umbilicus and the flanks. It is not a reliable sign in SAM. **See Fig 24.11**.

Skin turgor is normal in no dehydration status (goes back instantaneously on release without leaving any dimple). In some dehydration, the fold of skin starts going back on release of pinching fingers but a dimple at the region of pinch is visible as the skin goes back. In severe dehydration, the tenting produced by the skin pinch remains for a second or two after the pinching hand is removed. **See Fig. 24.11**, p 493 and note that the tenting of skin remains even after the pinching hand is removed.

Abdominal wall oedema: To demonstrate abdominal wall oedema, pinch the abdominal wall for 5 sec, release it, and look for pitting **(Fig. 17.12)**. Just pressure with stethoscope diaphragm or pressing with just one finger will also provide the same information.

Areas of Tenderness/Mass

Mention if there is any area of rigidity, tenderness or local rise of temperature. Tenderness over specific areas may point towards its origin. Examples are:

- Left upper quadrant: Perisplenitis.
- Right upper quadrant: Liver, gall bladder.
- Right lower quadrant: Appendicitis. Fullness over the right lower quadrant may be because of appendiceal mass and caecal mass. *Emptiness* over this area indicates that the caecum is pulled up as in intussusception (*sine de dance sign*).
- Left lower quadrant: Amoebiasis, inflammatory bowel disease.
- Periumbilical pain: Functional; small intestinal pain.
- Renal angle tenderness is seen in renal problems like pyelonephritis or perinephric abscess.
- Hypogastrium: Descending colon, sigmoid or urinary bladder. Urinary bladder, if distended, may be palpated and percussed above the symphisis pubis.
- Inguinal region: Feel for hernia, undescended testes, lymph nodes, etc.

In case any mass is detected, describe it: site, size, consistency, margins, surface, mobility, tenderness, movement with respiration, continuity with any organs, pulsations, ballotability, whether the mass appears more prominent while trying to get up from supine (parietal swellings become more prominent).

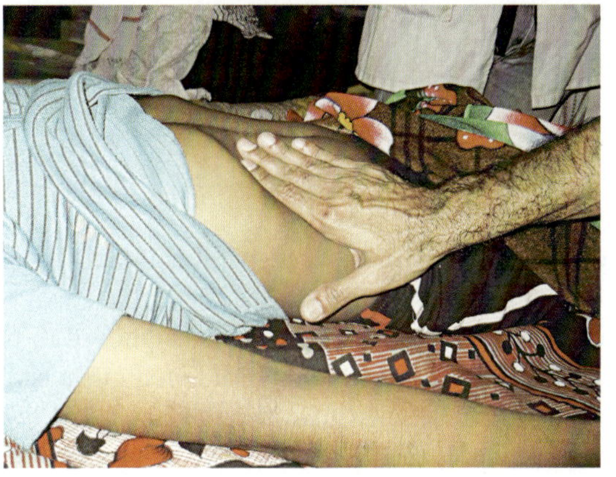

Fig.17.13 Palpation of liver with the hand parellel to the rib margin

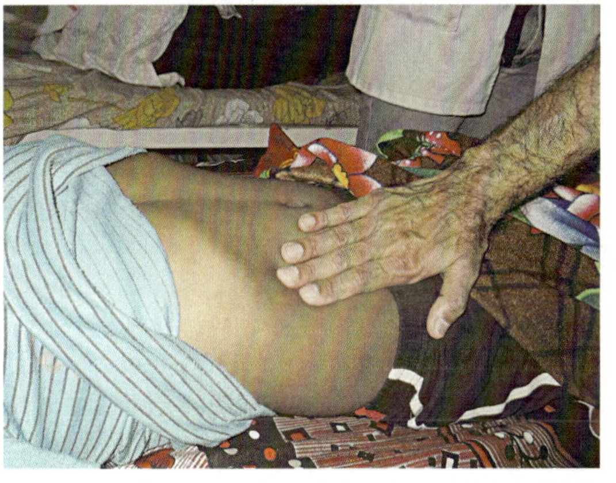

Fig.17.14 Palpation of liver with tip of fingers facing up

17

Liver

Standing on the right side (or better sit and be as close to the level of patient as possible), start palpating from the right lower quadrant, with the right hand below and parallel to the right subcostal margin. The tip (pulp) of fingers is more sensitive than the side of fingers. Hence while palpating, the finger up method is preferred (fingers pointing towards the ribs) **(Figs. 17.13, 17.14)**.

Another method as per "Hutchison's clinical methods" is palpating from above downwards placing both hands side by side in the right subcostal region with fingers pointing towards the ribs. If the liver is enlarged, a resistance is felt, and one can move down till the resistance disappears to find the lower edge of the liver.

This method may be of advantage where the liver is not normally palpable (as in adults) because then it avoids the discomfort of palpating up starting from the lower abdomen.

Normal liver is soft or soft to firm with smooth surface, regular rounded margins, moving with respiration, and fingers cannot be insinuated between the hepatic mass and the subcostal margin.

Points to be noted in examining the liver are:

- Size (measured in cm from costal margin, along the midclavicular line),
- Shape (may have an odd shape when there is a localized swelling like abscess/tumour or left lobe enlargement)
- Consistency (normal is soft, firm in cirrhosis, hard in malignancy)
- Border (sharp leafy border is supposed to be characteristic of Indian childhood cirrhosis)
- Surface (in cirrhosis the surface may feel nodular)
- Tenderness (rapid enlargement causing stretching of liver capsule causes pain, like viral hepatitis, congestive heart failure, etc)
- Pulsations (e.g., tricuspid regurgitation)
- Hepatojugular reflux (in CCF).

A truly soft liver is difficult to make out by palpation; it feels just as a difference in resistance from the rest of the abdomen. Rounded margin of the soft liver slips ("folds") under the examining fingers without giving a definite "edge" feel to the palpating fingers.

It is not true that acute events cannot produce a firm liver. In fact, in many cases of acute hepatitis, liver feels "firmish," due to the rapid enlargement of parenchyma within a less yielding liver capsule; the liver may then be tender as well. It is not true that once this tenderness goes off, the feel of the liver will return to soft; tenderness goes off as the capsule has somewhat adjusted to the stretched state, but the liver parenchyma inside is still remaining compressed and hence a "firmish" feel persists for days.

Firmish liver may be seen in fatty liver, congestive cardiac failure, hepatitis, IMN, typhoid, etc. Liver may be described as soft in some of these cases, but truly soft liver is seen only in the normal child. Any liver that is not definitely firm is best described as soft by the examination candidate. The term "firmish" is not relished by examiners!

Most often the feel of the liver in sick children will be somewhere between soft and firm. For example, an easily palpable liver that does not feel firm is actually not truly soft either, but a little firmer than the true soft one. Such 'soft to firm' livers usually have rounded margin that can be easily made out. Rounded margin, even when it is not feeling truly soft, will not resist the palpating finger but folds underneath it compared to the firm margin, which 'resists' the examining finger rather than slipping underneath.

Firm leafy margin is the description given to the edge of the cirrhotic liver, which has started shrinking at the margin; so much so, the palpating fingers can go underneath the liver edge, which is felt as a firm layer of liver tissue above the palpating fingers. Firm liver is characteristic of chronic conditions, e.g., cirrhosis, malaria, kala azar, chronic haemolytic anaemia, leukaemia, etc; truly hard liver is unlikely in paediatric practice, but may be seen in carcinoma of liver (hepatocellular carcinoma).

Nodular surface of the liver is almost never found in children as macronodular cirrhosis is uncommon in children (may be seen rarely in chronic viral hepatitis, Wilson disease, α_1-antitrypsin deficiency, etc).

Palpable liver may be because of:

- Visceroptosis: Here, the upper border of liver is displaced downwards and thus the liver span remains normal; spleen also may become palpable because of visceroptosis. Examples are rickets, PEM, etc.
- Pushed down liver (e.g., emphysema, pneumothorax, pleural effusion, etc): Here also liver span remains normal.
- True hepatomegaly (discussed elsewhere; see p 165).
- Upward enlargement of liver is seen in amoebic liver abscess. It may also be seen in some pulmonary conditions, which elevate diaphragm, e.g., collapse, pleurisy, etc.

When the liver edge is palpated, measure the size below the costal margin in midclavicular line dur ing quiet breathing. If it is palpable only on deep inspiration, that fact should be mentioned (e.g., 2 cm on deep inspiration).

Normal Values of Palpable Liver

- Up to 6 months: 2–3 cm
- 6 months to 4 years: 2 cm
- >4 years: 1–2 cm

Liver Span

Percuss along the midclavicular line (it is customary to start from 2nd space) and note the point where the liver dullness starts, normally at the 5th right intercostal space in the midclavicular line. Moving lateral to midclavicular line, the liver may be a bit down, at 6th rib; moving 2 cm medial to the midclavicular line, the upper border may be at 5th rib. The **"579 rule."** The upper border of liver dullness is in the 5th space in the midclavicular line, the 7th space in the mid axillary line, the 9th space in the scapular line. Once the upper border is percussed out, demonstrate that the dullness moves down with inspiration (tidal percussion).

Distance from this point to the lower edge of palpated liver is the liver span (if the lower border is not palpable as in cirrhosis, it also will have to be percussed out).

Table 17.1 Aproximate liver span of infants and children *(Modified from: Sheila Sherlock, 7th ed.)*

Birth	5.5 cm
1 year	6
2 years	6.5
3 years	7
4 years	7.5
5 years	8
12 years	9

The left lobe of liver should be looked for in the epigastrium, left lobe being particularly enlarged in amoebic liver abscess, chronic active hepatitis, cirrhosis and sometimes in portal hypertension. One may also consider localized tumour growths involving the left lobe. The left lobe, if unusually enlarged, it is measured from the xiphoid process in the midsternal line.

Riedl's lobe is sometimes seen as a downward projection from the right lobe of liver. It can be mistaken for gall bladder, but it is felt lateral to the site of gall bladder. The ***gall bladder*** is a pear-shaped cystic swelling and is palpable only if it is enlarged. The usual site of an enlarged gall bladder touching the anterior abdominal wall is at the lateral border of right rectus muscle near the costal cartilage. Sometimes turning the child to left lateral position facilitates its palpability. Even if not readily palpable, tenderness over the area described above should make one suspicious of gall bladder enlargement. Most often, it is the tenderness rather than palpability that clinches the diagnosis of enlargement of gall bladder. Although gall bladder enlargement is classically described in stone disease, it can occur in other situations as well, e.g., acute hydrops of gall bladder in typhoid fever and dengue fever.

Following could be suggestive of chronic liver disease.

- Long duration/recurrent episodes
- Family history suggestive of liver disease (e.g., Wilson)
- Firm non-tender liver
- Evidence suggestive of portal hypertension
- Ascites
- Bleeding tendency
- Features of fat soluble vitamin deficiency
- Biochemistry values, if available: liver enzymes only mildly elevated (liver enzymes elevated to thousands in acute liver disease); hypoalbuminemia; hypoprothrombinemia

17

Spleen

Spleen becomes palpable when it is enlarged to at least 2–3 times its normal size, but may be normally palpable in <3 months. This is because the initial enlargement of spleen is in superior and posterior direction. Palpate either in supine or right lateral position (Short's manoeuvre). In the right lateral position, palpate the spleen with the right hand (fingers pointing towards the spleen), with the left hand encircling the left lower ribs and pushing forward. To facilitate the palpability of spleen, taking a deep breath by the patient is useful. To avoid missing a large spleen, it is recommended to start palpating from right iliac fossa, the direction of enlargement of spleen being that way. However, there are situations where the spleen may enlarge in non-classical directions. This is especially true when it is a splenic "tumour" rather than splenomegaly in the usual sense (as in lymphoma). Here, the odd-shaped enlargement may be because the growth occurs from one part of the spleen rather than a generalized splenic enlargement. In IMN, when repeated palpation is to be avoided and in situations where spleen is not readily palpable, one may use percussion sign of Castell. The most inferior interspace in left anterior axillary line (Castell point) is always resonant in the normal and dull in splenic enlargement. Percussion of the lower intercostal spaces in the anterior axillary line from 9th to 11th rib normally should produce resonance (normal splenic dullness does not extend anterior to the mid-axillary line). On splenic enlargement, percussion may be dull in this area, especially during full inspiration.

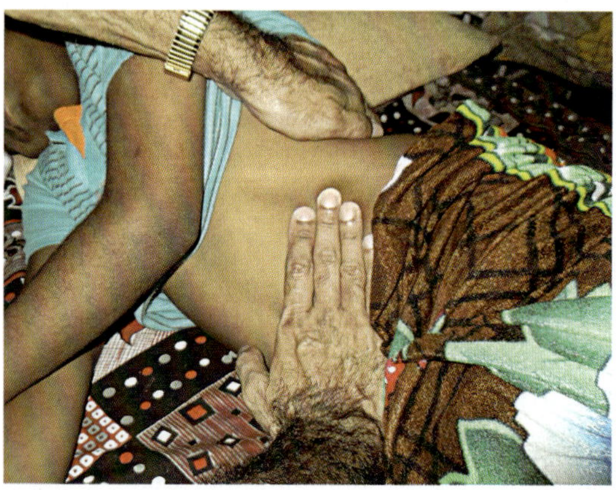

Fig.17.15 Palpation of spleen

Spleen can also be palpated starting from the costal margin and then going down to the abdomen (as in case of palpation of liver, this method is endorsed by Hutchison's).

Characters to be noted in splenic swelling are:

- Size,
- Consistency (e.g., soft in IMN, typhoid, etc; firm in portal hypertension, leukaemia, etc),
- Surface (look for splenic notch on the medial border in massive splenomegaly) and
- Tenderness (note that spleen is usually not tender but may be so in rare cases).

It moves freely with respiration (the direction of movement is down and to the right) and fingers cannot be insinuated between the costal margin and the mass.

Rarely enlargement of left lobe of liver may be confused with splenic swelling. Its continuity with liver swelling will differentiate the two.

The spleen is measured from a point on the left costal margin in the midclavicular line along its long axis.

Grading of Splenomegaly

- Mild or tip splenomegaly: Spleen is around 2 cm (e.g., typhoid, endocarditis, etc).
- Moderate splenomegaly: Spleen measures several centimeters (3–7 cm), but does not cross the midline (e.g., portal hypertension).
- Massive splenomegaly: Spleen is hugely enlarged (>7 cm), crosses midline in the direction of right iliac fossa. It may be seen in Gaucher's disease, chronic myeloid leukaemia, tropical splenomegaly syndrome, *kala azar,* etc.

Kidney

Bimanual Palpation

Bimanual palpation is administered for kidneys. Palpate with one hand placed anteriorly while the other hand that is placed posteriorly pushes the kidney upwards (ballotable swelling). Try to approximate both hands and see if kidney can be felt in between. It may be felt best moving down between the examining hands in deep inspiration. Right kidney being placed lower than the left, is more likely to be palpable in the normal. Although it is conventional for all examinations to be done from the right side of the patient, it is more rewarding to palpate from the left side for the left kidney. In a newborn, bimanual palpation can be done with a single hand, the thumb anteriorly and the fingers placed posteriorly.

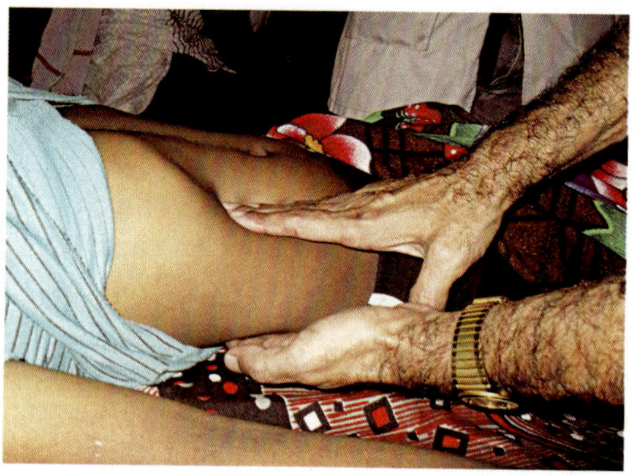

Fig.17.16 Bimanual palpation for kidney

Dipping Palpation

In the presence of ascites, if ordinary palpation fails to reveal the organs, one may resort to dipping palpation. The hand is placed on the abdomen and the fingers are suddenly dipped into the abdomen (by flexing at the metacarpophalangeal joint), which displaces fluid quickly for a short while giving time for the examining fingers to have a feel of the organs. 17

Rectal examination: In cases in which it is not indicated, it would suffice to say that it has not been done.

Other Palpable Masses

If any other mass is palpated, define its

- Location
- Size

Table 17.2 Difference between splenic swelling and kidney swellings

Spleen	Kidney
Finger insinuation between swelling and costal margin is not possible.	Possible to push the fingers between kidney swelling and the costal margin.
Splenic notch may be palpable.	No notch.
Better felt anteriorly, not pushed forward by the posterior hand. . (Non ballotable)	Bimanually palpable and ballotable mass.
Moves freely with respiration. Direction of movement is down and to the right.	Moves with respiration, but much less readily. Direction of movement is vertically down.
Renal angle is resonant.	Renal angle (angle between the 12th rib and the lateral margin of erector spinae muscle) may become dull.
Traubes space dull Long axis to the RIF.	A band of colonic resonance may be demonstrable anteriorly over the swelling.

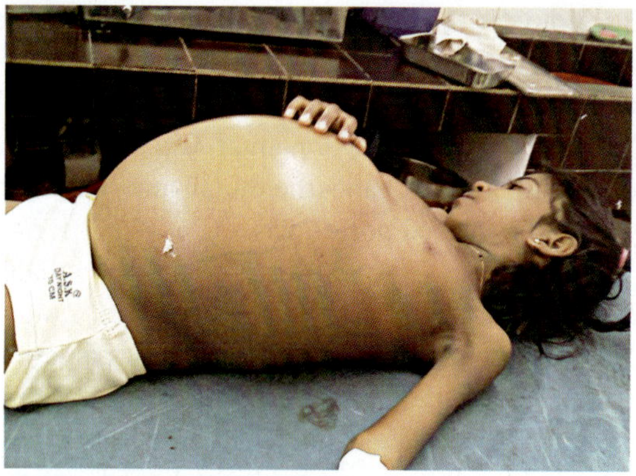

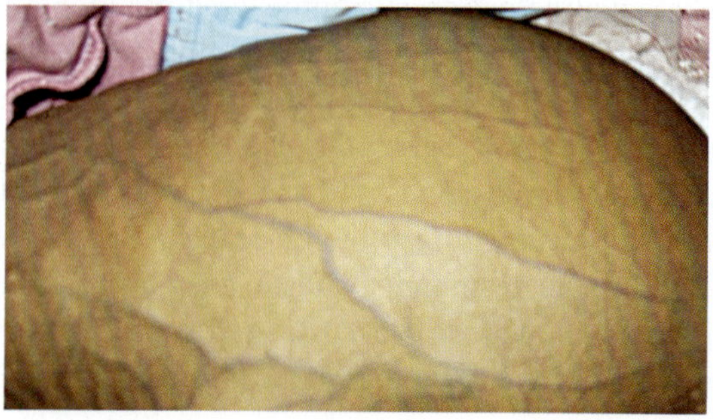

Fig.17.17 Gross ascites. Dipping palpation will be required in this case. Note the dilated veins.

- Shape
- Consistency (soft, firm, hard, cystic or varying consistency)
- Surface (smooth or irregularities)
- Tenderness
- Margins
- Movement with respiration (swelling arising from an organ in contact with the diaphragm moves with respiration.
- Cough impulse

Examples are liver and spleen. Kidney also moves with respiration but to a much lesser extent), intrinsic mobility of the mass (try moving the lump in various directions), etc. To differentiate the origin of intra-abdominal from parietal mass, ask the patient to try to get up from supine position. If the mass becomes less apparent, it is intra-abdominal; if it becomes more prominent, it is parietal. The mass of congenital hypertrophic pyloric stenosis is felt on the *right* side of the abdomen, to the *right* side of the *right* rectus muscle. If a mass palpated once had disappeared later, it could be urinary bladder, faecal mass, worm mass or rarely intussuception.

Demonstration of Direction of Flow in Distended Veins

Patient is best examined standing. Empty a segment of the vein, which does not have any branching points (to avoid errors due to filling through the tributaries), then release one finger. If it is not filling, try releasing the other finger and see if it is filling from the other side. However, in long-standing cases, due to incompetence of valves of veins, this method may fail to give the right information on direction of flow. In a normal child and in portal hypertension (e.g., cirrhosis), direction of flow is away from the umbilicus (radially away from the umbilicus, i.e., downwards in veins below the umbilicus and upwards in veins above the umbilicus). In extrahepatic portal obstruction (portal vein thrombosis), the flow can occasionally be towards the umbilicus if the blood is bypassed via the paraumbilical veins to the liver. In inferior vena cava obstruction, the distended veins are seen in flanks with direction of flow upwards (when inferior vena cava is obstructed, the veins drain via collaterals to the superior vena cava and hence the upward flow).

Note: In massive ascites, always look for dilated veins, which are very likely to be present because of obstruction by the pressure of ascites (if just due to ascites, these dilated veins will disappear when the ascites disappears).

Percussion

Percussion of liver, spleen, etc, have been discussed already along with its palpation.

Obliteration of liver dullness may be seen in pneumoperitoneum.

Normally, tympanitic note is obtained over the stomach. Abdomen is resonant (less tympanitic than stomach area) over most areas, except over the organs. Highly tympanitic note may be obtained in intestinal obstruction, paralytic ileus, etc. Dull note will be there over free fluid, solid organs, masses, etc. Fluid thrill will be elicitable in massive ascites, shifting dullness when lesser amount of fluid is present and puddle sign in minimal ascites.

Fluid Thrill

Place the patient's hand or a third person's hand vertically over the midline in the abdomen with the child supine. Now examiner places his one hand in one flank and taps the other flank with the fingers of other hand. The fluid wave generated by the tap by one hand can be felt by the other hand in the flank. The hand placed in midline blocks the false transmission of wave directly through the abdominal wall. This sign is elicitable only in massive ascites.

Shifting Dullness

Ask the child to void the bladder, then with the child in supine position, start percussing from the epigatrium downwards with the fingers perpendicular to the midline until an area of dullness if any (bladder) is reached. Now keep the pleximeter finger parallel to the midline and percuss laterally till an area of dullness is reached and ask the child to turn to the other side.b Give a minute for the fluid to shift to the other side (and intestines to float up) and then percuss the same area again. If it has now become resonant, it means that the fluid that was there to give the dullness has now shifted to the other side. Now demonstrate that the dullness has shifted to the other side by percussing till the dullness on the other side is reached. This demonstrates that the dullness has shifted to a new site.

Inability to demonstrate shifting dullness despite the presence of fluid is likely in a few rare situations. One situation obviously is massive ascites where there is no scope for shift. Loculated fluid is another reason for the inability of fluid to shift. Multiple adhesions (as in tuberculous peritonitis) preventing intestines from floating up may be another reason for the same.

Normal dull note at the extremes of the flanks being misinterpreted as fluid is another reason for "failure of demonstration of fluid shift." This dullness at extremes of flanks is common in obese individuals where the protrusion of the flanks is due to fat and not due to ascites.

17

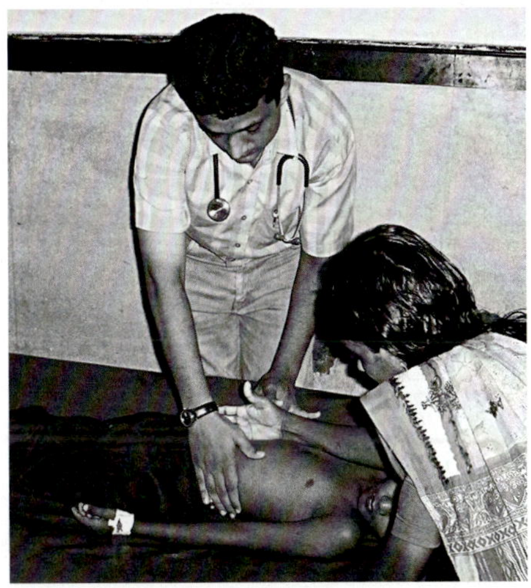

Fig.17.18 Fluid thrill

Puddle Sign

With the child in knee–elbow position or as shown in Fig. 17.19, percuss over the periumbilical region. Normally, it should be resonant, but with fluid in the abdomen, this area becomes dull. This is useful to detect minimal fluid (which in reality may not be minimal! Without percussion in the knee–elbow position, one may miss fluid collections as large as 300–500 mL in an adult, because of the large size of the abdominal cavity and its many recesses).

Auscultation

Bowel sounds are normally best heard a little to the right or left of umbilicus (frequency is highly variable, may be 6–8/min).

Bowel sounds increase in diarrhoea, empty bowel, intestinal obstruction, etc. It is absent in paralytic ileus, late intestinal obstruction, peritonitis, etc. It may not be audible in massive ascites due to mechanical blockade of sound transmission.

Borborygmi: Increased frequency and intensity of bowel sounds (gurgling sound), often audible to the unaided ear.

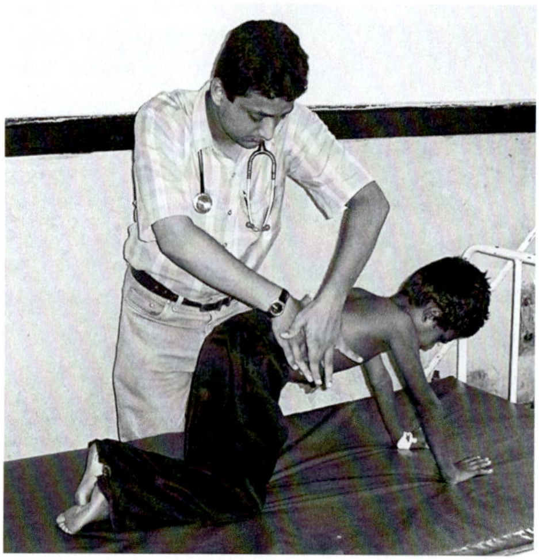

Fig.17.19 Puddle sign (in this case, knee-elbow position makes the trunk tilt down anteriorly & hence this position is considered more appropriate).

Auscultate for liver rub, splenic rub, etc (very rare; described in enlarged organs due to perihepatitis or perisplenitis).

A bruit over the renal artery may be heard with the bell of the stethoscope lateral to the umbilicus in patients with stenosis of renal artery as the cause of hypertension. In portal hypertension, cirrhosis, etc, look for venous hum, which may be heard rarely due to opening up of venous channels along the falciform ligament (auscultate in the midline between the umbilicus and the xiphoid).

GENITALIA

Look for micropenis, hypo/epispadias, phimosis, undescended testes, any evidence of orchitis, urethral discharge, etc; and look for secondary sexual characters in case of adolescents. Micropenis may be seen in hypopituitarism, Klinefelter syndrome, etc. Apparent micropenis may be seen in obesity, due to the penis being submerged in suprapubic fat. Here, the true penile length becomes obvious once the fat around the base of the penis is pushed down. A normal newborn penis is 4 cm (stretched length) and below 2.5 cm is considered small (as per Nelson's textbook, <1.9 cm only is considered small in newborn). Inappro-priately large penis for age may be seen in congenital adrenal hyperplasia. Here, the testes size will be normal (the excess hormones are coming from adrenal, not testes). In true precocious puberty, both penis and testes will be large. Prepubertal testis will measure about 1 cm.

- Chordee: Curved penis.
- Hypospadias: Urethra opening on the under surface of penis.
- Epispadias: Urethra opening on the upper surface of penis. May be associated with extrophy of bladder.
- Phimosis: The prepuce is not retractable. It is normal in newborn and infants.
- Empty scrotum: If the scrotum is empty, palpate the inguinal canal for testis. If it is palpable and can be brought down to the scrotum then it is retractile testes, not an undescended one.
- Large scrotum: Large scrotum may be because of hydrocele or hernia (hernia is reducible and not transilluminant in contrast to hydrocele).

If a painless hydrocele like mass is not transilluminant and not hernia, think of a tumour like gonadoblastoma. Look for scrotal oedema in gross ascites.

Large testes may be part of macro-orchidism of fragile X syndrome (macro-orchidism may be obvious only by puberty). Thickening of scrotal skin making it a large scrotum is seen in elephantiasis. Tenderness of scrotum may be due to local causes, torsion testes or obstructed hernia.

- Ambiguous genitalia: Genitalia that do not look like typical male or female are ambiguous. The pointers could be a large clitoris, fused labia, bifid scrotum, mass in the inguinal region in females, etc.

ANUS AND RECTUM

Look for perianal erythema (e.g., diarrhoea due to lactose intolerance), polyps (will be red and pedunculated), tags, scratch marks (pinworm), fissures (on rectal examination), haemorrhoids (dark red in colour), prolapse of rectum (seen in diarrhoea with malnutrition, whipworm, pertussis, etc). Perianal fistula may be seen in Crohn's disease. Empty rectum may be seen in Hirschsprung disease (here rectal examination will be followed by a gush of stool).

Digital rectal examination is indicated only rarely; like intussusception, Hirschsprung disease, polyp, etc.

In meningomyelocele, the anus looks patulous (Fig. 24.87, p 530. Normally, one will have to spread out the buttocks to visualize the anus; in meningomyelocele, the anus is quite obvious without having to separate the buttocks (due to weakness of gluteal muscles).

CHAPTER 18

Disorders of GIT: Case Sheet Formats

CHRONIC LIVER DISEASE WITH OR WITHOUT PORTAL HYPERTENSION

Chief Complaints

- Jaundice
- Abdominal distension/swelling of legs
- Altered sensorium/bleeding manifestations (hepatic encephalopathy)

History of Presenting Illness

- History of fever: Onset in relation to jaundice (prodrome of fever in viral hepatitis; once jaundice is well established, fever comes down in viral hepatitis), duration of fever.
- History of abdominal distension/leg oedema; enquire about progression, whether gradual/ sudden.
- History of pain abdomen (could indicate spontaneous bacterial peritonitis, a massive fluid collection can also cause pain). Non- GIT cause for abdominal pain may be lower lobe pneumonia, HSP, DKA.
- History of vomiting/decreased appetite.
- History of rectal bleeding, malena, colour of the urine/stool history of excessive itching (obstructive jaundice).
- History of altered sensorium (either hypotension following massive hematemesis or liver cell failure in case of intrahepatic portal hypertension).
- History of hypersplenism (whether child has been pale, any bleeding tendency, etc).
- Treatment details before the present episode, if any (gastritis producing drugs is important in hemetemesis).
- History of complications:
  - Jaundice (jaundice is not expected in extrahepatic portal hypertension. May be present in intrahepatic portal hypertension); viral hepatitis.
  - Bleeding manifestations: Hemetemesis, melaena.
  - Altered sleep pattern/seizures /involuntary movements (hepatic encephalopathy).
  - Complications due to malabsorption: Vitamin A, D, E, K deficiencies (chronic liver disease).
  - Decreased urine output (hepatorenal syndrome, leptospirosis).
- History of aetiology:
  - History of fever – viral hepatitis, sepsis (may cause thrombosis).
  - History of trauma, surgery.
  - History of umbilical infection or catheterization, dehydration, appendicitis (all can predispose to portal venous thrombosis).
  - History of urine colour and stool colour (cholestasis).
  - History of bone pains, bleeding (malignancy).
  - History of recent scholastic deterioration, involuntary movements, deterioration of handwriting (Wilson's disease).
  - History of drug intake (ATT, Valproate, alpha methyl dopa, methotrexate, ketoconazole) (drugs among ATT that DO NOT

cause jaundice: ethambutol, streptomycin).
- Recurrent respiratory infections (cystic fibrosis, α_1-antitrypsin deficiency).
- Features like rash/arthritis/nephritis/thyroiditis may point towards extra hepatic manifestations of autoimmune hepatitis.

- Relevant past history.

Antenatal, Natal, Postnatal History

- History of neonatal seizures: Could be due to hypoglycaemia, e.g., galactosemia/tyrosinemia.
- History of neonatal jaundice: α_1-antitrypsin deficiency, tyrosinemia, Niemann pick disease.
- Delayed passage of meconium: cystic fibrosis.
- History of umbilical vein catheterization in the neonatal period (extrahepatic portal hypertension due to portal vein thrombosis).
- History of umbilical sepsis (extrahepatic portal hypertension due to portal vein thrombosis).

Immunization: Hepatitis A&B vaccines.
Development: Delay possible in any chronic illness.

Nutrition

- Assess protein intake, qualitatively (non vegetarian diet has a higher bioavailability) and quantitatively.
- Any dietary modification advised previously (e.g., in Wilson's disease, inborn errors of metabolism). Examples of copper rich foods are liver, shellfish, nuts, chocolates, etc.
- Usage of copper utensils may be a pointer towards Indian childhood cirrhosis (obsolete now except for a few regions in Tamil Nadu).

Family History

Jaundice in other siblings/neuropsychiatric illness (Wilson).

Socioeconomic

Drinking water source, hygiene, etc (in CLD also the acute presentation could be due to viral hepatitis); school absence; effect on sibling and family income, etc.

Examination

- General comment on sensorium, posture and typical facies, if any.
- Anthropometry: Moderate malnutrition is common but may be obscured by oedema.
- Long standing CLD children are markedly wasted. So may comment on subcutaneous fat and muscle mass. Gluteal wasting is commonly missed due to not looking for it specifically.
- Vitals:
  - Pulse: Bounding pulse due to hyperkinetic circulation may be present.
  - Bradycardia in obstructive jaundice (postulated to be the effect of bile salts on SA node), tachycardia if there's a significant blood loss due to hemetemesis.
  - Tachypnea due to volume loss (due to bleeding) or secondary to the movement restriction by massive ascites.

Head to Foot Examination

- Hair loss in chronic liver disease.
- Typical facies, e.g., Alagille, GSD (chubby doll face), steroid facies due to prolonged treatment or hepatic facies.
- Hepatic facies: Sunken eyes, hollowed temporal fossa, pinched up nose with malar prominence, muddy complexion of skin, icteric tinge of conjunctiva.
- Eyes: Look for jaundice (comment on depth and colour, e.g., greenish yellow in obstructive jaundice).
  - Pallor: Nutritional or GIT blood loss in CLD or hemolysis in Wilson's disease or auto-immune hepatitis. Pallor is difficult to appreciate in eyes if deeply jaundiced.

18

- Cataract in galactosemia, Wilson's disease, prolonged steroid treatment for chronic active hepatitis bleeding manifestations.
- Features of vitamin A deficiency: Dryness of conjunctiva, Bitot spots.
- KF ring.

- Oral cavity: Bleeding manifestations; aphthous ulcer in IBD; fetor hepaticus in hepatic failure.
- Parotid enlargement may be present in older children.
- Chest: Evidence of rickets (rosary, sulcus, etc).
- Gynecomastia.
- Abdomen: Distension, dilated veins.
- Perianal region: Relevant only in inflammatory bowel disease. Anal fissure, fistulae, abscess, anal tags, etc.
- Limbs: Nails: Terry's nails (proximal 80% whitish, non specific), blue lunula (seen in Wilson's disease).
- Cyanosis, if present is due to pulmonary A-V shunts clubbing in liver cirrhosis and inflammatory bowel disease.
- Palmar erythema. Look for flapping tremor.
- Evidence of rickets (widening of wrist; bow legs); liver is involved in 25 hydroxylation of vitamin D and in addition chronic liver disease causes malabsorption of fat and hence fat-soluble vitamins. Erythema nodosum (chronic active hepatitis, inflammatory bowel disease).
- Joint swellings in inflammatory bowel disease (IBD).
- Skin: Paper money skin, bleeding manifestations (coagulopathy, thrombocytopenia of hypersplenism), spider nevi, xanthomas (between fingers and extensor surface of hands, eye lids), scratch marks; striae in massive ascites.
- Paper money skin: Skin covered with numerous small blood vessels mostly in the upper body, often in association with spider naevi; the name because of resemblance to the silk threads in a US dollar bill.
- Mention SMR in older children; testicular atrophy in chronic liver disease.
- Involuntary movements, if any: Wing beating tremor in Wilson disease.
- Asterixis/flap (hepatic encephalopathy).

Systemic Examination

I. Upper GIT

1. Gum: Look for any bleeding.
2. Teeth: Hygiene, caries, etc.
3. Tongue: Dry (dehydration), jaundice (look at the undersurface), cyanosis (hepato pulmonary syndrome in CLD).
4. Oral mucosa: Bleeds.
5. Tonsils: Normal or hypertrophied, inflamed, etc (e.g., in IMN).

II. Examination of abdomen

1. ***Inspection***
   - Shape of abdomen: Is it normal, distended or has any localized bulges.
   - Movement with respiration: Type of respiratory movement and whether all parts of abdomen are moving symmetrically. Restriction of mobility is expected in case of painful regions.
   - Skin over the abdomen: May look shiny in ascites; look for scars of surgeries (e.g., Kasai), liver biopsy marks, peritoneal tap marks. Dilated veins may be present in cirrhosis with portal hypertension; find the direction of flow in them (to make veins more prominent examine the child in standing position; valsalva manoeuvre can be done, if necessary).
   - Umbilicus: Normal or everted/transversely stretched (ascites).
   - Visible pulsation, peristalsis or visible mass (unlikely in hepatitis).
   - Flanks: Whether flanks appear full or not.

- Examine the hernial orifices and external genitalia (hydrocele and hernia in ascites of long duration).

2. ***Palpation***
   - Feel of abdomen: Softness, tenderness, guarding, etc.
   - Look for any area of warmth or tenderness.
   - Look for abdominal wall oedema or skin turgor if relevant to the case at hand (vomiting).
   - Organomegaly: Liver is enlarged, tender, soft or firmish (the usual consistency is between soft and firm) in viral hepatitis; in cirrhosis, liver is firm often have sharp borders (also look for left lobe enlargement); impalpable liver in a child could also indicate cirrhosis; gall bladder is rarely palpable. Spleen is rarely palpable in acute viral hepatitis (palpable in some 10% cases); hence always consider co-existing portal hypertension (cirrhosis) when spleen is significantly enlarged (do not get mislead into diagnosing abdominal distension due to massive hepatosplenomegaly as ascites). Bimanual palpation for enlarged kidney (cystic disease of kidney and liver). In IBD, matted loops may become palpable mass.
   - Rectal examination (not to be done routinely; haemorrhoids likely in CLD with portal hypertension; in IBD blood and pus on examining finger).

3. ***Percussion***
   - Percussion over the enlarged organs. Find out the liver span.
   - Shifting dullness (if ascites is present; ascites is due to hypoproteinemia plus intrahepatic portal hypertension). Clinically detectable ascites makes the diagnosis of acute viral hepatitis unlikely. Consider chronic hepatitis, intrahepatic portal hypertension.
   - Fluid thrill (it may be discussed as part of palpation or percussion).
   - Puddle sign for minimal fluid (only if indicated).

4. ***Auscultation***
   - Bowel sounds: Normal/increased or decreased (in sick child, there can be ileus).
   - Bruit: Especially over the renal artery/ over the enlarged organs (hepatocellular carcinoma). Murmur in the umbilical region suggests intrahepatic portal hypertension (Cruveilhier Baumgarten murmur).

5. ***CNS***
   - Assess concentration (connect the dots test), memory, speech and handwriting.
   - Dysarthria in Wilson.
   - Look for flap.
   - Ataxia (vitamin E deficiency due to malabsorption); diminished sensations and reflexes also possible with vitamin E deficiency.
   - Deep tendon reflexes may be exaggerated in initial stages of hepatic encephalopathy.
   - Extrapyramidal manifestations in Wilson. Choreo athetosis, dystonia, tremor, myoclonus, etc in Wilson. In newborn with jaundice and choreo athetoid movement consider kernicterus.

6. ***CVS***: Usually normal, cardiomegaly due to hyperdynamic circulation in long standing cases. Congenital heart disease in Alagille (pulmonary stenosis).
7. ***Respiratory***: In cases with ascites, look for pleural effusion. Lobar pneumonia.

Diagnosis

Case of chronic liver disease, decompensated or not, with/without portal hypertension probably due to .... (aetiology) with/without features of hepatic encephalopathy.

Aetiology of chronic liver disease.

"WATCH EGG," standing for Wilson disease, autoimmune hepatitis, α_1-antitrypsin deficiency, Alagille syndrome, tyrosinemia, chronic hepatitis B and C, cystic fibrosis, hereditary fructose intolerance, extrahepatic biliary atresia, galactosemia, glycogen storage disease.

Complications of Chronic Liver Disease "HEPATIC"

- Hepatorenal syndrome
- Encephalopathy
- Portal hypertension, hepatopulmonary syndrome
- Ascites
- Thrombosis of portal vein
- Infections (spontaneous bacterial peritonitis)
- Coagulopathy, cirrhosis, carcinoma (hepatocellular carcinoma)

Investigations for Chronic Hepatitis

- Serum bilirubin, total and conjugated.
- Liver enzymes, alkaline phosphatase, prothrombin time and albumin.
- Cultures (prone for sepsis).
- Metabolic screen ("WATCH EGG"; urine-reducing substance, serum ceruloplasmin, α_1-antitrypsin, etc).
- Thyroid function studies in newborn (hypothyroidism presents as prolonged jaundice in newborn).
- Ultrasonography.
- Liver biopsy (may be required for monitoring treatment of chronic active hepatitis).

Treatment

- The recommended diet for stable CLD (without encephalopathy) is high energy normal protein diet enriched with special formulas of branced chain amino acids (together, the protein intake becomes slightly higher than normal). If oral intake is not tolerated, consider total or partial parenteral nutrition.
- Fat soluble vitamin supplementation.
- Micronutrient supplementation (zinc, calcium phosphate, etc).
- Ascites management: Sodium restriction, spironolactone, frusemide after IV albumin.
- Specific treatment depending on specific diagnosis, if available.

PORTAL HYPERTENSION

The scheme of examination for chronic liver disease may be used for portal hypertension case.

Table 18.1 Classification of portal hypertension

	Pre hepatic (extra hepatic)	(Portal vein or splenic vein thrombosis)
Portal hypertension	Intra hepatic	Pre sinusoidal (e.g,.congenital hepatic fibrosis) Sinusoidal (cirrhosis, fatty liver, nodular hyperplasia) Post sinusoidal (veno occlusive disease, high dose chemotherapy etc)
	Post hepatic	Budd Chiari syndrome, tumor invasion of hepatic vein or inferior vena cava, membraneous obstruction of inferior vena cava or hepatic vein

Clinical Diagnosis of Extrahepatic (Prehepatic) Portal Hypertension

- Suggestive neonatal or other history (umbilical catheterization, GI tract infections, etc).
- Haemetemesis: Bleeding from varices, usually precipitated by intercurrent infections, drugs, increase in pressure due to coughing or no apparent reason.
- No jaundice.
- Liver is of normal consistency and size.
- Splenomegaly for which there is no other identifiable cause.
- Absence of any clinical signs of liver cell failure or chronic liver disease.
- Absence of ascites.

Differential Diagnosis of Extrahepatic Portal Hypertension

- Other causes of hemetemesis: Gastritis (aspirin, steroids, etc), peptic oesophagitis, tear following violent vomiting (Mallory-Weiss syndrome).
- Intrahepatic portal hypertension: Cirrhosis of various aetiologies is the example. Jaundice, firm liver with sharp margins, ascites, features of chronic liver disease (like spider angioma, palmar erythema, etc), bleeding tendency other than variceal bleed, etc.
- Post hepatic (supra hepatic) portal hypertension: Massive ascites, large hepatomegaly, abdominal pain due to hepatomegaly.

Investigations

- Liver function tests (abnormal in intrahepatic portal hypertension).
- During an acute episode of bleeding, blood counts, PCV, platelet count, renal function test (prerenal type of renal failure due to hypovolaemia). Coagulation profile (prothrombin time, APTT, etc may be abnormal in intrahepatic portal hypertension).
- Ultrasonography: Measure calibre of portal vein; demonstrate collaterals around the obstruction; Doppler examination of the hepatic vessels.
- Endoscopy to visualize varices. Barium swallow to demonstrate the oesophageal varices if endoscopy not available.

Treatment

Treatment of an Acute Episode of Bleeding

- Stabilization of ABC.
- Monitor BP, urine output, capillary refill time.
- Correction of circulatory shock, if any (normal saline, fresh blood transfusion).
- Vitamin K and/or fresh frozen plasma if the coagulation profile is abnormal.
- Octreotide infusion.
- Emergency endoscopic sclerotherapy.
- Sengstaken-Blackemore tube.
- Long-term management of portal hypertension.
- Avoid drugs like non-steroid anti-inflammatory agents, iron, etc.
- Oral propranolol daily for many months to years to reduce re-bleeding.
- Endoscopic sclerotherapy or banding.
- Surgical shunts (e.g., mesocaval or distal splenorenal shunts), TIPS.

18

VIRAL HEPATITIS

1. **Complaints**
   - Fever (consider other causes)
   - Yellow discolouration of urine and eyes
   - Anorexia, nausea, vomiting
2. **History of present illness**

   Associated symptoms to be inquired into:
   - History of abdominal pain (hepatic tenderness).
   - History of clay coloured stools, itching (obstructive phase of infective hepatitis).
   - History of drug intake (e.g., anti-TB drugs).
   - History of travel, contaminated water source and injections.
   - History of constipation (constipation can lead on to more ammonia absorption from GIT).

- History of arthralgia, rash, etc (extra-hepatic manifestations. Extrahepatic manifestations make hepatitis A less likely; hepatitis B more likely).
- History suggestive of complications:
  - Bleeding, malena.
  - Sleep disturbances, altered behaviour, convulsions.
  - Ascites, bipedal oedema.
- History of suggestive of leptospirosis (myalgia, hematuria, oliguria, redness of eyes).
- History of co-existing malaria is to be considered in case of travel to endemic areas.

3. **Past history**
   History of blood transfusions, injections.
4. **Antenatal, natal, post natal**
   History of jaundice/hep B in mother, history of exchange transfusion, umbilical sepsis, IU infections.
5. **Immunization, development & diet history**
   Hepatitis A/hepatitis B.
6. **Family & socioeconomic history**
   - History of jaundice in family/locality.
   - Drinking water source & sanitation.
   - Bathing in contaminated water.
   - History of abdomen surgery for gall stones.
7. **General examination and head to foot**
   Follow the standard case sheet format vitals:
   - Bradycardia: Vagal effect of bile acids.
   - Temperature: Fever is likely in the early phase (becomes afebrile once jaundice is well established).
   - Anthropometry
   - Growth failure is likely in chronic liver disease. Growth is normal in any acute hepatitis.
   - General comment: It is best to comment on the sensorium, which is most important in case of early hepatic encephalopathy.
     - Eyes: KF ring (Wilson), bitot spot (fat-soluble vitamin deficiency in chronic liver disease). Pallor unlikely in acute viral hepatitis, so consider differentials like autoimmune hepatitis, haemolytic anaemia, Wilson, etc.
     - Facies: Haemolytic facies, coarse face of hypothyroid (hypothyroidism may present as prolonged jaundice in newborn only).
     - Hair loss (chronic liver disease).
     - Look for any lymphadenopathy.
     - Gynecomastia (chronic liver disease).
     - White nails in chronic liver. Clubbing in chronic liver disease.
     - Hands: Look for flapping tremor.
     - Testicular atrophy in chronic liver disease.
     - Pedal oedema in chronic liver disease.
     - Skin: Scratch marks; bleeding; spider naevi. Look for signs of dehydration in case there is vomiting.
8. **Systemic examination**
   Refer under chronic liver disease.

Differential Diagnosis of Viral Hepatitis

Other hepatotrophic viral infections (Ebstein Barr, CMV, etc), drug toxicity and metabolic disorders (Wilson, α_1-antitrypsin deficiency, galactosaemia, etc).

Investigations

- Urine bile pigments, bile salts and urobilinogen are elevated.
- Both conjugated and unconjugated bilirubin are elevated.
- Transaminases (SGPT, SGOT) and alkaline phosphatase are elevated.
- Prothrombin time.
- Antibodies to specific viruses (chronic hepatitis B, C etc).
- In autoimmune hepatitis, autoantibodies are estimated like ANA, anti-LKM (liver kidney microsome), anti-mitochondrial, anti-smooth muscle, etc and Coombs test.

- Investigations for various entities of mnemonic "WATCH EGG" (p 410).

Treatment of Acute Hepatitis

- High carbohydrate, low fat diet with emphasis on frequent feeding. Normal requirements of proteins are allowed in uncomplicated hepatitis.
- Bed rest till the serum bilirubin is near normal.
- Isolation with precautions to prevent feco-oral spread and needle precautions.
- Withdraw any offending drug, withdraw them (e.g., INH, rifampicin, valproate).
- Paracetamol is avoided as far as possible. Sponging the best method.
- Lactulose to ensure regular bowel movements.
- Oral ampicillin for bowel sterilization.
- In case of vomiting, IV fluids may be given.

NEONATAL CHOLESTASIS

Name:
Age:
Sex:
DOB:
Consanguinity:

1. **Complaints**
    - Jaundice:
        - Onset of jaundice
        - Associated with high coloured urine +/- clay coloured stools (obstructive jaundice)
    - Abdominal distension:
        - Progressively increasing (organomegaly, ascites)
        - Is swelling confined to upper or lower abdomen?
    - Urine output and stool history (frequency & color)
2. **History regarding aetiology**
    - Maternal history of drug ingestion, jaundice/infection in pregnancy
    - Neonatal umbilical catheterization
    - Associated skin rash, petechie, fever, cardiac disease
    - Full term or preterm
    - Dysmorphic features
    - Constipation and lethargy (hypothyroidism)
    - Family history of haemolytic anaemia
    - History of giving sugar water/ fruit juice (fructose intolerance).
3. **History of complications**
    - Bleeding from any site
    - Altered sensorium
    - Ascites
4. **Examination**
    - *General examination:*
        - Dysmorphic features (chromosomal, Alagille)
        - Jaundice
        - Anaemia
        - Cataracts
        - Fundus for chorioretinitis
        - Signs for vitamin deficiencies (A, D, K)
        - Oedema, anasarca
    - Vitals & anthropometry: Failure to thrive is likely in neonatal hepatitis.
    - *Abdominal examination:*
        - Inspection: Localized bulge, distension (which quadrant is more affected).
        - Divarication of recti, hernial sites.
        - Palpation: Superficial palpation: Guarding, tenderness, rigidity
    - *Deep palpation:*
        - Hepatomegaly
            - Tender/Nontender
            - Surface: Smooth/Nodular
            - Span and Size
            - Border: Well felt/sharp/diffuse
            - Consistency: Soft/firm/hard
        - Splenomegaly
            - Size (grades of splenomegaly)
            - Consistency: Soft/firm
            - Splenic notch
        - Kidneys (bimanual palpation)

18

- Percussion: Shifting dullness/horseshoe dullness/fluid thrill; Puddle's sign
- Auscultation: Renal bruit, Venous hum

5. Other systems: Cardiac murmur, hydrocephalus, meningitis
6. Diagnosis:
   - Neonatal jaundice: With/without hepatosplenomegaly, with/without ascitis, with/without dysmorphic features, with/without anaemia, with/without associated anomalies. The most likely aetiology being: Neonatal hepatitis/Biliary atresia/Inborn error of metabolism//Chromosomal disorder

PROLONGED NEONATAL JAUNDICE

- See p 493. Persistent icterus beyond 2 weeks of age; clay coloured stools.
- Suspect biliary atresia in a healthy baby with persistent conjugated hyperbilirubinaemia.
- Suspect "neonatal hepatitis" in a sick baby or low birth weight baby with persistent conjugated hyperbilirubinaemia. Neonatal hepatitis means hepatic inflammation, not necessarily viral hepatitis; the aetiology can be one of the many other possibilities also, like galactosemia, α_1-antitrypsin deficiency, low grade *E. coli* sepsis, etc.

Investigations for Persistent Neonatal Jaundice

- Serum bilirubin, total and conjugated.
- Liver enzymes, alkaline phosphatase, prothrombin time and albumin.
- Bacterial cultures (blood & urine), especially for *E. coli* (Galactosemia).
- Metabolic screen (urine-reducing substance, serum ceruloplasmin, α_1-antitrypsin, etc).
- Thyroid function studies (hypothyroidism presents as prolonged jaundice).
- Ultrasonography (choledochal cyst is a differential for conjugated hyperbilirubinemia). Fasting (4hr) USG shows absent/ small GB, Triangular cord sign, polysplenia in biliary atresia.
- Hepatobiliary IDA (imidodiacetate) scan (detects failure of excretion of dye into the intestine in biliary atresia).
- Liver biopsy (in early stages can differentiate between neonatal hepatitis and biliary atresia). in EHBA shows intrahepatic biliary radicle proliferation with bile plugging.

Treatment for Neonatal Hepatitis/Biliary Atresia

- Surgery for biliary atresia (Kasai procedure within the first 2 months of life).
- Diet rich in calories and proteins.
- Replace the usual formula with a formula containing medium-chain triglycerides.
- Vit A 10,000 IU daily orally. (water soluble formulation)
- Vit D 4000 IU daily orally.
- Vit E 150–500 IU daily orally.
- Vit K 5 mg on alternate days orally in water soluble form.
- Vit B complex, twice the usual daily recommended allowance.
- Micronutrient supplementation (zinc, calcium phosphate, etc).
- Ursodeoxycholic acid (15 mg/kg/24 hrs).
- Hydroxyzine 2 mg/kg/day for irritability (due to pruritus).
- Ascites management: Sodium restriction, spironolactone, frusemide after IV albumin.
- Liver transplantation.

DIARRHOEA

Ask about the onset, duration and progress.

- **Onset**: Very acute onset could be food poisoning, so ask about food intake in the immediate past.
- **Duration**: Duration of diarrhoea helps to decide whether it is acute diarrhoea (usually <7 days), persistent diarrhoea (>14 days) or chronic diarrhoea (the term chronic diarrhoea

is reserved for non-infectious prolonged recurrent diarrhoeas like inflammatory bowel disease, celiac disease, malabsorption, etc).

- **Progress**: This should include inquiry into the quantity (large volume or small volume), quality (just watery or mixed with stool particles, blood/mucous, foul smell, etc) and frequency of stools (help to assess possible dehydration), and associated symptoms.

Appearance of Stool

- Watery stools with increased flatulence and *perianal excoriation* suggests lactose intolerance.
- Watery large volume stools is likely in secretory diarrhoea (e.g., cholera, entero toxigenic *E. coli* and other toxin-mediated diarrhoeas; rota virus diarrhoea is a combination of secretory and osmotic diarrhoea and the stool is watery; cholera stool is typically described rice-water stool).
- A greasy, bulky, foul-smelling stool that is difficult to flush is seen in fat malabsorption syndromes (steatorrhoea).
- Bloody stools indicates acute invasive diarrhoea (dysentery); rarely intususception (red-current jelly like bright red blood, sausage-shaped mass lateral to umbilicus, and exhausting cry in an infant of age group 6 months to 1 year). Also see hematochezia.
- Associated abdominal pain and tenesmus with blood in stools, if acute, suggests dysentery and if chronic, suggests inflammatory bowel disease, amoebiasis, etc. ***Note***: Tenesmus is the painful urgency to pass stools.
- Pea soup stool is seen in typhoid.
- Green stools do not have specific significance, except that it indicates rapid GIT transit so that bile comes out before having had the time to get absorbed.

Associated Problems

- Vomiting, fever, abdominal pain, etc are to be specifically asked for. Worm infested children may pass worms also during diarrhoea (enhanced intestinal peristalsis brings worms out).
- Decreased urine output indicates severity of dehydration. Hence always ask for urine output in diarrhoea cases.
- Abdominal distension (hypotonia of malnutrition, hypokalaemia).
- Weight loss indicates chronic diarrhoea (always think of HIV in chronic diarrhoea with weight loss).
- History of rectal prolapse is common in whipworm colitis, cystic fibrosis and malnutrition when diarrhoea occurs.
- Antibiotic-induced diarrhoea, food allergy (cow's milk, soy, wheat, etc) must be kept in mind and inquired into.
- Severe malnutrition per se may cause diarrhoea. Unabsorbed bile salts in the gut act as an irritant and cause secretory diarrhoea. Poor epithelial regeneration in PEM may cause osmotic diarrhoea due to unabsorbed food in the gut.
- In celiac disease, the diarrhoea starts a few months after introduction of wheat-containing weaning foods.
- Look for acrodermatitis (around orifices), as zinc deficiency causes diarrhoea (acrodermatitis enteropathica). Perianal excoriation may also be found in lactose intolerance.
- Specifically ask for diet during diarrhoea. There are beliefs that child must be fasted during diarrhoea.

General Examination and Vitals

- **General comment**: Whether child is irritable or thirsty, etc.
- **Vitals**
  - Pulse: Tachycardia may indicate dehydration and probably compensated shock

(look for the difference between central and peripheral pulses and capillary refill time)
- BP: Hypotension may be there if significant volume loss has occurred (actually it is a late sign - occurs when >30% volume loss has occurred).
- RR: Increased rate may be due to acidosis or associated illness like broncho-pneumonia (in yesteryears, this scenario of diarrhoea with systemic illness was used to be called parenteral diarrhoea).
- Temperature: Fever favours infective diarrhoea.

- **Growth assessment** (anthropometry):
  - Diarrhoea can lead to malnutrition and malnutrition can predispose to diarrhoea, so carefully record all parameters.
  - A significant short stature could be due to celiac disease, cystic fibrosis or IBD.

Head to Foot Examination

1. AF - depressed/not - as an indicator of hydration status (ideally examined in upright position in a calm child).
2. Eyes - Note if:
   - Sunken/tears present (if yes confirm with mother whether this has been a recent change) paradoxically a child can have puffy eyelids if the child has been fed with high osmolar ORS/ over enthusiastic IVF treatment/renal failure secondary to diarrhoea.
   - Pallor (cow's milk protein allergy can present with pallor and diarrhoea in an infant; worm infestation, celiac disease, inflammatory bowel disease, etc are a few other causes).
   - Evidence of vitamin deficiency (in chronic/ malabsorptive diarrhoea).
3. Oral cavity: Tongue - assess if dry - not reliable if child has been fed recently.
   - Look for angular stomatitis/glossitis.
   - Oral candidiasis - think of immuno-suppression in the context of chronic diarrhoea.
   - Look for the presence of tonsils (absent tonsils - immune defeciency).
   - Perioral pigmentation - Peutz-Jegher's polyps (rare possibility in a child presenting with features of intussusception).
4. Clubbing: IBD, celiac disease
5. Skin:
   - Skin turgor to assess hydration (pinch for 2 sec in abdominal area).
   - Doughy skin in hypernatremia.
6. Rectal examination: Perianal excoriation (common with lactose intolerence), rectal fistulae, fissures, and rectal prolapsed (common in malnutrition).

I. **Upper GIT**
   1. Eyes: Dry without tears if the child is dehydrated.
   2. Tongue: Dry (dehydration).

II. **Examination of abdomen**
   1. ***Inspection***
      - Shape of abdomen: Is it normal, distended or scaphoid.
      - Examine the anus. There can be perianal excoriation; in severely malnourished child, there may be prolapse of rectal mucosa. The same is possible with protracted diarrhoea.
   2. ***Palpation***
      - Feel of abdomen: Softness, guarding, etc. Surgical abdomen can also present with diarrhoea.
      - Look for any area of warmth or tenderness.
      - Look for skin turgor.
      - Organomegaly: Most normal babies will have palpable liver, hence make a mention of it.
   3. ***Percussion***
      - Percussion over the enlarged organs if any. Find out the liver span.

- Shifting dullness (if ascites is present). Occasionally, nephrotic syndrome children may present with diarrhoea in which case ascites is likely. Depending on the size of ascites, consider demonstration of fluid thrill/puddle sign.
- In case of abdominal distension due to ileus, abdomen may be tympanic in resonance.

4. ***Auscultation***
   - Bowel sounds: Normal/increased (usually increased in diarrhoea) or decreased (in ileus).

Diagnosis: Acute diarrhoeal disease or acute invasive diarrhoea or persistent diarrhoea with or without dehydration, with or without malnutrition.

Aetiology of Diarrhoea (ADD or AID)

- Virus (e.g., rotavirus, Norwalk, Coronavirus, etc)
- Bacteria (salmonella, shigella, *E. coli*, cholera)
- Protozoa (amoeba, giardia)
- Fungus (in HIV patients, cryptosporidium)
- Non infective causes: Lactose intolerance, antibiotic induced, inflammatory bowel disease, celiac disease, etc

Signs of Dehydration

To diagnose some dehydration, two or more signs are required of which at least one must be a star sign*. Severe dehydration is indicated by altered sensorium, inability to drink, decreased urine output, hypotension, etc.

- Restlessness or irritability*
- Increased thirst*
- Decreased skin turgor*
- Dry mouth and tongue
- Absent tears
- Sunken eyes

Investigations

No investigations are required in acute watery diarrhoea. Investigations may be considered in cholera, persistent diarrhoea and dysentery.

- Stool - Ova, cysts, trophozoites, leucocytes culture in dysentery and cholera
- Blood - Complete blood counts, blood smear for band cells
- Serum electrolytes
- Blood urea and creatinine

Treatment of Acute Watery Diarrhoea

- **PLAN-A if there is no dehydration**: Home available fluids and/or ORS after each stool (50–100 mL in <2 years of age and 100–200 mL in >2 years); continue normal feeding; bring back the child in case of dehydration (mother is counseled to identify dehydration).
- **PLAN-B if there is some dehydration**: 75 mL/kg of ORS within 4 hrs, administered as small quantity at frequent intervals. If the child vomits, the ORS may be stopped for 10–15 min and restarted as sips every few minutes. If on reassessment after 4 hrs, the child still has some dehydration, plan B treatment should be repeated. Children in PLAN B with high purge rate (>8 mL/kg/hr) or persistent vomiting (>3 times in 1 hr) may be given IV fluids.
- **PLAN-C if there is severe dehydration**: IV fluid (Ringer lactate or 0.9% saline) at 30 mL/kg in ½ hr. followed by 70 mL/kg in the next 2½ hrs (1 hr and 5 hrs, respectively in case of infants). No antibiotics are needed in ADD.

Treatment of Acute Invasive Diarrhoea (AID) (Dysentery)

- AID is diagnosed when there is *macroscopic* blood in stools.
- Fluids as above.
- Antibiotics: Co-trimoxazole (8 mg of trimethoprim/kg/day for 5 days) or nalidixic acid (50

mg/kg/day for 5 days). Present WHO recommendation: Ciprofloxacin 15 mg/kg twice a day for 5 days.

Treatment of Amoebiasis and Giardiasis

The diagnosis of amoebiasis and giardiasis are by the microscopic demonstration of corresponding *trophozoites* (not cyst) in stool. Treatment is with metronidazole 30 mg/kg/day × 10 days for amoebiasis and 15 mg/kg/day × 5 days for giardiasis.

Complications of Diarrhoea

- Dehydration
- Dyselectrolytemia: Hypokalemia (abdominal distention due to ileus, hypotonia, hyporeflexia), hyponatremia, hypernatremia, etc. Both hyponatremia and hypernatremia can produce seizures.
- Acidosis (deep and rapid breathing).
- Acute renal failure due to dehydration (oliguria/anuria).
- Venous thrombosis: Diarrhoea in tetralogy of Fallot, nephrotic syndrome, etc.
- Diarrhoea associated haemolytic uremic syndrome (HUS).
- Malabsorption especially lactose intolerance when the diarrhoea is persistent.
- Malnutrition in persistent diarrhoea.

Prevention

- Health education: Use freshly cooked food; Store food in clean containers; Avoid exposure of food to dust and flies; Wash and peel vegetables and fruits before giving to a child.
- Exclusive breast feeding till 4–6 months followed by proper complementary feeding practices.
- Improvement of nutritional status.
- Personal hygiene (e.g., hand washing before handling food; periodic trimming of nails)
- Safe drinking water.
- Good sanitation and sewage disposal
- Avoidance of disease carriers from food handling jobs.
- Vaccines: E.g., Rotavirus, cholera, typhoid, etc.

PYREXIA OF UNKNOWN ORIGIN

1. **Age**: Children <1 year may not have localizing signs because of poor immunological development; hence infections may present clinically as fever of unknown origin. Children >6 years of age may have a localized infection (abscess) or respiratory or genitourinary cause for fever. Kawasaki disease is more common in less than 5 years. Autoimmune processes are common in adolescents.
2. **Sex**: Autoimmune causes are likely in older female children.
3. **Presenting complaint**
   - H/o fever since——
   - History of present illness:
   - History must be tailored keeping in mind the most probable diagnosis in your area. Example could be infections (Viral: IMN, HIV; Bacterial: UTI, respiratory, typhoid, TB; Spirochetes: Leptospira; Protozoa: Malaria, leishmaniasis; ricketsiae: Scrub typhus), collagen vascular or malignancy.
   - Ask whether and how the fever was documented (many mothers attribute normal head warmth as fever). Note the onset (insidious/acute), duration and progression of fever. In typhoid, fever starts as low grade and progressively increases over many days. In contrast, malaria starts as high spiking fever. But the typical pattern of fever (e.g., step ladder pattern in enteric fever) may not be present in all cases as the course gets interrupted by antipyretics.
   - Enquire whether the fever was of high grade and was associated with chills and rigor (characteristically in malaria, urinary infection and pneumococcal pneumonia).

- Number of spikes of fever per day: Once daily spikes (quotidian) in JIA or tertian/quartan in malaria.
- Ask whether child was well and playful in between periods of fever and is unwell only during the period of fever (less chances of serious infections).
- H/o rash if any and the day on which rash appeared helps in diagnosing exanthematous fevers. It can be remembered by the mneumonic "Very Sick Person Must Take Double Tablets"
  - Very – Varicella (day 1)
  - Sick – Scarlet fever (day 2)
  - Person – Pox – small pox (day 3)
  - Must – Measles (day 4/5)
  - Take – Typhus (day 5)
  - Double – Dengue (day 6)
  - Tablets – Typhoid (day 7)

  Transient salmon coloured macular non-pruritic rash recurring with fever spikes may indicate systemic onset JIA.
- Ask for h/o associated complaints as symptoms referable to many organ systems may be present and a detailed history is a must.
  - Nervous system: Consider meningitis when there is irritability/drowsiness, refusal to suck, seizures in an infant or headache, drowsiness, projectile vomiting, in an older child. Cerebral malaria may be a close differential.
  - Respiratory symptoms like persistent cough, chest pain: Pleuritis due to tuberculosis/pneumonia. Ear discharge: Mastoiditis, meningitis (otitis media). Pain, nasal discharge, nasal obstruction, headache: consider sinusitis (frontal sinuses do not develop until a child is 7 years old); Sore throat: IMN.
  - Neck swellings: TB, lymphoma.
  - Cardiac: Child with a heart disease before or after surgery presenting with persistent fever think of infective endocarditis.
  - Abdomen: Abdominal pain, vomiting, constipation: enteric fever/dengue fever/TB abdomen.
  - Renal: Frequent micturition, dysuria, hypogastric pain, flank pain – UTI.
  - History of recurrent infection, oral thrush, significant loss of weight-HIV.
  - History of joint pain, rash, photosensitivity - autoimmune causes like SLE, JIA.
- History of pica can be a risk factor for Toxoplasmosis, Toxocara canis.
- History of contact with animals - Brucellosis, leptospirosis.
- Travel to endemic areas - Malaria, Kala azar, histoplasmosis.
- Drug history – Anticholinergics: Topical agents including eye drops can cause drug fever. Drug fever may follow many antibiotics.
- Endocrinological causes such as diabetes insipidus, thyrotoxicosis, Addison's disease are rare causes.
- History suggestive of malignancy or familial causes should also be kept in mind.
- Familial causes: Familial dysautonomia, hereditary periodic fever syndromes.

4. **Past history**
   H/o recurrent infections/unusual course/not responding to regular antibiotics may point towards immune deficiency.
5. **Natal & postnatal**
   Prematurity, LBW, prolonged rupture of membranes, maternal sepsis are high risk factors to development of sepsis in a young infant.
6. **Immunization history**
   Inquire about all vaccines particularly as for BCG, Hib, hepatitis A & B, measles, varicella.
7. **Growth and development**: Usually normal.
8. **Nutrition history**: As routine.

18

9. **Family history**: Contact with TB, h/o AIDS related illnesss in the parents.
10. **Socioeconomic history**
11. **General examination**
    Note the general appearance - whether toxic; note the sensorium of the child.
12. **Vitals**
    - Pulse: Tachycardia (could be due to fever: 1° rise in temperature approximately increases pulse by 10 beats; disproportionate tachycardia - think of toxemea). Bradycardia is occasionally seen in dengue, typhoid, leptospirosis.
    - BP: Hypotension may be seen in dengue, perform hess test. Hypotension is possible in the advanced stage of any serious illness.
    - RR may increase with fever.
    - Temperature: Record temperature in the appropriate manner for the age of the child at the time of examination.
13. **Head to foot examination**
    - **Eyes**
      - Look for pallor, icterus
      - Palpebral conjuctivitis: Measles
      - Bulbar conjuctivitis: Kawasaki disease, leptospirosis
      - Petechiae: Haemorrhagic fevers, infective endocarditis
      - Phlycten: TB
      - Proptosis: Thyrotoxicosis, metastasis, orbital infection
      - Uveitis: Connective tissue disorders
      - Fundus: Look for chorioretinitis/ choroid tubercles
      - Lack of tear, absent corneal reflex may indicate familial dys autonomia
    - **Nose**
      - Look for pus discharge
    - **Ear**
      - Discharge: Note the colour; whether foul smelling or not
      - Look for sinus tenderness
    - **Mouth**
      - Look for oral ulcers, dental hygeine, gingivitis
      - Throat: Bilateral enlarged tonsils, with/without exudates in IMN
      - Tongue: Coated tongue - enteric fever
      - Strawberry red tongue: Kawasaki disease, scarlet fever
      - Oral candidiasis (beyond newborn period): Immunosuppression
      - Thyroid enlargement: Thyroiditis or Graves disease
    - **Lymph nodes**
      - Matted lymph nodes: TB, generalized lymphadenopathy - IMN (look for epitrochlear nodes too), TB or malignancy.
    - **Skin**
      - Rash: Note the distribution (more in face or trunk, where it started first) and type (macular/papular/vesicular).
      - Fever blisters: pneumococcal, staphylococcal, streptococcal and rickettsial infections.
      - Bleeding manifestations - malignancy.
      - Absence of sweating (familial dysautonomia/anhidrotic ectodermal dysplasia).
      - Genitalia: Look for any local inflammation (often missed in exam).
      - Limbs: Pain may suggest deep vein thrombosis, especially in prolonged immobilization of a fat child.
      - Bone pain/muscle pain: Note if generalized or point tenderness (osteomyelitis abscess).
14. **Systemic examination**
    - Proceed to examine relevant system based on clinical clues from history and general examination.
    - Most often, a good general examination followed by abdominal examination is the

one needed. Hepatosplenomegaly is likely in IMN, typhoid, malignancy, etc.

Investigations

Investigations must be tailored depending on the differential diagnosis. The following is a general suggestion.

- Total WBC count (>15,000 is more likely to have bacterial infection), DC (shift to left/increased band counts suggest bacterial infection), Pl. count, ESR/CRP, blood film for abnormal cells and malarial parasites
- Urine routine, C&S
- Blood C&S
- Mx, X-ray chest
- Widal, dengue & leptospira serology
- HIV serology
- ANA, rheumatoid factor
- Bone marrow
- Imaging studies (USS, CT)
- Immunoglobulin assay

Treatment

Treatment depends on the diagnosis. Students are encouraged to consult "Manual of Pediatric Practice" by the same author for treatment details for individual conditions.

TYPHOID FEVER

Case sheet format for PUO and the format for examination of abdomen may be used.

- Prolonged fever
- Headache (mainly because of fever)
- Cough is a common early symptom (typhoid bronchitis)
- Diffuse non-localized abdominal pain
- Diarrhoea (early) or constipation (late, due to ileus)
- Abdominal distension (ileus)
- History of water source
- History of diarrhoea/constipation; dark stools (intestinal haemorrhage)
- Pallor
- Coated tongue
- Delirium
- Meningeal signs may be elicitable
- Look for rose spots
- Hepatomegaly and/or splenomegaly
- Gall bladder may become palpable

Differential Diagnosis

See causes for hepatosplenomegaly with fever (p 167).

Treatment

- Ceftriaxone followed by oral cefixime. Ciprofloxacin if not responding to third generation cephalosporin.
- Fever: Paracetamol and tepid sponging.
- IV fluids, if necessary.
- Laxatives and enemas must be avoided even when there is constipation.
- Surgical intervention for perforations.
- Individuals excreting the bacteria in stool for more than 3 months are carriers; those excreting for more than 1 year are chronic carriers.

Complications

- Intestinal haemorrhage. Dark stools or fresh blood in stool.
- Perforation and peritonitis. Tender distension of abdomen, vomiting and other signs of peritonitis.
- Toxic myocarditis.
- Other complications are anaemia, encephalopathy, pyelonephritis, meningitis, thrombocytopenia, jaundice, acute hydrops of gall bladder, etc.

Prevention

- Safe drinking water
- Toilet use and safe sewage disposal
- Vaccination

MALARIA

- Case sheet format for PUO and the format for examination of abdomen may be used.
- Usual presenting complaints are fever with chills and anaemia. Rare presentations are reddish urine (blackwater fever) or seizure (cerebral malaria or febrile seizure because of fever).
- Ask about rigor and chills along with fever; sweating with reduction of fever. Ask about the periodicity of fever (daily rise or alternate day, etc).
- There may be history of travel to endemic area.
- Examination will show anaemia, lemon yellow tinge icterus, splenohepatomegaly.

Investigations

- *Thick and thin blood smears.*
- *Qualitative buffy coat (QBC) test.*
- Rapid diagnostic kits detect antigens of malarial parasites like histidine rich protein-2 of *Pl. falciparum*, parasite-specific LDH, pan-malarial plasmodial aldolase, etc.

Treatment

- ***Specific treatment***
  - Treatment of vivax: A total of 25 mg of chloroquine base/kg over 3 days. The WHO recommends 10 mg of base/kg orally followed by 5 mg of base/kg 6 hrs later on the first day, and then 5 mg of base/kg on the second and third day. National Malaria Control Program recommends 10 mg/kg on the first and second day followed by 5 mg/kg on the third day. In addition, primaquine 0.25 mg base/kg daily orally for 14 days is also given for radical cure of vivax.
  - *Pl. falciparum*: Artesunate (4 mg/kg for 3 days) + Sulpha & Pyrimethamine (25 and 1.25 mg/kg, respectively as a single dose) + Primaquine (0.75 mg/kg as a single dose).
  - In *cerebral malaria* and when oral intake is not tolerated, parenteral quinine is used.
- ***Supportive treatment***
  - Fever: Paracetamol and sponging
  - Hydration: Oral or IV fluids
  - Severe anaemia: Blood transfusion

Complications

CABS: **C**erebral malaria, severe **A**naemia, **A**cidosis, **B**lackwater fever, **B**leeding (due to DIC), **S**hock ("algid malaria"), and low **S**ugar (hypoglycaemia).

Prevention

- Mosquito control measures (nets, larvicidals).
- Travel to endemic areas: Chloroquine 5 mg/kg once a week started 1 week before the entry and continued till 4 weeks after the exit.

INFECTIOUS MONONUCLEOSUS

Fever, enlarged tonsils, lymphadenopathy, splenomegaly; rarely maculopapular rashes (ask history of treatment with ampicillin).

Investigations

- Peripheral blood smear shows lymphocytosis and *atypical lymphocytes*.
- Heterophile antibodies (detected by Paul Bunnel test).
- Antibodies to viral capsid antigen (VCA) or early antigen or Epstein Barr nuclear antigen (EBNA).

Differential Diagnosis

Streptococcal pharyngitis (this is not associated with hepatosplenomegaly).

Refer p 166 for causes of hepatosplenomegaly and lymphadenopathy.

Treatment

- Paracetamol for fever.
- IV fluids for vomiting and poor oral intake.

- Rest to avoid trauma to abdomen.
- Steroids for airway obstruction due to lymph node enlargement.

Complications

Airway obstruction, thrombocytopenia, autoimmune haemolytic anaemia and CNS involvement.

CHRONIC DISSEMINATED TB

- Contact with an infected adult.
- Low grade fever of prolonged duration with multiple organ involvement.
- Fever, cough, loss of weight, loss of appetite and organ involvement are the usual scenario.
- Generalized lymphadenopathy.
- Lungs: In case of miliary TB, the classic finding is respiratory distress, very poor oxygen saturation, but not much auscultatory findings. Look for pleural effusion.
- Meningitis: Look for meningeal signs.
- Eyes: Look for choroid tubercles.
- Abdomen: Hepatosplenomegaly, ascites. Abdomen may feel doughy.
- Bone marrow suppression resulting in anaemia and bleeding tendency.

Diagnosis of TB

- History
- Suggestive physical findings
- Mantoux
- X ray
- Histopathology/AFB
- Newer methods: Read the "Manual of Pediatic Practice" from same author.

Treatment

As per NTEP regimen.

KALA AZAR

- Usual case is an emaciated, pale, hyper-pigmented child with distended abdomen and low grade prolonged fever.
- Headache and body ache are unusual, in contrast to usual fevers.
- Insidious onset prolonged fever. May be high grade initially, two spikes per day.
- Anaemia
- Splenomegaly, later massive spleen
- Hepatomegaly
- Bleeding manifestations (usually epistaxis or gum bleeds)
- Dry rough skin with hyperpigmentation
- Progressive weight loss
- Severe anaemia can cause cardiac failure and hypersplenism may cause cytopenia. Thus, look for clinical evidences for these.

Investigations

- Napier's aldehyde test (serology).
- Histopathology: Biopsy specimens, bone marrow.

Treatment of Kala Azar

- Parenteral pentavalent antimony compounds (sodium stibogluconate) for 28 days.
- Liposomal amphotericin B.

CHAPTER 19

Disorders of Haematological System: Case Sheet Formats

There is no definite scheme of examination for haematological system. The usual practice is general examination followed by examination of abdomen. General examination and examination of abdomen are already discussed in detail in Ch. 18 and so this chapter focuses on guidelines to examine a child with anaemia or bleeding.

The usual presenting symptoms/signs in a haematology case are anaemia, bleeding (e.g., purpura), lymphadenopathy or hepato-plenomegaly.

1. Age: Onset of clinical manifestations of β-thalassemia is after the first few months (may not be symptomatic until the total content of fetal haemoglobin falls; HbF at birth is about 70%, which drops down to 2% by 6 months). Iron deficiency anaemia is likely only after the first 6 months of life (usually around 9 months). Megaloblastic anaemia of infancy is usually by 4–7 months of age, somewhat earlier than iron deficiency. Fanconi anaemia, though congenital, presents clinically only by 6 years of life.
2. Sex: Hemophilia, G6PD deficiency, etc are X linked and hence manifest only in males.
3. Race: Thalassemia (Pujabis, Sindhis), sickle cell anaemia (certain tribal groups), G6PD (Parsis), etc are confined to certain ethnic groups in India as indicated within brackets.
4. Presenting complaints: The usual presenting complaints are pallor, bleeding (petechiae, echymosis, epistaxis, hematemesis, malena, hematochezia, etc), or fatigability (due to anaemia).

Anaemia (pallor) may be looked at:

- Conjunctiva (may not be reliable if the child has been crying or rubbing eyes)
- Tongue
- Hard palate
- Palm/sole
- Nail bed

In case of bleeding, always inquire about mucosal bleed, because mucosal bleed is considered forerunner of CNS bleed in thrombocytopenia. Specifically inquire about epistaxis, gum bleeds, malena, hematuria, etc. Recurrent epistaxis is quite common in von Willebrand disease.

Constellation of symptoms/signs give clue to the probable diagnosis.

- Pyrexia, purpura, pallor, and (bone) pain (4 Ps) point towards leukemia. Lymphadenopathy and hepatosplenomegaly gives additional support to this diagnosis.
  - Anaemia, lymphadenopathy and hepatosplenomegaly with optic atrophy could point towards osteopetrosis.
  - Lymphadenopathy and hepatosplenomegaly could also be due to storage disorders.
- Purpura (palpable purpura over the outer aspect of leg, thigh and gluteal region), abdominal pain, arthritis and nephritis (PAAN) point towards HSP.
- Painful crisis point towards sickle cell anaemia.

- Repeated blood transfusion, haemolytic facies and splenomegaly point towards congenital haemolytic anaemia (look carefully for icterus which is likely).
- Anaemia, splenomegaly and mild icterus without haemolytic facies or blood transfusions point towards hereditary spherocytosis (in addition, may have history of neonatal jaundice).
- Repeated blood transfusion without haemolytic facies and splenomegaly suggests aplastic anaemia.
- In case of anaemia without any readily demonstrable physical findings, consider:
  - Nutritional
  - Aplastic anaemia
  - Chronic renal failure (specifically look for short stature, rickets)
  - Hypothyroidism (being a readily treatable condition, always consider this). Anaemia, constipation, short stature and developmental retardation may be additional points in favour of hypothyroidism.
- History of repeated blood transfusions may be obtained in:
  - Thalassemia
  - Aplastic anaemia
  - Pure red cell aplasia
  - Osteopetrosis
- Sudden onset anemia could be due to:
  - Acute blood loss
  - Autoimmume haemolytic anaemia
  - G6PD deficiency
  - Aplastic crisis in haemolytic anaemia (like spherocytosis or sickle cell anaemia)
- Anaemia noticed over weeks could be due to:
  - Leukemia (usual history is less than a month in case of acute leukemia)
- Aplastic anaemia
- Anaemia developing over months could be:
  - Nutritional (e.g., iron deficiency)
  - Low grade chronic blood loss (e.g., hook worm)
  - Chronic illness (e.g., chronic kidney disease)

5. Past history:
   - In cases of anaemia:
     - History of any actual blood loss (as a cause for anaemia). Clues to obvious loss of blood are accidents, hematemesis, per rectal bleeding, malena, etc.
     - Drugs as a cause of anaemia (drugs like chloramphenicol that cause bone marrow suppression and drugs like primaquine that cause haemolysis in G6PD deficiency). Acquired haemolytic anaemia could be following viral infections or drugs.
     - History of pica is usually forthcoming in iron deficiency anaemia. There is a curious tendency to eat inedible things in iron deficiency anaemia. In addition, pica could be a source for lead poisoning. Malena could point towards hookworm infestation. Severe anaemia may have symptoms suggestive of cardiac failure (oedema, effort intolerance, tachycardia).
     - Chronic infections like TB is one cause for anaemia and hence must be inquired into. Chronic renal failure (anaemia, short stature, rickets; may have previous history suggestive of renal involvement), hypothyroidism, lead poisoning (may have history of pica), etc are rare causes of anaemia. Viral infections can cause acquired haemolytic anaemia or bone marrow suppression.
     - Acute onset anaemia, oliguria and bleeding in a toddler could be

haemolytic uraemic syndrome (may have a history of diarrhoea). Other causes of anaemia plus thrombo-cytopenia (hence bleeding) are Evans syndrome, micro-angiopathic haemolytic anaemia, malignancy, etc.
  - Other relevant past histories to ask for: jaundice (haemolytic anaemia, Wilson disease); blackish stools (hookworm or other causes of GIT bleeds, including cows' milk protein intolerance); history of blood transfusions.
- In cases of bleeding:
  - Drugs causing thrombocytopenia or affecting platelet function in case of bleeding disorders (NSAIDs). Recent viral infections could be a cause for thrombocytopenia (hence elicit history of viral infections in the preceding 1–4 weeks). History of trauma is relevant in cases of contusion or echymosis. In adolescents, excessive menstrual bleed may be inquired into.
  - History of excessive bleed from umbilicus in newborn period (coagulation disorders); excessive bleeding following shedding of teeth or dental extraction or circumcision; past history of joint bleeds (coagulation disorders).

6. Antenatal, natal and postnatal history: Iron deficiency anaemia is more likely in preterm babies, babies who had frank bleeds (e.g., from umbilical cord, cephalhematoma, etc), babies of mothers who themselves are iron deficient or not received iron-folic acid during their pregnancies (so ask this history). History suggestive of IU infection also is to be elicited as IU infection can present with anaemia, thrombocytopenia and hepatosplenomegaly. Closely spaced pregnancies and multiple gestation (twin to twin transfusion) could predispose to anaemia.
   In case of newborn bleeds, maternal drug history (antiepileptics, warfarin); history of vitamin K injection to newborn.
7. Immunization and development history.
8. Dietary history: Diet history must specifically focus on deficiencies of iron, B_{12}, and folic acid; exclusive milk feeds without any supplement beyond 6 months of age is the most common cause of iron deficiency anaemia. History must elicit dietary content of iron rich foods. Cow's milk allergy can cause intestinal blood loss if cow's milk in excess of 500 mL is regularly consumed. Goat's milk could predispose to megaloblastic anaemia (folic acid deficiency). Strict vegetarian diet, which excludes even milk, can cause B_{12} deficiency anaemia.
9. Family history: Consanguinity; family history of abdominal surgery (splenectomy, gall stones); history of bleeding tendency, jaundice, repeated blood transfusions.
10. General comment: Well child or unwell child. Child with leukemia or with joint pains may look unwell. Child with cardiac failure due to severe anaemia may also look ill.
    Look for features of hypothyroidism that may have caused anaemia.
11. Growth: Weight/height may be adversely affected in long standing diseases like thalassemia.
    Head circumference may be low in Fanconi; could be high in thalassemia due to expansion of skull bones. Puberty may get delayed in congenital haemolytic anaemias like thalassemia and sickle cell anaemia.
12. Hand to head and head to foot examination:
    - The candidate can adopt hand to head and head to foot examination; or stick on to the conventional head to foot examination with the examination of limbs included within that.

- Nail: Platynychia/koilonychia (iron deficiency); leuconychia (white nails in chronic liver disease), clubbing (cyanotic heart disease: cyanotic heart diseases may cause platelet dysfunction); splinter haemorrhage (subacute bacterial endocarditis). Nail ridging and dystrophy in dyskeratosis congenita. Hyperpigmentation of knuckles in megaloblastic anaemia.
- Pale palm and palmar creases in anaemia. Hyperkeratosis of palms and soles in dyskeratosis congenita **(Fig. 19.1)**
- Limb anomalies in TAR (radius absent, thumbs present), Fanconi (hypoplastic radius/thumbs), Diamond Blackfan (triphalangeal thumb), etc.
- Pulse: Could be low volume with tachycardia (blood loss and circulatory shock); high volume and tachycardia (compensatory mechanism in long standing anaemia).
- Epitrochlear nodes (this is often missed by candidate in exam).
- Blood pressure: Low in anaemia due to acute blood loss or in cardiomyopathy of transfusion hemosiderosis (chronic iron overload in thalassemia); BP may be high in anaemia due to chronic renal failure or HUS; wide pulse pressure in anaemia as a compensatory mechanism.
- Axillary, supra clavicular nodes and neck nodes.
- Head, face (note dysmorphism, haemolytic facies, etc).
  - Haemolytic facies in thalassemia; pigmentation may be there in thalassemia; subcutaneous nodules in leukemia; Cushingoid face may be seen if the child is on steroids.

    Haemolytic facies consists of a large head with frontal and parietal bossing, depressed nasal bridge, malar (maxillary) prominence, irregular maxillary teeth with resultant anterior overbite, sallow complexion, etc.
  - Eyes for squint, ptosis, nystagmus, icterus (look carefully for icterus in good daylight; light lemon yellow colour of haemolytic jaundice can be easily missed), pallor, subconjunctival haemorrhage, cataract (cataract could be an adverse event of long-term desferioxamine or steroids), fundus for haemorrhages in bleeding disorders. Pale fundus in severe anaemia. Optic atrophy in osteopetrosis.
    - Cataract in those on long-term deferoxamine.

19

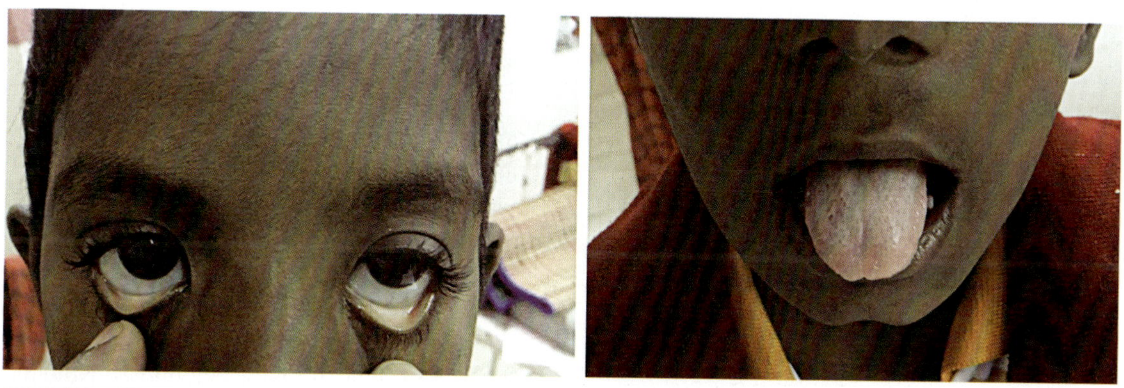

Fig.19.1 Pallor

- Opine if icterus is proportional to pallor, which is usually the case with haemolytic anaemias (deep jaundice is unlikely in haemolytic anaemia). If icterus is out of proportion consider primary hepatic causes with anaemia (e.g., Wilson's with haemolytic anaemia).

- Ears: Hearing assessment; sensorineural deafness is an adverse event in those on long-term deferoxamine.
- Look at oral mucosa, palate, etc for bleeds. Blue lines of gums is described in lead poisoning (may present as anaemia).
  - Ulcers/mucositis may indicate neutropenia.
  - Pale tongue with atrophic papillae in iron deficiency anaemia. Always look for features of other deficiencies, as iron deficiency may not occur in isolation.
  - Special emphasis on gums (leukemia).
- Neck: Lymph nodes, including supraclavicular nodes. Not to miss any node, follow the scheme described in p 101, JVP (cardiac failure).
- Chest and back: Look for bone tenderness over sternum/clavicle/spine, etc.
- Be sure to examine heart fully. Hemic murmurs are very likely; may have cardiac enlargement due to cardiomyopathy or anaemia.
- Abdomen (look for distension & organomegaly): Tender hepatomegaly with hepatojugular reflux in case of cardiac failure. Needle marks on abdomen could be due to desferioxamine subcutaneous injections.
- Surgical scars (splenectomy, gall stones).
- Testes: Testicular swellings are especially significant in leukemia. Priapism is a rare complication in sickle cell anaemia. Puberty gets delay-ed due to endocrinopathy in the mul-tiple transfused hemolytic anemia child.
- Perianal fissures and fistulae in Crohn disease. Altered stool colour in HSP or GIT bleed of any reason.
- Lower limb (including gait as there could be painful involvement of bone/joint in leukemia). Inguinal lymph nodes. Erythema nodosum. Dependant oedema in case of cardiac failure. Chronic leg ulcers in congenital haemolytic anaemia.
- Skin: See column 2.
- Note any bleeding or joint swelling or bone pain anywhere.
- In case any joint is involved, proceed examining the joint as described in Chapter 12. Joint swelling is possible in hemophilia, sickle cell anaemia, leukemia, inflammatory bowel disease, juvenile idiopathic arthritis (these can present with anaemia and joint pain), HSP, etc.
- Examine the mother (and the father if available at the time of examination) for splenomegaly (hereditary spherocytosis is autosomal dominant).

Summary

We suggest placing emphasis on "S" for examination of haematological system. This will cover almost every common entity related to hematological system. So after finishing the systematic examination, verify whether you have covered the entire "S" mentioned below.

- Sex: Hemophilia, G6PD deficiency, etc are X linked and hence manifest only in males.
- Skin: Petechiae, purpura, echymosis: Note its distribution (buttocks, outer side of thighs, legs

etc in HSP). Raised and/or tender petechiae indicates vasculitis. Non-raised, non-tender petechiae denotes platelet deficiency or dysfunction. Look for stigmata of well-defined diseases known to cause vasculitis (e.g., SLE). Big haemangioma could be a reason for consumption coagulopathy/thrombocytopenia (Kasabach–Merritt syndrome). Leg ulcers in sickle cell anaemia. Hyperpigmentation (knuckles in megaloblastic anaemia; generalized hyperpigmentation in Fanconi, Kala azar, etc). Cafe au lait spots in Fanconi's anaemia.

- Swellings: Lymph nodes, liver, or any other mass (example of abdominal mass is adrenal mass of neurobastoma).
- Spleen (leukemia, haemolytic anaemia, osteopetrosis, storage diseases).
- Sternum and spine and any other areas of bone tenderness.
- Syndromes: Look for dysmorphism: Fanconi anaemia, Diamond Blackfan, TAR syndrome, Dyskeratosis congenita, etc are examples. Haemolytic facies in congenital haemolytic anaemia.
- Skeletal system: Examination for musculoskeletal system if any joint is involved (joint tenderness/swelling). Examine the gait (antalgic gait due to pain; ataxic gait due to loss of posterior column sensations in B_{12} deficiency).

Note: Look for evidence of disorders of various cell lines: RBC (anaemia), WBC (history of infections; gingivitis) and platelets (skin and mucous membrane bleeds). Evidence of dysfunction of coagulation is deep seated bleeds (like bleeding into the muscles) or joint bleeds. Whereas thrombocytopenia causes skin & mucous membrane bleeds.

APPROACH TO A CASE OF PALLOR

The candidate must read the hematology case sheet format (see p 424) the following discussion focuses on what is specifically applicable to pallor with organomegaly.

1. **History**
   - Presenting complaint: Pallor/easy fatigability, yellowish discolouration of eyes or just come for blood transfusion (a child already diagnosed and on follow-up).
   - History of present illness (HOPI): History of pallor: noticed when (thalassemia usually presents at 6 months of life, hereditary spherocytosis can present whenever there is an increased stress, e.g., infection/intake of drugs, which precipitate hemolysis) whether the pallor is progressively increasing/episodic (G6PD).
   - History of easy fatigability in older children, irritability/decreased activity in infants.
   - History of jaundice: Differentiates between haemolytic anaemias (e.g., hereditary spherocytosis) from non-haemolytic anaemia.
   - History of fever: Fever can act as a trigger and precipitate haemolysis in congenial haemolytic anaemia, high grade fever, chills with pallor-malaria has to be kept in the differentials.
   - History of blood transfusion, if present how frequent (increasing need of BT indicates probable hypersplenism).
   - History of bleeding manifestations, history of bony tenderness/recurrent infections/ swellings over the body - to rule out malignancy (bone pain can also be due to deferasirox).
   - History of drug ingestion (sulphonamides, quinines, etc).
   - History of eating inedible substances (pica).
   - Use of foot wear while outside.
   - Malena or any other blood loss.
   - Goat milk (could cause folate deficiency).
   - Elicit history suggestive of complications:
     - History of cardiac failure (less common in chronic anaemia).

- Growth of the child as per parents (chronic anaemia leads to undernutrition).
- History suggestive of gall stones suggested by intermittent pain abdomen.

2. **Antenatal natal and post natal**
History of neonatal jaundice (hereditary spehrocytosis may have history of jaundice in newborn period).
3. **Immunization**
Enquire regarding optional vaccines (important if splenectomy has to be planned).
4. **Development history**
5. **Nutrition**
   - Assess iron intake.
   - Ingestion of goat's milk may lead to folate deficiency.
   - Strict vegetarian diet may predispose to B_{12} deficiency.
   - Thalassemia – whether the child is on restriction of foods with high iron content. Taking tea along with food is said to decrease iron absorption from the food.
6. **Family history**
   - History of pallor requiring transfusions among other siblings (thalassemia - AR inheritance) or history of pallor in parents (hereditary spherocytosis AD).
   - History of jaundice or splenectomy in siblings or parents points towards HS.
7. **Socioeconomic**
   - Whether beneficiary of any social schemes.
   - Effect of this child's illness on family expenses and care of siblings.
8. **Examination**
See Haematology Case Sheet Format, p 424–429.
Growth: Growth may be compromised in congenital haemolytic anaemias, except in a very few who are adequately transfused at adequate intervals. Tanner staging is needed as puberty may get delayed. In case of nutritional anaemia, there may be associated nutritional deficiencies, which may be looked for. Examples are B complex deficiency, iron deficiency, rickets, etc.
Aetiology of anaemia
   - Decreased synthesis could be due to aplastic anaemia. In congenital aplasia, one may see dysmorphic features. In acquired aplasia, drugs or infections are blamed.
   - Decreased synthesis due to restricted supply of raw material: Example could be iron or folic acid deficiency.
   - Increased destruction: Haemolysis: Could be congenital (thalassemia, G6PD deficiency, sickle cell anaemia, etc) or acquired (autoimmune haemolytic anaemia).

PANCYTOPENIA/APLASTIC ANAEMIA

Fanconi aneamia is the best recognized constitutional aplastic anaemia/pancytopenia. Acquired aplastic anaemia/pancytopenia may follow drugs, chemicals, toxins, infectious agents, radiation or autoimmune destruction. Clinically, the child *will not have* hepatosplenomegaly or lymphadenopathy.

FANCONI ANAEMIA

- Usually manifest by 6–8 years.
- Two or more cell lines are depleted. May have anemia, thrombocytopenia and leucopenia.
- Signs and symptoms: **CASH**: **C**hromosomal breakage, **C**afe au lait spots, **A**plastic anaemia, **S**hort stature, **S**mall head, **H**yperpigmentation, **H**ypoplasia of thumb or radial side of upper limb. See p 497–498.

Treatment

- For Fanconi, androgens (stanozolol).
- For acquired pancytopenia/aplastic anaemia, granulocyte macrophage colony stimulating factors (GM-CSF), anti-thymocyte globulin.
- Bone marrow transplantation.

IRON DEFICIENCY ANAEMIA

Common age group: 6 months to 2 years and adolescence.

Aetiology

- Poor dietary intake. Milk is a poor source of iron. Evaluate dietary history for deficiency of iron intake.
- Poor iron reserve as in case of preterm infants or severe maternal anaemia.
- Blood loss: Hookworm infestation; portal hypertension with bleeding, etc.
- Increased demand, e.g., during adolescence.
- Improper absorption of iron, as in malabsorption syndromes (e.g., celiac disease).

Clinical Features

Pallor, poor attention span, easy fatigability, koilonychia, glossitis, functional systolic murmurs due to hyperdynamic circulation, etc. Palpable spleen is rare in iron deficiency anaemia (in <10% cases).

Investigations

- Hypochromic microcytic anaemia with anisocytosis and poikilocytosis; increased red cell distribution width (RDW), meaning wide variations in red cell size. RDW is normal in thalassemia.
- MCV, MCH and MCHC are reduced.
- Bone marrow examination is never indicated but if done, will show normoblastic erythroid hyperplasia.
- Reticulocyte count is normal but gets transiently elevated in 5–7 days after starting iron therapy.
- Stool must be examined for hookworm infestation.
- Serum ferritin (iron storage protein) low, usually less than 10 ng/mL; serum iron is low.
- Investigations for any sources of blood loss (e.g., cow's milk protein intolerence).

Treatment

- Oral iron is 6 mg/kg/day of elemental iron. Ferrous sulphate distributed in national program has about 20% elemental iron.
- Anaemia cannot be corrected faster with parenteral iron and hence the only indication for parenteral iron is intolerance of oral iron.
- An increase of reticulocyte count is expected towards the end of first week of treatment. The anaemia gets corrected within 1 month. The treatment is continued for 3 months to replenish the stores.
- Packed RBC transfusion is considered only if there is haemodynamic compromise due to anaemia.

Prevention

- Promotion of breastfeeding (any milk is a poor source of iron. However, compared to cow's milk, breast milk iron is better absorbed).
- Treatment of hookworm infestation.
- Encourage the child to use sanitary latrine and to have footwear to protect against hookworm.
- Control of pica.
- Health education regarding iron rich foods, need for proper weaning after 4 months of age, methods of fortifying the infant cereals with iron rich food (e.g., jaggery), etc.
- Public health measures; e.g., fortification of salt with iron.

Prognosis

All changes of iron deficiency anaemia are reversible. Koilonychia may take a few months for getting corrected.

THALASSEMIA

Please read haematology case sheet format (p 424).

1. Name:

2. Age: Beta thalassemia clinically presents after the first few months of life (may not be symptomatic until the total content of fetal haemoglobin falls; HbF at birth is about 70%, which drops down to 2% by 6 months).
3. Sex: Males & females have equal chance of being affected (auto-somal recessive).
4. Race: Thalassemia (Punjabis, Sindhis)
5. Complaints:
   - Progressively increasing pallor
   - Abdominal distension (due to organomegaly)
   - Failure to thrive
   - Fatigability (due to anaemia)
   - Abdominal pain (gall stone)
6. History of present illness:
   - Increasing pallor: Easy fatigability, palpitation, fast breathing, oedema (heart failure).
   - Only symptoms pertaining to RBC is expected in thalassemia. Hence ask for bleeding, repeated infections, etc, which point towards the involvement of more than one element; so other diagnosis like aplastic anaemia, malignancy, etc becomes the differentials.
   - History of repeated transfusions: at what age was transfusions started, regularity and frequency of transfusions. This gives an idea of iron overload and the need for chelation.
   - History of receiving any regular injections/ medications (chelators, folic acid).
   - History of discolouration of skin.
   - History of not achieving adequate weight and height.
   - Older child: Ask for delayed puberty.
   - History suggestive of deafness (sensorineural deafness due to desferrioxamine toxicity or bony expansion of extra erythropoesis compressing the eight cranial nerve).
   - History suggestive of complications of blood transfusion: Hepatitis B, C or HIV; iron overload.
   - History of any actual blood loss to account for anaemia.
   - Viral infections or drugs, which could account for anaemia.
   - Chronic infections.
   - Jaundice and anaemia are suggestive of haemolytic anaemia.
7. Antenatal, natal, post natal:
   History suggestive of IU infection.
8. Immunization:
   Special emphasis on hepatitis B. Additional immunizations like pneumococcus and *H. influenzae* as child may be a candidate for splenectomy in future.
9. Development history:
   As with any other chronic illness, some delay in development is likely.
10. Diet history:
    - To check the iron consumption in food.
    - Rest of the history as usual.
11. Family and socio-economic history:
    - Sibling/relatives receiving transfusions; history of jaundice.
    - Effect of the disease on family and sibling.
    - Assistance from social security schemes.
12. General examination:
    - Overall general comment
    - Vital parameters
    - Growth parameters (anthropometry)– Height, weight with percentiles, HC
    - Tanner staging for puberty in older children
13. Head to foot examination:
    - Facial features: Frontal bossing/parietal bossing/chipmunk facies/maxillary overgrowth/dental malocclusion/prominent malar eminence/broadened nasal bridge.
    - Head & neck: Conjuctival pallor, scleral icterus, cataracts (desferrioxamine).
    - Teeth: Dental malocclusion.

- Endocrine abnormalities: Chvostek's and Trousseau's signs (hypoparathyroidism).
- Hearing (sensorineural deafness)
- Neck: Goitre
- Hands: Finger tip pricks (blood sampling) /pallor, pigmentation, also examine nails, palm (pallor).
- Peripheral stigmata of chronic liver disease (hepatitis likely in multitransfused child).
- Pulse: Slow (hypothyroid), irregular (cardiomyopathy), pulsus alternans (CCF), hyperdynamic (anaemia).
- Chest: Full precordial examination to detect cardiomyopathy, CCF, haemic murmurs.
- Abdomen: Distension, splenectomy scar. Injection sites over the abdomen: Desferrioxamine/Insulin; Hepatosplenomegaly.
- Lower limbs and gait: Leg ulcers, ankle oedema (CCF), bony tenderness.
- Gait examination for long tract signs due to vertebral bony expansion and cord compression.
- Delayed ankle jerk relaxation (hypothyroidism).
- Back examination for lordosis, tenderness.
- Skin colour, pigmentation, pallor, jaundice.

Clinical Features of Thalassemia Major

- Family history
- Transfusion requiring anaemia after 4–6 months of age
- Hepatosplenomegaly
- Haemolytic facies (prominent forehead, maxillary and malar prominence)
- Retardation of physical growth
- Aplastic crisis resulting in profound anaemia may occur following parvovirus infection. A shut down of RBC production in the bone marrow for a few days following parvo virus infection will result in profound anaemia as the life span of RBC is shortened in haemolytic anaemias including thalassemia.

Differential Diagnosis

- Other congenital haemolytic anaemias (hereditary spherocytosis, sickle cell, G6PD).
- Acquired (autoimmune) haemolytic anaemias, (sudden onset anaemia following a febrile illness).
- Iron deficiency anaemia.

Investigations

- CBC: Haemoglobin level is low. Peripheral smear shows microcytic hypochromic anaemia and evidence of haemolysis (target cells, polychromasia and nucleated forms of erythroid series). Reticulocyte count is increased (around 8%).
- Osmotic fragility is decreased (microcytes can accommodate more fluid before it bursts).
- Serum bilirubin is slightly elevated.
- Urinary urobilinogen is elevated.
- Hair-on-end appearance on lateral view of the X-ray of skull.
- Haemoglobin electrophoresis: Hb A2 and Hb F are increased and Hb A is almost absent in the homozygous β-thalassemia.
- Ultrasound of abdomen: To detect pigmentary gall stones (in older child).
- Monitoring: Monitor weight and height periodically. Monitor liver function every 3 months and serum ferritin every 6 months.
- Parents may be screened for microcytosis and elevated Hb A2. This may be the only evidence in thalassemia minor/trait (carrier parent).

Treatment

- Transfusion of packed RBCs to keep haemoglobin always above 10g/dL ("hyper transfusion"); usually requires transfusions once in 3–4 weeks.
- Folic acid (1 mg/day).

- Iron chelation is started when serum ferritin values is >1000 ng/mL. and/ or a liver iron concentration is 2500µg/gm dry weight. Chelation is done by continuous IV or subcutaneous administration of desferrioxamine 5–7 days a week or deferisirox orally twice daily.
- Splenectomy when there is hypersplenism (transfusion requirement >180–240 mL/kg of packed cells/year). Candidates for splenectomy must be over 5 years and vaccinated against pneumococci, *H. influenza* and preferably meningococci. They should be on continuous penicillin prophylaxis after splenectomy even if vaccinated (vaccine does not cover all serotypes). Chelation must be continued after splenectomy
- Hepatitis vaccine if not taken under national schedule, must be advised as multiple transfusions is a risk for hepatitis B.
- Bone marrow transplantation is the only curative treatment at present.

Prevention

- Parental screening and genetic counselling accordingly.
- Prenatal detection.

HEREDITARY SPHEROCYTOSIS

Clinical Features

- Family history of surgery for splenectomy or gall stones or anaemia
- History of neonatal jaundice
- Mild anaemia, mild icterus, splenomegaly
- Abdominal pain due to gall stones in older child
- Examine parents for splenomegaly (autosomal dominant inheritance)

Investigations

Blood picture shows haemolytic anaemia (refer under thalassemia) and *spherocytes*. *Reticulocyte count* is markedly elevated (10–20%). *Osmotic fragility is increased. The direct Coomb's test is negative* (it is positive in autoimmune haemolytic anaemia, another condition where spherocytes are seen).

Treatment

- Folic acid (1 mg/day).
- Not transfusion dependent but transfusion may be required in aplastic crisis.
- Splenectomy will be curative (done after 5 years of age).

SICKLE CELL ANAEMIA

In thalassemia, the *quantity* of β chains formed is decreased but in sickle cell anaemia, adequate number of β chains are synthesized but they are *qualitatively* abnormal (see p 569).

Clinical Features

The child is asymptomatic in the first few months of life due to the presence of Hb F (Hb F does not contain β chains).

- Anaemia
- Vaso-occlusive (painful) crisis

Vascular occlusion may cause painful hands and foot; may affect other organs also. Pulmonary infarcts (*acute chest syndrome*), priapism (persistent painful erection >30 min), progressive renal impairment (concentration defect presenting as polyuria), osteomyelitis following ischaemic necrosis, splenic infarct resulting in *auto splenectomy*, cardiomyopathy, etc.

- Aplastic crisis
- Hyper haemolytic crises
- Sequestration crisis
- Cerebrovascular accidents
- Auto splenectomy: Spleen becomes non-palpable and non-functional due to infarction. Presence of Howell Jolly bodies in peripheral blood indicates non-functional spleen.

Investigations

- Sickling can be demonstrated after exposing blood to reducing agents like sodium meta bisulphate.
- Haemoglobin electrophoresis will identify the Hb S and confirm the diagnosis.

Treatment

- Folic acid.
- Aplastic, sequestration and hyper haemolytic crises may require blood transfusions.
- Hydroxyurea by its ability to increase HbF content, is useful for treatment.
- Bone marrow transplantation may be curative.

G6PD DEFICIENCY

- Being X linked, only males are affected.

Clinical Presentation

- May present as neonatal jaundice.
- Haemolysis is seen within a day or two of exposure to oxidative agents (e.g., infections, primaquine, fava beans). Fava bean induced haemolysis is called favism.
- Chronic haemolysis with chronic anaemia and splenomegaly is an unusual presentation.

Investigations

- Urine: Haemoglobinuria
- Peripheral smear: Evidence of haemolysis
- Serum haptoglobin is reduced as it is used up binding the free haemoglobin in plasma. Serum may appear pink due to the presence of free heamoglobin indicating intravascular haemolysis.
- Heinz bodies (denatured haemoglobin) may be demonstrable by special stains.
- Quantitative estimation of G6PD enzyme. Estimation is best done 1 month later. Young RBCs have high levels of G6PD so that soon after a hemolysis falsely normal value may be obtained.

Treatment

- Stop administering the offending agent.
- Maintain high urine output by IV fluids and frusemide (to prevent renal damage due to haemoglobinuria) plus alkalinization of urine using $NaHCO_3$.
- Transfusion if anaemia causes haemodynamic instability.
- Folic acid 1 mg/day.
- Advise regarding the drugs to be avoided.
- Prenatal diagnosis is possible with G6PD assay of amniotic fluid cells or DNA analysis of chorionic villus biopsy.

IMMUNE THROMBOCYTOPENIC PURPURA (ITP)

The disease is due to the immune destruction of antibody bound platelets. However, unlike many other autoimmune diseases, the immune destruction is limited to platelets.

Clinical Features

- The most common age of presentation is 1–4 years.
- There may be a history of preceding viral infection about 1–4 weeks back.
- Skin bleeds: Petechiae and echymosis in an otherwise healthy child (***Note***: Deep muscle bleeds and joint bleeds indicate coagulation problem and not platelet abnormality).
- Mucous membrane bleeds: Look in oral mucosa, conjunctive, etc. Rarely, there may be haematuria, epistaxis, GIT bleeds, etc.
- Ask history of other cell line deficiencies, like easy fatigability tachypnea, edema, repeated infections, etc.
- Hepatosplenomegaly and lymphadenopathy will not be there. It is in sharp contrast to autoimmune haemolytic anaemia where splenomegaly is almost invariably seen. Platelet count is decreased but other elements in blood are normal. When there is hepatosplenomegaly in what appears clinically as ITP, one must think of

secondary causes of thrombocytopenia, like leukemia, IMN, etc.
- Examine fundus for retinal bleeds.

Investigations

- CBC: RBC & WBC are normal. Platelet count usually is < 50,000 in children with petechiae.
- Platelets may be of larger size due to the immature ones coming to circulation to replace the platelets that are destroyed.
- Bone marrow examination shows normal or increased number and size of megakaryocytes (indicating increased activity), immature megakaryocytes and marrow eosinophilia.
- Bleeding time may be prolonged in ITP but coagulation studies are normal (APTT, PT).
- In adolescent child, ANA, dsDNA, etc may be considered to rule out SLE. In at-risk population, HIV screening may be done. Direct Coomb's test may be done when there is significant anaemia to rule out Evans' syndrome (thrombocytopenia + anaemia).

Differential Diagnosis

- *Leukemia*: Constellation of Ps—Pyrexia (fever), Pallor, Purpura, Pain (bone pain) plus hepatosplenomegaly and lymphadenopathy.
- *Henoch Schonlein purpura*: Palpable purpura with typical distribution over the outer surface of thigh and legs. There may be oedema and pruritus.
- *Aplastic anaemia:* There is reduction of RBCs (anaemia) and WBCs (infections) in addition to platelets. DIC comes as a differential diagnosis in a very sick child.
- *Others*: HIV, SLE, Bernard Soulier disease (platelet functional disorder), von Willebrand disease (both coagulation abnormality plus thrombocytopenia), Wiskott Aldrich syndrome (immune deficiency, eczema and thrombocytopenia), thrombocytopenia absent radius (TAR) syndrome, etc.

Complications

Intracranial bleed is rare and occurs only in <1%. IC bleed is likely when the platelet count is very low (<20,000). Significant mucous membrane bleeds and retinal bleeds are warning signs of impending intracranial bleed.

Treatment

- Avoid IM injections and physical activities that are likely to cause trauma.
- Avoid drugs affecting platelet function (e.g., aspirin and other NSAIDs) and the ones likely to cause bone marrow depression.
- Prednisolone 2 mg/kg/day (1-4 mg/kg/day) in divided doses orally till the platelet count improves (max 2–3 weeks). Then it is rapidly tapered off. Steroids enhance vascular stability, decrease the production of antibodies and decrease the clearing of opsonized platelets by the RE cells.
- IV Ig 400 mg/kg/day for 5 days is equally effective. IgG occupies the Fc receptors of the RE cells preventing destruction of opsonized platelets.
- Platelet transfusion is of limited value as the transfused platelets also get destroyed within a short time. However, to tackle emergencies like IC bleeds, a combination of high dose steroids, IV Ig and platelet transfusion may be considered.

Prognosis

Majority will recover in 2–3 months with no further recurrences.

A small proportion with persisting symptoms and thrombocytopenia beyond 1 year is termed chronic ITP. Splenectomy is an option in chronic ITP beyond 5 years of age.

The other options for chronic ITP may be monthly pulses of methyl prednisolone, monthly IVIg pulses, azathioprine, dapsone, rituximab, etc.

HEMOPHILIA

Points to be noted during examination:

- Prolonged bleeding following injury
- Prolonged bleeding following tooth shedding
- Haematoma following immunization
- Palpable subcutaneous echymosis
- Joint bleeding
- Deep muscle bleeding
- Ask about average clinically significant bleeds per year; usual precipitants of bleed; any previous life-threatening bleeds
- Draw family tree indicating affected individuals
- Must do joint examination (may have arthropathy following joint bleeds)
- Evidence of diseases like HIV, hepatitis
- Investigations:
  - Prothrombin time: Normal
  - Bleeding time and platelet count: Normal
  - Activated partial thromboplastin time (APTT): Prolonged.
  - Whole blood clotting time is generally not done as aPTT is much more sensitive.
  - Estimation of factor VIII level: Level reduced; in severe variety, to <1% of normal; in case of hemophilia B, estimate factor IX level.
- Treatment:
  - Avoid trauma.
  - Avoid anti-platelet drugs like NSAIDs.
  - In case of joint bleed, **RICE**, meaning, **R**est the joint, apply local **I**ce, local **C**ompression and **E**levation.
  - Specific factor: Factor VIII or IX as the case may be. Read 'Manual of Pediatric Practice' by the same author.
  - Anti-fibrinolytic agents like epsilon amino caproic acid (EACA) or tranexamic acid is an add-on drug in addition to factor VIII in case of oral bleeds.
  - Desmopressin (DDAVP) releases factor VIII from the endothelium and hence is useful in minor bleeds.
- Prevention:
  Prenatal diagnosis is possible by chorionic villus sampling, analysis of fetal blood or amniocentesis.

ACUTE LYMPHATIC LEUKEMIA

- Acute lymphatic leukemia (ALL) is the most common malignancy in children.
- The peak age of presentation is 2–6 years; males are more commonly affected.

Clinical Features

Constellation of Ps: Pyrexia (fever), Pallor, Purpura, Pain (bone pain) plus hepatosplenomegaly and lymphadenopathy.

19

Investigations

- CBC: Anaemia, thrombocytopenia and high WBC counts.
- The peripheral blood shows blast cells.
- Bone marrow aspiration will show increased number of blasts (normal <5%).
- Chest X-ray: Mediastinal lymph nodes in T cell leukemia.
- CSF should be examined for leukemic cells.
- Uric acid level may be raised as the turnover of leukemic cells is high.
- Chromosome analysis help in the prognostication (e.g., hyperploidy, that is chromosome number more than normal, predicts good response to chemotherapeutic agents).
- In majority of ALL, the lymphoblasts are PAS positive (cytoplasmic glycogen stains with periodic acid Shiff), but myeloperoxidase and Sudan black negative (these are strongly positive in myeloblasts).

Differential Diagnosis

- Conditions with hepatosplenomegaly, e.g., IMN.
- Conditions with pancytopenia, e.g., aplastic anaemia (lymphadenopathy and hepatosplenomegaly are not seen in aplastic anaemia).

Treatment

- The standard risk patients are the ones in the age group of 1–10 years, with a WBC count less than 100,000 and immunophenotypically belonging to the B progenitor group cell line.
- Induction of remission: Vincristine once a week IV, prednisolone daily orally and L-asparaginase biweekly IM for 4 weeks. A fourth drug (anthracycline) is added in high risk cases.
- CNS prophylaxis: Hydrocortisone, methotrexate and cytosine arabinoside (triple drug intrathecal treatment) every week for the period of induction and then every 2 months for 2 years.
- Consolidation of remission: It is periodic intensification of induction, for about 6 months; e.g., inj vincristine once every 2 weeks, inj cyclophosphamide once every 2 weeks, inj Ara C (cytosine arabinoside) 3 days every 2 weeks and oral 6-MP 7 days every 2 weeks.
- Systemic continuation therapy: Oral 6-mercaptopurine daily and methotrexate orally, IV or IM weekly.
- Periodic reinforcement: This consists of vincristine once a month IV and prednisolone orally for 7 days every month.
- Supportive therapy: Blood components, prevention and treatment of infections, care to nutrition, psychological support, etc.

CHAPTER 20

Disorders of Genitourinary System: Case Sheet Format

20

Genitourinary system examination involves general examination plus examination of the abdomen. Examination of upper gastrointestinal tract (GIT) is not necessary.

1. **Age and sex**: Minimal change nephrotic syndrome is common at 1–8 years and AGN in school age child (5–12 years). Congenital nephritic syndrome is clinically obvious in the newborn or the first 6 months of life. Beyond infancy, UTI is more common in girls.
2. **Presenting complaints**: Primary complaints could be oliguria, haematuria, oedema, painful micturition, enuresis or fever. Other complaints could be abdominal pain (p 163), abdominal swelling (mass/ascites), growth failure (CKD, RTA) or anaemia (pallor).
3. **History of the present illness**
    - Oedema: Renal oedema starts at periorbital area; better noticed in the morning. Oedema starting with eyelids and progressing to massive oedema suggests nephrotic syndrome. Must elicit history to rule out other causes of oedema (p 169).
    - Haematuria may indicate UTI or AGN or stone disease or trauma or rarely coagulation disorders. Red urine need not be haematuria, hence ask about drug intake (e.g., rifampicin, furazolidone, etc); dark urine along with high fever, chills and pallor could be blackwater fever of falciparum malaria. Cola coloured urine is suggestive of glomerular origin of haematuria. Fresh blood colour or clots suggests bleeding from lower urinary tract, often from bladder.
    - Oliguria: Although it is almost impossible to get a quantitative measurement of urine output from the history, parents do frequently notice decreased urine output. Some renal disorders, like tubulointerstitial nephritis and RTA, actually may present with polyuria.
    - Frequency, urgency and pain during micturition suggests lower UTI. Inquire the change of frequency of urination compared to the child's previous routine. Polyuria may be seen in renal tubular acidosis or chronic renal failure.
    - High fever and chills could point towards pyelonephritis.
    - Abdominal pain: Pain during micturition in urethritis; suprapubic pain in cystitis; loin pain in pyelonephritis; loin to groin colicky pain in renal colic due to stone disease; generalized pain and tense abdomen could be due to peritonitis.
    - Palpable mass could be urinary bladder, polycystic kidney, hydronephrosis, Wilm's tumour, renal vein thrombosis, etc. Renal vein thrombosis classically presents abdominal pain, renal mass and haematuria.
    - Dyspnoea and cough could be due to left ventricular failure (acute pulmonary oedema) in AGN; dyspnoea in nephrotic

syndrome may be because of pleural effusion or indirect effect of massive ascites.

- Headache, vomiting, altered sensorium, seizure, etc could be due to hypertensive encephalopathy in AGN or venous thrombosis in nephrotic syndrome.
- Bony deformities, if present may be due to renal rickets of chronic kidney disease. Failure to thrive, anaemia and sometimes polyuria are indicators of CKD.

4. **History of past illnesses**: Past history of similar illness (nephrotic syndrome and UTI can recur); sore throat/pyoderma (AGN); past history of jaundice (hepatitis B, C); hearing impairment (Alport). A history of recent upper respiratory/skin infection or GI infection suggests postinfectious glomerulonephritis or haemo-lytic-uraemic syndrome, respectively. Rash and joint complaints may suggest HSP nephritis or SLE nephritis.
5. **Antenatal, natal & postnatal history** Oligamnios could point towards renal disease in infant; history of delay in passage of urine or poor stream.
6. **Immunization history**: Children with nephrotic syndrome may have been advised additional vaccines like pneumococcal vaccine.
7. **Development history**: Growth and development will be retarded in CKD.
8. **Dietary history**: Child may be on dietary restrictions for renal impairment and this also may be mentioned in addition to dietary listing of intakes before the illness. Important to assess diet for salt intake and iron-rich items.
9. **Family and socio-economic history**: Family history of renal disease, early onset hypertension or hearing impairment could point towards hereditary nephritis (Alport); polycystic kidney disease could be autosomal dominant or recessive.

GENERAL EXAMINATION

1. General Comment

Altered sensorium could be due to uraemia in CKD or hypertensive encephalopathy in AGN.

2. Vital Signs (compare with normal values for age)

- Pulse rate, respiratory rate, blood pressure and temperature. BP may be high intrinsically due to the renal disease or as a result of steroids. RR may be increased in cases of CKD/RTA as a compensation for the metabolic acidosis.

3. Assessment of Growth (Measurements or Anthropometry)

Generally, weight and height will be below normal in chronic kidney disease and renal tubular acidosis. In nephrotic syndrome with multiple relapses, growth failure due to steroid is likely. No growth failure is expected for acute illnesses like AGN.

4. Assessment of Development

Could be below normal in any chronic illness and chronic kidney disease is no exception. Assessment of development from history is enough; one need not objectively evaluate unless the child has another reason for developmental retardation.

5. Head to Foot Examination

- Face: Potter facies is typical in oligamnios due to renal dysplasia. The facial features could be remembered if one can visualize tight socks being pulled over the face (p 514). Cushingoid facies in those on long-term steroids. Turner pheno-type may have associated horse-shoe kidney. Several malformation syndromes are associated with renal disease, e.g., VATER association (vertebral body anomalies, anal atresia, tracheoesophageal fistula, and renal dysplasia), Hirsutism (due to steroids or cyclosporin A).

- Eyes: Subcapsular cataract and glaucoma secondary to steroid intake; look for pallor.
- Fundus: Hypertension is expected in AGN and hence fundus examination is a must. Look for pallor and eyelid oedema.
- Malar rash: SLE.
- Mouth: Look for residual throat infection that may have initiated AGN. Oral ulcers in SLE. Uremic breath in CRF.
- Ear: Hearing impairment in Alport.
- Neck: JVP; may have cardiac failure secondary to fluid retention and hypertension.
- Nail: If white nails are found, it could be due to chronic hypoalbuminemia (however, chronic hypoalbuminemia is a feature of chronic liver disease and hence white nail is more likely in CLD).
- Chest: Findings suggestive of rickets (CRF; note: in rickets of CRF, bony findings are mostly in lower limb). Cardiomegaly in hypertension.
- Skin: Look for scars of pyoderma; rash (e.g., HSP, SLE); striae of steroid-induced Cushing; scratch marks (CRF).
- Spine: Any local lesions resulting in neurogenic bladder.
- Genitalia: Anatomic abnormalities of the external genitalia may be associated with renal disease. Look for phimosis, hypo/epispadias. There can be scrotal oedema in nephrotic syndrome.
- Lower limbs: Findings suggestive of rickets and peripheral neuropathy (sensory blunting, posterior column sensations, depressed deep tendon reflexes, etc) in CRF. Steroid induced myopathy or osteoporosis (hence fracture).

Examination of Abdomen

1. **Inspection**
   - Shape of abdomen: Is it normal, distended or has any localized bulges; whether flanks appear full or not. Wrinkled abdominal wall due to absence of anterior abdominal wall muscle may be seen in prune belly syndrome (associated renal anomaly likely). See p 513.
   - Movement with respiration: Whether all parts of abdomen are moving symmetrically.
   - Skin over the abdomen: May look tense stretched and shiny in ascites; look for striae due to steroid intake, look for previous scars - surgery, peritoneal dialysis, etc.
   - Dilated veins: If present, find the direction of flow in them.
   - Umbilicus: Normal/everted/transversely stretched.
   - Visible pulsation, peristalsis or visible mass.
   - Flanks: Whether flanks appear full or not.
   - Examine the hernial orifices and external genitalia. Nephrotic syndrome can have scrotal/vulval oedema. Look for phimosis in UTI. Any inflammation or discharge at urethral orifice (urethritis).
2. **Palpation**
   - Feel of abdomen: Softness, guarding (in peritonitis), etc.
   - Look for any area of warmth or tenderness. Look for abdominal wall oedema by pinching.
   - Organomegaly: Liver, spleen, kidney; rarely urinary bladder, or other masses may be palpable. Kidneys must be palpated bimanually (the hand on the anterior abdominal wall is pushed inwards towards the kidney during expiration and kept there steady without allowing it to move up with inspiration; kidneys if enlarged, become palpable). If any mass is found, describe in detail. Full bladder is seen as a rounded swelling at hypogastrium (suprapubic area) and pressing over the swelling produces a sense of urgency to urinate. If the bladder swelling persists when palpated

after urination, it means some obstruction to bladder emptying (e.g., posterior urethral valve).

- Tenderness of the renal angles may be elicitable in pyelonephritis (press at renal angle with the thumb; patient preferably sitting). Abdominal tenderness may be found in peritonitis in nephrotic syndrome and intussusception secondary to HSP.

3. **Percussion**
   - Percussion over the enlarged organs. Find out the liver span. Full bladder is dull to percussion. If any mass is found, percuss the mass as well.
   - Shifting dullness (if ascites is present).
   - Fluid thrill (it may be discussed as part of palpation or percussion).
   - Puddle sign for minimal fluid (only if indicated).
   - Dullness of the renal angles.
4. **Auscultation**
   - Bowel sounds: Normal/increased or decreased.
   - Bruit: Especially over the renal artery/over the enlarged organs.

Other Systems

- CVS: Hypertension and cardiomegaly or cardiac failure in AGN and chronic renal disease; pericardial effusion or pericardial rub in uraemia; hemic murmurs.
- Respiratory system: Pleural effusion in nephrotic syndrome; basal crackles of pulmonary oedema in AGN (increased intra-vascular volume plus hypertension together causes leakage of fluid into the interstitium and hence pulmonary oedema).

  Check for pleural effusion, evidence of pneumonia.
- CNS: May be examined in case of hypertensive encephalopathy. Look for focal neurological deficits: cerebral venous thrombosis, hypertensive bleed. Assess behaviour: steroid psychosis; lower limb: peripheral neuropathy (both lateral column and posterior column sensations could be blunted in chronic renal disease; depressed DTR).
- In case of skeletal changes due to rickets, examine as per examination of musculoskeletal system. Examine spine in case of neurogenic bladder.

NEPHROTIC SYNDROME (Minimal Change Nephrotic Syndrome)

- See case sheet format above.
- Diagnostic features: History of recurrent episodes (may be precipitated by some febrile illness), massive oedema (may be ascites), massive proteinuria, hypoalbuminemia.
- Rarely hypertension, oliguria.

Investigations

- Urine: Proteins 3+ or 4+ (4+ indicates >1 g/dL proteinuria). Microscopy: hyaline casts.
- 24-hr urine protein (>40 mg/m^2/hr).
- Urine culture: UTI may precipitate a relapse.
- Blood: Serum albumin <2.5 g/dL.
- Serum cholesterol is high.
- Blood urea, creatinine and electrolytes are normal.
- C3 level is normal.
- Total serum calcium is low (decrease in the albumin bound fraction due to hypoalbuminemia).
- Mantoux test and X-ray chest to rule out TB before steroids. X-ray also for hydrothorax.

Differential Diagnosis

Acute glomerulonephritis and various other causes of oedema, see p 169.

Treatment

- Restriction of physical exertion in the phase of massive oedema.

- Intake and output chart.
- Daily urine albumin, weight, abdominal circumference and BP charts.
- Fluid restriction till the oedema subsides: Fluid allowance is previous day's output plus insensible loss (400 mL/m^2/day).
- Diet: Proteins intake is maintained at high normal daily requirement. Cholesterol-rich food is restricted (e.g., egg yolk).
- Steroids for first episode: Prednisolone 2 mg/kg/day in divided doses or single dose for 6 weeks. Followed by 1.5 mg/kg on alternate day morning as single dose for the next 6 weeks.
- Steroids for relapse: Induce remission with prednisolone (2 mg/kg/day). Continue till urine is albumin free for 3–5 days. Then prednisolone 1.5 mg/kg/day once daily on alternate day morning for next 4–6 weeks followed by abrupt stopping or rapid tapering and stopping.
- Immunization against pneumococci and *H. influenzae* while in remission.
- Drugs for nephrotic syndrome can be remembered by the mnemonic **'CLAMP,'**– **C**yclophosphamide (steroid-resistant nephrotic syndrome), cyclosporin A, **L**evamisole (steroid-dependant nephrotic syndrome), **A**CE inhibitors (ACEI reduce glomerular hyperfiltration), **M**ycophenolate mofetil (usually for SLE associated nephrosis), **P**rednisolone (for all types of nephrotic syndrome; all other drugs are "add on" to prednisolone).

Complications

- **Relapse**: Proteinuria of nephrotic range plus oedema is considered a relapse. Treated with prednisolone 2 mg/kg/day till remission (urine protein free for 3 consecutive days) and then 1.5 mg/kg on alternate day morning for 1 month and then stopped.
- **Frequent relapse**: 4 or more relapses in 1 year is frequent relapse. Cyclophosphamide is the usual add on drug after renal biopsy.
- **Steroid dependence**: Two or more consecutive relapses while on alternate day steroid therapy or within 28 days of stopping steroids. Levamisole is the usual add-on drug in steroid dependence.
- **Steroid resistance**: Remission is not attained even after 8 weeks of steroid therapy (likely to be non-minimal lesion nephrotic syndrome; needs renal biopsy).
- **Severe oedema**: E.g., ascites interfering with respiration; lid oedema causing inability of opening the eyes; massive scrotal oedema. Management is by infusion of albumin followed by frusemide. Scrotal support for scrotal oedema. 20
- **Infections**: Nephrotics are more prone to infections like pneumococcal peritonitis, UTI, pneumonia, sepsis, etc.
- **Thrombosis**: Hemoconcentration due to hypovolemia, and urinary loss of anti-thrombin III predispose to thrombosis; e.g., renal vein thrombosis, cerebral thrombosis, etc.
- **Shock**: Hypovolemic shock is more likely if diuretic is administered.
- **Renal failure**: Prerenal renal failure due to hypovolemia.
- **Respiratory distress**: Due to abdominal distention, pleural effusion or pneumonia.
- **Diarrhoea**: Oedema of the intestinal wall interferes with absorption.
- **Hypocalcaemia**: Decrease in protein bound calcium due to hypoalbuminemia.
- **Growth retardation**: Protein loss, steroid treatment.

Prognosis

Despite multiple relapses over a long period, MCNS does not leave permanent renal damage.

ACUTE POST STREPTOCOCCAL GLOMERULONEPHRITIS

- See case sheet format, p 439.

- Diagnostic featues: History of preceding skin or throat infection; oedema (first appear over lids), oliguria, haematuria, hypertension.

Investigations

- Urine: 1+ or 2+ proteinuria; RBC casts.
- Urine culture to rule out UTI.
- Blood: Blood urea, creatinine and potassium are elevated.
- *ASO* titre is elevated in cases of AGN preceded by pharyngitis.
- *C3 levels* are low in the first 2 weeks but normalizes in 8 weeks (continued depression of C3 indicates that AGN is not post streptococcal).
- X ray for cardiomegaly.
- ECG for changes of hyperkalaemia.
- Ultrasound: Bilateral enlarged kidneys with increased parenchymal echogenicity.

Differential Diagnosis

- Nephrotic syndrome.
- Haemolytic uraemic syndrome (after 2–3 days of diarrhoea, the child deteriorates to oliguria, pallor and bleeding. There will be evidence of microangiopathic haemolytic anaemia and thrombocytopenia in peripheral smear).
- IgA nephropathy (usually nephritis comes along with a respiratory infection and not after a latent period as in PSGN; there will be history of recurrences, which is very unlikely in post-streptococcal nephritis).
- Hereditary nephritis (Alport syndrome - There may be family history of renal disease or deafness).
- SLE (other features of SLE may be there).
- Consider other causes of oedema and haematuria (see p 169, 172).

Treatment

- Restriction of physical exertion till hypertension and gross haematuria settles.
- Intake and output chart.
- Daily urine albumin, weight, and BP charts.
- Diuretics: Furosemide 2 mg/kg/dose if there is oliguria.
- Diet:
  - Salt restriction till diuresis begins.
  - Potassium restriction: Potassium-rich foods are fruits, green leafy vegetables, meat, fish, chocolates, nuts, etc.
  - Fluids restriction to the previous day's output plus insensible loss (400 mL/m^2/day) till diuresis begins.
  - Protein restriction: Restriction to less than 1 g/kg/day is needed if blood urea is high.
  - No restriction to carbohydrates and fats.
- Procaine penicillin (injection) or oral penicillin for 10 days if there is residual streptococcal infection.

Complications

- Acute renal failure: Treatment is diurctic and peritoneal dialysis.
- Pulmonary oedema and acute left ventricular failure: Cough, dyspnoea, orthopnoea and basal crackles. Therapy consists of oxygen, furosemide, ventilation and dialysis.
- Hypertension: Frusemide, nifedipine.
- Upper limit of normal BP: 90+(2 × age in years).
- Hypertensive encephalopathy.
- Persistent acidosis (pH < 7.2): If it persists despite standard management, PD must be considered.
- Cardiac failure: Diuretics; peritoneal dialysis. There is no role for digoxin.
- Uraemia: Symptomatic uraemia needs peritoneal dialysis.
- Hyperkalaemia:
  - 10% calcium gluconate 0.5 mL/kg/dose IV over 10 min monitoring the heart rate (if the heart rate falls by >20 beats/min, stop and wait for the heart to pick up before pushing more of calcium).

Calcium reduces potassium induced myocardial irritability.
- 7.5% sodium bicarbonate 2 mL/kg/dose IV (shifts potassium into the cell thus reducing the serum level).
- 50% glucose 1 mL/kg IV slowly with regular insulin 0.1 unit/kg (1 unit/5 g of glucose) (shifts potassium into the cell).
- b_2 agonist inhalation by nebulization.
- Ion exchange resins orally to remove potassium from the intestinal tract.
- Sufficient carbohydrate intake to reduce the catabolism and hence the potassium load.

- Rapidly progressive glomerulonephritis (RPGN): Extremely uncommon in PSGN. Needs renal biopsy for confirmation. Treatment involves immunosuppressives like cyclophosphamide or IV methyl prednisolone.

Prognosis

PSGN, has excellent prognosis; no recurrence is likely. No need for antibiotic prophylaxis.

URINARY TRACT INFECTIONS (UTI)

- Burning pain on micturition: Urethritis.
- Suprapubic pain, frequency: Cystitis.
- High fever with vomiting, flank pain: Pyelonephritis.
- Ask for predisposing factors for UTI
  - Perineal hygiene
  - Phimosis
  - Poor urinary stream in male: posterior urethral valve
  - Pinworm infestation.
  - Constipation (loaded colon pressing on the bladder creates pockets of stagnant urine).
  - Voiding dysfunction (incomplete voiding due to detrussor sphincter dys-synergy).

Investigations

- Urine microscopy and culture.
- Blood investigations, USG and other studies for pyelonephritis.

Summary of work-up of children with first episode of UTI

>1 year:	USG, DMSA and MCU
1–5 years:	USG and DMSA
>5 years:	USG (ultrasonogram)

If any abnormality is found in any investigation or if there is recurrent UTI, full work-up with all the above investigations may be warranted.

Treatment

- For lower urinary tract infections, (urethritis, cystitis): Co-trimoxazole for 5–7 days.
- For pyelonephritis: Cefotaxime IV for 7–10 days.
- Investigations for urinary tract abnormalities and uroprophylaxis are needed for under five children. This may be read from 'Manual of Pediatric Practice' by the same author.

20

CHAPTER 21

Disorders in Endocrinology: Case Sheet Format

1. Endocrine case examination involves general examination with special emphasis on presence of typical profile features of specific diseases, SMR staging and anthropometric measurements. Gender-specific growth chart should be part and parcel of the case sheet.
2. Age and sex: Date of birth should be asked in small children and age should be recorded in years & completed months, as it is essential for recording height, weight and BMI in growth chart. There could be few cases where the sex of rearing & chromosomal sex/gonadal sex are different; in those cases the case sheet should have a mention of that.
3. Presenting complaints: Could be varied depending on the case. Common ones are concern regarding:
   - Not growing well/shortest in class (GHD, hypothyroidism);
   - atypical genitalia, increased pigmentation, (especially of nipples and genitalia), vomiting with dehydration/shock, failure to thrive (CAH);
   - small phallus, cryptorchidism, midline defect (hypopituitarism);
   - coarse facies, constipation, prolonged jaundice, umbilical hernia, developmental delay, mental retardation, fatigue, facial puffiness, decreased scholastic perform-ance, midline swelling in the neck (hypothyroidism);
   - excessive weight gain, black pigmentation and swelling over nape of neck, striae, tall/short stature (obesity exogenous/endocrine);
   - appearance of breast buds in a girl <8 years, pubic hair in a boy <9 years (precocious puberty);
   - seizures, tetany, short stature (hypoparathyroidism);
   - polyuria, weight loss, fatigue, admission with fast breathing (diabetes mellitus).
4. History of the present illness: Evolution of presenting symptoms are important; a child who was not growing well since infancy may be having congenital hypothyroidism, while growth failure that appeared later could be due to GHD or acquired hypothyroidism. In a child with hypothyroidism, presence of mental retardation indicates congenital onset while short stature and slowness of activity occurs in acquired hypothyroidism. A rapid progression of pubic hair development and increase in the size of phallus in a young boy points to a adrenal tumour as the cause of his precocious puberty while a 2-year-old girl with breast buds not increasing in size (static) is suggestive of an isolated premature thelarche. In an obese child with mild dysmorphism, if there is history of feeding difficulty and failure to thrive during infancy Prader Willi syndrome should be considered during examination. A sedentary child, overweight since early childhood, taking a lot of fried foods with obese parents, exogenous obesity may be the diagnosis. An infant with recurrent seizures and dysmorphic features

with otherwise normal birth history and history of a heart murmur could be suspected to have hypoparathyroidism (secondary to DiGeorge syndrome).

5. History of past illnesses: Asking for medical history sometimes may help you to not to diagnose a child with DKA as a case of abdominal pain or pneumonia.

   In a child with ambiguous genitalia, episodes of hospital admissions with dehydration and shock indicates salt losing variety of CAH; increasing pigmentation, virilisation, etc indicates inadequate treatment or poor compliance. A child treated for malignancy with radiotherapy could be short due to acquired GHD.
6. Antenatal, natal & postnatal history: History of breech presentation, prolonged labour, etc could be there in a case of hypopituitarism. Admissions during the initial weeks of life with lethargy and poor feeding may be due to salt losing type of CAH.
7. Immunization history: Vaccine preventable diseases could be more dangerous in children with CAH, diabetes and Cushing compared to normal children.
8. Development history: Developmental delay in congenital hypothyroidism, syndromic obesity.
9. Dietary history: Find out whether a diabetic child is taking a healthy diet and also whether he is taking his insulins as per the correct temporal relation with food. Detailed diet history in obesity.
10. Family and socioeconomic history: Family history of young onset diabetes prompts one to consider the possibility of MODY; neonatal deaths in the siblings, infertility in aunts, etc are important in cases of suspected CAH; family history of thyroid disease, type 2 diabetes, and obesity are relevant in respective cases.

GENERAL EXAMINATION

1. General Comment

- Extreme short stature, morbid obesity, etc may be included in the general comment.

2. Vital Signs (Compare with normal values for age)

- Pulse rate, respiratory rate, blood pressure and temperature.

3. Assessment of Growth (Measurements or Anthropometry)

- Height of children above 2 years is taken using a stadiometer; recumbent length in children <2 years using an infantometer. Weight is taken using a bathroom scale with zero error corrected if beam balance or electronic balance is not available.. These two measurements are of utmost importance in a paediatric endocrine case because most of the time an excess or deficiency of either will be one of the presenting complaints. These should be recorded in a standard gender-specific growth chart (author prefers WHO chart upto 5 years and an Indian chart for older children). Also, the midparental height should be recorded in the same growth chart. These recordings should be marked as dots in the intersecting lines of the chart carefully after calculating the age in years and completed months.
- In children with obesity if height centiles are also correspondingly high, most probably the case is exogenous obesity; if short more chance of an endocrine cause.
- US:LS ratio: Refer to discussion under short stature, p 449.
- Arm span.

4. Assessment of Development

- Intellectual impairment is a feature of conditions like hypothyroidism, syndromic obesity, etc and hence a good development history supplemented by objective assessment is a must. For example, in addition to getting a reliable history, the student may test if the child can perform specified tasks (e.g., pick up a pellet from floor).

21

5. Hand to Head to Foot Examination

Overall Profile Appraisal

- Have an overall look at the child. Common diagnosis could be suspected by the very appearance; e.g., congenital hypothyroidism, short/tall stature, Cushing syndrome, LMBB syndrome, etc.

Hand to Head and Head to Toe Examination

- Pulse: Weak femorals (Turner with CoA); bradycardia (hypothyroidism).
- BP: Hypertension in Cushing syndrome, CAH due to 11 β-hydroxylase deficiency, pheochromocytoma, adrenocortical tumours, etc.
- Look for typical facies like coarse face in florid hypothyroidism, immature face in growth hormone deficiency (immature facies, prominent forehead, prominent eyes, depressed nasal bridge, small mandible and chin), moon face in Cushing (rare in children), etc.
- Midline defects like cleft lip, cleft palate, bifid uvula, bifid epiglottis; a single central incisor, crowded teeth, etc could be features of hypopituitarism.
- Fingers:
  - Nails: Hypoplastic nails (GHD); hyperconvex nails in Turner syndrome.
  - Clinodactyly of fifth finger in Down, Russel Silver, and Seckel; trident hand in achondroplasia.
  - Short 4th metacarpal/metatarsal in pseudohypoparathyroidism and Turner syndrome.
  - Polydactyly in Lawrence Moon Biedl. Wrist: Widened wrists (suggestive of rickets); madelung deformity in Turner syndrome.
  - Limitation of movements of small joints of fingers in a diabetic child (prayer sign) is an indication of poor glycaemic control.
- Lower limb: Bowing (rickets, metaphyseal dysplasia, obesity); oedema of dorsum of feet may be seen in newborns with Turner (not in the grown up Turner and hence unlikely to find it in a short stature child).
- Head: Triangular facies in Russel Silver with assymetry between the sides (small face with micrognathia, making the normal skull appear big apparently: the whole thing makes it look triangular face); frontal/parietal bossing in rickets.
- Eyes: Look for hypertelorism, epicanthic folds, etc; partial ptosis (Turner and Noonan), blue sclera in osteogenesis imperfecta, cloudy cornea (plus short stature & coarse facies) in MPS, cataract in CRS, changes of diabetic retinopathy like micro aneurysms in diabetes, visual field defects in craniopharyngeoma; fundus: retinal pigmentation in LMB.
- Mouth: Delayed dentition in hypothyroidism, delay in falling of milk teeth and crowded teeth in GHD.
- Ears: Low set in Turner, Noonan, Seckel, etc; posteriorly rotated ear may be seen in Turner and Russel Silver.
- Neck: Low posterior hairline (Turner, Noonan); short neck (Turner, Noonan). Goitre may be seen in hypothyroidism, palpate for nodules and regional lymphadenopathy. Taking a neck circumference is a crude method to assess whether the size of goitre is increasing on follow-up.
- Chest: Pectus excavatum (Noonan, Turner); wide spaced nipple (Turner); shield-shape chest (Turner); rachitic rosary (rickets); lipomastia in obese children; gynaecomastia in Klinefelter and androgen insensitivity syndrome.
- Abdomen: Distension could be because of weak muscles due to malnutrition; or celiac disease; or ascites; or organomegaly (e.g., chronic haemolytic anaemia). Pink striae over the abdominal wall and easy bruisability may be seen in Cushing. Look at injection sites for the presence of any lipohypertrophy or atrophy in diabetic children. Fatty liver/hepatomegaly due to glycogen excess occurs if control of diabetes is not optimal.
- Skin: Pigmentation of nipple, areola, umbilicus and genitalia in CAH; cafe-au-lait spots in

Russel Silver, Mc Cune Albright; candidial infections in diabetes, hypoparathyroidism.

- Skin sensations helps in identifying early stages of diabetic neuropathy.
- Genitalia: Micropenis in hypopituitarism, hypogonadism; buried penis in obesity (stretched penile length is to be measured from the pubic bone after depressing the pubic pad of fat using a plastic scale). In a young boy, increased penile size with small testes (prepubertal size is <4 mL) indicates peripheral precocious puberty CAH/adrenal tumour. Increased penile size with testes >4 mL indicates central (GnRH dependent) precocious puberty.
- In atypical genitalia, one should describe the size of the phallus, location of the urethral meatus, degree of fusion of the labioscrotal folds/ scrotal development and presence of palpable gonads. Pigmentation of the genital skin also is to be noted.
- ***Tanner staging***: Advanced Tanner stage is seen in precocious puberty [both in peripheral (CAH) and central (gonadotropin dependent)]. Delayed Tanner stage (in relation to the present age of the child) may be seen in growth hormone deficiency, hypothyroidism, chronic illnesses and constitutional delay (late bloomers). In constitutional delay, pubertal changes get delayed; so much so the fusion of epiphysis also get delayed; so child has more time to achieve height and so ultimate height achieved will be almost normal.

SHORT STATURE

- Enquire birth parameters. IUGR due to chromosomal anomalies is likely to mature into a short adult.
- ***Nutritional status***: Take a good diet history. In the developing world, severe malnutrition is the most common cause of short stature. Assess muscle mass, fat (mid arm circumference, skin fold thickness) (see p 50, 50). Obese short child is always abnormal; could be syndromic or endocrine problems. Chronic severe undernutrition affects height in addition to weight (short, under weight child).
- **Anthropometry**
  - Wt, Ht (grossly underweight short child may be suffering from severe malnutrition. Obese short child must be having an endocrine problem). Arm span. Head circumference (large head in achondroplasia; small head in IU infection, and syndromes like Seckel).
  - US : LS ratio (deter-mine whether the short stature is disproportionate or proportionate). If US : LS ratio is more, most often it suggests short limbs (and not longer trunk). Example of short limb is achondroplasia. In hypothyroidism, the infantile proportions are retained longer than usual, so that at a given age, the limb may appear shorter than expected. In rickets, because of poor mineralization and hence bending of limbs, the limbs may be short. On osteogenesis imperfecta, multiple fractures make the limb short.
  - Short arm span occurs in skeletal dysplasias like achondroplasia.
  - Mid parental height.

21

Overall Appraisal

The candidate must show the child what he is expected to do and then ask them to do the same.

- View from the front: Examine with the child standing with arms by the side and palms facing forward.
  - Look for asymmetry between the sides (Russel Silver).
  - Look for cubitus valgus (over 15° in Turner).
  - How far the fingers of UL will reach. Normally, it reaches distal thigh. If fingers can reach only above the mid thigh, the limb is short.

If the trunk is short, the fingers may reach up to the knee.
- Palm up: Look for numerous findings possible (clinodactyly, simian crease, etc to mention a few; see p 119, 130).
- Palm down: Make a fist to detect short 4th metacarpal (pseudohypoparathyroidism, p 504). Trident deformity of achondroplasia is best displayed with hands down position. Hypoplastic nails of Ellis-van Creveld and hyperconvex nails of Turner, Noonan are examined for in this position.
- Joints: Look for joint laxity or stiff joints (restricted joint mobility or increased joint mobility).
- Tip of thumb on shoulder test (demonstrate how to do it, p 459). If the thumb overshoots, there is proximal segment shortening (rhizomelic); e.g., achondroplasia.
- Shoulder approximation test for cleidocranial dysostosis (p 502).

- View from the side: look for
  - Prominent forehead (achondroplasia, rickets, hydrocephalus, haemolytic anaemia)
  - Flat occiput
  - Proptosis (craniosynostosis)
  - Micrognathia
  - Prognathism
- View from the back:
  - Neck: Standing at the back, look at the back of neck for short neck, webbing, low hair line, etc.
  - Spine: Have the child bend forwards to touch the toes, to detect scoliosis (true scoliosis will persists even after bending down, whereas the positional scoliosis disappears).
- Skin:
  - Pigmentation (Addison; Fanconi)
  - Cafe-au-lait spots (neurofibromatosis I, Fanconi)

Hand to Head and Head to Toe Examination

- Nails: Clubbing in cystic fibrosis; hyperconvex nails in Turner; bluish nails in cyanotic congenital heart disease; leukonychia in chronic liver disease (all chronic disorders will cause deceleration of height velocity).
- Palms: Palmar erythema in chronic liver disease, changes of Down syndrome if the case is Down.
- Clinodactyly of fifth finger in Down, Russel Silver, and Seckel.
- Trident hand in achondroplasia.
- Short 4th metacarpal in pseudohypoparathyroidism, occasionally Turner.
- Polydactyly in Lawrence Moon Biedl.
- Wrist: Widened wrists (suggestive of rickets); changes suggestive of rheumatoid arthritis (like deviation of wrist).
- Pulse: Radiofemoral delay (coarctation may be seen in Turner); bradycardia (in hypothyroidism).
- BP: Hypertension in chronic renal failure, Cushing, etc.
- Head:
  - Dysmorphism (look at head, hand and heart whenever dysmorphism is suspected). Syndromes are Down, Turner, Noonan, Russel Silver, fetal alcohol syndrome (mid facial hypoplasia in FAS), etc.
- Triangular facies in Russel Silver (small face with micrognathia, making the normal skull appear big apparently: the whole thing makes it look triangular face); frontal/parietal bossing in rickets.
- Mid-line defects may be seen in hypopituitarism. Anosmia in Kallmann syndrome.
- Eyes:
  - Look for hypertelorism, epicanthic folds, etc.
  - Partial ptosis (Noonan).
  - Pallor (in chronic renal disease; thalassemia); Jaundice (chronic liver disease).

- Blue sclera in osteogenesis imperfecta.
- Photophobia in cystinosis (due to cysteine crystal deposition in cornea).
- Cloudy cornea in IU infections; cataract in congenital rubella.
- Visual field defects in craniopharyngeoma.
- Fundus: Chorioretinitis in IU infections.

- Mouth: Delayed dentition in hypothyroidism.
- Ears: Low set in Turner, Noonan, Seckel, etc; posteriorly rotated ear may be seen in Russel Silver.
- Neck: Low posterior hairline (Klippel Feil, Turner, Noonan); short neck (Klippel Feil, Noonan). Goitre may be seen in hypothyroidism.
- Chest: Pectus excavatum (Noonan, Turner); wide spaced nipple (Turner); shield-shape chest (Turner); rachitic rosary (rickets). Auscultate the chest (e.g., bronchiectasis in cystic fibrosis) and heart (congenital heart disease).
- Abdomen: Distension could be because of weak muscles due to malnutrition; or celiac disease; or ascites; or organomegaly (e.g., chronic haemolytic anaemias). Striae over abdominal wall may be seen in Cushing.
- Look for organomegaly.
- Cafe au lait spots (in neurofibromatosis, Fanconi, Russel Silver)
- Back: Scoliosis (Klipper Feil)
- Genitalia
- ***Tanner staging***: Advanced Tanner stage in precocious puberty. Delayed Tanner stage (in relation to the present age of the child) may be seen in growth hormone deficiency, hypothyroidism, chronic illnesses, and constitutional delay (late bloomers, meaning pubertal changes get delayed; so much so the fusion of epiphysis also get delayed; so child has more time to achieve height and so ultimate height achieved will be normal).
- Micro penis in hypopituitarism.
- Tanner stage is advanced in precocious puberty; retarded in hypothyroidism and all chronic illnesses.
- Lower limb: Bowing (rickets, metaphyseal dysplasia); oedema of dorsum of feet may be seen in newborns with Turner (not in the grown up Turner and hence unlikely to find it in a short stature child).
- Erythema nodosum (in IBD).
- Delayed relaxation of ankle jerk in hypothyroidism.
- Gait (muscle weakness in Cushing; UMN signs with spastic gait in intracranial tumours).
- Look for features of endocrine disorders: Hypothyroidism, Cushing, growth hormone deficiency; see p 545 for achondroplasia and p 503 for osteogenesis imperfecta.

21

Aetiology of Short Stature

Proportionate Short Stature: "NICE"

- **N**ormal variants: Familial/genetic, constitutional delay.
- **N**utritional: PEM.
- **I**nfections (chronic): Tuberculosis, malaria, HIV, etc.
- **I**atrogenic: Long-term use of steroids.
- **C**hromosomal/dysmorphic: Turner, Down, Russel Silver, etc.
- **C**hronic systcmic diseases (chronic diseases of various systems):
  - CVS: Congenital heart diseases, cardiac failure.
  - Respiratory: Poorly controlled asthma, bronchiectasis.
  - Renal: Chronic renal failure, renal tubular acidosis.
  - Hepatic: Cirrhosis, chronic active hepatitis.
  - Gastrointestinal: Malabsorption syndromes, inflammatory bowel disease, persistent diarrhoea, etc.
  - Haematology: Thalassemia, Fanconi anaemia, etc.

- CNS: Cerebral palsy, mental retardation, etc.
- **E**motional deprivation
- **E**ndocrine: Hypothyroidism, growth hormone deficiency, Cushing syndrome, etc.

Also read short stature from p 175.

Disproportionate Short Stature

- Achondroplasia (short limbs)
- Vertebral anomalies (short trunk)

Investigations

- Blood counts (Fanconi anaemia), ESR (inflammatory bowel disease/collagen vascular disease)
- Blood urea, serum creatinine (chronic kidney disease)
- Serum electrolytes, blood pH (renal tubular acidosis, Bartter)
- Liver function tests for chronic liver disease
- Bone age: X-ray wrist up to 6 years of age; Over 6 years, X-ray wrist and elbow.
- Thyroid function test.
- Tissue transglutaminase for celiac disease
- Karyotyping (Turner syndrome).
- Growth hormone assay.
- MRI of head (pituitary tumour).

THYROID DISORDERS

- US/LS ratio in small children. Because of delayed maturation, infantile proportions may be maintained longer than usual.
- Development retardation in hypothyroidism.
- Vitals: Bradycardia in hypothyroidism, tachycardia in hyperthyroidism.
- BP: Pulse pressure may be wide in hyperthyroidism.

Head to Foot Examination

- Dry hair; alopecia due to autoimmune association.
- Coarse facies **(Fig. 6.15b, p 87)**.
- Eyes: Prolonged jaundice in newborn.
  - Loss of outer third of eyebrows in hypothyroidism.
  - Pallor in hypothyroidism.
- Quality of voice (hoarseness).
- Neck: Thyroid swelling. Percuss chest for retrosternal extension of thyroid swelling.
- Hands: Cool in hypothyroidism.
- Tanner staging: Delay in puberty in hypothyroidism.
- Slow relaxation of ankle jerk in hypothyroidism.
- Look for exophthalmos, lid lag, lid retraction, tremor, sweating, palpitation, etc in hyperthyroidism. Subtle proximal myopathy in hyperthyroidism (test "stand after squat").
- Look for other autoimmune diseases like Addison, (hyperpigmenation of skin and oral mucosa in Addison), vitiligo.

Clinical Features of Hypothyroidism

In infants and toddlers – "THYROIDS"

- **T**one is poor (hypotonia); **T**ongue is protruding
- **H**ypothermia, **H**ernia (umbilical), **H**oarse voice
- **Y**ellow colour (prolonged neonatal jaundice)
- **R**ough dry skin, '**R**ough' face (course facies with protruding tongue and open mouth)
- **O**pen fontanellae beyond the age of expected closure
- **I**ntellectual retardation
- **D**elay in development
- **S**hort stature (see p 541)

Investigations in Hypothyroidism

- Thyroid function studies (T3, T4, TSH).
- X-ray for bone age; lateral X-ray spine may show beaking.
- Serum cholesterol (likely to be elevated).
- USG of thyroid gland.
- Anti-TPO and anti-Tg antibodies in auto-immune thyroiditis.
- FNAC in case of autoimmune thyroiditis.
- Radionucleotide studies.

Treatment of Hypothyroidism

- L-thyroxine orally daily.

OBESITY

- Any drug intake, which could contribute to obesity
- Vitals
- Hypertension in Cushing or as a complication of obesity
- Intellectual retardation in PW, Bardet-Biedl (Laurence–Moon–Bardet–Biedl), etc
- Anthropometry:
  - Short and obese is almost always pathological; endocrine cause is likely.
  - Tall and obese is generally exogenous obesity. Mention birth parameters and family history to see if it is familial obesity.
- Profile description:
  - Distribution of obesity (e.g., truncal). Obliteration of supraclavicular hollow in Cushing. Buffalo hump in Cushing.
  - Morbid obese ones may appear sleepy (Pickwickian).
  - Large head may indicate hydrocephalus due to tumour.
  - Dysmorphic face (e.g., Pradder Willi, Bardet-Biedl).
  - Rounded immature looking face in hypopituitarism.
  - Moon face in Cushings.
  - Coarse face in hypothyroidism.
  - Midline defects like cleft lip, palate, single incisor, etc in hypopituitarism, Kallmann.
  - Anosmia in Kallman.
  - Almond-shaped eyes, squint in PW.
  - Visual acuity is reduced in Bardet-Biedl, Frohlich, Alstrom.
  - Bitemporal hemianopia in pituitary tumour.
  - Cataract in Cushing.
  - Fundus: Retinitis pigmentosa in Bardet-Biedl, papilledema in pituitary tumour, changes of hypertension in Cushing.
  - Delayed dentition in hypothyroidism.
  - Oral candidiasis in Cushing (steroid effect).
  - Neck: Goitre; JVP in right heart failure in Pickwickian.
  - Hands: Short small hands in Pradder Willi, short forth metacarpal (McCune Albright); Cyanosis in Pickwickinan; Polydactyly in Laurence Moon Bardet Biedl.
  - Hypotonia in PW.
  - Chest: Gynecomastia in Klinefelter. However, more often breast enlargement is fat deposition as part of obesity. CVS examination for right heart hypertrophy.
  - Back: Buffalo hump in Cushing. Kyphosis/scoliosis due to osteoporosis in Cushing. Spinal tenderness also may be there if there is osteoporosis.
  - Abdomen: Hepatomegaly due to right heart failure in Pickwickian.
  - Tanner staging: Do not be mislead by the penis embedded in supra pubic fat.
  - Hypogonadism in PW, Bardet-Biedl, Frohlich, Kallmann, Klinefelter, etc. Rare cases of hypothyroidism may present with precocious sexual maturation.
  - Lower limb: Look for gait. Look for lower limb shortening as avascular necrosis of femoral head and slipped capital femoral cpiphysis arc common in the obese. Stand from squat (proximal myopathy of Cushing).
  - Skin: Cafe-au-lait spot in McCune Albright; Hirsutism and striae in Cushing **(Fig. 21.1)**.

Investigations

- Fasting and 2-hour post prandial blood sugar with corresponding insulin level.
- Fasting lipid profile.
- Thyroid function test.
- Bone age (delayed bone age in obese child is pathological. In exogenous obesity, bone age is normal or marginally advanced).

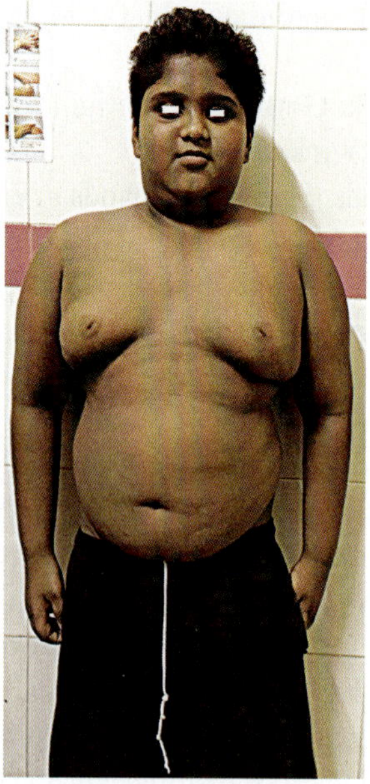

Fig.21.1 Exogenous obesity

- Serum cortisol at 8 am and 8 pm (for circadian rhythm).
- MRI brain, if indicated.
- Investigation for PCOD, if indicated (ultrasonogram, fasting insulin).
- Karyotyping, if indicated.

Treatment

- Calorie-restricted diet and aerobic exercise (30 min/day) to bring down the weight slowly and steadily.
- Medications (sibutramine, orlistat, metformin. etc) in rare cases.
- Syndromic obesity responds poorly to management programs.

AMBIGUOUS GENITALIA

The students are advised to read "Manual of Pediatric Practice" by this same author to get a basic understanding on the subject.

Approach to a Newborn with Ambiguous Genitalia

- The possibilities are that the infant is a virilized female (female pseudo hermaphrodite) or under virilized male (male pseudohermaphrodite) or a true hermaphrodite.
- If there is no palpable gonads then clinically it is taken as a virilized female (female pseudohermaphrodite).

  The reason for virilization is androgen; either from maternal medications or maternal androgenic tumours or due to congenital adrenal hyperplasia (CAH is the most common cause; usually associated with hyperpigmentation of skin due to excess ACTH secreted in response to lack of cortisol). When there is a deficiency of some enzymes for the synthesis of cortisone (most common is 21 OH-lase) or aldosterone, all the precursors are diverted to the production of testosterone. The most common enzyme deficiency is that of 21-hydroxylase, the severe deficiency resulting in salt losing manifestations (severe dehydration with vomiting and diarrhoea). The immediate precursors like 17-hydroxy progesterone will be increased in the serum.
- If there are palpable gonads then clinically it is an undervirilized male (male pseudohermaphrodite).

  The reason for ambiguity in male pseudohermaphrodite is *lack of testosterone action* (excess estrogen cannot cause ambiguity in a male). It may be due to deficiencies of enzymes of testosterone synthesis or lack of conversion of testosterone to DHT (5α-reductase deficiency) or resistance of peripheral tissues to testosterone action (testicular feminization syndrome). Usually CAH is a condition of excess testosterone and *hence cannot cause ambiguous genitalia in a male.* CAH is clinically missed in a male infant, as there is no ambiguity.

- Rarely, external genital ambiguity may be associated with true presence of internal sex organs of both sexes - the true hermaphrodite.

  Another situation where one sees both sex organs in the same infant is the mixed gonadal dysgenesis where the underdeveloped ovaries and testes may be there, but they are functionally abnormal.

History and Examination

- Family history of similar problems, unexplained deaths, infertile members in the family, etc. Unexplained male infant deaths could be due to unrecognized congenital adrenal hyperplasia. History of consanguinity (CAH).
- Maternal drug history, (hormones). Examine mother for virilization (e.g., virilizing tumours).
- Measure the size of phallus/clitoromegaly; find out where the urethral orifice is (orifice at the tip of phallus is more suggestive of penis); look for midline fusion of what is probably labia/scrotum (single raphae more in favour of scrotum).
- Palpate for testes, in the normal position and in the inguinal canal.
- Grossly, assess if the available phallus can be fashioned to be a functional penis (normal stretched length of newborn penis is 2.5 cm).
- Monitor for dehydration, vomiting, failure to thrive (in CAH; especially likely by the end of first week of life or second week when the protective effect of maternal hormones wanes).
- Hypertension (11-hydroxylase deficienty) or hypotension (21-hydroxylase deficiency).
- Look for hyperpigmentation of genital skin, lips, areola, nipples and umbilicus (indicates increased ACTH production due to cortisol deficiency, supporting a diagnosis of CAH).

Investigations

- Blood examination for hyponatremia, hyperkalaemia and hypoglycaemia; if it is normal in the newly born, retest after 10 days.
- Urinary 17-keto steroids are increased in congenital adrenal hyperplasia.
- Chromosome analysis either from the peripheral blood or bone marrow aspirate.
- Serum 17-OH progesterone: If it is high, the diagnosis is congenital adrenal hyperplasia.
- Sonogram of abdomen and inguinal canal to assess the internal sex organs and adrenals. If inconclusive, consider CT or MRI.
- If 17-OH progesterone is normal, then CAH is unlikely; now classify whether it is a male or a female pseudohermaphrodite or a true hermaphrodite based on chromosome analysis and internal sex organs. 21
- Urinary 17-keto steroids are increased in congenital adrenal hyperplasia.
- FSH, LH, testosterone, estrogen and cortisol, testosterone/dihydrotestosterone ratio (a high T/DHT ratio suggests 5α-reductase deficiency).
- MRI is very useful to visualize Wolfian and Mullarian structures and also the gonads.
- Genitography: This is needed for surgeon to decide and plan surgery.

Management

- All pseudohermaphrodites due to CAH are assigned the same sex for rearing as their chromosomal sex.
- Genetic males with total end organ resistance to androgens (testicular feminization syndrome) are reared as females. They cannot be reared as males as their end organs will not respond to testosterone. The testes, wherever it is situated, must be removed.
- For male pseudohermaphrodites, the sex of rearing depends on whether the penile size is good enough for future sexual function. Religious circumcision must not be done as the foreskin may be precious for creating a urethra.

A stretched penile length less than 2.5 cm in the newborn is likely to be inadequate.

- Male pseudohermaphrodites with 5α-reductase deficiency (this is heritable, autosomal recessive) must be reared as males only. It is because at puberty they will take a male gender role under the influence of testosterone.
- True hermaphrodites may be assigned the sex of rearing depending on the sexual and reproductive capacity of external genitalia; most often a female sex is assigned.
- The final decision on sex of rearing must be left to the parents after explaining all the pros and cons.
- CAH: Oral hydrocortisone, fludrocortisone, and additional salts to normal foods; in case of circulatory shock, resuscitation with normal saline and glucose plus high dose hydrocortisone.
- Therapy is monitored by assessing growth, bone age and 17-OH progesterone.
- Surgical correction of external genitalia at around 1 year of age or later.

CHAPTER 22

Examination of Joints

Arthritis means swelling (effusion) of the joint *plus* pain or tenderness *plus* limitation of range of passive movements. Also, there may be local warmth/ redness. Pain without swelling is just arthralgia and not arthritis.

Pain may at times be misleading. Pain in the knee may be referred pain from hip. Bone pain of malignancy is not arthritis but can be localized to the bone near the joint. Muscle pain may be confused with arthritis. Muscle pain may be there in viral fevers, leptospirosis, trichinosis, etc.

HISTORY

- Mode of onset and progression (e.g., fleeting joint involvement in rheumatic fever).
- History of preceding events: Sore throat or scarlet fever (rheumatic fever), gastrointestinal symptoms (reactive arthritis of GIT infections like salmonella or inflammatory bowel disease), urethritis (Reiter's disease), viral infections (arthritis may be part of some viral infections like rubella), recent immunization (rubella), viral myositis (pain can be really severe, at times the child even crawling), trauma or pyoderma (septic arthritis).
- Monoarticular (septic or tubercular) or polyarticular (migratory in rheumatic fever).
- Large joint or small joint involvement.
- Cardiac symptoms: Exertional dyspnoea, chest pain, palpitation (rheumatic carditis).
- Long duration with remissions and exacerbations (rheumatoid arthritis).
- Pain that is worse on activity is indicative of musculoskeletal pain or destructive joint disease such as osteoarthritis of adults. Pain and stiffness early in the morning and improving with activity is indicative of inflammatory disease like juvenile rheumatoid arthritis. Pain of infection is generally fixed, day and night. Non-specific "growing pains" of leg occur at night, usually bilateral, improve with massage and disappear in the morning. Joint pain of arthritis get worse on massaging.
- Low backache or temporomandibular joint involvement (rheumatoid arthritis).
- Visual problems (may be uveitis of rheumatoid arthritis).
- Bleeding disorder in the family (coagulation disorders like haemophilia).
- Sickle cell anaemia (swelling of hands and feet due to sludging of circulation producing infarction; it is called hand-foot syndrome of sickle cell disease).
- Any rashes (erythema marginatum in rheumatic fever; evanescent macular rash with fever in systemic onset rheumatoid arthritis; butterfly rash of malar area in SLE; nodular rash of erythema nodosum in inflammatory bowel disease).
- Family history of tuberculosis (joint symptoms can be due to Poncet's allergic arthritis or TB arthritis in older child).

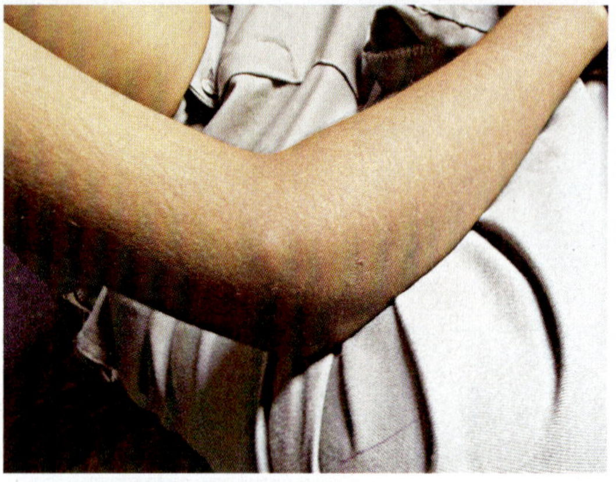

Fig.22.1 Subcutaneous nodule over the elbow

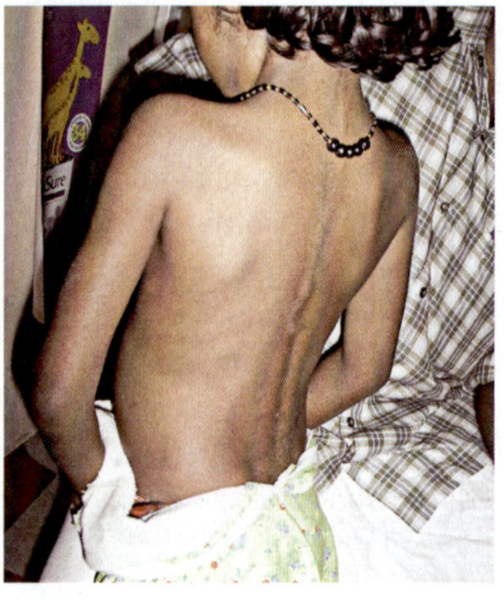

Fig.22.2 Subcutaneous nodule over the spine

GENERAL INSPECTION

- General inspection consists of examining the patient in front, back and side profiles followed by observation of gait.
- Inspection begins by observing the patient in the standing position for postural abnormalities, symmetry between the sides and any swellings.
- Let the child stand on one leg, while the examiner holds one hand. Note whether the child holds on to examiner's hand more firmly when standing on the affected leg. This may detect subtle differences between the sides.
- Let the child walk on heel and then on toes to bring out any subtle weaknesses and pain. Let the child stand on everted and then inverted foot, to bring out any pain.
- Ask the child to sit on floor and then to stand up. Proximal muscle weakness (pelvic girdle muscle weakness) makes this difficult. One may even see typical Gower's sign (p 186).
- If the child has trouble squatting down, suspect some joint problem. If the trouble is in getting up from squat, suspect muscle weakness.
- Squat on floor and walk like a duck while still squatting. Normal duck walk makes significant ankle, knee or hip disease unlikely. When squatting, the heel will touch the buttocks unless prevented by bulky calf muscles.
- Inspected from the back, the shoulders must be at the same level in a normal child. Prominence of scapulae must be of same magnitude on both sides. Compare the iliac crests to know if there is a tilt of pelvis. The best way is to mark the spinal dimples and then observe their relative levels looking from the back, with the child standing. (In case of different levels, suspect leg length discrepancy.) Compare gluteal creases. It is asymmetrical in neglected congenital dislocation of hip. Look for any central abnormalities like tuft of hair, lipoma, dimple, naevus, angioma, etc (may indicate underlying spinal or vertebral anomaly).
- In the side profile, look for the normal curvatures of cervical, thoracic and lumbar region; any flattening of lumbar area could be due to acute pain (e.g., vertebral osteomyelitis) or chronic pain (e.g., ankylosing spondylitis).
- Gait: Have the patient walk toward and away from you and observe the gait. Ill-fitting shoes may cause abnormalities in gait and hence let the child walk without shoes if there is a complaint about the gait.
- Check mechanics of walking: Push off, follow through till the heel strike. Push off is

avoided when there is pain in forefoot or Achilles tendon insertion. Heel strike is avoided in case of painful heel.

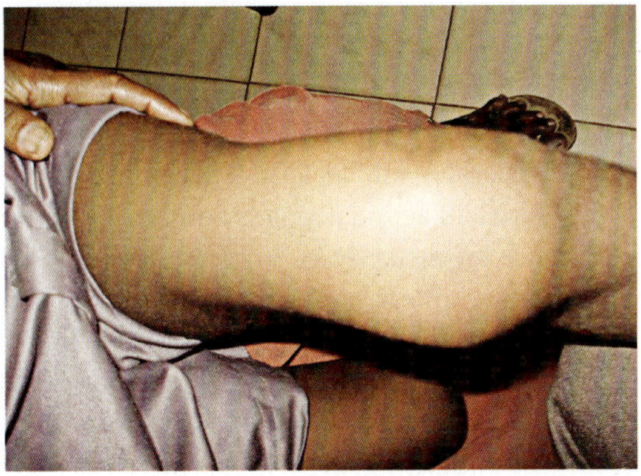

Fig.22.3 Muscle wasting proximal to long duration arthritis

- Look for muscle wasting (expected in long standing joint disease, see Fig. 22.3), look for evidence of steroid side effects, deformity of joints, etc.
- Look for subcutaneous nodules (rheumatic fever or rheumatoid arthritis), hepatosplenomegaly (SLE, rheumatoid arthritis); alopecia, mouth ulcers, weight loss, etc may be additional symptoms of SLE.
- Range of movement around all the major joints can be tested as is described in the testing of power under CNS examination (p 213). Range of movement in each joint may be compared with that of the examiner.

MEASUREMENT OF LIMB LENGTH

- Actual leg length: From the anterior superior iliac spine to the heel or medial malleolus, with both lower limbs in equal degree of abduction from midline.
- Apparent leg length: From umbilicus to the heel or medial malleolus.
- Leg length and thigh length may be measured separately by taking knee joint as the cut-off point.
- Upper limb: Arm length is from acromion to olecranon. Total limb length is from acromion to the tip of middle finger.
- Proximal segment shortening as in achondroplasia can be easily detected by testing as shown in Fig. 22.4; ask the child to touch the shoulder with thumb as shown in the picture; normally it touches exactly but if the thumb overshoots the shoulder, there is proximal segment shortening (Fig. 22.6).

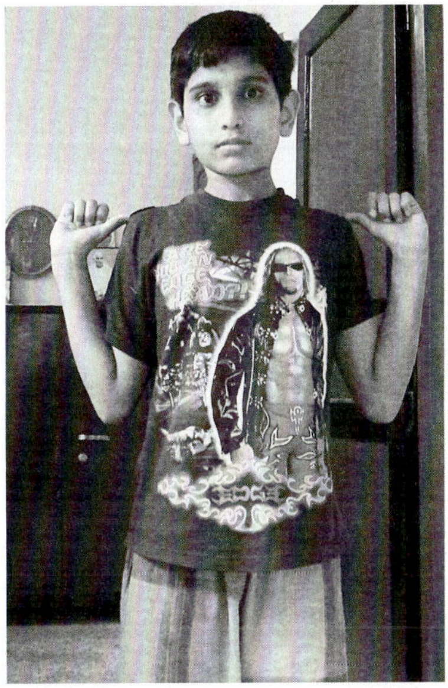

Fig.22.4 Testing for rhizomelic shortening

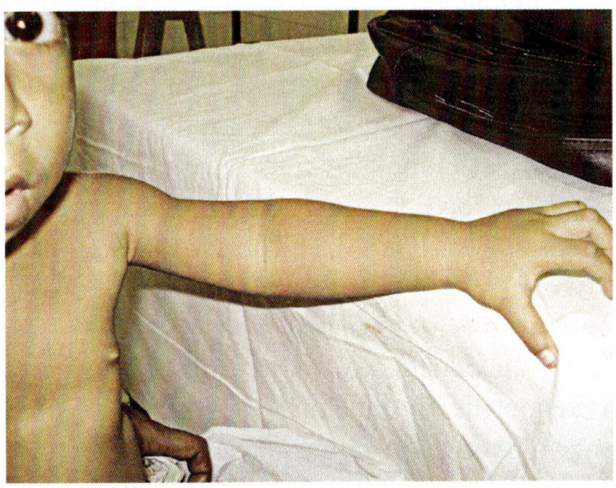

Fig.22.5 Rhizomelic shortening

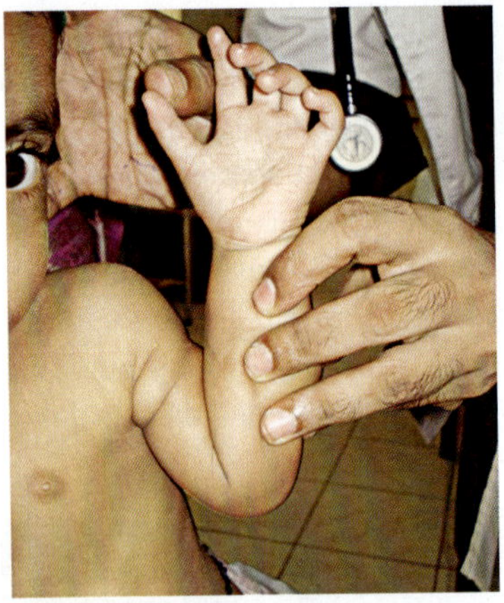

Fig.22.6 Rhizomelic shortening; the thumb overshoots the shoulder.

EXAMINATION OF JOINTS

The suggested order of examination of joints is from hand to head and from head to toe (Ref. 14); i.e., hand, wrist, elbows, shoulders, temporomandibular joints, cervical spine, thoracolumbar spine, hip, knee, ankle and feet. **If your dept wants you to use pGALS for examination, do follow that advice. (See pGALS p 480)**.

The patient can sit on the examining table facing the examiner (infants may remain in mother's lap). Examining with the patient standing is also equally acceptable. Each joint is assessed individually by **inspection, palpation and range of movements**. Inspection is for swelling, erythema or deformity and asymmetry between the two sides (including muscle wasting around the affected joints compared to the normal side). Palpation is for tenderness, warmth, synovial thickening ("boggy" swelling), crepitus or effusion; do not forget to palpate areas expected to have enthesitis. Range of motion, active and passive, are assessed; active first because a passive movement that causes inadvertent pain will make the child immediately uncooperative. Passive movements need be attempted only on joints, which fail to have full range of motion on active movement. Tenderness or pain is usually elicited when testing for range of movement (always watch the child's face during the manoeuvre for early evidence of discomfort). Sometimes, passive movements to the extreme range of motion brings out mild tenderness that is otherwise missed. Whether the range of movement is normal or not is to be decided by comparing with the examiner's corresponding joints. Also palpate part of the bone just proximal and distal to the joint, because tenderness in some disease like leukaemic deposits and osteomyelitis are found at the metaphysis. Bony tenderness close to a joint may appear as if it is joint pain or tenderness. Bone tenderness is best localized by asking the child to point to the area of tenderness with fingertip and then palpating the area involved. A feeling of induration and tenderness over the muscles is seen in dermatomyositis and trichinosis. Here again careful localization by palpation will differentiate it from joint pain.

Tenderness is likely in trauma, osteomyelitis and subperiosteal leukaemic deposit.

HAND TO HEAD AND HEAD TO FOOT EXAMINATION

The suggested flow of examination is hands, wrist, elbows, shoulders, temporomandibular joint, cervical spine, thoracolumbar spine, hips, knees, ankles, feet (including Achilles tendon insertion point).

Hand

- Examine distal interphalangeal (DIP), proximal interphalangeal (PIP) and metacarpophalangeal (MCP) joints (inspection, palpation and range of movement as described above). Bimanual palpation using thumb and index finger of both hands is preferable. Note that MCP joints are just distal to the knuckles and not exactly over the knuckles. Swollen MCP joints obliterate the depression between the knuckles.
- Making a good fist gives good assessment of flexion of small joints of hand. Passive movements also may be assessed in addition because this may detect stress pain at the extreme range of joint movement.

- MCP joints normally flex up to 90° and extend to 30° on active movement. PIP joints flex to 120° and extend 0°. DIP joint flex to 90° or a little less and extend to 0–10°. Squeezing each small joint individually should bring out tenderness of the small joints of the fingers.
- Pain, swelling and limitation of range of movements can occur in tenosynovitis (inflammation of tendon sheaths) also. To identify this, palpate along each tenosynovial sheath for swelling, tenderness, crepitus, nodules, etc.
- Stress pain at extremes of joint movements may be elicited by passive movements.

Wrist

Movements of wrist: Flexion, extension, radial deviation and ulnar deviation. Inspect, palpate and test range of movement. Inspect for any deformity. For example in JRA, ulnar deviation of wrist is a common residual deformity. Volar subluxation of wrist joint is a rare deformity in long standing poorly treated cases of JRA. Full extension of wrist is tested by "namasthe" position: ask the patient to press the palms together and elevate the forearms parallcl to thc floor. In the same position, full flexion of both wrists can be tested (see Figs. 22.7, 22.8). The joint line of wrist joint is normally a bit depressed compared to the proximal and distal regions. Swelling at joint line indicates wrist joint effusion. Swelling of dorsum of hand, distal to the wrist joint indicates tenosynovitis of extensor tendons rather than wrist joint swelling. Swelling of tenosynovitis moves as the child opens and closes the fist. When the child extends the affected finger actively, the distal margin of swelling moves proximally to produce a bulge.

Characteristic changes of the hand in adult type of rheumatoid arthritis include *(Harrison's Textbook of medicine, 17th ed., section 314)*:

- Radial deviation at the wrist with ulnar deviation of the digits, often with palmar subluxation of the proximal phalanges (**"Z" deformity**).
- Hyperextension of the proximal interphalangeal joints, with compensatory flexion of the distal interphalangeal joints (**swan-neck deformity**).
- Flexion contracture of the proximal interphalangeal joints and extension of the distal interphalangeal joints (**Boutonniere deformity**).
- Hyperextension of the first interphalangeal joint and flexion of the first metacarpophalangeal joint with a consequent loss of thumb mobility and pinch.

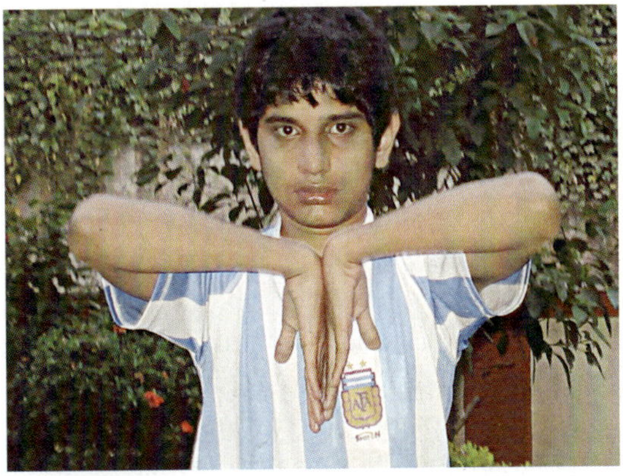

Fig.22.7 Wrist flexion

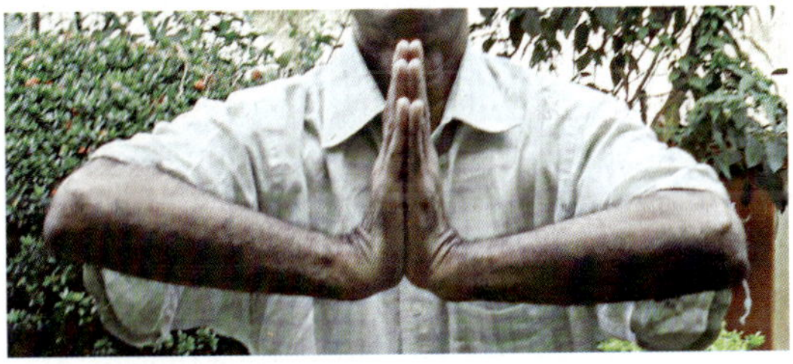

Fig.22.8 Extension of wrist

Forearm and Elbow

- Supination-pronation is tested with the arm by the side and elbow flexed at 90°.
- Normally, supination is 90° and pronation nearly 90°. A pencil held in the closed fist can simplify the assessment of 90° supination/pronation.
- Movements of elbow: Flexion, extension.

22

Elbow flexes 135–150°, extends to neutral position (i.e., 0°); however, 5–10° hyper-extension is within acceptable limits. Extend the elbow to reduce the joint space so that joint effusion, if any, may bulge out in the lateral and medial depressions. Palpate for any rheumatoid nodules (painless, and usually mobile; commonly found near the proximal part of ulna, but may be seen over other pressure points, joints, tendon sheaths and occiput).

Shoulder

- Movements of shoulder: Abduction, adduction, flexion, extension, internal and external rotation. Hands above the head tests abduction, hugging movement tests flexion and adduction and moving arm backwards tests extension.
- The normal rounded contour of shoulder is lost in joint dislocation or deltoid muscle atrophy. Effusion of shoulder joint may show up as an anterior prominence just lateral to the coracoid process.
- Shoulder is an uncommon joint to get affected in JRA; limited external rotation is the first restriction in JRA of shoulder.
- Range of motion is now checked as follows (demonstrate and then ask the child to do the same):
  - *Raise the arms over the head pressed against the ears*: Ask the child to raise and keep the arm pressed against the ear. Normal is 180°.
  - *Shoulder adduction*: Normal is 90° from horizontal.
  - *External rotation*: Clasp the hands behind the neck to test external rotation.
  - *Internal rotation*: From the above position, ask to scratch the middle upper back in the midline with both hands to check internal rotation. Or ask the child to pronate forearms and then "keep your hands behind your back."
  - *If active movements are very restricted, one can assess by passive movements.* Keep the shoulder abducted at 90° and elbow flexed 90°. Now pulling the forearm up rotates the shoulder externally and pulling the forearm down rotates shoulder internally; range of both these movements in the normal being 90°.
  - Proximal musculature of shoulder is evaluated for strength with the patient abducting both shoulders parallel to the floor and resisting the examiner's downward pressure.
- Along with the shoulder joints, the contiguous joints may also be examined now: gleno-humeral, acromioclavicular, sternoclavicular and costochondral. Sternoclavicular swellings are easily visible.
- Look for *temporomandibular joint* swelling just anterior to the tragus of ear (swelling of TM joint is so small and localized that it will not be confused with parotid swelling). Palpation is done with the mouth closed, and then open (feel for the crepitus). To elicit tenderness over the temporomandibular joint, put one finger into the external auditory meatus and push forward (anteriorly).
- Look for micrognathia as the jaw growth may be affected if TM joint has been affected for a long time. Facial asymmetry may be there if there is long duration unilateral TM joint involvement. Palpate the mandibular condyles for pain and try to appreciate the normal rounded contour of condyles (the shape may be lost in long standing TM joint affection). Crepitus may be felt if the cartilage between condyles and temporal bone is eroded.
- With the mouth wide open, interdental distance of at least 3 cm (3 finger width of the child) is expected in a normal child. When opening the mouth, the jaw may appear to be deviated to the affected side if there is mandibular growth retardation on the affected side.

Cervical Spine

Inspect in lateral profile and look for the normal cervical lordosis. Palpate the paravertebral muscles for spasm or spinal tenderness.

Test the range of motion. Normal extension allows the child to look directly at the ceiling. Flexion of neck in normal child will allow the chin to touch the chest. Limited extension is an early sign of cervical spine involvement in JRA (flexion may remain normal early in JRA). Child with limited extension of neck will be seen trying to look at the ceiling by elevating his eyes to compensate the loss of extension. Normal neck flexion and extension are about 45° each. To test rotation, ask the child to look towards each shoulder and try to touch the chin to shoulder; normally, it is just less than 90, may be 80° (i.e., the chin will nearly touch the shoulder). Ask the child to bend the neck laterally to touch the ear to the shoulder; normally, it is possible with a helping elevation of ipsilateral shoulder (normal lateral flexion is about 45°).

If any torticollis is noticed, look for facial asymmetry, which may occur in untreated long standing torticollis. Make sure that the torticollis is not secondary to pelvis abnormality (hence examine for congenital dislocation of hip). Other causes of torticollis are discussed in p 85.

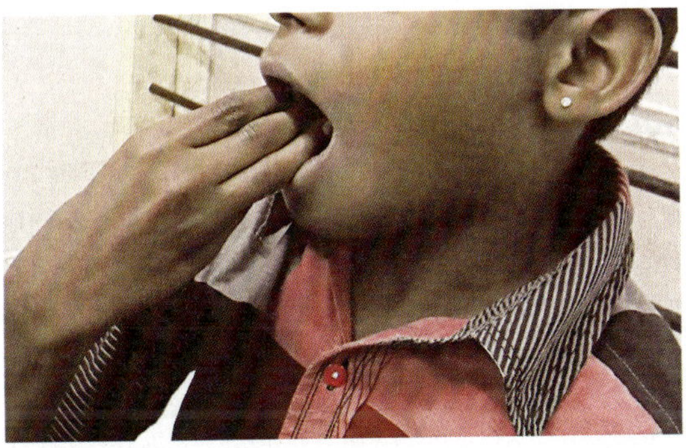

Fig.22.9 Interdental distance

Thoracolumbar Spine

Palpate the spine, sacroiliac joints and feel for any paravertebral muscle spasm. This is best done with the child prone, but examination in standing posture is also acceptable.

Look for scoliosis. In non-structural scoliosis, the lateral curve corrects itself when the child bends laterally to the convex side. With structural scoliosis, such a correction cannot happen. Structural scoliosis produces prominence of ribs on the convex side of the bend. Asking the child to bend forward at waist without bending the knees will bring out even subtle rib cage asymmetry in case of scoliosis.

Examination of Scoliosis

- Have the child bend and try to touch the toes. Postural scoliosis will disappear with this. Fixed scoliosis will remain with a rib hump on one side.
- In a small child, holding the child by the axilla will eliminate the postural scoliosis.
- Re-evaluate after making the child sit. Sitting will eliminate contribution of unequal leg length to scoliosis.

Those with scoliosis may have secondary curvatures above or below, to keep the head upright (hence one must look for it).

Child with scoliosis must be examined for neurofibromatosis; also a thorough neurologic examination must be done to rule out a neurological cause for scoliosis.

Kyphosis is found in thoracic region and appears as excessively rounded back. Kyphosis due to poor posture disappears while prone. When the child bends, the lumbar spine must form a smooth curve from thorax to sacrum. Instead, if there is flattening in the lumbar region, one may suspect local pathologies like ankylosing spondylitis, osteomyelitis, tumour deposits, etc that prevent the movement of lumbar vertebrae.

The standing child may be asked to try to touch his toes without bending the knees. Normal children can either touch the toes with their fingertips or can nearly touch (those having difficulty may be allowed to keep their legs a little apart to help this manoeuvre). This tests the flexion of thoracolumbar spine. Extension is tested by asking the child to arch backwards (about 30° at lumbar area).

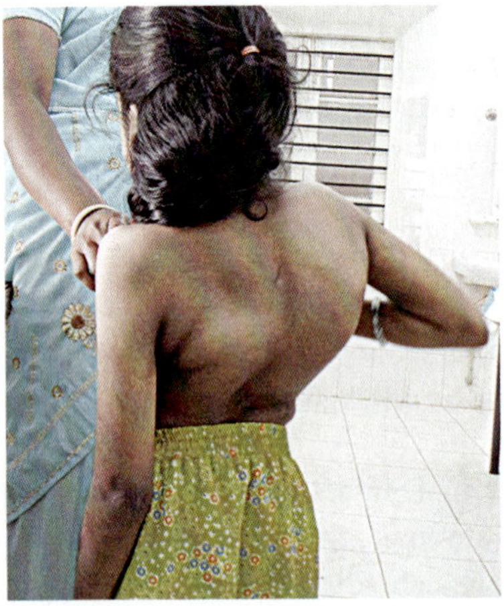

Fig.22.10 Kyphoscoliosis

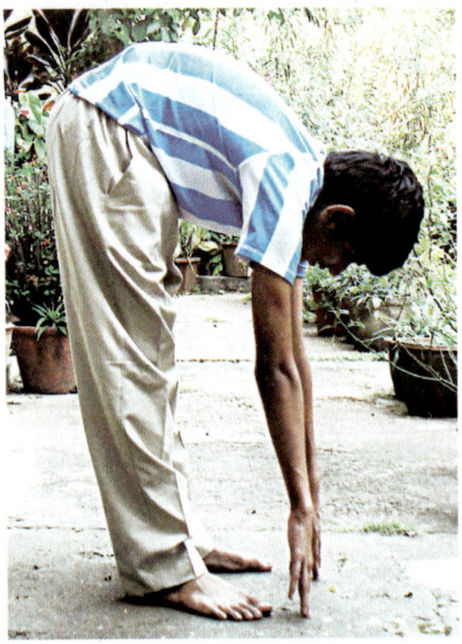

Fig.22.11 Spine flexion

With the child standing, test the lateral flexion (bend laterally without bending forwards; normal is about 45°). Normally, the fingers must be able to reach below the side of the knee, to the level of head of fibula. To test the rotation of spine, make the child straddle a chair to stabilize the pelvis and cross the arms across the chest to stabilize the shoulder girdle and then ask the child to rotate the trunk. But rough idea may be obtained by just asking a standing child to rotate the trunk to either side.

Sacroiliac joints: Palpate over the joints for tenderness. Press pelvis from each side towards the midline to assess for pain.

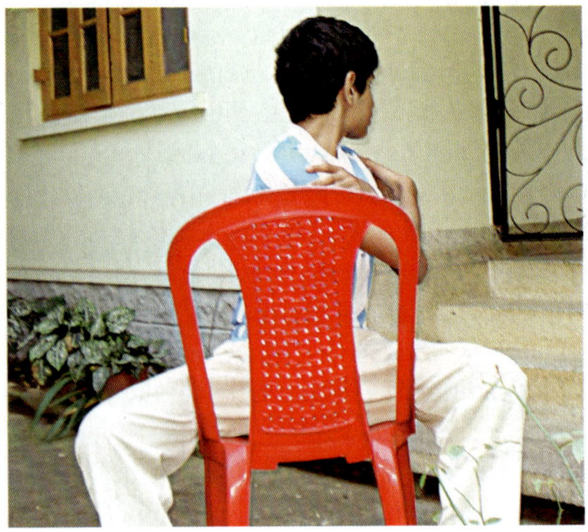

Fig.22.12 Spine rotation

Hip

Measure the leg length (see p 459).

The patient now lies down for examination of the lower extremities. Position at rest in supine position gives valuable information: flexed and externally rotated hip indicates hip disease. Hip pain may be referred to anterior thigh or even to knee. Palpation is of value in the greater trochanter area. Tenderness suggests trochanteric bursitis. Then the following manoeuvres are carried out on the hip. While assessing the range of hip movements, the examiner must place his hands on child's pelvis to stabilize it. When a movement of pelvis is noted, it means the end of independent hip movement has been reached and any further movement is because of pelvis rotation.

- *Abduction*: Fix the pelvis by placing your hand on the pelvis and concentrate on the side not being tested for any movement of pelvis. Abduct the leg maximally. When you feel movement of pelvis, it means maximal abduction is reached.

  Normal is about 40–50°. Abduction must be done individually for each side, because when testing them together the compensatory spinal curvature will give false impression of normal abduction.

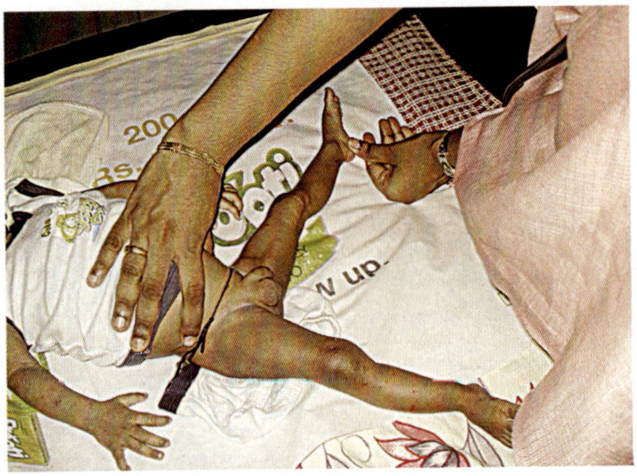

Fig.22.13 Hip abduction (excessive abduction)

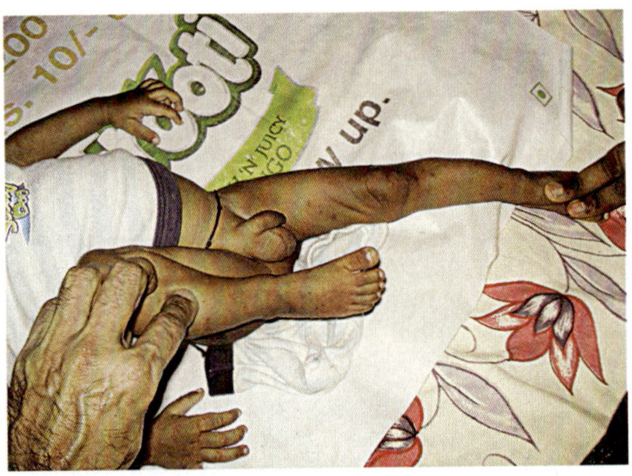

Fig.22.14 Normal hip flexion

- *Adduction*: Normal range of adduction is 25°.
- *Flexion*: Flex the hip with knee bent (normal, 120°) and then with the knee straight (normal, 90°).
- *Internal and external rotation tested as shown in Fig. 22.15.* Normal internal rotation is about 35–40° and external rotation is equal or a bit more, 45°. Loss of internal rotation is often the first sign of hip inflammation (leg lies externally rotated while supine). External and internal rotations are best tested with hips at 90° flexion (patient supine) though testing as shown in figure is equally acceptable if the child is in bed.
- *External rotation*: The rotation can be tested actively by supine patient also. Ask the patient to rotate the lower limb and try to touch the bed with fifth (small) toe. The opposite motion, i.e., to try to touch the bed with big toe, tests internal rotation.
- With the child supine, one may test rotation passively also; place hands on the thigh and rotate it internally and then externally noting any resistance or pain.
- *Flexion contracture*: Hip flexion contracture is tested for as follows: Have the patient lie supine. Opposite hip is flexed until the lumbar lordosis has flattened. Now ask the child to put down the other leg as far as it goes. If the back of thigh does not touch the bed, there is some flexion contracture at that hip. The thigh should be extended fully (flush with examining table), if there is no contracture. The angle between the thigh and the table quantifies the contracture.

Adduction and abduction can be tested as discussed under nervous system. With the child prone and with knees at 90° flexion, rotate the femurs holding on the legs. When the heels cross over, the external rotation of hip is being tested and when the heels go away from one another, the internal rotation of hip is being tested (Fig. 22.15).

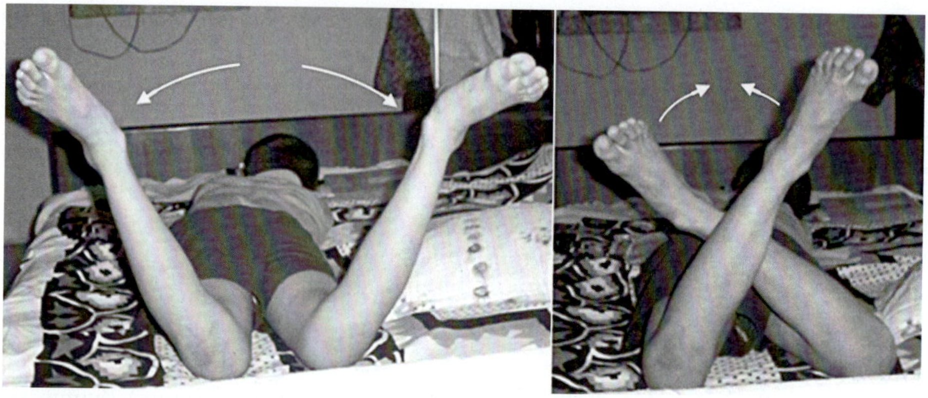

Fig.22.15 Rotation of hip

Straight leg raising: With the patient supine and the leg straight, flex the hip (this produces stretch on the sciatic nerve). 90° flexion is normally possible in children without any discomfort. At least 70–80° must be possible. If hip is normal, pain in hamstrings and below the knee indicates nerve root disease. The angle of elevation of the leg from the table at the point where the pain is produced is recorded. The leg is lowered a little now till the stretching pain just disappears; at this angle if the ankle is dorsiflexed the pain is again felt in case of root compression (Bragard's sign). In performing SLR, sciatic pain in the leg produced between 0–30° indicates nerve root compression, pain between 30 and 60° indicates sacroiliac disease and pain produced beyond 60° indicates lumbosacral conditions.

Trendelenburg Gait in Hip Disease or Hip Girdle Weakness

- Normally, when we stand on one leg, the gluteus medius of same side pulls the hip down so that the opposite hip moves up a bit (because pelvis moves as a single unit and so if one side is pulled down, the other side goes up). When the child with weak proximal muscle stands on one leg, the gluteus medius of the affected side is unable to pull down the hip of same side; so much so the opposite hip cannot tilt up, but instead drops a bit.

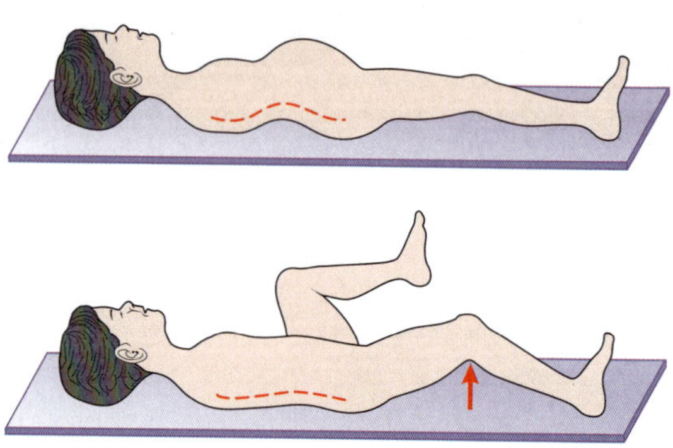

Fig.22.16 Hip examination. The top drawing is of normal hip. The middle one shows masking of flexion deformity of hip by exaggerated lumbar lordosis. The bottom drawing shows unmasking of hip flexion deformity when the lumbar lordosis is obliterated by flexion of the other hip.

- To test objectively, squat in front of the standing child, place hands in each side of pelvis and ask the child to raise one foot while observing for any up/down tilt of other side of pelvis.
- Ortolani test is for newborn and small infants. In older infants and children with untreated DDH, Ortolani result will be negative because the dislocated femoral head cannot be reduced to the acetabulum (acetabulum has failed to grow in depth as femoral head was not inside it; so now it cannot accommodate the femoral head). So in grown up children the signs of DDH will be painless limp, asymmetric posterior skin folds at thigh-buttock junction, limited abduction of hip, and shortened thigh length (because femoral head is not in acetabulum).

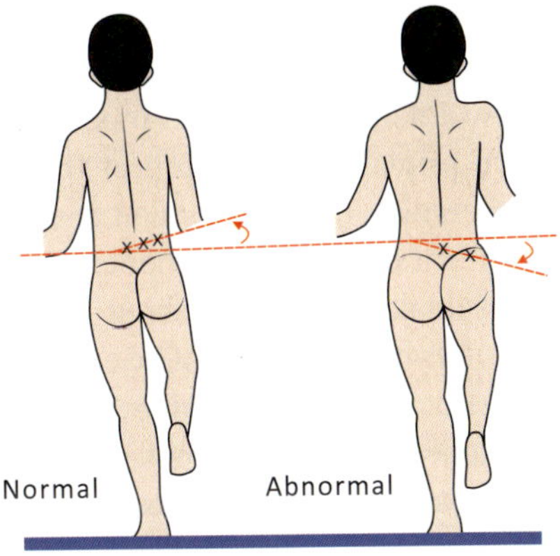

Fig.22.17 Trendelenburg gait

Knee

The knee examination is next. Inspection is carried out for discolouration, swelling, and deformities, particularly lateral angulation (genu valgum) or medial angulation (genu varum) (see p 130). A slight genu recurvatum due to ligament laxity is generally only a variation of normal. Note any increased skin temperature or swelling and determine if the swelling is due to synovial proliferation or thickening as opposed to an actual effusion.

The first sign of knee effusion is loss of normal concavity along the medial side of patella. Compare the knee joint, especially its medial and lateral borders with the normal side to see if there is any subtle swelling. As the effusion enlarges, it may extend in a horse-shoe shape to the suprapatellar pouch.

Bulge sign: This helps to detect small effusion. Milk the fluid out of medial recess into the suprapatellar pouch. Then stroke the lateral recess down wards which will move the fluid back to medial recess, creating a fluid bulge on the medial aspect of knee between patella and femur. Positive patellar tap indicates large effusion. Effusion in the knee joint floats the patella so that a sharp tap gives the feeling of patella touching the underlying bone. 22

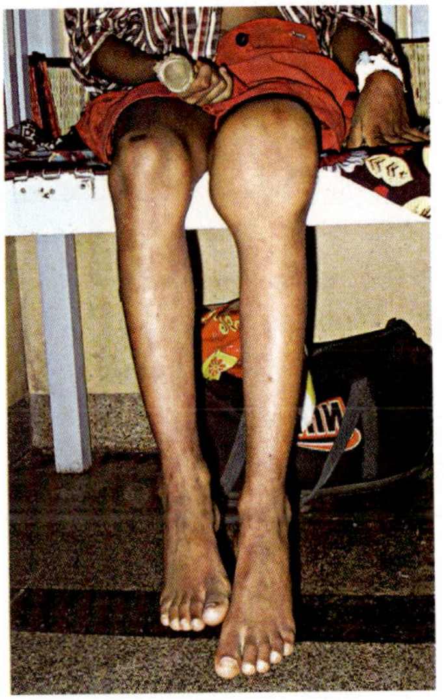

Fig.22.18 Haemarthrosis: Note the swelling of left knee joint

Empty fluid from suprapatellar pouch by pressing firmly on the supra patellar pouch downwards with one hand, and with fingers of the other hand, sharply press down the patella to elicit patellar tap.

Synovial thickening can be appreciated by a doughy feel and in superficial joint like the knee, the edge of thickened synovium can be rolled by fingers. If the swelling involves only one side of the joint, periarticular swelling is to be considered as a close differential.

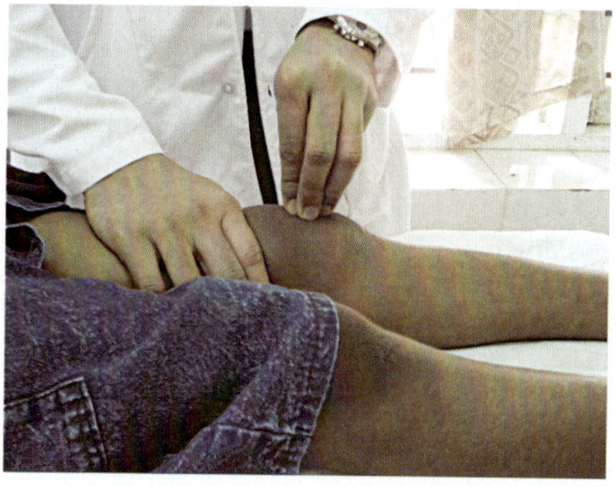

Fig.22.19 Patellar tap

With knee flexed to 90°, palpate for joint line tenderness. Tenderness along the entire joint line indicates synovitis. When associated with thickened synovium, the normal bony landmarks may be obscured. Tenderness localized to only medial or lateral aspect suggests meniscal injury. Palpate for tenderness at insertion of patellar tendon to tibial tuberosity (enthesitis).

Then the following manoeuvres are carried out on the knee:

- *Flexion*: Note the degree of flexion, which should be at least 135°.
- *Extension*: Note any deficit in ability to fully extend to 0°.
- *Cruciates*: Test the stability of anterior and posterior cruciates by holding the femur in a fixed position with the knee flexed at 90° and attempting to pull and push the tibia forward and backward on the femur. Correspondingly forward movement indicates a defect in the anterior cruciate ligament, whereas backward mobility indicates a defect in the posterior cruciate ligament.

It is advisable to measure muscle bulk of thigh and leg at a point 10 cm above and below a bony point like the superior aspect of patella or tibial tuberosity.

Ankle

The *ankles* are examined next. Observe for discolouration and swelling and palpate for tenderness. Ankle swelling is indicated by the obliteration of the depressions around the malleoli (between Achilles tendon and medial/lateral malleoli). Palpate the Achilles tendon for any tenderness, especially at the insertion.

The ankles normally have a dorsiflexion and plantar flexion of about 20 and 50°, respectively.

- *Dorsiflexion*: The patient is asked to pull the toes up toward the knee.
- *Plantar flexion*: Ask the patient to push the feet down as far as they can go.
- *Eversion* (away from the midline) and *inversion* (toward the midline): Eversion and inversion are primarily a function of the subtalar and mid tarsal joints. Inversion and eversion independent of ankle joint movement (occurring at subtalar joints) are about 10°.
- Other joints of foot need not be examined as a routine. But if needed, the following joints may be examined. Mid tarsal joints (talonavicular and calcaneocuboid) can be tested by stabilizing calcaneus with one hand and adducting or abducting the fore foot with the other hand (abduction 10° and adduction a little more like 20°). First metatarso phalangeal joint may be tested, as it may be selectively involved in spondyloarthropathies. Normal plantar flexion is around 45° and dorsiflexion around 70°.

Feet

Lastly, the feet are inspected for abnormal colouration and localized areas of swelling. Look for obvious abnormalities in the longitudinal arch, pes planus (flat foot), or pes cavus. Flat foot is best made out by wetting the leg and then looking at the footprints on the floor. If there is pes cavus (p 130), make sure that neurological examination is done, as many neurological conditions like Friedreich ataxia, Charcot-Marie-Tooth disease, spinal dysraphism, etc cause pes cavus.

The first metatarsophalangeal joints are observed for lateral angulation, so-called hallux valgus. The metatarsal heads are observed on the plantar surface for formation of callosities over pressure points. Compression of metatarsals elicits pain when there is inflammation of metatarsophalangeal joints.

Palpate individual interphalangeal joints of the toes for signs of synovial inflammation and restricted range of motion.

Flex and extend the I-P joints (active and passive) and look for any decreased mobility or pain.

Hypermobile Joints

Joints will be having range of movements more than what is normal for each joint (see above). Some of the examples are: more than 10° extension of elbow or knee (Figs. 22.20, 22.21); more than 90° *passive* extension of metacarpophalangeal joints of hand (Fig. 22.22); ability to rest palms *flat on the floor* on forward flexion of trunk with knee extended (normally one will be able to touch the floor with finger tips, will not be able to rest the whole of palm flat on floor).

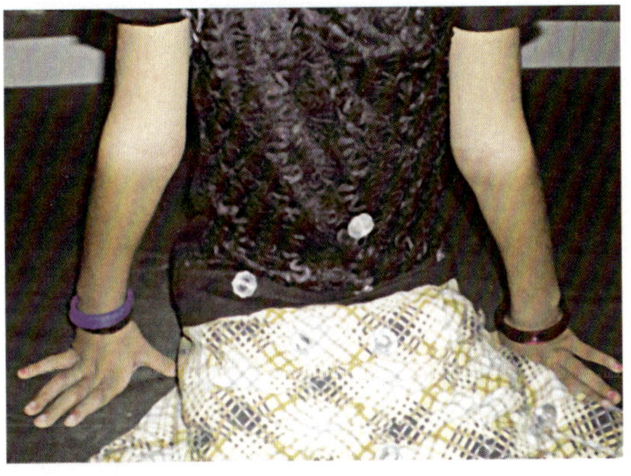

Fig.22.20 Hyperextension at elbow

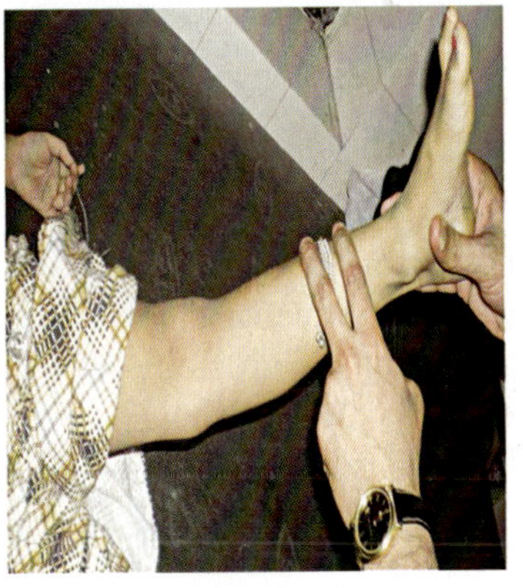

Fig.22.21 Hyperextension of knee

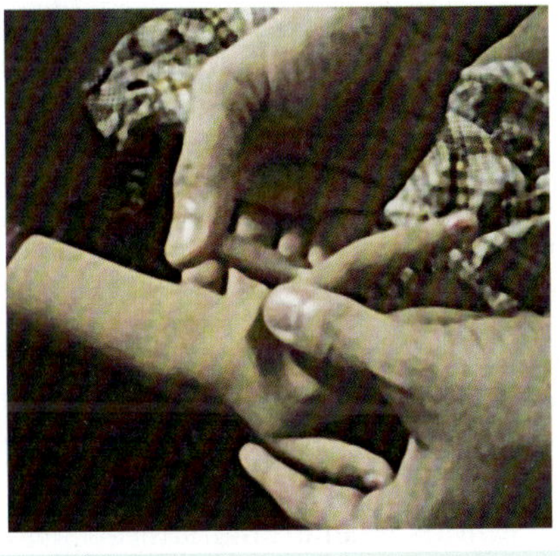

Fig.22.22 Hyperextension of fingers

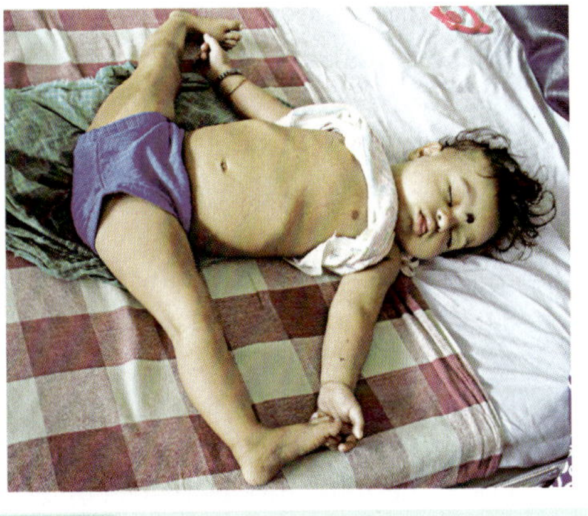

Fig.22.23 Extreme joint hypermobility in a hypotonic child (Down)

CHAPTER 23

Disorders Related to Rheumatology: Case Sheet Formats

Age and sex may be important; e.g., in classifying the type of juvenile rheumatoid arthritis; SLE is more likely in adolescent females.

Complaints

Usual complaints are:

- Fever
- Joint pain:
  - Ascertain if it is arthritis or arthralgia (p 457).
  - Polyarthritis or monoarthritis; in polyarthritis, whether the joint involvement is additive or previous joint gets better when another joint gets involved.
  - Predominantly large joint or small joint involvement; whether the axial skeleton is involved.
  - Acute, subacute or chronic (>6 weeks).
  - Pain more in the morning and getting better as daily activity progresses (rheumatoid arthritis).
  - Pain worse with activity (septic arthritis, rheumatic arthritis, musculoskeletal pains like sprains).
  - Pain manifesting only at the end of the day (non specific "growing pain"); massage soothens growing pains but worsens pain of inflammations.
  - Nocturnal pains: Common in rheumatoid arthritis; during sleep muscle spasm that keeps the joint surfaces apart gives way and hence the pain.
  - History of trauma.
  - Associated symptoms/signs subcutaneous nodules, fever, rash (see below), etc.

    Note: Since rheumatologic diseases are chronic ones, it may be advantageous to draw a line graph to represent periods of symptoms and symptom-free intervals to denote fever, joint pain, rash, symptom-free period, etc.
- Muscle pain:
  - Myalgia: Unaccustomed exertion, non specific, associated symptom of viral fevers, post traumatic.
  - Myositis: Viral polymyositis, dermatomyositis (myositis plus rash plus muscle weakness).
  - Pain during exertion (claudication on walking due to vascular compromise, seen in smoker adults; McArdle glycogen storage disease).
- Bone pain:
  - Pain usually over metaphysis. Osteo-myelitis or leukemia.

Other complaints to ask for:

- Limping:
  - If the clinical presentation itself is with limp in a previously well child, one will have to decide if it is due to joint, bone or muscle problem (or neurological problem). In rheumatology, limping is usually due to arthritis (rheumatoid arthritis, SLE, etc) or muscle weakness (dermatomyositis, polymyositis).

- Skin rash:
  - Purpura (leukemia; palpable purpura in HSP).
  - Systemic onset JRA shows very transient maculopapular "salmon rash" over trunk and proximal limbs (usually related to fever periods).
  - Other rashes possible are erythema marginatum (p 524), erythema nodosum (p 533), malar butterfly rash of SLE, heliotrope rash of eyelids in dermatomyositis (p 546), etc.
  - History suggestive of photosensitive rash (SLE).
- General health: Loss of weight, sleep disturbances, loss of self esteem, etc.
  - Ask about activities of daily living (ADL) to assess level of functioning (EDTA: eating, dressing, toilet, ambulation): examples are eating (restriction of jaw opening in temporo-mandibular joint involvement, in rheumatoid arthritis); walking (also ask if the child is using any devices to help walk); dressing; writing; squatting (toilet); missing of school days; limitation of play activities, etc.
- Chest pain: Pleurisy, pericarditis, costochondral pain, etc.
- Bowel symptoms: In inflammatory bowel disease.
- Eye symptoms: Uveitis is of foremost importance (p 93). Most often uveitis is asymptomatic and so must ask about redness.
- Neurological symptoms like personality change, seizure, etc (of importance in SLE).
- Side effects of drugs: Vomiting, abdominal pain, cushingoid features.
- Compliance with treatment: This is an issue in any chronic illness. If compliance is poor ask reasons for the same.
- **Past history**: Rarely chronic joint symptoms may start with some viral illnesses like rubella or chikungunya. Exacerbations and remissions of chronic rheumatological condition over a time period may be described (best done with a line graph).
- **Antenatal, immunization and development history as per routine format.**
- **Dietary history**: Take a good diet history. Poor nutrition could be an additional contributing factor to poor growth in any chronic illness; specific stress on calcium and vitamin D.
- **Socioeconomic history**: Impact of the disease on family; how the chronic illness affects the care of siblings; social support groups or financial assistance for management, etc.

General comment

Vitals

Anthropometry is of importance as growth may be impaired in any chronic illness. Also bear in mind that limb length discrepancies are also possible due to chronic arthritis (measurement, p 459). There may be wasting of muscles around joints with chronic arthritis. Overweight could be due to steroid therapy.

Overall Profile Appraisal

Any gross joint swellings, contractures, etc can be noticed on this gross inspection.

The candidate himself must show the child what he is expected to do and then ask the child to do the same.

- View from the front: Examine with the child standing with arms by the side and palms facing forward.
  - Look for asymmetry between the limbs (long standing JIA can have growth retardation of limbs).
  - Look for specific deformities described in the text (see p 461).
  - Joints: Examine as described in the text (p 461).
- View from the side: look for
  - Micrognathia (micrognathia due to growth impairment in JIA)
  - Any deformities

- View from the back:
  - Neck: Standing at the back, look at the back of neck for short neck, webbing, low hairline, etc (p 87).
  - Spine: Have the child bend forwards to touch the toes (p 464), to detect scoliosis (true scoliosis will persists even after bending down, whereas the positional scoliosis disappears).
- Skin: Rashes (p 471); subcutaneous nodules (juvenile rheumatoid arthritis); subcutaneous calcification in dermatomyositis (elbow, knee, buttocks; i.e., sites exposed to trauma); pits of calcinosis cutis; any area of lipodystrophy (loss of subcutaneous fat in dermatomyositis); tight skin (scleroderma, mixed connective tissue disorders); depigmentation (scleroderma).
- Gait: p 458, 183.

Hand to Head and Head to Toe Examination

- Nails: Pitting in psoriatic arthritis; sub ungual haemorrhage (SLE); telengiectasia of nail beds (dermatomyositis)
- Palms:
  - Digital ulcers/scars of vasculitis.
  - Nodules over flexor tendons (scleroderma); flexor tenosynovitis (juvenile rheumatoid arthritis).
  - Raynaud's phenomenon (also ask history of blueness while dipping in cold water; persistently cold extremities; throbbing pain of hands, etc). Raynaud's phenomenon may be demonstrable in SLE, mixed connective tissue disorders, scleroderma, and polyarteritis nodosa.
  - Gottron papules over knuckles (dermatomyositis).
- Wrist: Changes of rheumatoid arthritis (see p 461).
- Elbow region: Look for nodules.
- BP: Hypertension is likely in SLE nephropathy; also due to steroid therapy.
- Test joints as discussed in text (p 460); also palpate muscles for tenderness; test for muscle weakness and reflexes now (e.g., dermatomyositis).

  Do look for contractures that may rarely be present. In case muscle weakness is detected, a full examination of motor system and reflexes must be carried out and presented as such to the examiner after completing the hand to head to foot examination.
- Axilla and neck for lymphadenopathy.
- Neck: Look for lymph nodes (SLE, Kawasaki, mixed connective tissue disorders, systemic onset rheumatoid arthritis). At this point, look for lymph nodes elsewhere in the body also, lest the candidate may forget to do so later.
  - Look for neck flop by lifting the shoulders off the couch (in dermatomyositis).
- Hair: Alopecia in SLE or due to drugs like cyclophosphamide.
- Face: Look for any cushingoid features due to drugs.
- Eyes:
  - Look for heliotrope rash (violacious or purplish oedematous discolouration of eye lids; seen in dermatomyositis).
  - Look for pallor.
  - Glaucoma or cataract in long-term steroid therapy.
  - Dry eyes in Sjogren's.
  - Mention that iridocyclitis may be missed on clinical examination and hence need slit lamp examination by ophthalmologist.
  - Roughly assess vision (child may be on hydroxychloroquine).
- Fundus: Especially important if the child is on hydroxychloroquine.
- Mouth: Inflamed mucous membranes; oral ulcers in SLE.
- Dysphonia in dermatomyositis. Muscle weakness may lead on to impaired swallowing and impaired speech. Rarely hoarseness due to rheumatoid nodules in larynx.
- Chest: Tenderness; CVS examination for cardiomegaly, murmurs, pericarditis, etc. Cardiac murmurs are expected in rheumatic fever. Examine respiratory system, pleural effusion

is rarely seen in certain rheumatologic conditions like SLE.

- Abdomen: organomegaly, tenderness (serositis of SLE, enteritis of IBD).
    - Ask child to get up unsupported from supine to test truncal weakness.
- Lower limb:
    - Do neuromuscular assessment; inspect gait (if not already done during front profile examination).
    - Proximal muscle weakness (usually symmetrical) in dermatomyositis, polymyositis, steroid toxicity, etc (ask to stand from squat).
    - Palpate muscles for tenderness. Test joints as discussed in the text (p 464).
    - Erythema nodosum (in IBD).
    - Limb length measurement in relevant cases (p 459).
- Motor system and reflexes:
    - In case muscle weakness is detected, a full examination of motor system and reflexes must be carried out. Full CNS examination is possibly not necessary.
    - Most examiners expect the candidate to comment on functional assessment based on activities of daily living (EDTA - eating, dressing, toilet, ambulation): examples are speech and swallow (muscle weakness, e.g., dermatomyositis); chew (arthritis temperomandibular joint); sitting (soft tissue calcification of buttocks); squat at toilet, climb stairs (proximal muscle weakness of myositis); other examples are brushing teeth, feeding self, combing hair, etc. Show the child (imaginary) and ask him to repeat some movements; e.g., turn the door handle (imaginary), comb hair, brush teeth, hang out washed clothes, scratch the bottom (toilet), squat, pick an object from the floor, etc.
    - At the end of examination, do a mental sum up and be ready with the following inferences in addition to the differential diagnosis:
        - Number of joints involved over the period of illness.
        - Symmetry (relatively symmetrical in juvenile rheumatoid arthritis; asymmetrical in psoriatic arthritis).
        - Whether the disease is active or not at present (pain, warmth and redness of joints).
        - Effect on activities of daily living.

JUVENILE IDIOPATHIC ARTHRITIS

23

Students may please read and follow the rheumatology case sheet format. The following is a repetition of that, with emphasis on JIA.

1. Chief complaint:
    - Joint pain since...
    - Fever
    - Restriction of movements
2. History of presenting illness:
    - History suggestive of joint pain:
        - Ask for pain on movement/swelling of joints/restriction of movements/ history suggestive of morning stiffness getting better as the day progresses.
        - Onset and duration (acute onset- consider septic arthritis).
        - Number of joints (to determine the subtypes; not more than 4 joints must be affected in the first 6 months of the disease to call it oligoarticular).
        - Type of joints (small/large; to subclassify JIA).
        - Symmetrical, asymmetrical (relatively symmetrical in juvenile rheumatoid arthritis; asymmetrical in psoriatic arthritis).
        - Pattern of progression: Migratory, additive, intermittent.
        - Axial/peripheral joints.
        - Deformities.

Also note the functional level of each joint.

- History to elucidate the aetiology:
  - History suggestive of fever, rash-
    - Quotidian fever, evanescent salmon coloured rash - JIA
    - Malar/discoid rash over face - SLE.
    - Erythema marginatum - Rheumatic fever.
    - Gottron papules - JDM.
    - Rashes with blebs that leave dark residual patches - Chikungunya.
  - Purpura, abdominal pain - HSP.
  - History s/o viral infections - Post viral arthralgia.
  - History suggestive of bleeding manifestations/pallor - Leukemia.
  - History suggestive of UTI/diarrhoea - Reactive arthritis.
  - History suggestive of rheumatic fever (preceding sorethroat, migratory polyarthritis, involvement of large joints, etc).
  - History suggestive of tuberculosis (when the presentation is as monoarthritis).
  - Travel to endemic areas - Tick bite, lyme disease.
  - Recurrent infections - Common variable immunodeficiency.
- History to find out complications:
  - Restriction of activity/schooling and absenteeism
  - Deformities
- History suggestive of red eye or blurring of vision (most often uveitis is asymptomatic; persistent uncontrolled uveitis result in cataracts. Keratopathy leading to blindness); drug toxicities, e.g., side effects of steroids, oral ulcers due to methotrexate.
- Past history: Exacerbations and remissions are part and parcel of rheumatoid arthritis. Consider if there is history suggestive of rubella or chikungunya.
- Immunization: BCG, optional vaccines.
- Growth and development - Usually not affected; growth may be decreased in a chronic case. Chronically affected limbs may be shorter.
- Nutrition history: As routine. Poor nutrition could be an additional contributing factor to poor growth in JIA; specific stress on calcium and vit D.
- Family history: History of arthritis and/or psoriasis in the family (in a first-degree relative) - if present enquire the age at onset and progression.
- Socio-economic history: Socio-economic status, impact on the family, attitude towards the disease and treatment.

3. General examination:
   - Mention the posture/gross deformities, if any.
   - Comment on profile appraisal (see p 471)
   - May be of advantage to complete skin examination here
     - Skin: Note if scleroderma is present;
       - Purpura - HSP, leukemia
       - Mention the site and type of rash if present: Salmon coloured rash over the trunk and proximal extremities in SOJIA.
       - Rash over the eyes and knuckles (juvenile dermatomyositis), face (SLE).
       - History of rash appearing along the line of trauma (e.g., along scratch marks) (Koebner phenomenon).
4. Note vital signs - PR, RR, BP, temperature and JVP. As the child may be on steroids, BP may be high.
5. Head to foot examination:
   Note: For a quick assessment of joints it is best to follow PGALS (p 480).

- It is of advantage to follow **hand to head and head to foot** examination schedule not to miss any points. During case presentation, this may be formatted to fit in with head to foot scheme if that is the one your medical school follows.
- Nails: Look for nail pitting/gangrene/look at nail fold capillaries (use ophthalmoscope if you have one).
- Rheumatoid nodules: Look over flexor tendon sheaths.
- Test joints of hand as discussed in text (p 460).
- Wrist: Look for deformities, boutanairre, swan neck, mallet finger.
- Elbow: Look for any nodules.
- Examine for tender muscles (myositis).
- Shoulder: Assess if primarily a muscle or joint problem. If active movement is painful but passive posssible - rotator cuff is affected. If both are difficult - joint involvement.
- Axilla and neck for lymphadenopathy; lymph node enlargement is common in JIA.
- Examine the hair: Note the texture and if alopecia is present (alopecia areata in rheumatoid arthritis).
- Face: May have Cushingoid features due to steroids.
- Eyes: To look for features of pallor, cataract, uveitis (pain, redness, etc), non-purulent conjuctivitis, icterus, etc. Assess vision and fundus (child may be on hydroxy chloroquine).
- Mouth: Painless erosions/mucositis (SLE or due to methotrexate)/strawberry tongue.
- TMJ: Pain on opening the mouth/chewing.
- Feel the joint for crepitus when opening the mouth (p 462).
- Normally should be able to insert three fingers inside the open mouth (Fig. 22.9).
- Neck: Cervical spine movements- forward, backward, sideward and lateral rotation (p 463).
- Chest: Assess the heart for cardiomegaly, pericarditis, etc.
- Abdomen: Hepatosplenomegaly may be present in JIA.
- Hip: Internal rotation of hip affected in JIA.
- Knee joint: Examine suprapatellar bursae; in addition, look for evidence of active arthritis in all joints - pain on movement, swelling of the joint.
- Palpate muscles for tenderness.
- Toe deformities - Hallux valgus, splaying, widening of metatarsal joints.
- Look for evidence of enthesitis by palpating achilles tendon, calcaneum and head of metatarsals.
- Note limb length discrepancies, if any.
- Back: Thoracolumbar spine - if not examined during profile examination.

Diagnosis

JIA - oligo/polyarticular (mention how many joints are affected over how much period of time) - with/without active joint involvement now, possible aetiology and complications if present.

Investigations

There are no tests to confirm the diagnosis.

- Total count, ESR and CRP may be elevated during the active phase of the disease.
- RF and ANA.
- X ray may show osteoporosis, narrowing of joint space and erosion of articular surface.
- Ultrasonogram to detect effusions, synovitis, etc.
- MRI detects early changes in joints.
- Joint fluid aspiration and synovial biopsy when the diagnosis is in doubt.

- Slit lamp examination for uveitis.
- Bone mineral density studies in long standing cases.
- HLA typing to classify JIA (e.g., HLA–B27).

Treatment

- Rest the joints during the acute stage.
- Physiotherapy once the acute stage is over: Passive stretching of muscles to preserve the range of motion. Swimming is the best active exercise after the pain subsides.
- Walk assist devices, hard bed to sleep, etc.
- Follow-up for asymptomatic iridocyclitis.
- NSAID: Naproxen is the first-line drug.
- Local steroid injections to the affected joint if feasible.
- Disease-modifying antirheumatic drugs: When control with NSAID is unsatisfactory, add methotrexate once a week. Need monitoring of blood count and liver function monthly.
- Systemic steroids: When the symptoms are not controlled on NSAIDs, and methotrexate, steroid will be needed. In addition, during acute stage to get symptoms rapidly under control, short course steroid may be needed.
- Biologic reaction modifiers (e.g., etanercept, infliximab): For use when all the above fails.

Monitoring of Disease Activity

- Clinical symptoms (fever/joint/eyes)
- ESR
- Degree of anaemia
- MRI

Complications

- Iridocyclitis: May progress to visual impairment.
- Growth retardation, osteopenia and fractures: Due to the disease interfering with bone growth and due to steroid treatment.
- Macrophage activation syndrome. Rarely in SOJIA, macrophages start destroying body's own blood cells in bone marrow (histiophagocytosis) to produce pancytopenia and the complications of that may kill the patient. Will need immunosupressive therapy.

Prognosis

- Repeated exacerbations are likely but ultimately 75% of patients will have long-term remission.
- Long-term complications: Visual loss due to iridocyclitis; permanent joint damage.

Criteria for Diagnosis of Juvenile Rheumatoid Arthritis *(Ref: Nelson's textbook)*

- Age of onset <16 years
- Arthritis of more than or equal to one joint. Arthritis is diagnosed by swelling or effusion or presence of two or more of the following:
  - Limitation of range of motion
  - Tenderness or pain on motion
  - Heat over the joint
- Duration of disease > 6 weeks.
- The subtype of rheumatoid arthritis is defined by the type and number of articular involvement in the first 6 months after the onset.
- Exclusion of other aetiologies for the arthritis (see differential diagnosis).

Differential Diagnosis of Arthritis

- Septic arthritis: Here, the child will appear toxic with systemic symptoms. Excruciating pain and bright erythema of a single joint favour a diagnosis of septic arthritis.
- Tubercular arthritis: Contact history, positive Mantoux.
- Rheumatic arthritis: Jone's criteria; fleeting nature of arthritis and prompt response to aspirin; arthritis is not chronic.
- Osteomyelitis: Pain and swelling are maximum over the metaphysis and not the joint.
- Transient synovitis: This may be due to non–specific viral infections or specific viral infections (e.g., rubella) or GIT infections (e.g., Yersinia) or trauma.

- SLE will have other manifestations (see below).
- Malignancies: Leukemia may have bone pain, which on careful examination will be seen to be localized to metaphysis, not joints.
- Hemophila: family history and previous history in a male child with swollen joints (hemarthrosis).

Types of JIA (old name was JRA)

- Pauciarticular JIA (oligoarticular JIA):
  - Pauciarticular means not more than 4 joints are affected during the first 6 months of disease.
  - When a cumulative total of < 5 joints are involved throughout the disease course it is subclassified as Persistantoligoarticular. When a cumulative total of 5 or more joints get affected after the first 6 months, it is subclassified as extended oligoarticular JIA.
  - Onset: 1–5 years.
  - Usually girls are affected.
  - Large joints are involved (e.g., knee, elbow, ankle, etc). But hips and sacroiliac joints are spared.
  - Rheumatoid factor is negative.
  - ANA will be positive in 50% cases of oligoarticular JIA.
  - Asymptomatic iridocyclitis (painless red eye) is common.
- Enthesitis-related arthritis
  - This is the equivalent of spondyloarthropathies of adults.
  - Pauciarticular arthritis.
  - Enthesitis (inflammation of regions of tendon insertion): Painful patella, heel pad, tibial tuberosity, etc.
  - Hip and sacroiliac joints may be affected; in addition, peripheral arthritis is also associated.
  - Onset: Older childhood (>8 years).
  - Slightly more common in boys.
  - Rheumatoid factor is negative.
  - ANA is negative. HLA-B27 may be positive in up to 80% of cases.
  - Family history of spondylo arthropathy, inflammatory bowel disease or HLA B 27 positivity.
  - Iridocyclitis (uveitis) usually is symptomatic (painful red eye).
- Psoriatic arthritis
  - Chronic inflammatory arthritis with asymmetric involvement of small joints of fingers (dactilitis); knee and ankle also may get involved.
  - Age of onset is mid childhood.
  - Nail pitting.
  - Rash of psoriasis (may manifest only later).
  - Asymptomatic (painless) uveitis similar to oligoarticular JIA is possible but much less.
- Systemic onset JIA (SOJIA; Still's disease)
  - Onset at any age.
  - High-grade intermittent fever for many weeks.
  - Evanescent (fade within hours) pale-red, non-pruritic macular rash (salmon pink macules) usually in and around the trunk during periods of fever. The rash may extend linearly along a scratch mark (Koebner phenomenon).
  - Hepatosplenomegaly and lymphadenopathy.
  - Arthritis is polyarticular, affects small and large joints and will be evident within the first 6 months of febrile onset of disease.
  - Serositis like pleural effusion, pericarditis, etc.
  - Iridocyclitis (uveitis) is absent.
  - Rheumatoid factor (RF) is negative.
  - Antinuclear antibodies (ANA) will be negative.
  - Diagnostic criteria of SOJIA: Quotidian fever for at least 2 weeks plus evanescent rash plus arthritis. In the absence of

23

arthritis, diagnosis of SOJIA may be considered if any of the following two is present along with quotidian fever (two spikes per day) and evanescent rash: generalized lymphadenopathy/hepatomegaly/splenomegaly/serositis.

- Polyarticular JIA, RF negative:
  - This subtype is almost same as adult type rheumatoid arthritis, except that it has an earlier onset and RF is negative.
  - Small joints of hands are involved.
  - > 5 joints are involved in the first 6 months.
  - Onset could be at any age. Usually at an younger age compared to RF positive subgroup.
  - Temperomandibular joint involvement may result in micrognathia as the child grows.
  - RF is negative.
  - ANA may be positive.
- Polyarticular JIA, RF positive:
  - This subtype is almost same as adult type rheumatoid arthritis.
  - Onset at older age group and there is likely persistence of disability into adulthood.
  - Subcutaneous rheumatoid nodules may be seen over the elbow, heels, first metatarsophalangeal joint, extensor surface of fingers, knuckles, etc.
  - Swan neck deformity is common (i.e., hyperextension of proximal interphalangeal joints and flexion of distal interphalangeal joints).
  - RF is positive.

SYSTEMIC LUPUS ERYTHEMATOSIS

Basic Considerations

SLE must be suspected when the disease involves multiple organ systems, vasculitic rashes and arthritis in adolescent females. Unexplained fever, fatigue and weight loss are common presentations. American College of Rheumatology Criteria for the diagnosis of SLE (clinical and lab). Mnemonic:

SOAP BRAIN MD

Serositits (pleuritis, pericarditis, etc)
Oral ulcers
Arthritis
Photosensitivity
Blood: Autoimmune haemolytic anaemia or leucopenia or lymphopenia or thrombocytopenia.
Renal: Persistent proteinuria or cellular casts. Acute nephritic syndrome or nephrotic syndrome or hypertension in later stages.
ANA: Positive
Immunological: Anti-dsDNA or anti-sm or antiphospholipid antibody.
Neurological: Seizures stroke or psychosis.
Malar rash
Discoid rash (Fig.23.a & b)

***Note**:The new criteria for SLE is the SLICC (Systemic Lupus International, Collaborating Clinics) criteria. In this Low complements and positive DCT in absence of hemolytic anaemia have been included under the immunologic criteria.*

Investigations

- Haemoglobin, complete blood count, ESR.
- Urine routine and microscopy, and 24-hr protein or protein-creatinine ratio.

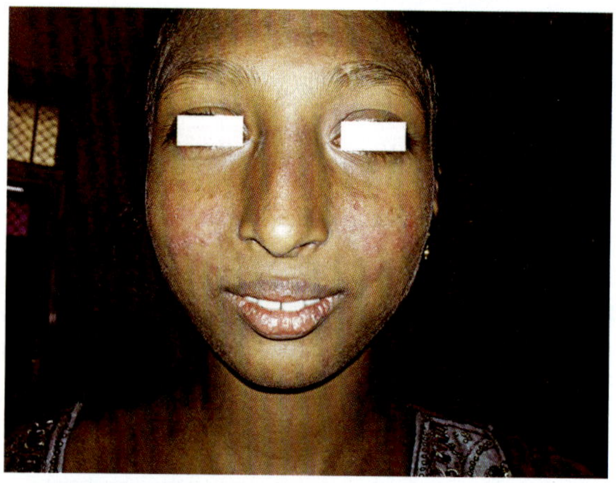

Fig.23.a Malar rash

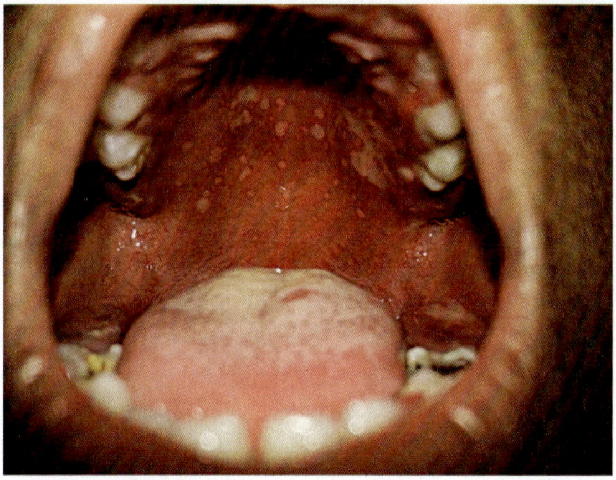

Fig.23.b Multiple oral ulcers

- Serum chemistry (urea, creatinine, liver function tests, lipid profile).
- Chest X-ray.
- ANA, anti-dsDNA, C3, C4.

Management

- Educate the patient about the disease.
- Avoidance of sun exposure.
- NSAIDs.
- Hydroxychloroquine (when NSAID alone is not effective; Hydroxychloroquine is useful for photosensitive cutaneous manifestations and joint manifestations).
- Systemic steroids when the above treatments are not sufficient.
- Immunosuppressives like cyclophosphamide pulses.
- Azathioprine
- Calcium and vitamin D (physiological dose) to retard steroid induced osteoporosis.

Students desirous to have more management details may read Manual of Pediatric Practice by the same author.

JUVENILE DERMATOMYOSITIS

- Proximal muscle weakness of limbs; weakness of neck muscle and palatal/pharyngeal muscles; muscle tenderness, periorbital violaceous (heliotropic) erythema, arthralgia and low-grade fever.
- Sequel (muscle atrophy, contractures, calcinosis).

Investigations

- Blood count, ESR elevated.
- Muscle enzymes [creatine kinase (CPK), sGOT, LDH, aldolase, etc].
- ANA elevated.
- Myositis specific autoantibodies [anti-Jo-1 antibody (myositis specific antibody), anti-SRP antibody (signal recognition particle), etc].
- EMG shows myopathic pattern [Brief small amplitude polyphasic potentials (BSAPP)].
- MRI with suppression of fat signals helps in demonstrating muscle oedema and inflammation.
- Muscle biopsy: If MRI, is done muscle biopsy may not be needed. Muscle histology will show degeneration and regeneration with mononuclear cell infiltration.

Management

- Use sunscreen when going outdoors.
- Vit D and Ca may be supplemented at physiological doses to compensate for blocking sunlight and osteoporotic effects of steroids.
- Steroids (prednisolone 1–2 mg/kg/day orally); long-term treatment will be needed.
- Hydroxychloroquine may be used as an add-on drug.
- Those not responding may need methotrexate or cyclophosphamide.

The following pictures summarizes the maneuvers in pGALS (pediatric gait, arm, leg and spine screaning) which is now the recommended standard for examination of joints.

23

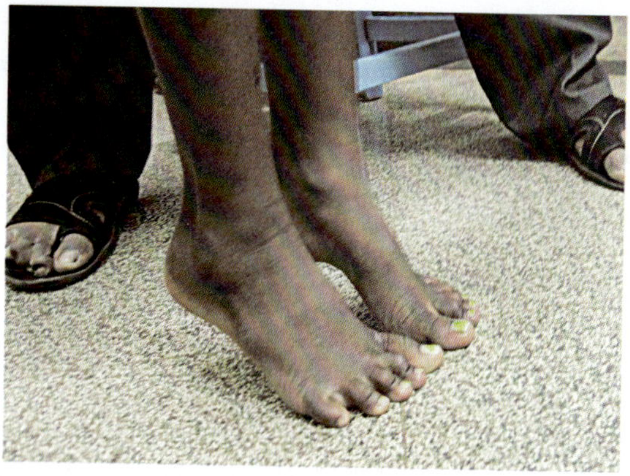

Fig.23.1 pGALS. Gait (1) - Walk of toes

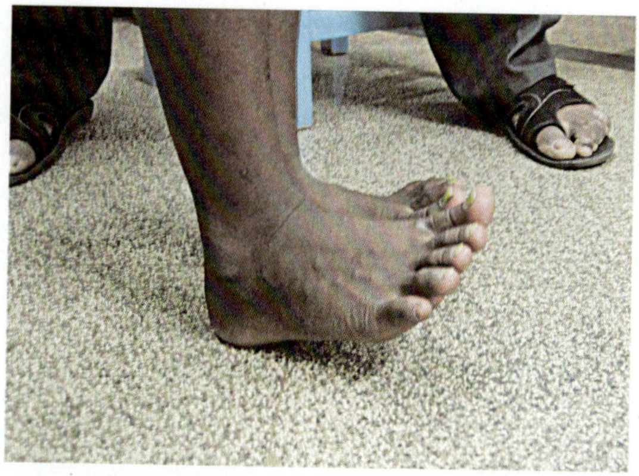

Fig.23.2 pGALS. Gait (2) - Walk on heels

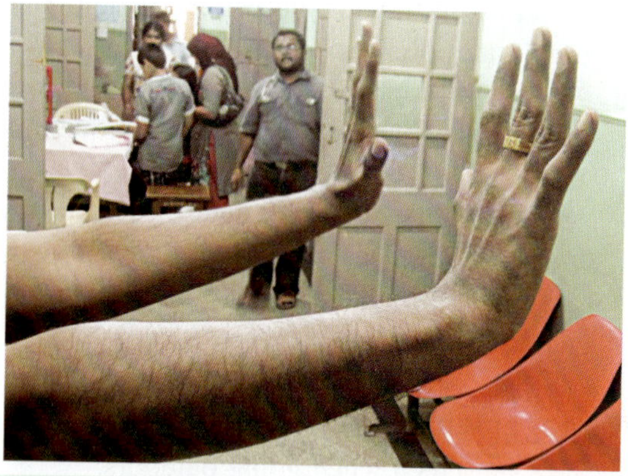

Fig.23.3 pGALS. Arms (1). Put arms in front; forearm pronated; then extend the wrist. Extension of elbow, wrist and fingers.

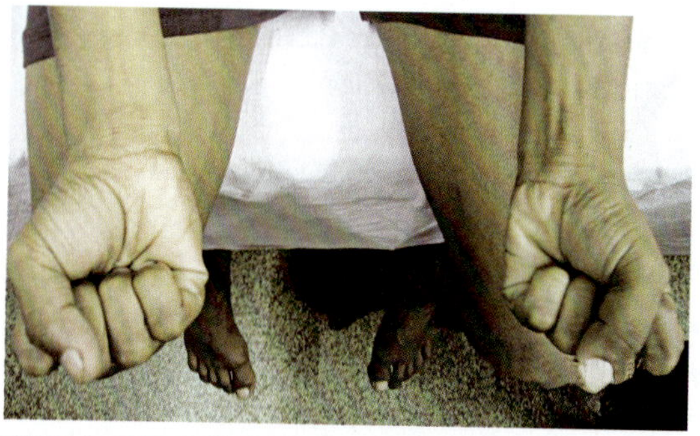

Fig.23.4 pGALS. Arms (2). Now turnover the hands (supinate). Make a fist. Assess supination of wrist; elbow and flexion of small joints of fingers are also assessed by this.

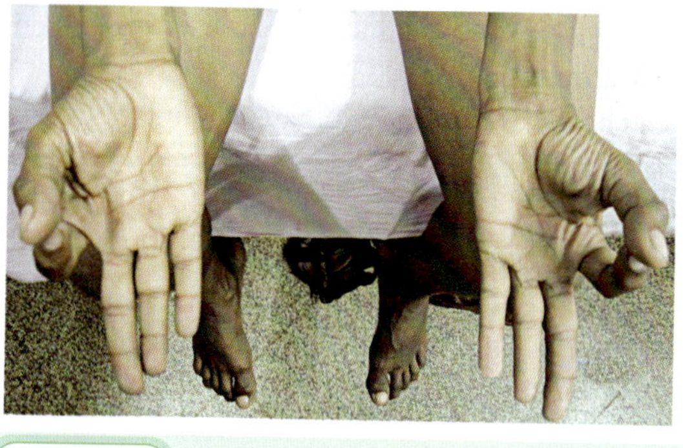

Fig.23.5 pGALS. Arms (3). Touch thumb with tips of each fingers.

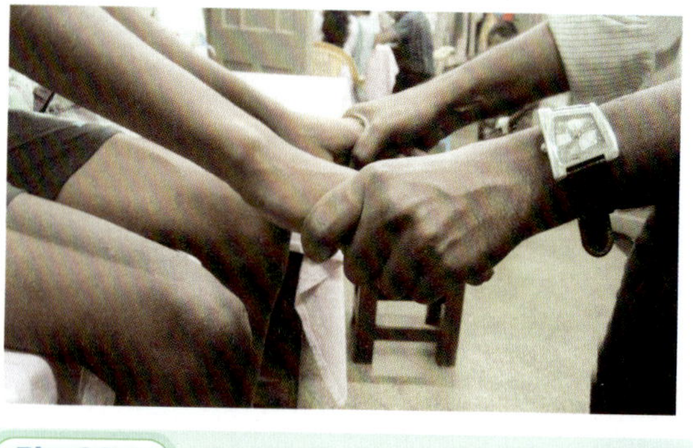

Fig.23.6 pGALS. Arms (4). Squeeze metacarpo phalangeal joints.

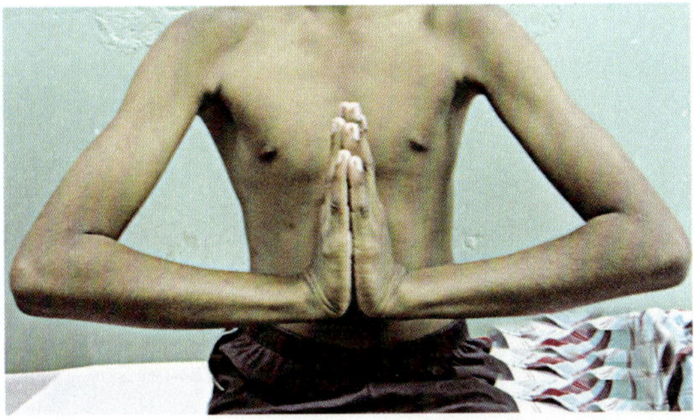

Fig.23.7 pGALS. Arms (5). Namaste position. Extension of small joints of fingers and wrist, flexion of elbow.

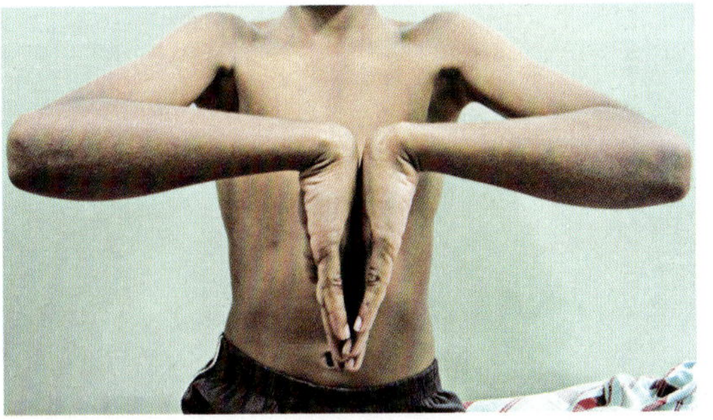

Fig.23.8 pGALS. Arms (6). Reverse namaste position. Flexion of wrist.

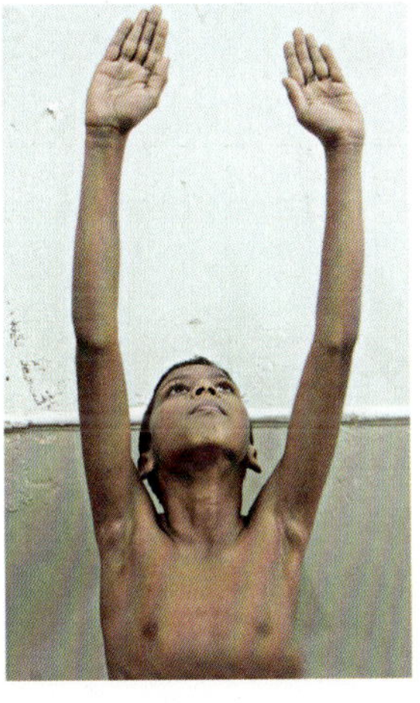

Fig.23.9 pGALS. Arms (7). Look at the ceiling and try to touch the ceiling. Elbow, wrist and neck extension, shoulder abduction.

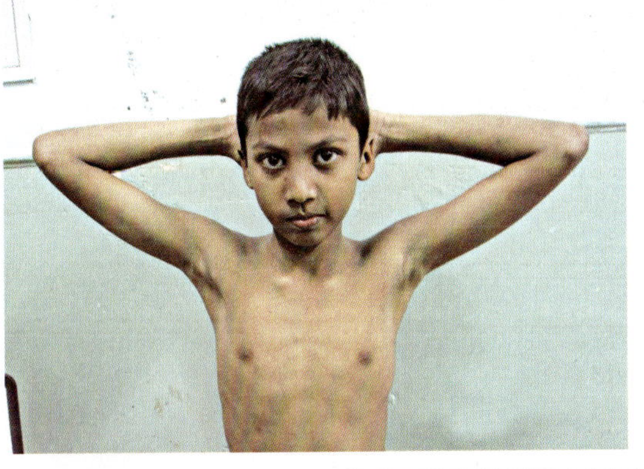

Fig.23.10 pGALS. Arms (8). Put hands behind your neck. abduction and external rotation of shoulders, flexion of elbows

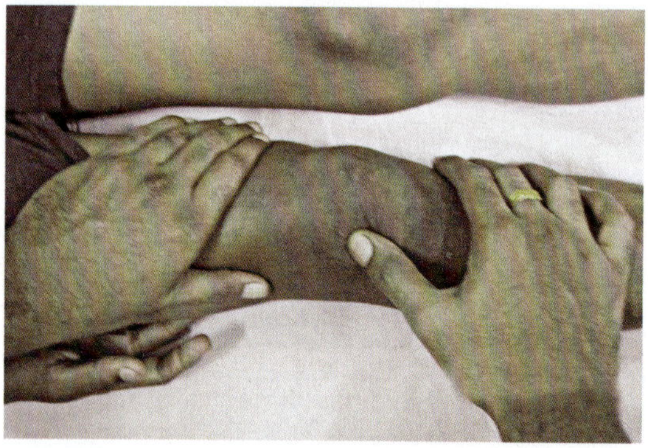

Fig.23.11 pGALS. Legs (1). Feel for effusion by patellar tap and cross fluctuation. Check muscle wasting contractures.

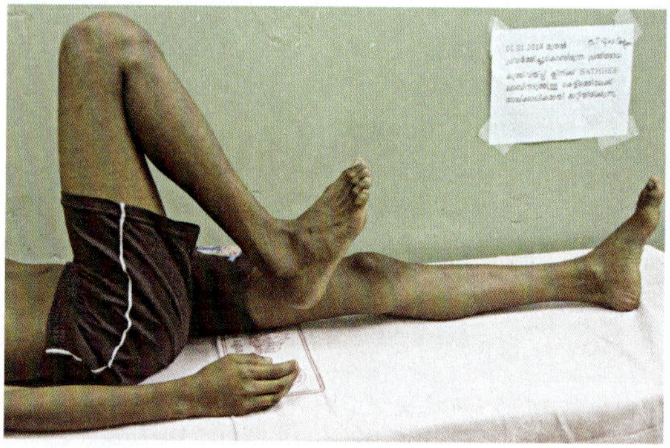

Fig.23.12 pGALS. Legs (2). Active flexion and extension knee as shown.

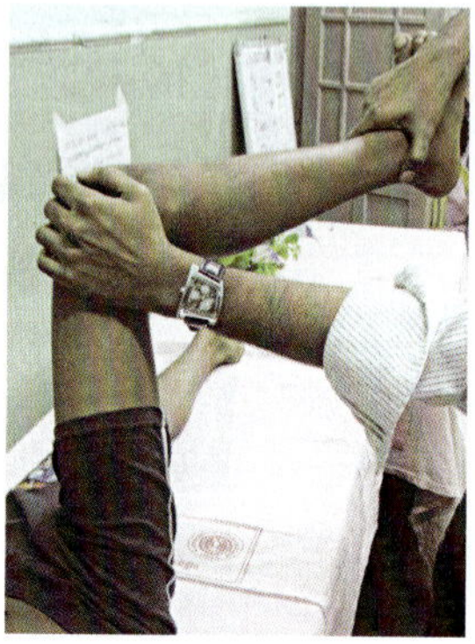

Fig.23.13 pGALS. Legs (3). Passive flexion internal rotation hip with knee at 90°.

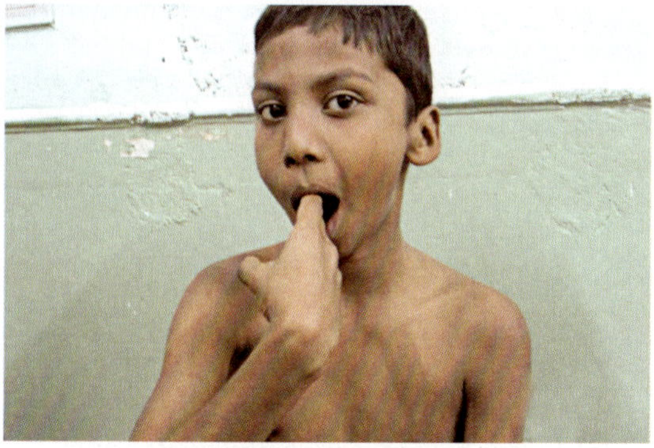

Fig.23.14 pGALS. Spine (1). Put 3 fingers in mouth - Tempero-mandibular joint.

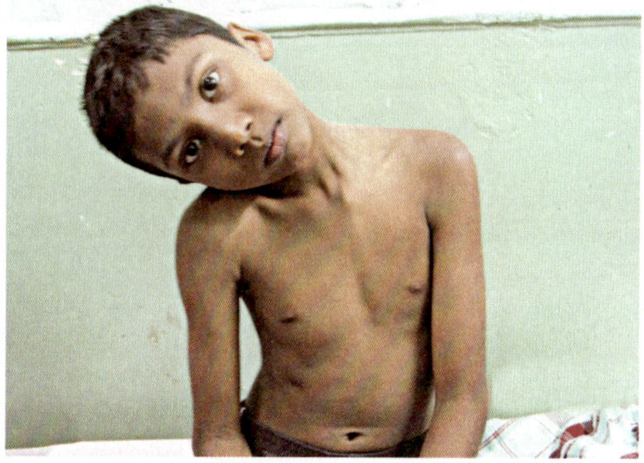

Fig.23.15 pGALS. Spine (2). Try to touch shoulder with ear. Lateral flexion of cervical spine.

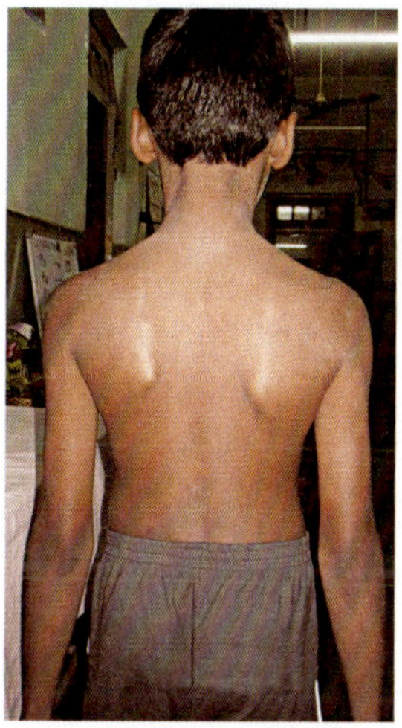

Fig.23.16 pGALS. Spine (3). Observe from behind; rashes, deformity, scoliosis, wasting, swelling, nodules, etc.

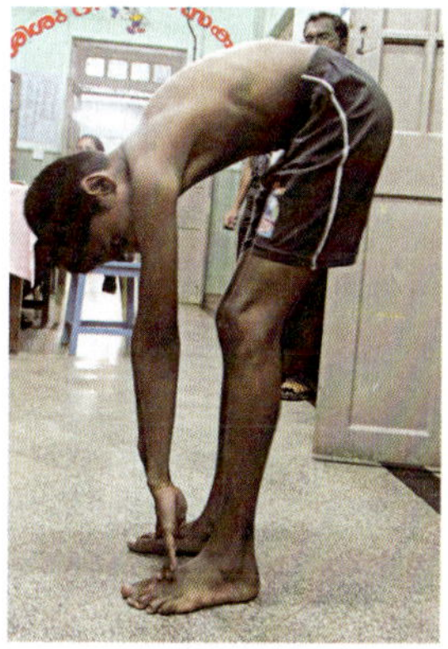

Fig.23.17 pGALS. Spine (4). Touch the toes without knee flexion. Flexion of thoraco lumbar spine. Check for scoliosis. Observe from behind and side.

Acknowledgement: pGALS pictures are provided by Dr Sajikumar *(Ref: Nelson's Textbook, 19th ed., p 2331).*

CHAPTER 24

Image Gallery I : Short Cases & Spotters

In postgraduate examinations of western countries, short cases and spotters are an integral part of the assessment of the candidate. This trend has started in India also, especially in the DNB examinations. In the following section, a few short cases and spotters that are important in examination are discussed. Long cases are discussed in detail along with case sheet formats of individual systems. The students may use the index to locate the topics that they want to refer.

The undergraduate student may skip the topics that are not important for their examination. ***Questions marked * are generally for postgraduates.*** *Mark alongwith discussion conveys that the marked feature is important in the diagnosis. The following is the usual list of *long* cases kept for undergraduate examination:

- CVS: Rheumatic heart disease (MR, AR, MS); congenital heart disease (TOF, VSD, PDA).
- Respiratory: Consolidation, bronchopneumonia, asthma, pleural effusion, pneumo/hydropneumothorax, etc.
- GIT: Hepatitis, hepatosplenomegaly.
- Genitourinary system: Nephritis, nephrotic syndrome.
- Haematology: ITP, leukemia, lymphoma, etc.
- Endocrinology: Only for postgraduates (short stature, hypothyroidism, ambiguous genitalia, etc).
- CNS: Cerebral palsy (various types), meningitis (usually TBM), acute flaccid paralysis (usually GBS), transverse meylitis, hydrocephalus, Duchenne muscular dystrophy, etc.
- Rheumatology: Juvenile idiopathic arthritis. SLE will be kept for postgraduates only.
- Dysmorphic syndromes: Down.
- Nutritional disorders: PEM, rickets.
- Newborn: Normal newborn, icterus, premature baby or minor problems like cephalhaematoma.

The undergraduate students should not propose a rare diagnosis and get themselves in deep trouble. In the following discussion, you will find a lot of rare cases; however, always remember that you are only rarely correct with a rare diagnosis. Consider the diagnostic priorities as given below when you decide to offer a rare diagnosis: Think if the clinical scenario of the patient can fit in with the following, the priority being in the following order:

- Common presentation of a common disease.
- Uncommon presentation of a common disease.
- Common presentation of an uncommon disease.
- Uncommon presentation of an uncommon disease.

List of cases in alphabetical order:

6. Angelman syndrome (p 505)
7. Anhidrotic ectodermal dysplasia (p 500)
8. Apert syndrome (p 538)
9. Aplasia Cutis Congenita (p 549)
10. Asthma (p 486)
11. Ataxia telangiectasia (p 523)
12. Beckwith-Wiedemann syndrome (p 506)
13. Benign pustular melanosis (p 553)
14. Blueberry Muffin spots (p 550)
15. Brushfield spots (p 509)
16. Cerebral palsy (p 528)
17. Chickenpox (p 525)
18. Cleidocranial dysplasia (p 501)
19. Colloidon baby (p 506)
20. Congenital complete heart block (p 553)
21. Cornelia de Lange syndrome (p 507)
22. Crouzon's syndrome (p 538)
23. Cushing syndrome (p 540)
24. Down syndrome (p 507)
25. Duchenne muscular dystrophy (p 535)
26. Edward's syndrome (p 504)
27. Ehlers-Danlos syndrome (p 502)
28. Ellis-van Creveld syndrome (p 509)
29. Encephalocele (p 531)
30. Erb's palsy (p 535)
31. Erythema marginatum (p 524)
32. Erythema nodosum (p 543)
33. Examination of upper limb (p 545)
34. Extrahepatic biliary atresia (p 493)
35. Facial nerve palsy (p 533)
36. Fanconi pancytopenia (p 497)
37. Farber's disease (p 545)
38. Floppy infant (p 536)
39. Follicular Hyperkeratosis (p 551)
40. Fragile X syndrome (p 539)
41. Friedreich ataxia (p 531)
42. Goldenhar syndrome (p 510)
43. Henoch-Schonlein purpura (p 498)
44. Holt-Oram syndrome (p 472)
45. Horner's syndrome (p 537)
46. Hydrocephalus (p 532-533)
47. Hypoglossal palsy (p 534)
48. Hypomelanosis of Ito (p 579)
49. Hypothyroidism (p 541)
50. III nerve palsy (p 533)
51. Incontinentia pigmenti (Bloch-Sulzberger disease) (p 519)
52. Infant of diabetic mother (p 505)
53. Juvenile dermatomyositis (p 546)
54. Juvenile rheumatoid arthritis (p 496)
55. Kawasaki disease (p 544)
56. Klinefelter syndrome (p 505)
57. Klippel-Trenaunay-Weber syndrome (p 524)
58. Laurence-Moon-Biedl syndrome (p 575)
59. LEOPARD syndrome (p 537)
60. Lowe syndrome (p 546)
61. Marfan syndrome (p 511)
62. McCune-Albright syndrome (p 543)
63. Measles (p 547)
64. Meningomyelocele (p 529)
65. Mucopolysaccharidosis (p 499)
66. Mumps (p 525)
67. Neonatal varicella (p 551)
68. Nephrotic syndrome (p 495)
69. Neurofibromatosis (p 522)
70. Noonan syndrome (p 572)
71. Oedema of hands and feet (p 497)
72. Osteogenesis imperfecta (p 503)
73. Palatal palsy (p 534)
74. PEM (p 487)
75. Pierre Robin sequence (p 573)
76. Poland sequence (p 503)
77. Prader-Willi syndrome (p 575)
78. Proboscis cyclopia (p 552)
79. Prune belly syndrome (p 573)
80. Rheumatic Fever (p 552)
81. Rickets (p 490)
82. Rubinstein-Taybi syndrome (p 516)
83. Russell-Silver syndrome (p 576)
84. Scabies (p 426)
85. Severe dehydration (p 493)
86. SLE (p 496)
87. Staphylococcal scalded skin syndrome (SSSS) (p 526)
88. Striae (p 553)
89. Sturge-Weber syndrome (p 520)

1. A 5-year-old child had rhinitis for a few days followed by cough and now fever. Previous history shows that the child had many episodes of prolonged cough following upper respiratory infections. Examination showed good air entry bilaterally with rhonchi and crepitations. As an infant, this child had reddish rash over both cheeks, which settled after a few months. What is the most probable diagnosis? His chest X-ray is shown below.

A: Asthma. Upper respiratory infection is one of the most common precipitating factors for

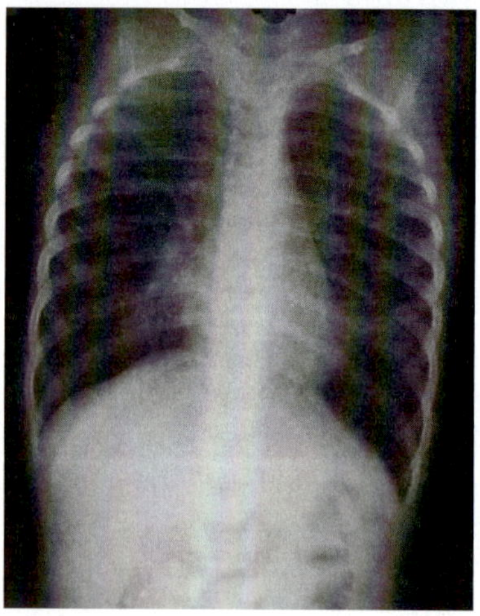

Fig.24.1

asthma. Here, the history of rhinitis is followed by cough and fever comes after that; it is unlike pneumonia where fever is likely to be a much earlier symptom. Crepitations per se do not diagnose bronchopneumonia (see discussion under respiratory system). Here, it seems that stagnated secretions due to bronchospasm were infected and hence the fever. So one may modify the diagnosis as wheeze-associated lower respiratory tract infection (WLRI), which is now the accepted term for this situation. Mild fever can be there in uncomplicated asthma also because of heat generation due to the effort of breathing. The rash seems to be atopic dermatitis (see Fig.6.151, p 138). Acute bronchiolitis becomes a differential diagnosis only in an infant and not at 5 years. History of many recurrences is also against the diagnosis of acute bronchiolitis.

Clinical Points on Asthma

- Family or personal history of eczema and/or allergic rhinitis*
- History of recurrent episodes* (3 or more)
- History suggestive of rapid response to treatment (like nebulization)*
- History suggestive of trigger-induced exacerbation*: E.g., viral infections, exposure to allergens/cold, smoking, weather, exercise, dust, pollen, animals, drugs (e.g., aspirin) etc. (Mnemonic: **AEIOU**; **A**llergens (e.g., dust, pollen, cockroach), **E**xercise/Environment, **I**nfection (e.g., URI)/irritants (e.g., smoke), **O**nset of lunar days (full moon/new moon) or seasonal variations, **U**se of drugs like NSAIDs).
- If the child has a well-controlled asthma, growth and development will be normal. Steroid facies may be there if the child is on long-term steroids. Hand tremors may be there as the child will be on salbutamol.
- Look for chest deformity; e.g., Harrison's sulcus, pectus carinatum/excavatum,

hyperinflation with increased anteroposterior diameter, etc. Look for features suggestive of allergy (see p 356).

- Respiratory rate may be increased.
- Trachea and apex will be in normal position.
- Chest expansion will be symmetrical.
- Percussion note will be resonant or may show increased resonance (if air trapping is there).
- Breath sounds are vesicular with prolonged expiratory phase (when the child is symptomatic). Asymmetric air entry in various areas may be found and goes well with a diagnosis of asthma because bronchospasm may not be affecting all areas equally. However, persistent localized chest signs may point towards a foreign body or lymph node obstruction as in tuberculosis. Hence, ask for suggestive history.
- Wheeze and crepitations may be there.
- Check single breath count test to know the respiratory reserve (this is more practical than peak flow rate in small children).
- Grade asthma as mild, moderate or severe (p 382–385).

X-ray in asthma shows hyperinflation, flattened diaphragm (bilaterally) and prominent bronchovascular markings.

2. What skin lesion is shown? What is wrong with the skin and the eyes? (see Fig. 24.2–24.5)

A: Crazy pavement dermatosis, flaky paint dermatosis and keratomalacia of the eye. The most probable condition associated with crazy pavement dermatosis and oedema is kwashiorkor.

SAM long case is discussed in detail in p 68–72.

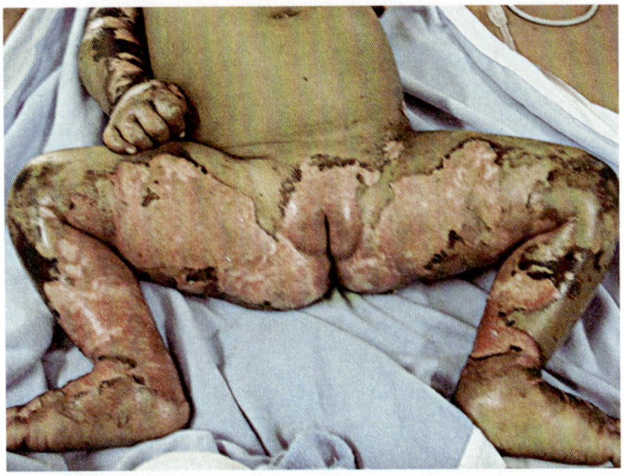

Fig.24.2 Flaky paint dermatosis

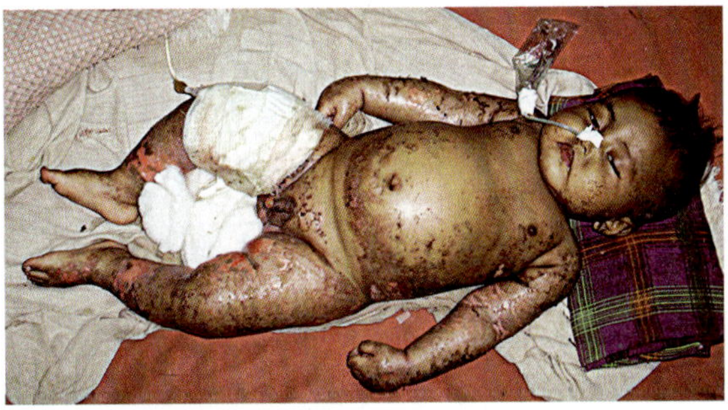

Fig.24.3 Kwashiorkor

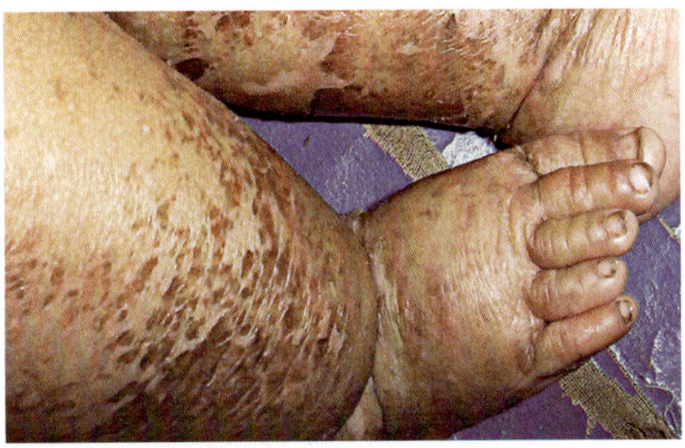

Fig.24.4 Crazy pavement dermatosis. Also see p.70, Fig. 5.1

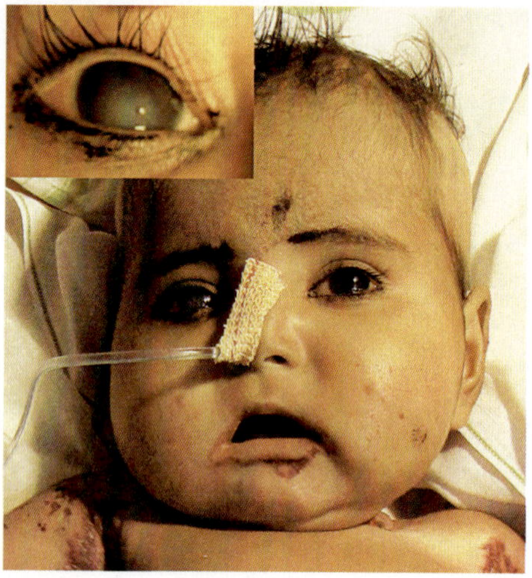

Fig.24.5 Keratomalacia *(Courtesy: Dr Abhilash)*

WHO Classification of Vitamin A Deficiency

- X1A - Conjunctival xerosis
- X1B - Bitot's spots
- X2 - Corneal xerosis
- X3A - Corneal ulcer, involving <1/3rd surface
- X3B - Corneal ulcer, involving >1/3rd surface
- XN - Night blindness;
- XF - Xerophthalmic fundus;
- Xs - Corneal scar.

PEM

Usual complaints are FTT, oedema, etc. The presentation may be due to the precipitating causes like diarrhoea, respiratory infection, measles, etc. If not, one must ask for history of these.

- Low birth weight delivery, inadequate feeding, maternal anaemia, etc, are significant. Look at the nutritional status of the mother. If she appears poorly nourished, it indirectly indicates that the child also may not be getting adequate nutrition. If the sibling is well nourished, then the cause of poor weight is unlikely to be poor diet.
- Maternal education, income, water supply details, whether working mother or not, addictions, etc, help to trace a reason for poor dietary input. Take the breastfeeding history in detail. Was weaning too rapid? If given cow's milk/milk substitute, is the dilution right? (it is best to ask how many days a 500 g tin will last; it lasts for about a week only, if given correctly), Birth spacing: Is the delivery of a second child contributing to PEM of the elder one?
- History of contact with tuberculosis is worth asking for.
- Immunization history must be taken in detail. Look for BCG scar. Remember that many severely malnourished children are under-immunized also.
- Development is usually retarded because of PEM per se. However, with nutritional supplementation it can be reversed.
- Look for potbelly; a wasted marasmic child with potbelly may have coeliac disease; so see if the failure to thrive can be related to the time of weaning.
- Scabies, pyoderma, ear discharge, worm infestation, pica, respiratory infection, diarrhoea, etc, may be associated and must be meticulously inquired into and looked for even when it is not the complaint. When looking for oedema, do not forget to look for oedema over the sacrum and scrotum.
- Take all the anthropometric measurements and do the necessary calculations like weight for height etc. Calipers may not be available in exam hall, but the student should at least make a rough assessment of subcutaneous fat by taking it between the thumb and index finger (usual sites are mid arm, axilla, subscapular region, etc). A similar rough assessment of muscle bulk can be made at biceps or quadriceps.
- Vital signs: Look for peripheral perfusion,

dehydration (look for dry tongue as skin turgor is unreliable), BP (blood pressure is likely to be low). Pulse/temperature/respiratory rate, etc, may be low or high, irrespective of whether there is infection or not. For example, a severely malnourished child with bronchopneumonia may have hypothermia and the respiratory rate may not be fast at all.

- General examination: Fontanel may be open. Give a detailed description of hair, like lusterless, brittle, straight, sparse, lightly pigmented, easily pluckable, etc. Look for flag sign, although it is uncommon to find one.
- Give a detailed description of skin changes. Crazy pavement dermatosis: look at extensor (e.g., shin) aspect for cracks that look like dried paddy field (hypopigmented skin covered with dark patches). Flaky paint dermatosis is more on flexural areas, the hyperpigmented layer of skin coming off like paint leaving behind raw red areas (note the raw areas and hyperpigmented areas in the picture). Also, look for any bleeds, ecchymosis, etc. One may find scabies, pyoderma, fungal infection, bedsores, perianal excoriation, etc, without the mother ever complaining of any of these things. Shiny skin may be because of oedema. Redundant skin folds will be present in marasmus. See p 45 for grading.
- Look carefully at the nail for any flattening/clubbing, etc. Transverse ridge in nail may indicate a period of arrested growth.
- Look for associated deficiencies, like vitamin A (Bitot's spot, dry conjunctiva, etc), vitamin B (angular stomatitis, cheilosis, glossitis, skin rash of extremities, which may be part of pellagra), vitamin K (bruising), vitamin C (bleeding gums, painful limbs), vitamin D (see rickets), iron (pallor). Note that manifestations of vitamin C, D deficiencies are rare in severe PEM. Rickets manifests only when the growth starts.
- GIT: Look at the oral cavity; caries tooth, gum bleeds, penetrating ulcers, etc, may be seen.
- Liver may be enlarged (fatty liver); doughy feel of abdomen may indicate tuberculosis of abdomen.
- Respiratory: Respiratory infections are usually associated and hence look for it.
- CNS: In CNS examination, look for altered sensorium, hypotonia, etc. See if the child is irritable (marasmus) or apathetic (kwashiorkor). Gait abnormality is usually due to hypotonia and weakness, but can rarely be due to deficiencies of vitamin B_{12}, E, etc.
- CVS: Examine heart carefully before committing as normal. There may be a haemic murmur. Microcardia or cardiomegaly with failure may be there. Cardiac failure is especially likely when there is associated B_1 deficiency or severe anaemia.
- Look for organic causes of FTT, like CRF (UTI), poorly controlled asthma, cleft lip or mental retardation affecting feeding, congenital heart disease, etc (see section on Failure to Thrive, p 174).

Notes:

- Anaemia in PEM may be due to deficiencies of iron, micronutrients, protein, suppression of bone marrow by infections, decreased transferrin levels, infections like hookworm, malaria, etc.
- Oedema in PEM could be due to hypoalbuminaemia, anaemia, fluid retention due to ADH, etc.
- Malabsorption in PEM may be due to short atrophied mucosa.

- Hypothermia may be due to decreased BMR, decreased skin fold thickness, decreased substrate like fat for thermogenesis, decreased peripheral perfusion, hypoglycaemia, etc.
- The diagnosis must be given as PEM grade —(kwashiorkor or marasmus if clinically suggestive) acute, on chronic or acute or chronic as evidenced by _________, with complications namely _________ with vitamin _________ deficiencies. The malnutrition is possibly now precipitated by _________ (diarrhoea, respiratory infections, measles, chronic diseases, etc). Etiology being _________ (? faulty feeding)

Investigations

- Blood counts for any evidence of infection, anaemia, malarial parasite, etc.
- Serum albumin may be reduced.
- Electrolytes: Low potassium and magnesium is expected.
- Blood sugar for hypoglycaemia.
- If serum bilirubin is increased, the prognosis is likely to be poor.
- Blood/urine culture: Infections may be there without obvious manifestations.
- Stool for worms, lactose intolerance (pH, reducing substance).
- Be on the look out for tuberculosis and HIV.
- Chest X-ray: Pneumonia may exist without clinical manifestations. In addition, TB has to be ruled out.

Treatment:

- Treat complications (see p 71)
- For hypothermia wrap, place under warmer, frequent feeds, aluminum foil, etc
- Nutrition (see p 71)
- Deworming
- Antibiotics
- Various vitamins, zinc, iron
- Follow-up care in *anganwadis* under ICDS

3.* A child of 1 year old is weaned off breast milk and developed diarrhoea and lesions around mouth and orogenital areas. What is the diagnosis?

A: Vesicobullous and eczematous lesions of perioral and perineal regions suggest the diagnosis of acrodermatitis enteropathica. It may be an autosomal recessive disorder of reduced intestinal absorption of zinc. FTT, diarrhoea and erythematous rash over mucocutaneous junctions are the diagnostic clues for acrodermatitis enteropathica.

4. What clinical finding is demonstrated here?

A: Rosary. It is easier to appreciate the rosary if the arms are elevated as shown in Fig 24.6. Rosary is commonly is associated with rickets. Figure 24.7 shows an unusually prominent rosary. Sharp angulation is expected in scorbutic beads. This is because in scurvy, there is displacement at the joint so that the

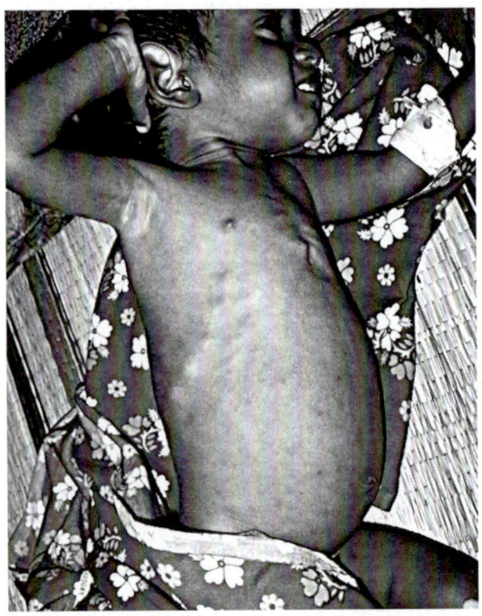

Fig.24.6

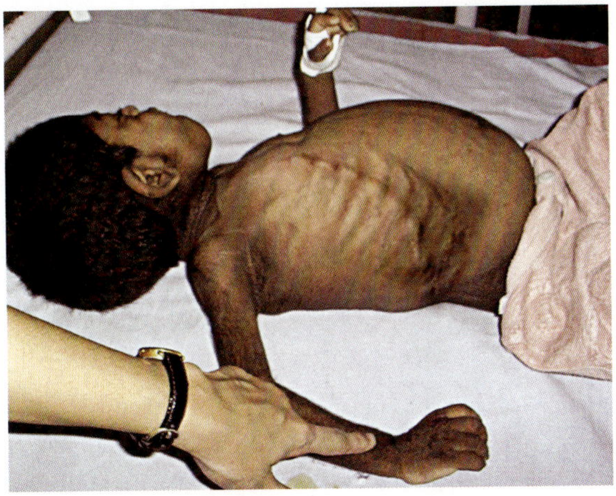

Fig.24.7 Note the rosary

sternum goes down away from ribs to produce a sharp angulation. Rosary of scurvy is painful.

Following is a brief examination-oriented case discussion on rickets can be found in p 72.

Rickets:

The usual complaints may be bowlegs. The student is cautioncd that many a time the child may be having complaints that may not be directly related to rickets. Like the child may come for failure to thrive, PEM, prolonged diarrhoea, respiratory infection, etc, and hence the importance of looking for manifestations of rickets in such cases.

History:

- Milk intake (if not breast milk, whether fortified or not), intake of egg, liver and other meat items.
- Exposure to sun.
- Birth history, whether premature or not (osteopenia is common in prematures).

Note: Now, the student may be confronted with the question as to what is osteopenia. Osteopenia is decreased bone size/mass. In contrast, rickets is failure of mineralization of growing osteoid in the growing bone. Osteomalacia is demineralization of fully grown bone. Naturally, osteomalacia is not osteopenia as the fully grown bone cannot lose its size, but can only lose its mineral!

- History of repeated respiratory infections is obtained very frequently in rickets.
- Excessive forehead sweating is supposed to be common in rickets, the reason for which is not clear.
- History of polyuria or other renal complaints (rickets could be renal).
- History of jaundice/other hepatic diseases/ clay-coloured stools (hepatic rickets is partially due to malabsorption and partially due to the defect in hepatic metabolism of vitamin D).
- History of steatorrhoea/prolonged diarrhoea (malabsorption causing rickets).
- History of tetany (usually history may be as convulsions). Note that it is rare to have tetany in nutritional rickets.
- History of medications (medicines like phenytoin can cause rickets). Some quack medicines may cause renal damage and ultimately Fanconi-like syndrome and hence rickets.
- Bone pain may indicate oncogenous rickets.

Examination:

- From head to foot look for various evidences of rickets.
  - Skull: Craniotabes, bossing, late closure of fontanels, etc
  - Delayed tooth eruption
  - Wrist widening
  - Harrison sulcus
  - Pigeon chest
  - Rosary (discussed elsewhere)
  - Protuberant abdomen, visceroptosis (hence palpable liver, spleen, etc)

- Look at the spine for kyphosis, scoliosis, etc
- Bowlegs; knock knee
- Double malleoli
- Hypotonia

- Look for associated deficiencies like A, B, D, K, etc. It is unlikely that isolated deficiency of only one vitamin occurs.
- Anthropometry is important for the same reason as the child may be malnourished.
- A smart student may look for Trousseau sign/Chvostek's sign.
- Alopecia and onset in early infancy may point towards type II vitamin D dependant rickets.

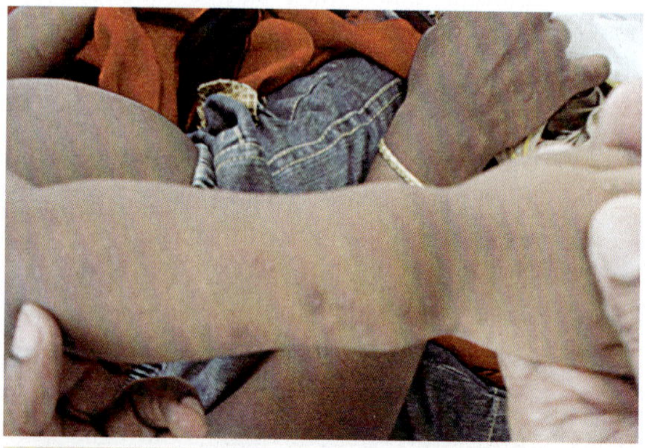

Fig.24.8 Widened wrist

- Manifestations of hypophosphataemic rickets start by the end of first year of life (when tubular function matures to excrete enough phosphate to produce hypophosphataemia) and the signs are usually confined to the lower limbs.

Investigation

- Serum Ca is low normal, phosphorus low and alkaline phosphatase is elevated.
- X-ray changes in rickets is discussed elsewhere (p 567.
- If rickets is not due to nutritional cause, consider RFT, LFT, etc.

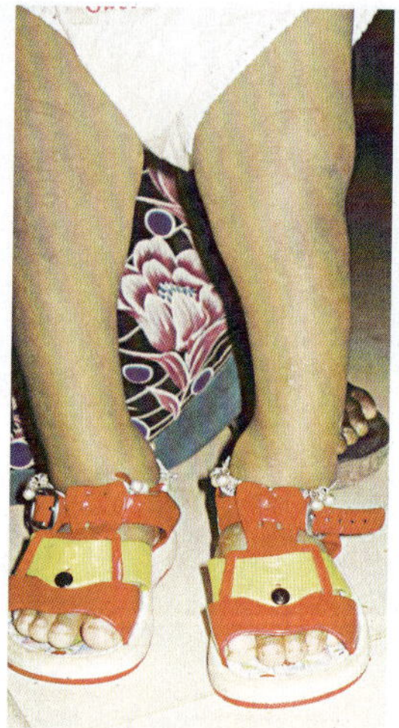

Fig.24.9 Double malleoli

Treatment:

- Vitamin D (see p 75)
- Treat associated vitamin deficiencies, PEM, anaemia, etc
- Dietary/sun light exposure advice
- If breast-fed child develops rickets, supplement mother's diet with vitamin D and calcium.

5. What sign is demonstrated? What is the most common cause of it? How do you treat? (Fig.24.10)

A: There is a rough, dry, wrinkled, grey patch on the temporal side of bulbar conjuctiva. The diagnosis is Bitot's spot. The most common pathological cause of it is vitamin A deficiency. Bitot's spots take a very long time to disappear after treatment.

Treatment

Oral vit A 2 lakh, 2 doses 1 month apart (CSSM) or 2 lakh units each on first 2 days & a third dose of 2 lakh at day 15 (WHO). Keratomalacia requires water soluble vit A 5000 U/kg/day IM for 5 days followed by oral preparation in oil (Nelson's Textbook). WHO Classification of Vitamin A Deficiency (see p 488).

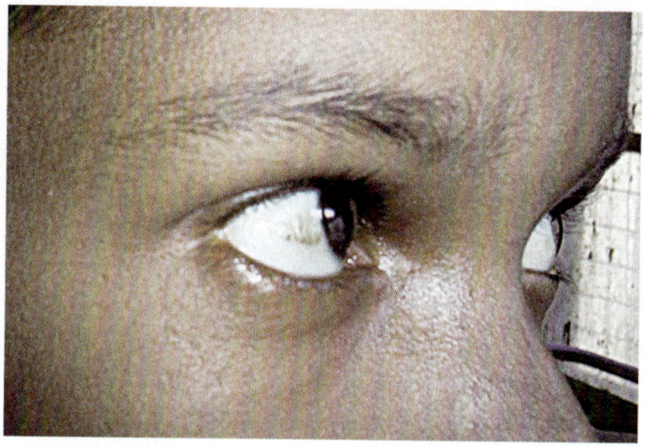

Fig.24.10 Note the lesion in bulbar conjunctiva

6. What clinical sign is demonstrated? (Fig.24.11)

A: Loss of skin turgor. It is a sign of dehydration. It is one of the three star signs of dehydration, the others being restlessness (altered sensorium) and increased thirst. The WHO treatment protocols depending on plan A, B or C can be found in p 417–418 (Fig. 6.28 shows sunken eyes due to dehydration).

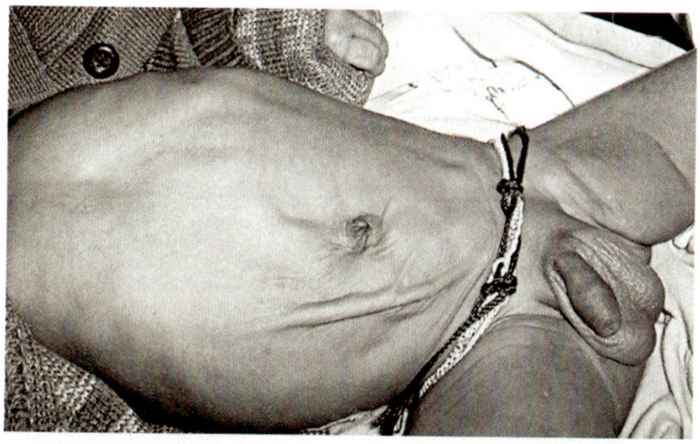

Fig.24.11

7.* An infant of 1 month with a normal birth history, presents with slowly increasing icterus but otherwise perfectly well. The child has hepatosplenomegaly and passes pale stools. What is the diagnosis? What is AIIMS scoring index?

A: See p 413. Progressively increasing jaundice at 1 month of age with hepatosplenomegaly and pale stools put the diagnosis as the so-called neonatal cholestasis. Since the child's general condition is OK, it is most likely to be extrahepatic biliary atresia rather than the neonatal hepatitis syndrome.

- Birth weight: usually small in neonatal hepatitis, but normal birth weight in EHBA.
- Jaundice, usually starting as a prolongation of physiological jaundice.
- Pale stools.
- Look for dysmorphism (Alagille syndrome, Zellweger syndrome, TORCH).
- Look for features of hypothyroidism (it is important because it is an easily treatable cause of prolonged jaundice).
- Failure to thrive and cachexia as the duration of jaundice increases.
- Clubbing and leuconychia.
- Palmar erythema, spider naevi.
- Cyanosis rarely may be there if pulmonary venous shunting is present.
- Excoriations: Deposited bile pigments cause itching. Remember that small infants do not scratch!
- Xanthomata over extensor surfaces and sites of pressure.
- Fat-soluble vitamins: Look for signs of vitamin D deficiency: rachitic rosary and epiphyseal widening. Bruising due to vitamin K deficiency. Xerosis due to vitamin A deficiency.
- Distended abdominal veins.
- Hepatomegaly usually is present but may not be present in advanced cirrhosis.
- Eyes: Cataract (galactosaemia), chorioretinitis (TORCH).
- Splenomegaly usually is present and suggests portal hypertension or it could be part of intrauterine infection.
- Ascites is usually there.

24

- Ask for history suggestive of encephalopathy (altered consciousness).
- Look for CVS findings (e.g., congenital rubella syndrome, Alagille syndrome, etc).

Causes of Neonatal Cholestasis Syndrome

- Extrahepatic biliary atresia (pale stools, deep jaundice but the child looks well). If the child looks ill, think of metabolic or infective cause (see p 414).
- Metabolic: Galactosaemia, hereditary fructose intolerance, α_1 antitrypsin deficiency, tyrosinaemia, etc.
- Choledochal cyst
- Total parenteral nutrition
- Viral hepatitis
- Alagille syndrome
- *E. coli* infection

8.* A 7-year-old child is admitted with history of a second episode of jaundice. He has pallor and hepatosplenomegaly. His viral marker screening is negative. There is history of jaundice to father in the remote past who is now on treatment for neuropsychiatric illness.

A: Wilson disease (hepatolenticular degeneration). History of recurrent jaundice in a child with pallor and family history of jaundice makes one think of haemolytic anaemia. However, family history of neuropsychiatric illness turns the diagnosis strongly in favour of Wilson disease. Pallor with evidence of haemolysis in peripheral smear may be seen in Wilson disease, but pallor is mild and is never to the extent seen in haemolytic jaundice.

AIIMS scoring index is a reliable bedside scoring system to differentiate Biliary atresia from neonatal hepatitis.

Clinical finding		Score
Age	<6 weeks	2
	>6 weeks	1
Jaundice	Fluctuating, mild to moderate	2
	Severe (>8mg/dl)	1
Stool	Normal or light yellow	2
	Clay coloured	1
Urine	Normal or light yellow	2
	Dark yellow	1
Liver	Soft and smooth	4
	Firm	1
Minimum score = 5, Maximum = 12, Total score > 10 suggests Neonatal hepatitis, and <10 Biliary atresia		

- Jaundice
- Family history of jaundice or psychiatric behaviour. Wilson disease is autosomal recessive in inheritance; gene is on chromosome 13.
- Anaemia (low-grade haemolysis) Coombs negative
- Kayser-Fleischer ring (Fig. 6.58, p 104)
- Hepatomegaly or hepatosplenomegaly.
- Look for stigmata of chronic liver disease
- CNS abnormalities: Slurred speech; choreoathetosis, tremor, dystonia, etc; CNS manifestations are very rare in children below 7 years. Change in personality and psychotic behaviour; poor scholastic performance.
- Wilson's disease is a disorder of copper metabolism with reduced biliary copper excretion, low plasma ceruloplasmin and raised urinary copper excretion.

9. This 1½-year-old child (Fig. 24.12) has presented with similar clinical picture twice before. Urine is of normal colour; the child had less frequent urination during daytime, but had been having increased bedwetting at night. What is the diagnosis?

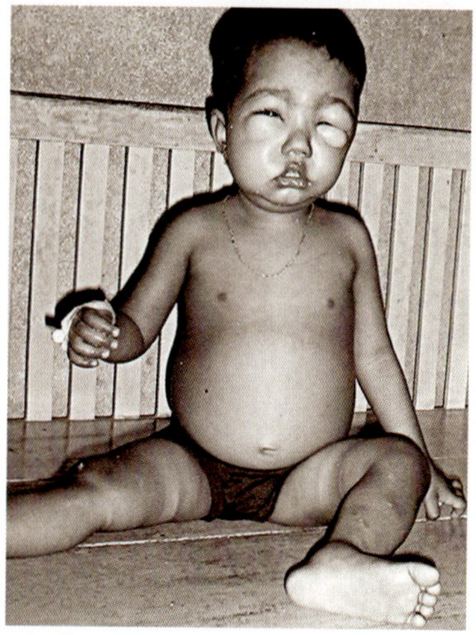

Fig.24.12

A: Nephrotic syndrome. See p 442. The oedema is predominantly over the face and lids with protuberant abdomen, which may indicate ascites. Predominant oedema over the face with history of recurrent episodes is in favour of nephrotic syndrome rather than glomerulonephritis. Also, ascites is uncommon in glomerulonephritis. The differential diagnosis of oedema is discussed elsewhere (p 169). Reason for nocturia: When lying supine, the element of gravity pooling the oedema to the dependant areas is taken off and the oedema fluid from dependant areas gets back to the vascular compartment and gets excreted as urine. Nocturia is more pronounced in cardiac failure where oedema is predominantly dependant. It is rather unusual in nephrotic syndrome, but does occur occasionally as in this case.

- Oedema: Periorbital oedema in younger children. Along with facial oedema, oedema around the ankle and legs is common in older children; do not forget to look for sacral and scrotal oedema.
- Abdominal distension: Ascites and/or hepatomegaly may be present. Hepatomegaly is more common after initiation of treatment with steroid (fatty change).
- Examine the chest carefully; there may be respiratory infection or pleural effusion.
- Check BP: It is normal in most children; there may be postural hypotension; mild hypertension is likely in a minority.
- White bands across the nails, if present, may indicate chronic hypoalbuminaemia.
- Proteinuria (the candidate may be required to check urine himself if this diagnosis is suspected).
- In history, relevant points to differentiate various types of oedema must be brought out (p 169). History suggestive of secondary nephrotic syndrome also must be sought (e.g., SLE, hepatitis B, malaria,

etc). Usually, nephrotic syndrome makes its appearance during an infection. Hence, look for any focus of infection. Severe abdominal pain may indicate peritonitis (classically pneumococcal). Look for steroid side effects like Cushingoid features, striae, etc.

- During remission, the child should be offered optional vaccines like Hib, pneumococcal vaccine, hepatitis B, etc.

10. This child had been suffering from stiff joints, especially in the morning for many months. There are no other complaints.

A: There is swelling and deformity of small joints. Since the duration is many months and definite morning stiffness is obtained in the history, the diagnosis to be considered is juvenile rheumatoid arthritis (juvenile chronic arthritis). The student is encouraged to see p 473–478 for detailed discussion on rheumatoid arthritis **(Fig.24.13)**.

Examine the joint for swelling, warmth and limitation of movements. Examination of joints is discussed in Ch. 22.

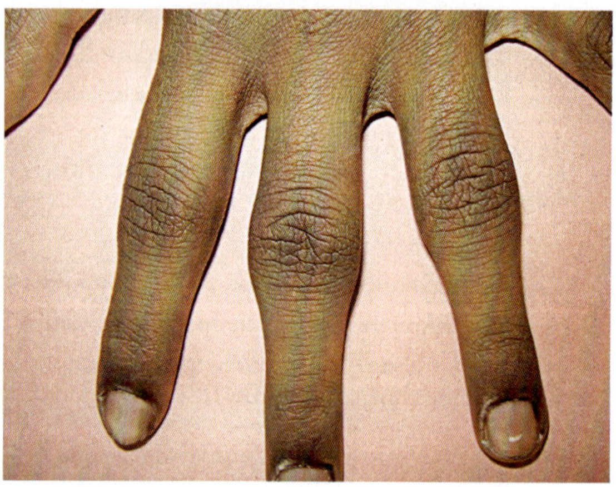

Fig.24.13 Swelling of joints and deformity

Look for the following

- General: Comment on general appearance and growth. Note that joints symptoms of JRA are more troublesome in morning (morning stiffness). The arthritis is non-migratory. Look for wasting of interosseus muscles.
- Skin: Nail pitting (psoriasis); fine red–pink macular rash changing from hour to hour; rheumatoid nodules (look for firm, non-tender, subcutaneous nodules, especially over the extensor tendon of digits).
- Eyes: Iridocyclitis (usually asymptomatic, detected on slit lamp examination) or its sequelae like irregular-shaped pupil (p 93).
- Systemic examination: Look for cardiomegaly, pericarditis, pleuritis, hepatosplenomegaly, lymphadenopathy.
- Limbs: Observe for and comment on: chronic joint deformity; muscle bulk and power; gait.
- Systemic onset rheumatoid arthritis: High spiking fever, intermittent rash and polyarticular arthritis.
- Pauciarthritis (four or less joints are affected when followed up for 6 months) affects mainly toddler girls; larger joints like knee are affected.
- Polyarticular: It is like the typical ones seen in an adult; i.e., small joints are affected.
- Refer to the section on differential diagnosis of arthritis (p 476).

11.* This 12-year-old girl has the rash shown, joint pain, alopecia and red urine. What is the diagnosis?

A: SLE. See p 478 for a brief discussion on SLE.

- General: Peak incidence in childhood is >12 years, with a female preponderance (female : male = 8:1). Various autoantibody associations: antinuclear antibody is positive in most active cases, but anti-dsDNA

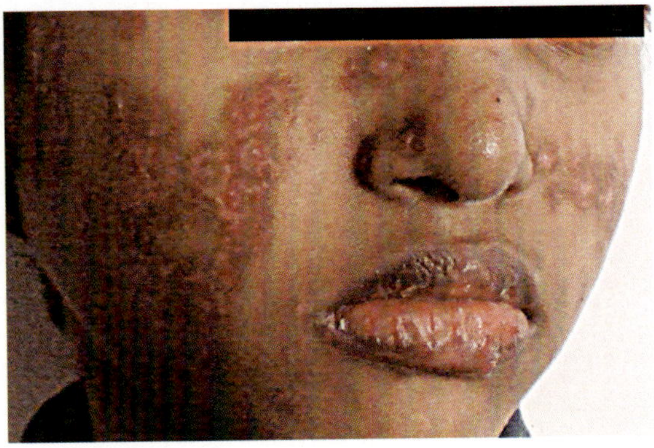

Fig.24.14 Malar rash

is more specific. Constitutional symptoms: Fever, weight loss, fatigue.

- Skin: Various rashes seen, including erythematous rash over malar eminences ('butterfly rash'); maculopapular rashes; ulcers of skin and mucous membranes (usually painless); patchy alopecia; rashes are photosensitive. SLE can be drug induced (e.g., hydralazine).
- Arthritis and/or arthralgia: It is often symmetrical and can involve any joints; arthritis is usually non-deforming. Myositis can occur and may be more painful than the joints.
- Respiratory: Pleurisy (check for 'rub') and pleural effusion.
- CVS: Pericarditis-check for evidence of pericardial rub; hypertension (secondary to renal), endocarditis (Libman-Sacks).
- CNS: Cognitive impairment, chorea, seizures, focal deficits, psychosis, etc.
- Renal: Check urine for haematuria and proteinuria.
- Haematological: Haemolytic anaemia, leucopenia, thrombocytopenia.
- Drug therapies used: Antimalarials, NSAIDs, steroids, azathioprine, cyclophosphamide.

12.* Name two conditions that may result in what is shown in picture (Fig. 24.15)

A: IV fluid extravasation, dactylitis of sickle cell disease, cellulitis, etc. Oedema of hands and feet in a female newborn could point towards Turner's syndrome. Dactylitis has also been described in childhood tuberculosis **(see Fig.24.15)**.

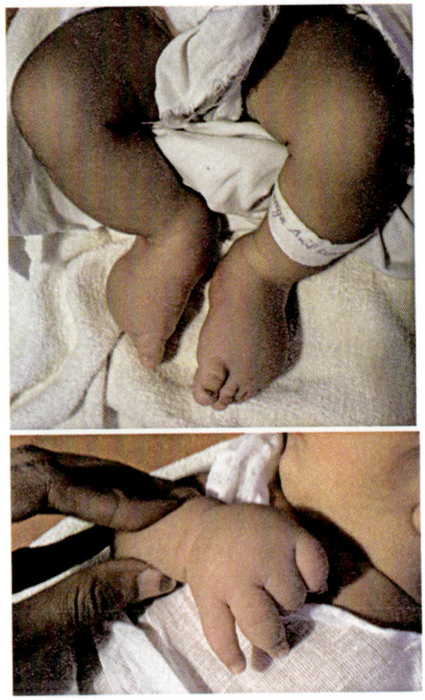

Fig.24.15 Oedema of hands and feet

13.* This child with microcephaly and short stature is being investigated for petechiae and pallor (Fig. 24.16). There is no hepatosplenomegaly or lymphadenopathy. What is the probable diagnosis?

A: Fanconi pancytopenia. The picture shows rudimentary thumb. The associated excess radial deviation could be due to radial hypoplasia **(see Fig.24.16)**. See p 430.

- Pancytopenia, usually occurring beyond 5 years of age*.
- Short stature

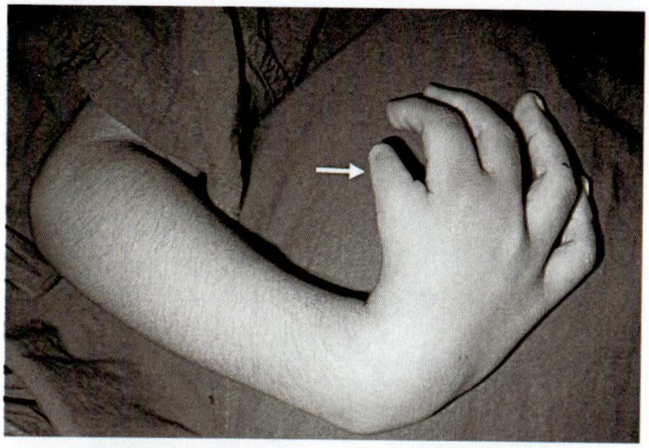

Fig.24.16 Thumb hypoplasia

- Microcephaly
- Strabismus, nystagmus, ptosis, cataracts, small iris.
- Generalized hyperpigmentation* (trunk and neck), cafe-au-lait or hypopigmented patches Fig 6.71, p 108).
- Abnormal thumbs*: Absent, rudimentary or bifid; absent or abnormal radii (hypoplasia of radius is clinically evident by the abnormal radial deviation of hand).
- Hypogenitalism, undescended testes, micropenis, renal anomalies, etc.
- Learning difficulties and developmental delay.
- Autosomal recessive inheritance.
- Enhanced chromosomal breakage. Diagnosis is made by chromosome breakage studies (induced by di epoxy butane).
- May develop malignancy in later age.
- This syndrome resembles thrombocytopenia absent radius (TAR) syndrome. In TAR syndrome, thumbs are *always* present (even when the radius is absent and humerus is severely hypoplastic, the thumb still is present). Holt-Oram syndrome may have similar hand abnormalities, but the associated heart disease clinches the diagnosis.
- Dyskeratosis congenita is different from Fanconi's syndrome. Here, congenital malformations of Fanconi are not there. Dyskeratosis congenita is characterized by hyperpigmentation of skin, leukoplakia of mucous membranes, dystrophic nails and pancytopenia.
- In Wiskott-Aldrich syndrome (affects males as it is X-linked), there is a combination of thrombocytopenia, eczema and recurrent pyogenic infections.

14. This child has reddish spots and abdominal pain (Fig. 24.17). What is the diagnosis?

A: Henoch-Schonlein purpura

- *Palpable* purpuric rash, most commonly on buttocks and extensor surfaces of legs and elbows.
- "PAAN": Purpura, abdominal pain, arthritis and nephritis.
- There may be oedema and excoriations from itching.
- No lymphadenopathy or hepatosplenomegaly.
- May follow an acute infection.

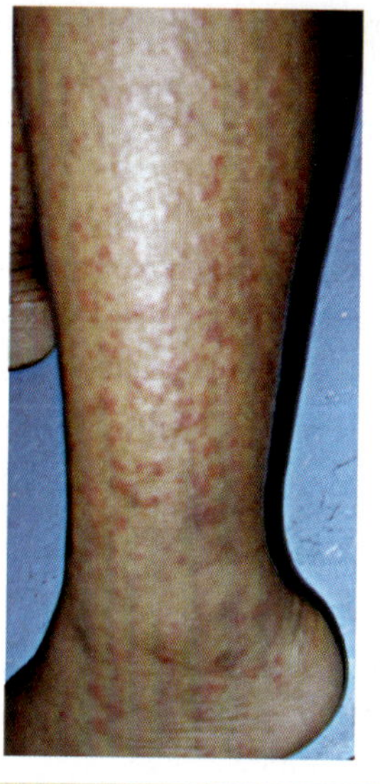

Fig.24.17 Note the elevated purpura

- Normal platelet count.
- Immune complex, type III hypersensitivity reaction.
- Self-limiting in majority of cases.
- Gastrointestinal haemorrhage, intussusception, haematuria and renal failure are complications.

HSP has to be differentiated from idiopathic thrombocytopenic purpura (ITP), which is much more common. The key features of ITP are given below.

- May have preceding viral infection in the 2 weeks before onset.
- Bruises or purpuric rash anywhere on body; purpura is not palpable. Purpura is not blanchable unlike mosquito bite lesion.
- Mucosal bleeding (uncommon but may be a forerunner of CNS haemorrhage).
- Retinal haemorrhage is rare (hence the importance of fundus examination).
- No lymphadenopathy or hepatosplenomegaly.
- Platelet count will be low.
- Gastrointestinal bleeding and haematuria are uncommon in ITP.
- 90% recover spontaneously.
- Immune complex formation and complement deposition on platelets may be the explanation.
- Differential diagnoses include any cause of bone marrow infiltration (e.g., malignancy), bone marrow failure (aplastic anaemia), etc.

15.* This child (Figs. 24.18–24.20) was normal at birth and his height and weight were above normal in the first few months of life. He is now brought because of his odd features and failure to maintain his initial tempo of growth and development.

A: Mucopolysaccharidosis.

Hypothyroidism is a close differential diagnosis. Corneal clouding, hepatosplenomegaly and stiff joints are not expected in hypothyroidism. Given below are the typical features of Hurler syndrome.

- Short stature (deceleration of growth starts by 6–18 months and not at birth)
- Mental retardation (again retardation starts after 6 months of age or later)
- The typical features are due to deposition of mucopolysaccharide and hence it occurs a few months after birth and not at birth.
- Macrocephaly
- Corneal clouding (usually by end of 1 year)
- Coarse facies: Depressed nasal bridge, bulbous nose, prominent supraorbital ridges, large tongue and lips, small widely spaced teeth, large tongue
- Hirsutism
- Hepatosplenomegaly
- Inguinal and umbilical herniae
- Joint contractures, especially the phalanges, elbows, shoulders and hips
- Kyphosis; thoracolumbar gibbus due to anterior wedging of vertebra, which are also short.

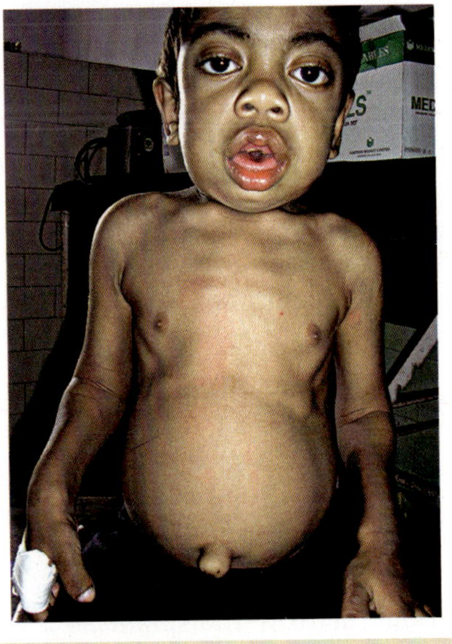

Fig.24.18 Note the face, abdomen and joints

24

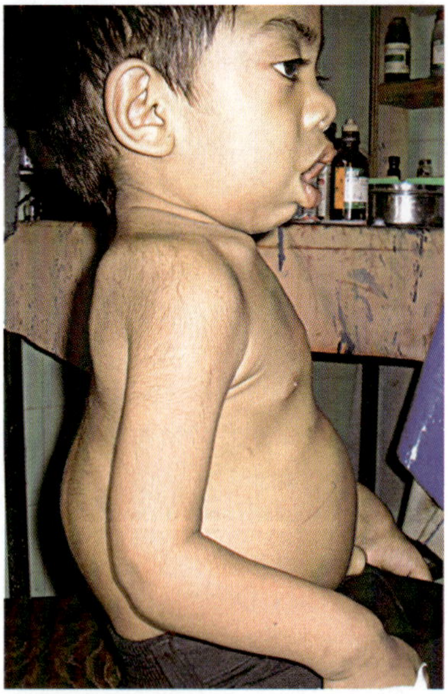

Fig.24.19 Side view

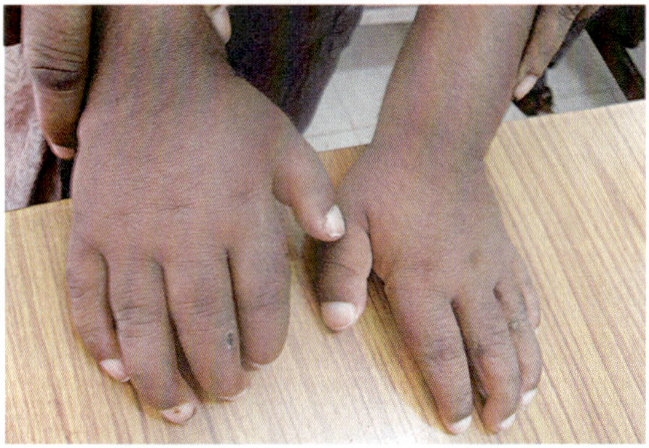

Fig.24.20 Short stubby hands

- Broad irregular bones, especially at metaphysis (see X-ray: p 568).
- Elongated J-shaped sella turcica.
- Cardiac failure from mucopolysaccharide deposition. Cardiac and respiratory decompensation leads to death before 10 years of age in most patients.
- Autosomal recessive.
- Bone marrow transplant as a curative treatment is experimental.

Other Mucopolysaccharidosis (MPS)

- Scheie syndrome: It is like Hurler, but mental retardation is not there.
- Hunter syndrome: Features of MPS is there. However, here the inheritance is X-linked and so only males are affected. There is no corneal clouding and no gibbus (mnemonic: Hunters are males with good vision!).
- Morquio syndrome: Relatively normal intellectual development. Severe joint deformities with visibly enlarged joints, chest deformities and spine deformities. Truncal shortening, kyphoscoliosis, exaggerated lumbar lordosis. X-ray: Conical bases of widened metacarpals, osteoporosis, widened metaphysis and anterio-superior wedging of thoraco lumbar vertebra.

16.* This child was referred because of his recurrent high fever and abnormal dentition. Spot the diagnosis (Fig. 24.21, 24.22).

A: Anhidrotic ectodermal dysplasia. The picture shows conical incisors, sparse hair, prominent forehead, depressed nasal bridge, etc.

- Absent or sparse scalp hair, fine dry and hypochromic; eyelashes also may be affected.

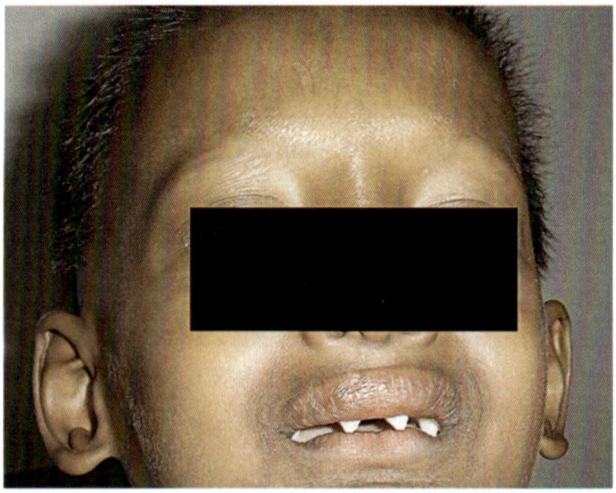

Fig.24.21 Note the hair, eyebrows and teeth

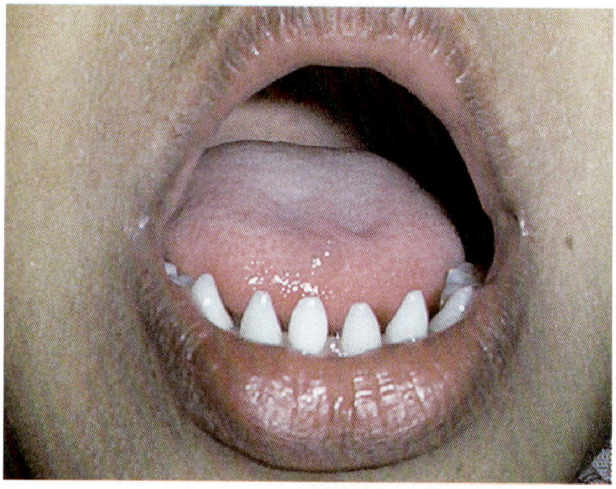

Fig.24.22 Conical incisors

- Cone-shaped incisors
- Delayed eruption of teeth or absent teeth
- Saddle-shaped nose (low nasal bridge)
- Prominent forehead
- Brittle nails
- Usually X-linked recessive inheritance, carrier females may show dental involvement (conical teeth).
- Sweat glands are greatly reduced in number; so, fever is difficult to control and the patient is susceptible to hyperthermia.
- Treatment is symptomatic; artificial tears to prevent corneal damage; regular dental care; prevention of overheating; fever is best controlled with cold sponging.

17.* Spot the diagnosis. Note the striking feature shown in the picture and note that the child is using a hearing aid (not shown in picture).

A: Waardenburg syndrome; there is hardly any other syndrome with localized white hair in forelock. Patches of hypopigmentation of skin seen in the forehead of this mother is also described in this syndrome.

- Heterochromia
- White hair in forelock*
- Sensorineural deafness
- Autosomal dominant inheritance

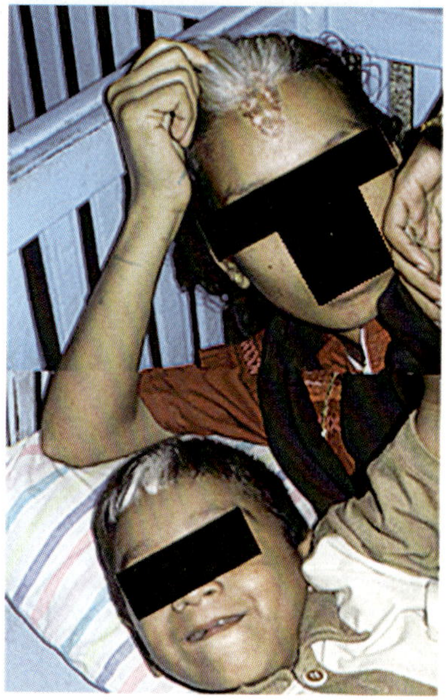

Fig.24.23

18.* Spot the diagnosis.

A: Cleidocranial dysplasia. There is hardly any other condition where shoulders can be approximated in front.

- Defects of clavicle* (partial or complete aplasia; so there is hypermobility of the shoulders so that shoulders can be approximated in front).
- Large cranium with delayed closure of fontanels and sutures*; Frontal and parietal bossing; Brachycephaly.
- Hypoplasia of the maxilla.
- Midfacial hypoplasia.
- Delayed dentition*.
- Narrow upper thorax and drooping shoulders.
- Long second metacarpals and tapering distal phalanges.
- Normal intelligence.
- Autosomal dominant inheritance with a variable expression or new mutations.
- Radiologically, wormian bones may be seen.

24

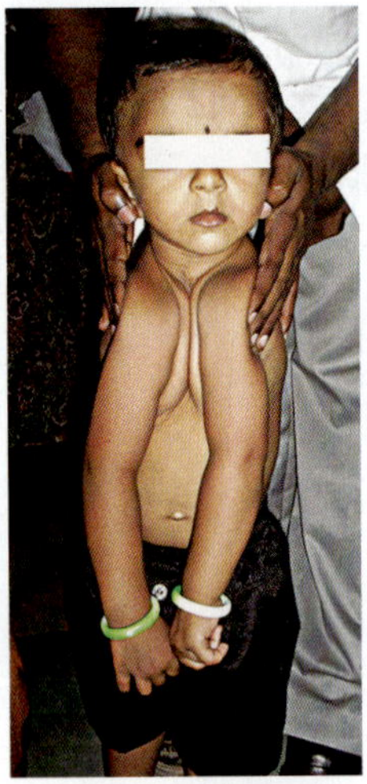

Fig.24.24a Approximation of shoulders is possible due to absence of clavicle

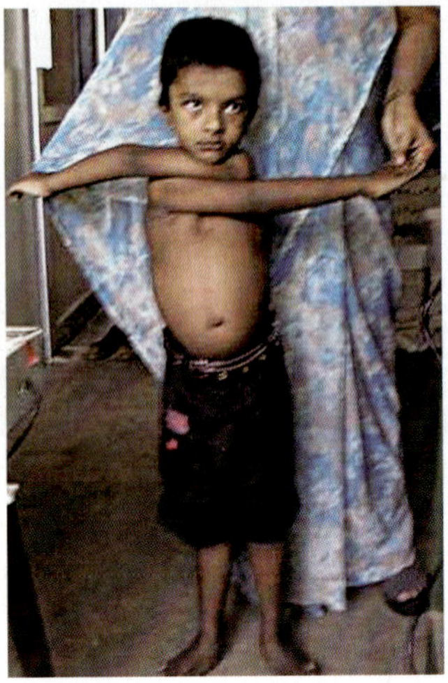

Fig.24.24b Cleidocranial dysplasia

19.* **What sign is being demonstrated? In which syndrome is it seen? What clinical feature does this syndrome have in common with osteogenesis imperfecta?**

A: Hyperextensibility of skin. Ehlers-Danlos syndrome. Blue sclera is found in both Ehlers-Danlos syndrome and osteogenesis imperfecta.

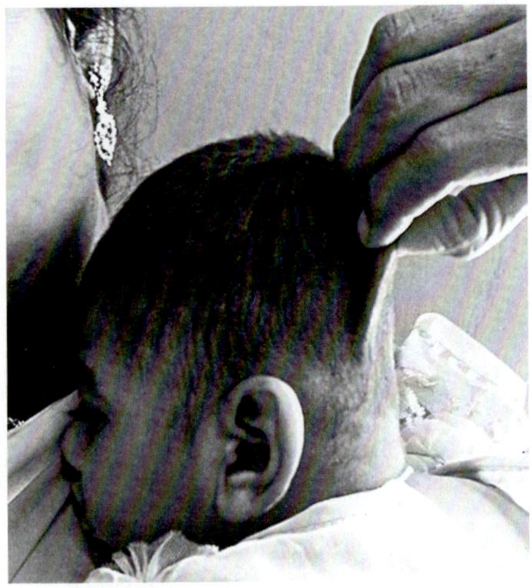

Fig.24.25 Elastic skin

- Marked skin hyperextensibility (but no redundant folds).
- Hyperextensibility of joints (hypermobility of joints).
- Increased skin fragility; slow-healing leaves 'cigarette paper'-like scars. Skin looks velvety.
- Very elastic and pliable ears
- Easy bruisability: May have skin and soft tissue haemorrhage.
- Small movable subcutaneous spherules may be palpable over the knees and elbows.
- No mental retardation.
- In cutis laxa, there is widespread redundant folds of lax skin (obvious without the examiner pulling the skin; in Ehlers-Danlos, the skin is not lax when left alone, but is hyper-extensible when pulled). Hypermobility of joints is not there in cutis laxa.

20.* This child is now brought with fracture lower limb. The child has history of many previous similar episodes. What is the diagnosis? What is an important complication apart from the bony lesions?

A: Osteogenesis imperfecta. Recurrent fractures without apparent reason hardly has any other differential diagnosis. Deafness is an important complication.

There are four major types of osteogenesis imperfecta. Type 1 is inherited as autosomal dominant; biochemically, there is a defect in the production of type I procollagen. Type II is the severest form and often is stillborn or has early neonatal death. Type III is autosomal recessive.

Type IV is autosomal dominant with normal sclerae but similar bone disease to type I. Type I is the most common and the following discussion is mainly on type I.

- Blue sclera.
- Fragile bones that are prone to fractures. The picture shows deformity of long bones due to old fractures.
- Hypermobility of joints, especially small joints of hands and feet.
- In type IB there is opalescent, often a yellow–brown coloured teeth that is easily cracked or worn (dentinogenesis imperfecta). Teeth in type IA are normal.
- Hearing is often impaired (usually conductive but can be mixed).

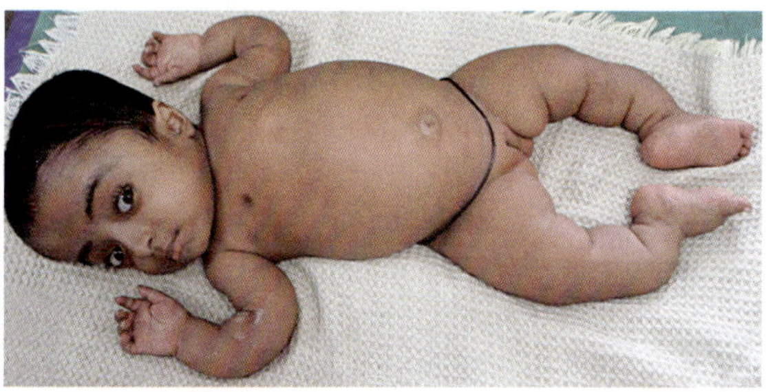

Fig.24.26 Note the abnormality of the limbs

- There may be tendency to easy bruising.
- X-rays may show wormian bones in skull and generalized osteopenia. The skull is large for body size with large fontanels.
- Aortic regurgitation and mitral valve prolapse may occur.
- Majority have had fractures before 5 years of age; 10% have fractures at birth.
- Life span is normal.
- There is no mental retardation.

21.* What is the abnormality demonstrated?

A: There is flattening of the right chest and hypoplasia of nipple. These abnormalities plus syndactyly is the classical feature of Poland sequence. 24

- Ispilateral aplasia or hypoplasia of pectoralis major. Ipsilateral aplasia of breast tissue or ribs may be there.
- Unilateral hand malformation: Syndactyly/oligodactyly.
- Most cases are sporadic.

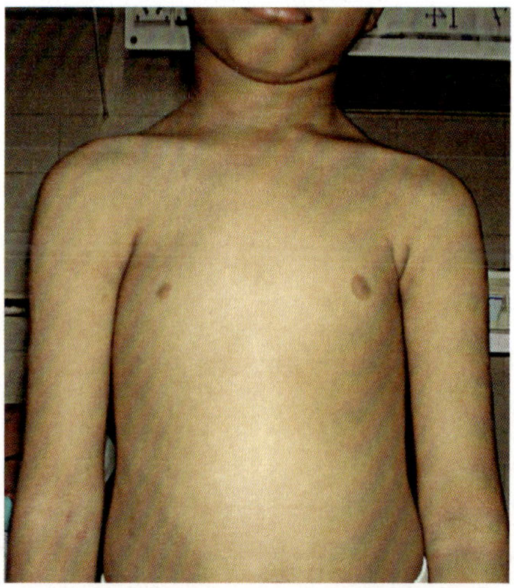

Fig.24.27 Compare the two sides of the chest

22.*What abnormality is demonstrated (Fig.24.28)? In which condition is this finding likely to be associated?

A: In the picture of the hand, the ring finger is shorter than the index finger (normally the reverse is true). Both the ring and little finger appear to be placed more proximally than the other fingers. It could be due to shortening of the 4th and 5th metacarpals. This is typical of Albright hereditary osteodystrophy (pseudohypoparathyroidism).

- Short stature.
- Mental subnormality.
- Round face and short neck.
- Obese.
- Metacarpal and metatarsal shortening, especially the 4th and 5th; this may result in dimpling on dorsum of hand see X-ray: p 535.
- Subcutaneous calcifications; ectopic calcification of basal ganglia may be seen in CT.
- May have delayed tooth eruption and enamel hypoplasia.
- Cataract.
- Hypocalcaemia may or may not be there. Hypocalcaemic tetany may be there.
- Autosomal dominant inheritance.
- Treatment is with oral calcium supplements and vitamin D analogue.
- Pseudospseudohypoparathyroidism: Patients have the clinical features but not the biochemical abnormalities.

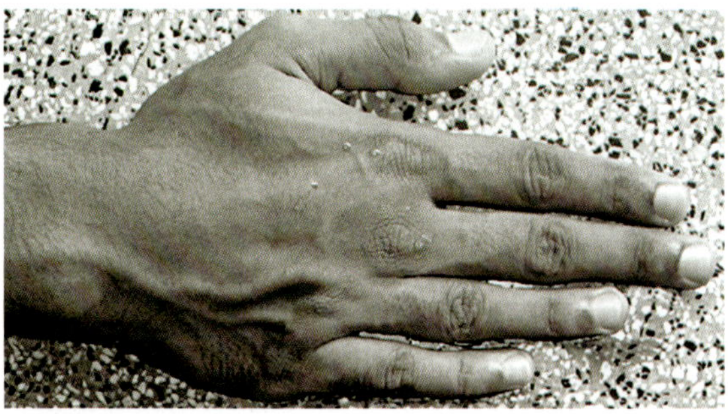

Fig.24.28 Make a note of finger lengths

23. * The picture is of a child who expired in the neonatal period. What is the abnormality shown? What is the basic anatomic defect that produces this? Which syndrome is it associated with?

A: Abnormality shown in **Fig. 24.29** is rocker bottom feet. It is classically described in Edward's syndrome (trisomy 18). The basic anatomic defect is vertical talus. **Fig. 24.30** shows over- riding toe.

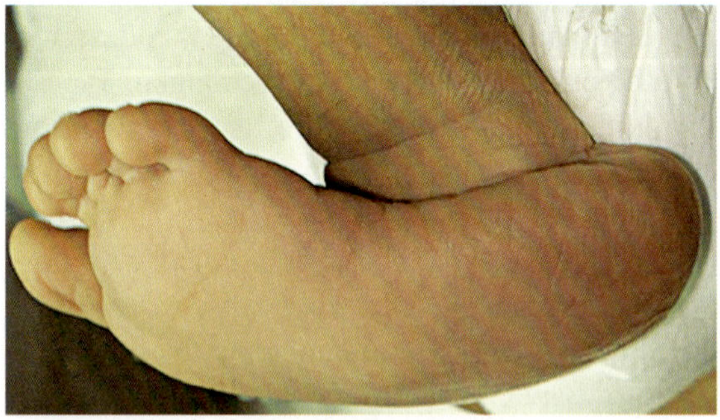

Fig.24.29 Note the shape

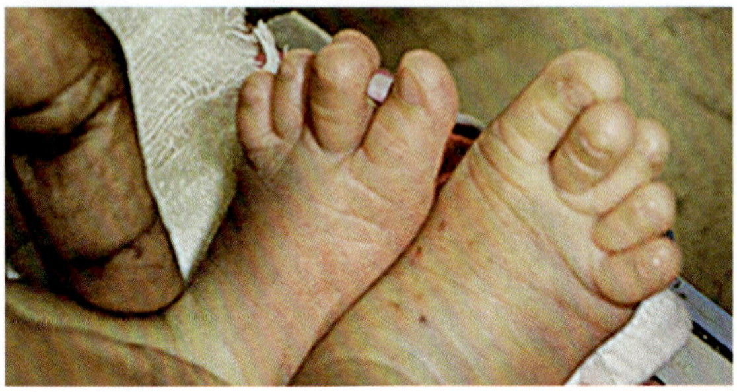

Fig.24.30 Overriding of toes

The other features of Edward's syndrome are:

- Low birth weight
- Microcephaly
- Decreased subcutaneous fat*
- Prominent occiput*
- Hypertonia*
- Rocker bottom feet*
- Small palpebral fissure
- Low set malformed ear

- Micrognathia
- Clenched hands with overlapping digits*
- Short dorsiflexed hallux*
- Cardiac anomalies
- Like all non-dysjunction trisomies, trisomy 18 is also more common with advanced maternal age.

24.* A tall adolescent boy with gynaecomastia and delayed puberty has presented himself for evaluation. What is the most probable diagnosis?

A: Eunachoid habitus, gynaecomastia and delayed puberty points towards Klinefelter syndrome (XXY). They have long limbs and hence have a reduced upper/lower limb ratio. They have hypogonadism (infertile); prone for carcinoma of breast. The extra X chromosome may be from father or mother. Depending on whether the dysjunction is maternal or paternal, advanced maternal or paternal age may be a risk factor for its occurrence.

25.* This child is brought for evaluation of mental subnormality, unsteady walk and bursts of uncontrollable laughter. Spot the diagnosis.

A: The presentation is typical of Angelman (happy puppet) syndrome. It is not the photo that clinches the diagnosis, but the presentation.

- Happy appearance but on careful observation one will find that the laughter is inappropriate.
- Characteristic arm posture (arm upheld and flexed at elbow and wrist, resembling a puppet) and jerky ataxic movements and gait.
- Prognathism
- Maxillary hypoplasia (midface hypoplasia)
- Large mouth with tongue protrusion
- Widely spaced teeth
- Microbrachycephaly
- Hypopigmented hair

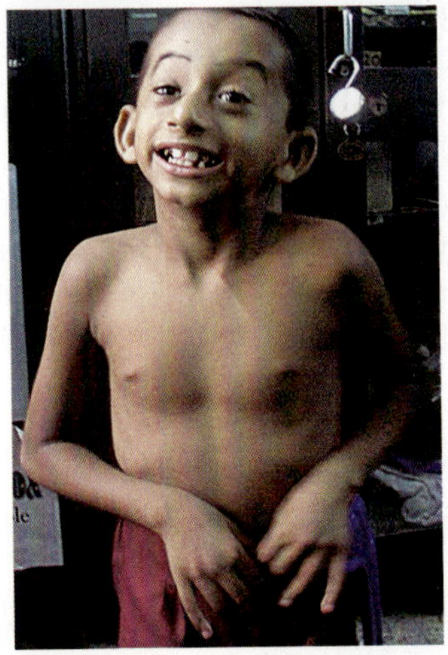

Fig.24.31 Angelman syndrome *(Courtesy: Dr PAM Kunju)*

- Deep set eyes
- Hypotonia
- Growth and developmental retardation
- Seizures
- Inheritance is by an absence of maternal contribution to chromosome 15 (15q11–13) due to either a deletion or paternal uniparental disomy (i.e., the child inherits both chromosome 15 from father and none from mother). In Prader-Willi syndrome, the same deleted segment is paternal in origin.

26.* A baby with a birth weight of 4.2 kg is brought with convulsions on the first postnatal day. What maternal history must be inquired into? What is the possible diagnosis and what is the reason for convulsions?

A: Infant of diabetic mother. The most common pathological cause for a very large birth weight is poorly controlled maternal diabetes. Such children may develop hypoglycaemia (may develop seizures) soon after birth.

The features of infant of diabetic mother are:

- Neonatal macrosomia*

24

- Hairy pinna **(Fig. 24.32)**.
- Caudal regression syndrome (hypoplasia of sacral region and lower limbs).
- Neonatal fetal complications are high, like hypoglycaemia, hypocalcaemia, polycythaemia, etc; complications due to the big size include birth trauma and birth asphyxia.

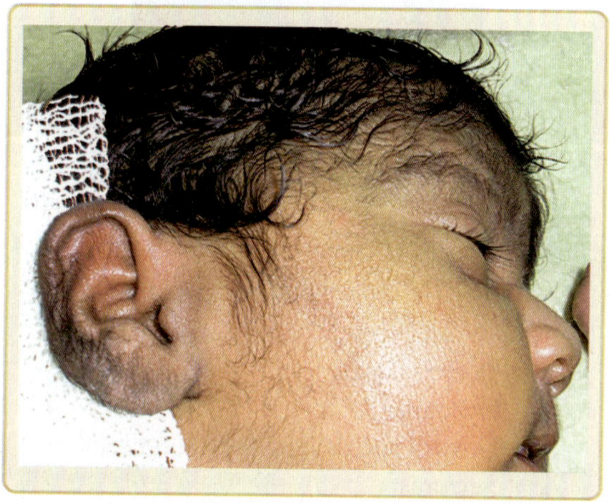

Fig.24.32 Hairy pinna

27.* Spot the diagnosis of this child who had a birth weight of 4.2 kg and developed neonatal hypoglycaemia.

A: Beckwith-Wiedemann syndrome. The picture shows gross macroglossia, horizontal fissure of ear lobe and capillary nevus of central forehead **(Fig.24.33)**.

- Neonatal macrosomia*
- Macroglossia,* which gets leveled off as the child grows
- Linear horizontal ear lobe crease*
- Capillary naevus flammeus of central forehead or eyelids
- Organomegaly
- Neonatal hypoglycaemia may result in mental retardation
- Has a tendency for the development of malignancy like hepatoblastoma and gonadoblastoma and hence has to be followed up with ultrasound of abdomen and α-fetoprotein.
- May have abdominal wall defects like diastasis of recti, umbilical hernia, omphalocele,* etc.

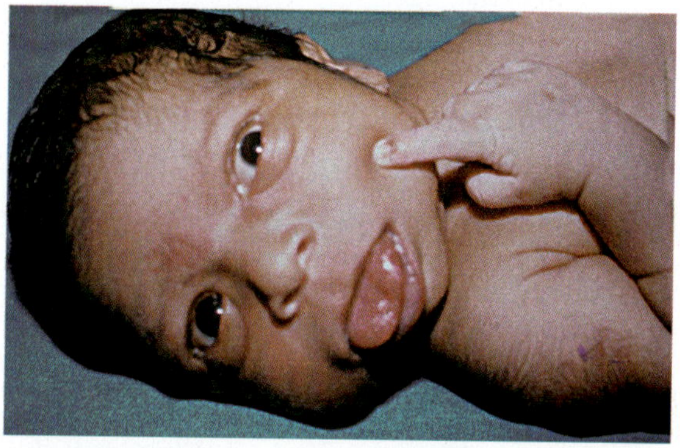

Fig.24.33 Note the facial features

28. What problem is this newborn baby having? (Fig. 24.34).

A: This is a collodion baby, a serious form of icthyosis. The baby is covered at birth by a thick taut membrane resembling oiled parchment or collodion. It may crack with initial respiratory efforts, failing which the baby will have severe distress. The membrane sheds

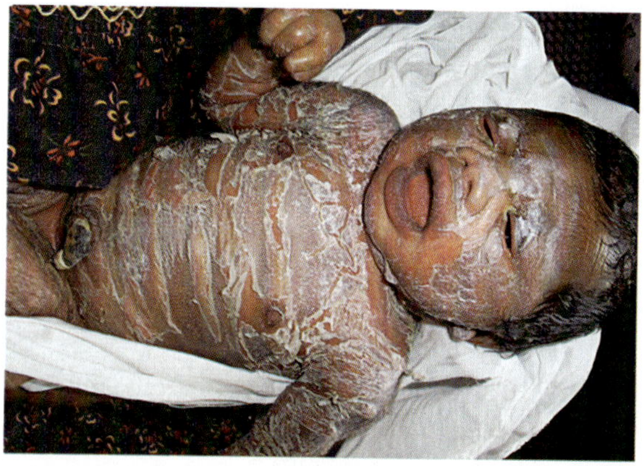

Fig.24.34 Note the skin changes

after several weeks, and gets replaced with new membranes of less extensive nature. Rarely, near normal skin may ensue.

29.* What is the diagnosis?

A: Cornelia de Lange syndrome. The picture shows small nose with anteverted nostrils, depressed nasal bridge, long philtrum, thin upper lip, limb malformation (like lobster hand), synophrys, etc. **(Fig. 24.35)**

- Prenatal onset growth retardation (short stature)
- Microbrachycephaly
- Generalized hirsutism with hair whorls over arms and posterior trunk
- Synophrys* (eyebrows meet in midline) with bushy eyebrows; long curly eyelashes
- Small nose with anteverted nostrils and depressed nasal bridge
- Long philtrum
- Thin upper lip; down turned corners of mouth*
- Micrognathia
- Late erupting hypoplastic teeth
- Limb malformation*
    - Micromelia
    - Phocomelia and oligodactyly/syndactyly
    - Proximal implantation of thumbs
- Simian crease
- Clinodactyly
- Abnormal genitalia
    - Hypoplasia
    - Undescended testes
    - Hypospadias
- Mental retardation
- VSD
- Inheritance is usually sporadic

30. Spot the diagnosis.

A: Down syndrome. Down may have up-slanting palpebral fissures and epicanthic folds. Other features in this picture are low set ears, depressed nasal bridge and hypertelorism. The clue to the diagnosis is typical flat facial profile, which to an experienced clinician strikes at first sight. Flat facial profile is better appreciated on lateral view **(Fig.24.40)**. Single crease, hypoplasia of middle phalanx of little finger **(Fig.24.37)** and deep crease between 1st and 2nd toe **(Fig.24.38)** are also shown. The clinical features can be memorized from hand to head and head to toe as follows.

Hands → back of head (flat occiput) → top of head (wide fontanels) → inside head (mental retardation) → nasal bridge (flat) → eyes → ears → mouth (protruding/furrowed

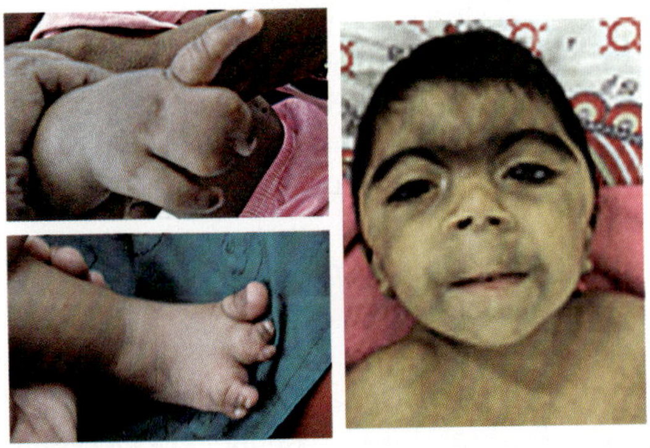

Fig.24.35 Note the facial features and the limb

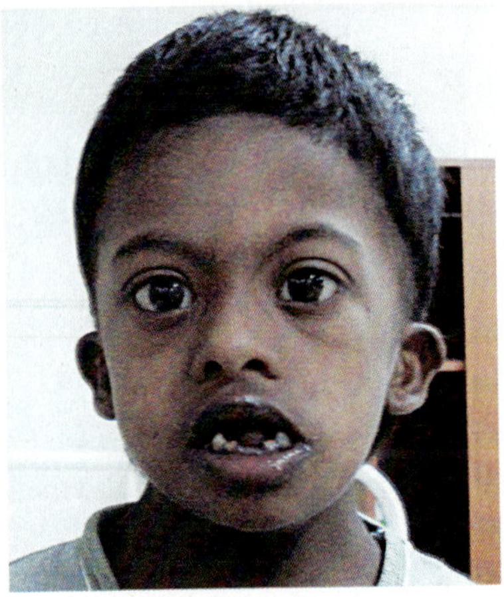

Fig.24.36

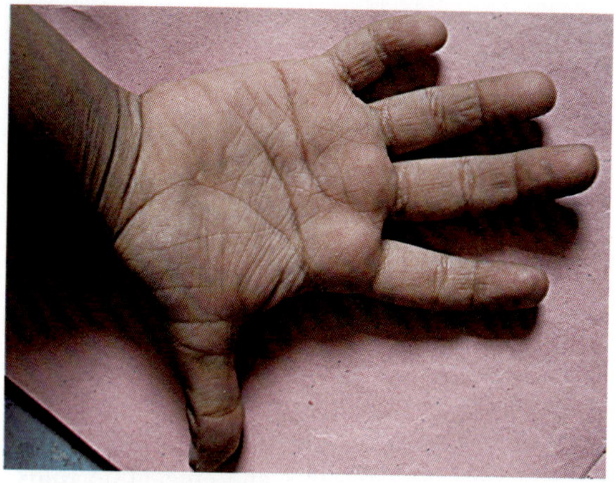

Fig.24.37 Note the little finger

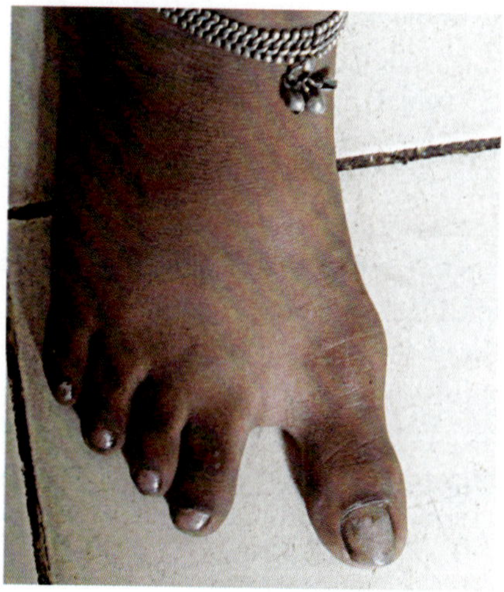

Fig.24.38 Sandal space

tongue) → neck (thyroid, atlanto-axial instabitity) → chest (heart diseases) → abdomen → feet.

- Mental retardation*
- Hypotonia*
- Short stature
- Upslanting palpebral fissures*
- Epicanthic folds (look at the medial canthus)
- Brachycephaly. Flat occiput is better appreciated when looked at in a lateral profile
- Brushfield spots (look for speckled iris). Note that it is rare in Indians **(Fig.24.41)**.
- Cataracts: Often they are in the periphery, not obstructing the vision; fine opacities may need slit lamp for identification and hence often missed in clinical examination.
- Mouth held open with protruding tongue. It seems tongue protrudes out due to relative lack of space in the small oral cavity. Tongue may be furrowed.
- Flat nasal bridge (hence there may be an apparent hypertelorism).
- Ears apparently low set; may be malformed.
- Single palmar crease (Simian crease, **Fig.6.128a, p 130**). Sometimes, two creases may be there but unlike the normal, the proximal one extends to full width of palm (Sidney line).
- Short broad hands. Distal triradius (p 129).
- Clinodactyly or curved fifth finger. Often the 5th middle phalanx bone is shortened and hence its occurrence.
- 'Sandal' gap between first and second toes. Deep crease between the two (Kennedy crease, shown in **Fig.24.39**, **6.128b**).
- Congenital heart disease: AV canal defect is characteristic. VSD is almost equally common. Specifically look for features of pulmonary hypertension as Down children are prone for early development of pulmonary hypertension; rarely tetralogy of Fallot.
- Increased risk of leukaemia (AML and ALL).
- Premature dementia (Alzheimer's disease).
- Duodenal atresia, anal atresia (in newborn).
- Hypothyroidism.
- Atlantoaxial instability.
- Types of Down: Trisomy 21 (95%), translocation (4%), mosaic (1%).

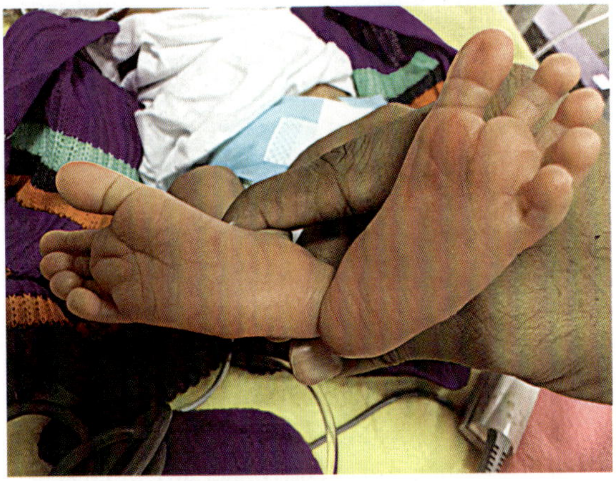

Fig.24.39 Kennedy crease

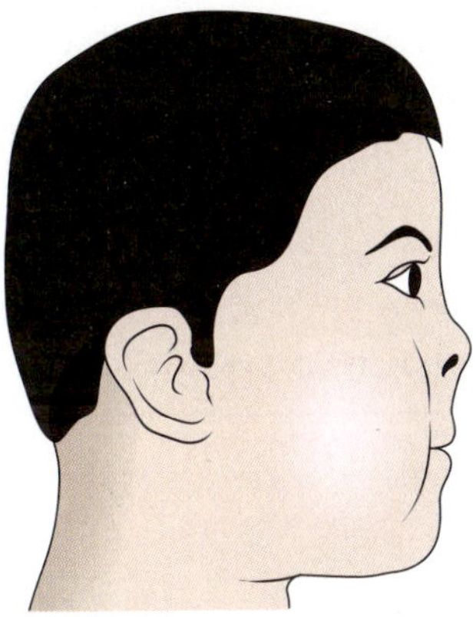

Fig.24.40 Flatness of face and occiput are best appreciated on side profile

- Increased risk with increasing maternal age—approximately 1 in 350 at 35.
- Antenatal diagnosis: Serum α-fetoprotein and unconjugated cortisol are decreased and HCG and inhibin-A are increased. This is quadruple test done at 16–20 weeks. Triple test avoids inhibin-A. Ultrasound: Nuchal fat pad thickness 1st trimester tests (11–12 weeks) include fetal USG (increased nuchal translucency), decreased pregnancy associated plasma protein A (PAPP-A) and elevated β-HCG.
- 2nd trimester: major and minor anomaly markers.
- See case discussion p 146.

31.* Identify the clinical sign that is demonstrated.

A: Brushfield spots. Described in Down syndrome (see p 508). It can rarely occur in otherwise normal child. **(Fig.24.41)**

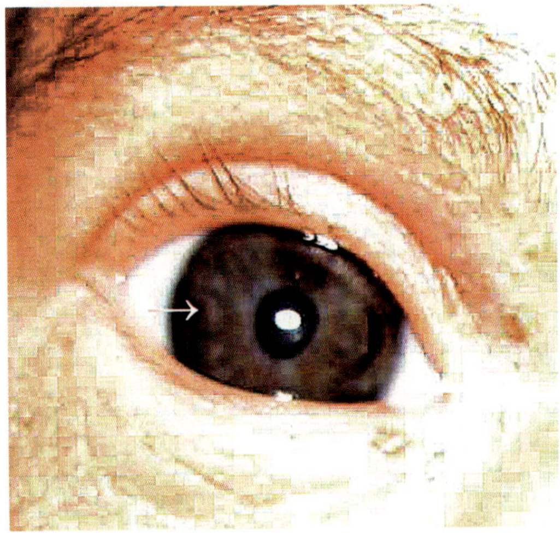

Fig.24.41 *(Courtesy: Dr Sheela Nampoothiri)*

32.* What abnormalities are seen in the hands, mouth and chest?

A: Ellis-van Creveld syndrome. The picture shows polydatyly of both limbs and a narrow thorax. Figure 24.43 shows multiple frenulae. **Note:** Although not related to this case, it is worth mentioning here that lack of frenulum and single incisor tooth may be indicative of holoprosencephaly.

- Short limbs*; short stature of prenatal onset.
- Small thorax; small thorax may cause respiratory embarrassment **(Fig. 24.42)**
- Postaxial polydactyly* (Fig. 6.100, p 120)
- Hypoplastic nails*
- Multiple frenulae **(Fig. 24.43)**

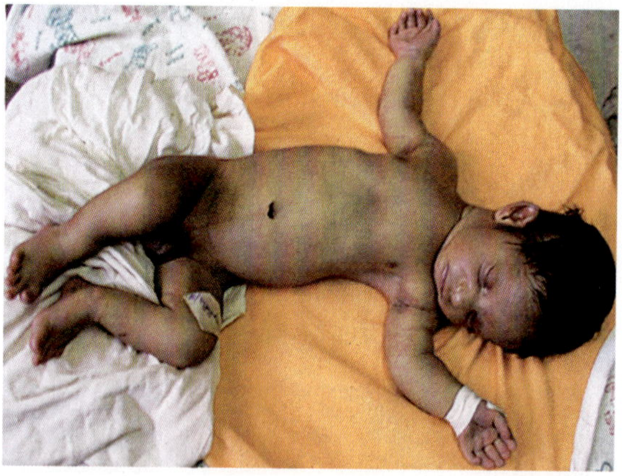

Fig.24.42

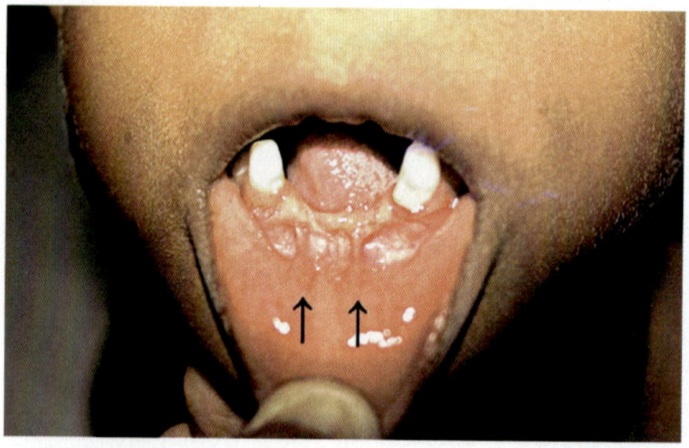

Fig.24.43

- Delayed eruption of teeth, neonatal teeth or anodontia.
- Intelligence is normal.
- Congenital heart defects (present in 40%; atrial septal defect is the most common). Single atrium also may be associated.
- Autosomal recessive inheritance

33. * What is the diagnosis?

A: Goldenhar syndrome (facio-auriculo-vertebral spectrum; first and second branchial arch syndrome). The picture shows malformed ear, skin tag, cleft-like extension of corner of mouth and epibulbar dermoid.

- Facial defects are predominantly unilateral (hemifacial microsomia; there is hypoplasia of facial musculature, usually unilateral).
- Lateral cleft-like extension of corner of mouth (macrostomia).
- Malformed pinna.
- Preauricular skin tags or pits; usually found in a line from tragus to the corner of mouth.
- Epibulbar dermoid
- Microphthalmia
- Coloboma of eyelid (upper lid). In Treacher Collins syndrome, coloboma is in the lower lid.

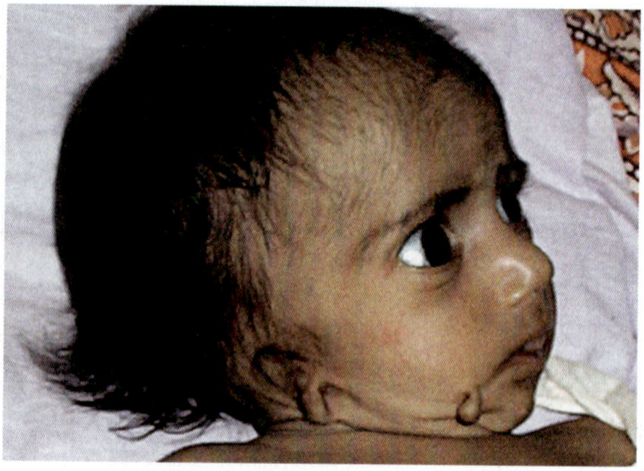

Fig.24.44

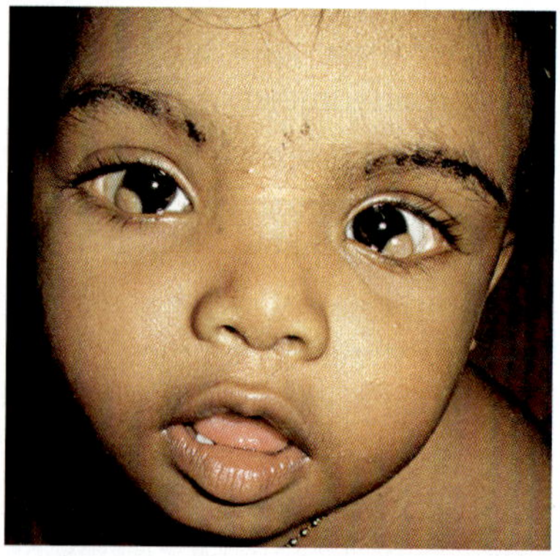

Fig.24.45 Epibulbar dermoid

- Hypoplasia of malar (hypoplastic zygomatic arch), maxillary and/or mandibular regions.
- Deafness, which may be conductive or sensorineural.
- Cardiac malformations including ventricular septal defect, PDA and Fallot tetralogy.
- Vertebral anomalies (hemi/hypoplastic vertebrae).
- Cleft lip and palate.
- No mental retardation.
- Inheritance is sporadic.

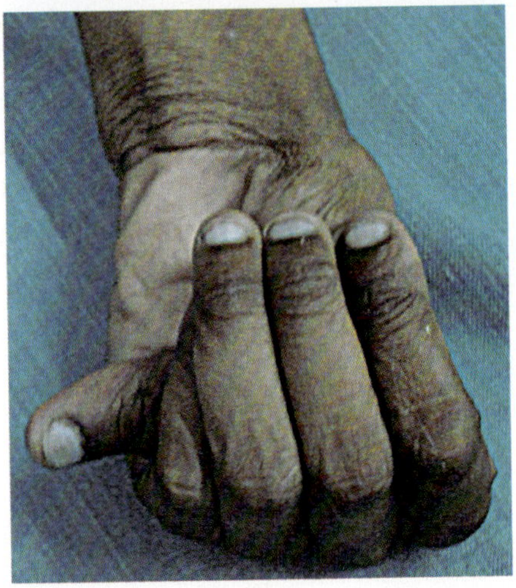

Fig.24.46 Steinberg sign

34.* What are these signs called and in which condition are these signs positive?

A: Steinberg's sign **(Fig.24.46)**. This sign is seen in Marfan syndrome, although *very rarely* it may be demonstrable in a normal child.

- Tall and slim with very little subcutaneous fat.
- Arm span > height.
- Long thin arms (dolichostenomelia).
- Long and tapering fingers (arachnodactyly).
- Thumb and 5th finger overlap around wrist with the complete overlap of distal phalanx of the 5th finger on the distal phalanx of the thumb (wrist sign, **(Fig. 24.47)**; this complete overlap will exclude normal children with apparently positive wrist sign.
- Thumb extends beyond the ulnar border of hand when opposed across palm (Steinberg's sign).
- Joint laxity, which may result in recurrent dislocation.
- Pectus excavatum or pectus carinatum.
- Kyphoscoliosis.
- High-arched palate.
- Eyes: Ectopia lentis (upward subluxation of lens); usually wears myopic glasses. Clinically present with symptoms of refractory error. Mnemonic to memorize the direction of lens dislocation: visualize a child urinating; urine goes down; thus it is easy to remember that in homocystinuria the lens goes down! Marfan is very tall; now associate tallness with the upward displacement of lens in Marfan!

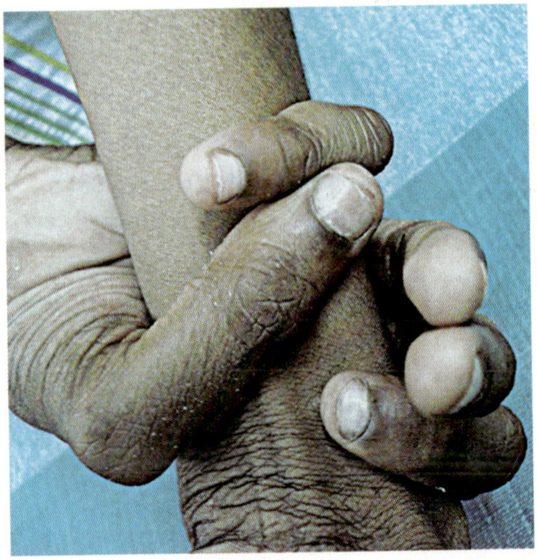

Fig.24.47 Wrist sign

- CVS: MVP or AR or MR.
- Autosomal dominant with variable expression. Mutation in fibrillin gene in

chromosome 15q21.3. Advanced paternal age is suspected to be associated.

- Distinguished from homocystinuria by direction of lens subluxation, absence of mental retardation and lack of homocystine in urine. Homocystinuria mimics Marfan morphologically, but in homocystinuria the dislocation of lens is downward (inferior and nasal), has tendency to multiple thrombotic episodes and has mental retardation.

35.* Note the facial features of this 5-year-old boy who has been referred for evaluation of an ejection systolic murmur with a click at pulmonary area. He has no CVS related symptoms. Mother has history of some congenital heart disease, which was operated at around 20 years of age. What is the probable diagnosis?

A: Noonan's syndrome. The features obvious in the picture are partial ptosis (also note the raised eyebrows due to frontalis acting to keep the lid elevated), hypertelorism and down slanting palpebral fissure. Mother's heart disease may have been ASD or PS, both of which being asymptomatic may result in delayed surgery by the patient. **(Fig.24.48)**

- Short stature
- Epicanthic folds
- Downward slanting palpebral fissure
- Partial ptosis
- Hypertelorism
- Short webbed neck
- Low hairline posteriorly
- Pectus excavatum or carinatum
- Shield chest
- Cubitus valgus
- Small penis, cryptorchidism
- Oedema of dorsum of hands and feet (rarely)

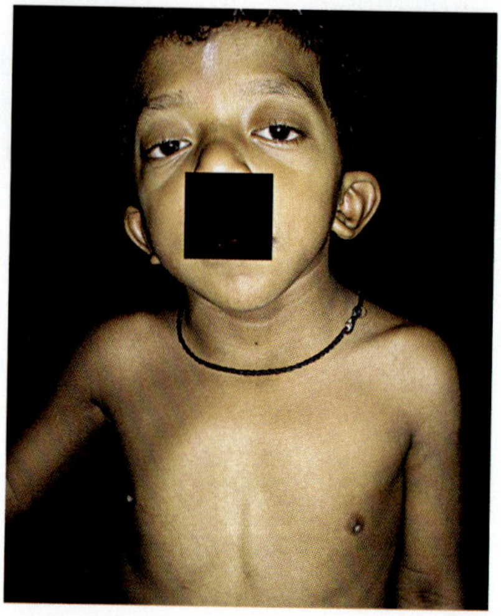

Fig.24.48 Note features in face & chest

- Congenital cardiac defects (80%): Pulmonary stenosis, HCM, atrial septal defect.
- Mild mental subnormality (Turner has normal intelligence).
- Karyotype is normal (XO in Turner). Usually, sporadic inheritance; can be autosomal dominant with variable expression; occurs in males and females (Turner occurs in females only). However, it is prudent to exclude Turner syndrome mosaic in female Noonan. Normal sexual maturation is expected; with a possible mild delay (Turner is sterile).

36.* What heart disease is this child likely to have?

A: ASD; this abnormality of hand is due to the absence or severe hypoplasia of radius, which along with ASD will fix a diagnosis of Holt-Oram syndrome (refer to p 536 for a short discussion). Note that the thumb on one side is finger like and the thumb is absent on the other side. In contrast, in TAR syndrome thumb will always be present despite of radial hypoplasia.

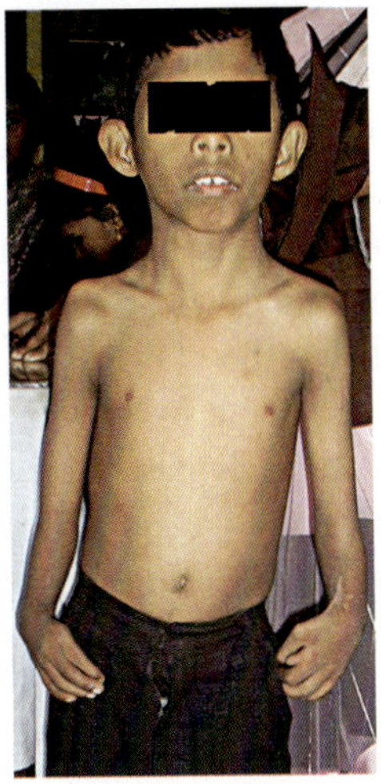

Fig.24.49 Note the hands

37.* This child is admitted in newborn ICU for respiratory and feeding difficulty. The child has a cleft palate as well. What is the diagnosis?

A: Pierre Robin sequence. Please refer to case with VACTERL association for explanation of the term "sequence" (p 514). Feeding problems are due to the cleft palate and the airway obstruction is due to the tongue falling back into the pharynx.

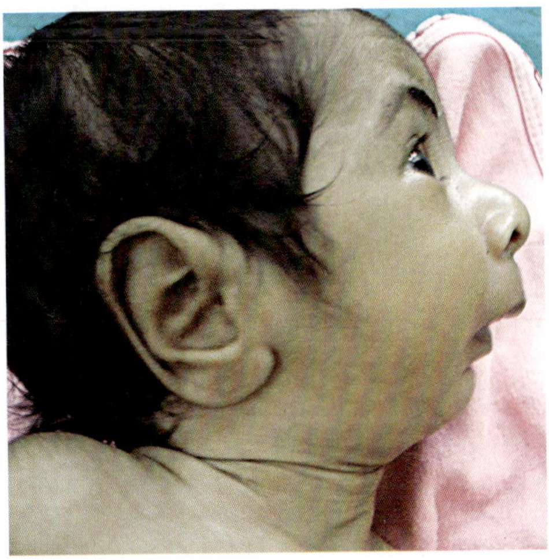

Fig.24.50 Pierre Robin sequence

- Micrognathia
- U-shaped cleft palate (the usual cleft palate is V shaped) **(Fig.24.51).** The U shape is produced by the tongue that is falling back.
- Congenital heart disease may be an association.
- Sporadic inheritance.

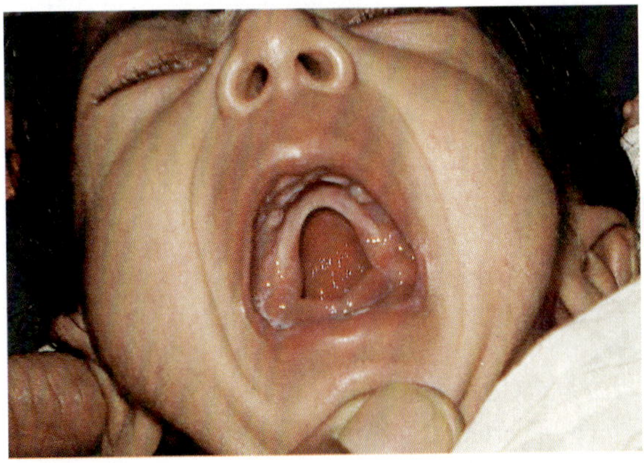

Fig.24.51 U-shaped cleft palate

38.* What is the abnormality seen in this picture?

A: Wrinkled abdominal wall stands out in sharp contrast to the rest of the body. Diagnosis is prune belly syndrome. Sex is not clear from the picture but it should be male. To understand how prune belly looks like, visualize the

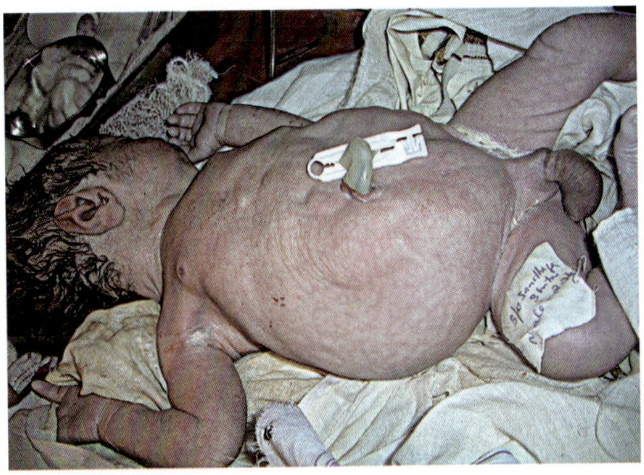

Fig.24.52

wrinkled surface of dried grapes. Prune belly looks exactly like that but feels totally soft, very different from dried grapes.

- Skin hangs in wrinkled folds because of deficient abdominal wall musculature.
- Various urinary tract abnormalities and constipation are usually associated. Kidneys may be palpable due to hydronephrosis.
- Cryptorchidism.
- Usually sporadiac in occurrence.

39. * The child shown here was operated for anorectal malformation. The picture shows limb anomalies and marked scoliosis. Auscultation of heart reveals a murmur. What is the diagnosis?

A: VACTERL association

V—Vertebral: hemi or bifid vertebrae (see Fig. 25.45); Hypersegmentation (13–14 ribs/thoracic vertebrae; 6–7 lumbar vertebrae); marked scoliosis in the above picture could mean vertebral anomalies.

A—Anal; anorectal malformation

C—Cardiac; ventricular septal defect, tetralogy of Fallot

T—Trachea; tracheo-oesophageal fistula

E—Oesophageal: oesophageal atresia

R—Renal; hydronephrosis, renal dysplasia, vesicoureteric reflux

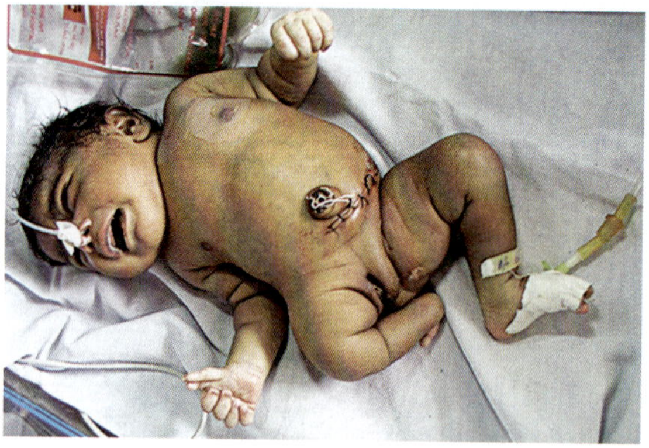

Fig.24.53

L—Limb: radial dysplasia

VATER anomaly is without cardiac and limb components.

Note: Associations refer to non-random but significant grouping of malformations without known aetiologies (e.g., VACTERL association). It may be that at some point of intrauterine life some insults result so that totally unrelated body parts under development at that particular time get affected. Syndrome is a pattern of malformations that are recognized to result from a specific cause. (e.g., trisomy 21). Sequence refers to a cascade of multiple deformities, all developing because of a single initiating abnormality. For example, in Pierre Robin sequence, the basic abnormality is small mandible, which in turn results in small chin, backward displacement of tongue, cleft palate, obstruction of airway, etc.

In Potter sequence, the initiating event is oligohydramnios. Thus, face gets compressed as though a nylon stocking has been pulled through the face. Because of oligohydramnios, there is not enough fluid to fill up the lung and hence there is pulmonary hypoplasia. As fluid is too little to allow the fetus to move around, there will be joint contractures.

The term 'malformation' implies a structural defect due to a developmental abnormality; the part was never normal. For example, anencephaly, duodenal atresia, congenital heart disease, etc. Deformation means abnormal form or position of a body part that was initially formed normal, deformed by mechanical forces. Examples are clubfoot, DDH, etc. Disruption means interference with the originally normally formed body part (e.g., amniotic band).

Below are given the features of **CHARGE** association:

- **C**oloboma of retina, choroids, lens or optic nerve

- **H**eart defect, e.g., patent ductus arteriosus, atrial septal defect, ventricular septal defect
- **A**tresia choanae (unilateral or bilateral)
- **R**etarded growth/development or both
- **G**enital anomalies in males (cryptorchidism, micropenis, etc.)
- **E**ar anomalies or deafness
- Facial nerve palsy/other cranial nerves
- Mental retardation
- Micrognathia

40.* An obese school-aged child presents for evaluation. Her birth weight was low, had poor feeding and failure to thrive during infancy. After infancy, the child started to have increased appetite and put on weight. Her school performance is below normal. She is short for the age and the obesity is mainly central with tapering extremities. What is the diagnosis?

A: Prader-Willi syndrome. Failure to thrive in infancy followed by obesity later is the typical natural history of Prader-Willi syndrome. If the obesity is due to simple overeating, the child should have been tall and obese, not short and obese. The distribution of obesity of this child is unlike the obesity of Cushing's syndrome. Mental subnormality is not a feature of either Cushing or exogenous obesity.

- Obesity beyond infancy; usually there is hyperphagia; obesity is especially over the lower abdomen, buttocks and thighs.
- Short stature
- Small hands and feet
- Mental retardation
- In neonates and infants, the major sign is hypotonia; it results in poor feeding and may even lead to failure to thrive. Obesity manifests later when the child is 1 year or later.
- Birth weight is normal or low. Reduced fetal movements and breech presentation are common.

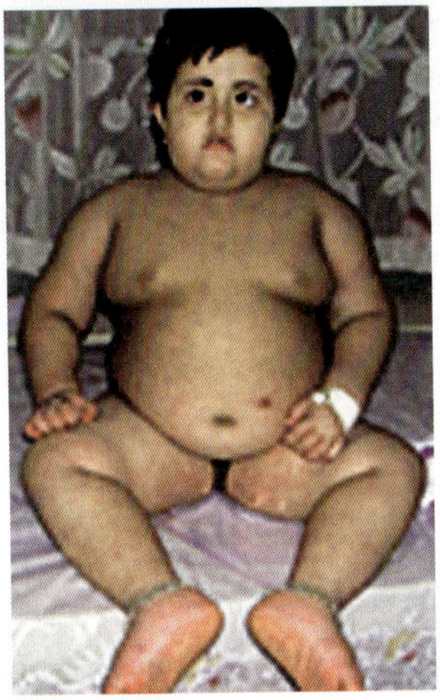

Fig.24.54

- Almond-shaped palpebral fissures.
- Hypogonadism/cryptorchidism.
- Prone for diabetes mellitus in later life.
- Inheritance due to absence of paternal contribution to chromosome 15 (15q11–13), as a result of either deletion or maternal uniparental disomy (also refer to Angelman syndrome, p 505).

41.* A short obese child with polydactyly is referred to child psychologist for assessment of IQ because of mental retardation. See Fig. 24.56 & 24.57. What is the probable diagnosis?

A: Laurence-Moon-Biedl syndrome. Polydactyly gives the clue to the diagnosis.

- Short stature.
- Obesity: Obesity may not present until after infancy (same is the case with Prader-Willi).
- Polydactyly.
- Hypogonadism (deficiency of gonadotrophins).
- Visual impairment usually is late to manifest and starts as difficulty in night vision (retinitis pigmentosa).
- Mental retardation.

42.* This child with mental subnormality was brought for evaluation. The picture shows mild ptosis (compensated by the frontalis action), strabismus, posteriorly rotated ears, broad nasal bridge and broad thumbs. What is the diagnosis?

A: Rubinstein-Taybi syndrome. It is essentially the broad thumbs that clinch the diagnosis (Fig. 24.55).

- Short stature
- Broad thumb and first toe
- Clinodactyly of 5th finger
- Microcephaly
- Downward slanting palpebral fissure
- Ptosis
- Strabismus
- Prominent 'beaked' nose
- Broad nasal bridge
- Hypertelorism
- Posteriorly rotated ears
- High-arched palate
- Proportionate short stature
- Mental retardation
- Cardiac anomalies, e.g., ventricular septal defect, patent ductus arteriosus
- Poly/syndactyly (rare)
- Inheritance is sporadic

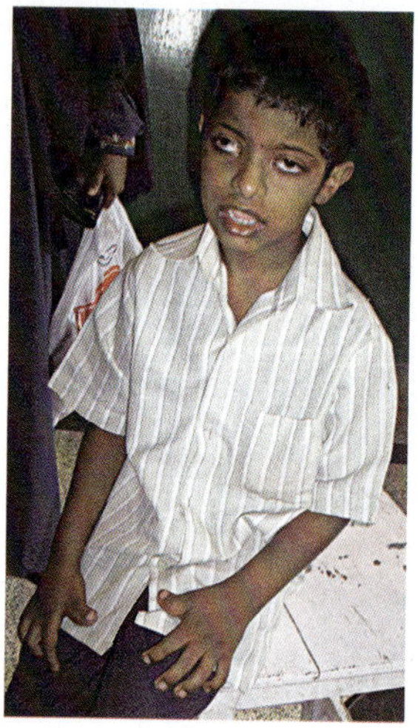

Fig.24.55 Note the thumbs.

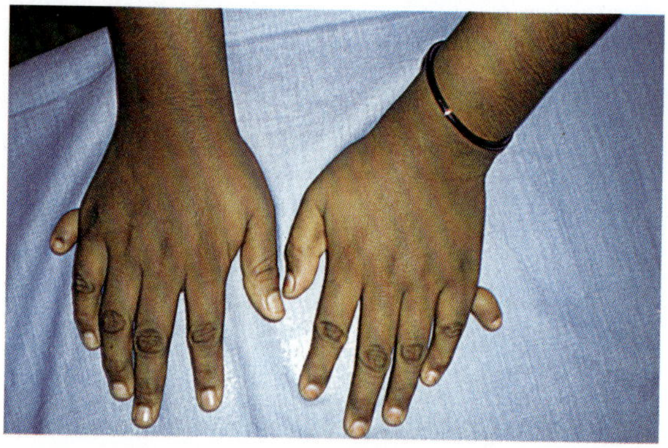

Fig.24.56 LMB syndrome *(Courtesy Dr Raji RP)*

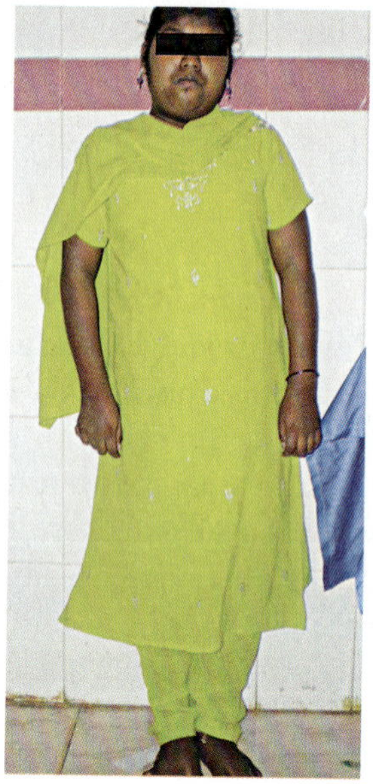

Fig.24.57 Laurence Moon Biedl syndrome

43.* A child is brought for evaluation of severe short stature but normal intellect. He was small at birth and continues to be small. He has a triangular facies, clinodactyly of 5th finger and cafe-au-lait spots.

A: Russell-Silver syndrome tops in the list of differential diagnosis. Hypothyroidism has mental subnormality as one component, especially when the onset is early in infancy. Mention of clinodactyly of 5th finger and cafe-au-lait would not have been there in the question if growth hormone deficiency or hypothyroidism were the diagnosis.

Russell-Silver Syndrome

- Short stature of prenatal onset, growth slowly improves as the child matures.
- Small triangular face with down-turned corners of mouth. Because of the small face, the upper head may appear large although the head circumference is normal.
- Thin lips.
- Clinodactyly of 5th finger.
- Syndactyly of second and third toes (see p 121).
- Skeletal asymmetry—can involve entire one side of body or be limited, e.g., to a limb.
- Cafe-au-lait spots.
- Normal intelligence.
- Inheritance is usually sporadic; some familial dominant cases have been described.
- Seckel syndrome simulates it in some aspects; but in Seckel, the short stature is severe, there is mental retardation, microcephaly, dental abnormalities (anodontia/ enamel hypoplasia) and prominent nose.
- Cockayne syndrome: Growth is normal in infancy; then it falters. There is loss of subcutaneous fat in face to give "old man" look. There is mental retardation, visual defects, photosensitive dermatitis, etc.

44.* Spot the diagnosis.

A: Treacher Collins syndrome. The picture shows malar hypoplasia, downslanting palpebral fissure, lower lid coloboma, absence of lower lid eyelashes and preauricular skin tag.

- Downward slanting palpebral fissures*
- Lower lid coloboma*
- Partial or total absence of lower eyelashes
- Malar hypoplasia*
- Mandibular hypoplasia (view the side profile)
- Dysplastic auricles, often with skin tags or fistula*
- External ear canal defects (conductive deafness may be there)
- Cleft palate
- Majority of cases have normal intelligence
- Inheritance is autosomal dominant with variable expression; 50% of cases represent fresh mutations

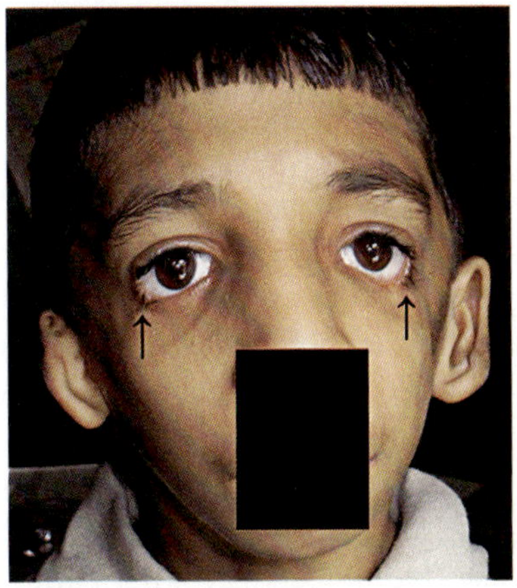

Fig.24.58

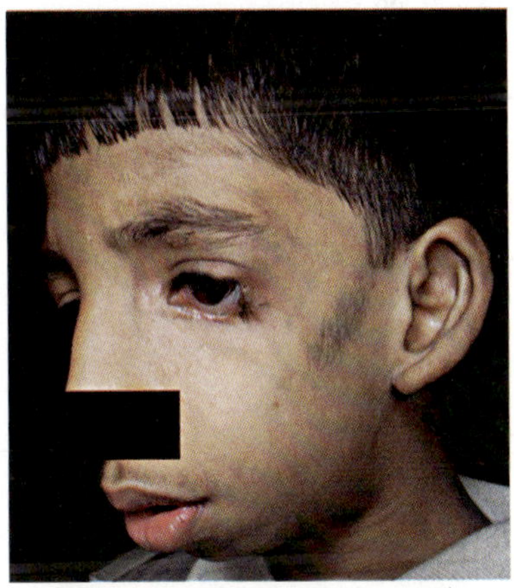

Fig.24.59

45.* Spot the diagnosis.

A: Turner syndrome. The picture shows short webbed neck, broad chest with widely spaced nipples, pectus excavatum and ptosis. Note the frontalis overaction to compensate for ptosis. This patient has downslanting eyes also, more commonly described with Noonan than Turner. For long case discussion, see p 148.

- Short stature in a female child*
- Low posterior hairline
- Short webbed neck
- Broad chest (shield-like chest)
- Wide-spaced, often hypoplastic nipples
- Narrow maxilla
- Small mandible
- Cubitus valgus
- Narrow, convex and deep set nails (note that this is not clubbing; hyperconvex nails may be seen in Noonan's syndrome as well).
- Renal anomalies, most commonly horseshoe kidney.
- Cardiac defects (20%): Coarctation of aorta, bicuspid aortic valve, valvular aortic stenosis. Check femoral pulses and four-limb blood pressure to rule out coarctation of aorta.

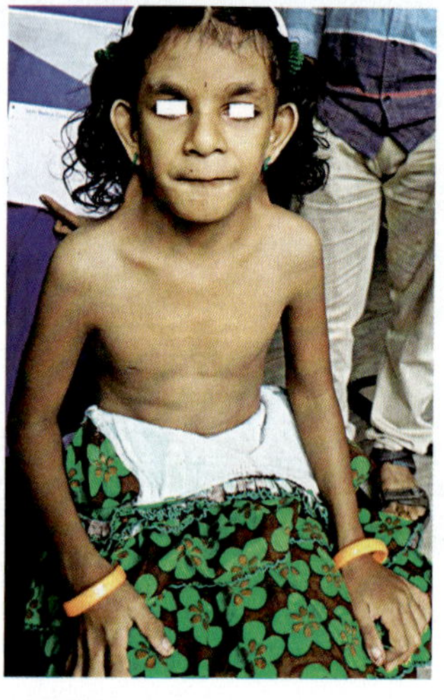

Fig.24.60 Webbing

- Ovarian dysgenesis (hence failure of puberty; Turner's is sterile).
- No mental retardation.
- Clinical clues in the newborn: Loose skin of the neck in infancy (shown in picture below); congenital lymphoedema of dorsum of fingers and toes in neonates.
- Incidence is 1 in 3000 live births.
- Karyotype is 45 XO but mosaics may occur about 50% of the time.
- Untreated adult height is less than 145 cm. Treatment with oestrogen replacement and growth hormone improves the secondary sex characteristics and the adult height. If affordable, growth hormone replacement may be started from early childhood to improve the height. Oestrogen replacement is started by around 13 years, not earlier, to allow maximum height gain (sex hormones will cause fusion of epiphysis and hence block further height gain). Estrogen also prevents osteoporosis. Premarin 0.3–0.625 mg OD for 3–6 months will induce puberty. Then oestrogen 1–23 days and progesterone 10–23 days will result in withdrawal bleed.
- XO/XY mosaicism has increased risk of gonadoblastoma and therefore gonads are surgically removed.

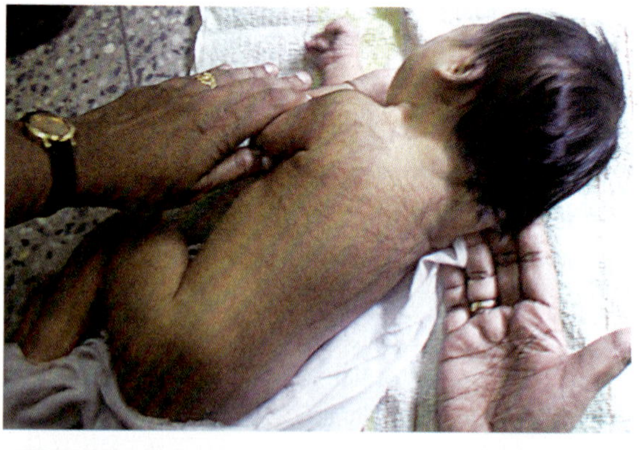

Fig.24.61 Note the webbing of neck

- Periodic thyroid function tests are recommended.

46. * These skin lesions were noted in a child who had seizures (Fig. 24.62). What is the possible diagnosis?

A: Hypomelanosis of Ito. Skin lesions and seizure point towards a neurocutaneous syndrome. Of the various neurocutaneous syndromes, the irregular whorled depigmented patches seen here fits in best with a diagnosis of hypomelanosis of Ito.

- Irregular, streaked, whorled or mottled depigmented patches on the trunk and limbs.
- May have associated seizures, mental retardation, etc.
- Sporadic. Familial cases may be autosomal dominant.
- It is also called incontinentia pigmenti achromians, meaning the skin lesions are like incontinentia pigmenti, but are achromic (hypopigmented).

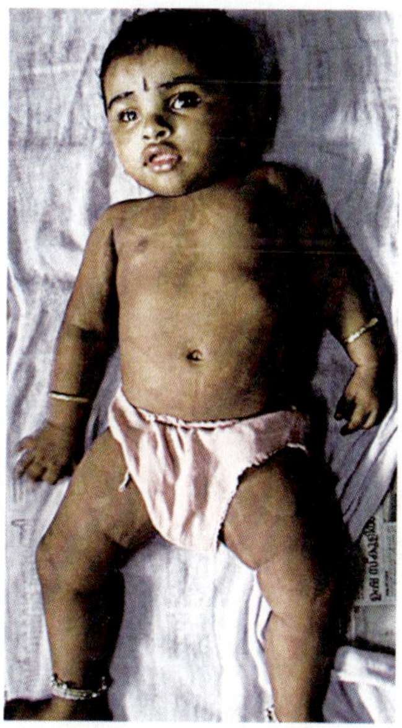

Fig.24.62 *(Courtesy: Dr PAM Kunju)*

47.* These skin lesions are noted in a child with seizures and developmental retardation. What is the diagnosis?

A: Incontinentia pigmenti (Bloch-Sulzberger disease). Skin lesions and seizure points towards a neurocutaneous syndrome and these lesions fit best with this diagnosis.

- Females are affected. Inheritance possibly is X-linked dominant, the affected males possibly getting aborted or die early in life.
- Brownish gray bizarre whorled macular pigmentation, the distribution as though splashed on the skin with a paintbrush*. Skin lesions in newborn period may be linear streaks of blisters or vesicles **(Fig.24.64)**.
- Look for dystrophic changes in hair (e.g., patchy alopecia of scalp), teeth, nail, etc.
- Skin lesions fade with age. Hence, even if lesions are not there in the mother, ask for history of similar lesions in the mother when she was a child.
- CNS: Microcephaly, spastic cerebral palsy, seizures, mental retardation, etc, may be associated.
- Eye: Microphthalmia, cataract, strabismus, optic atrophy, etc, may be associated.

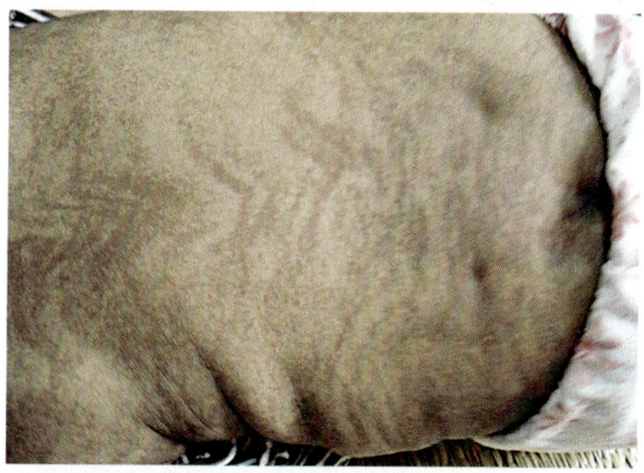

Fig.24.63

24

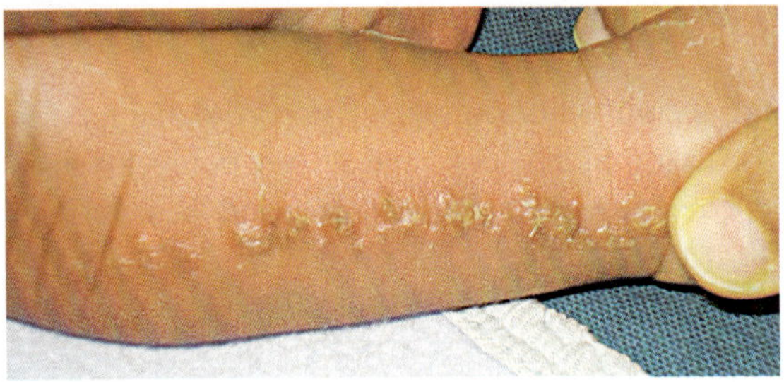

Fig.24.64 Incontinentia in the newborn period

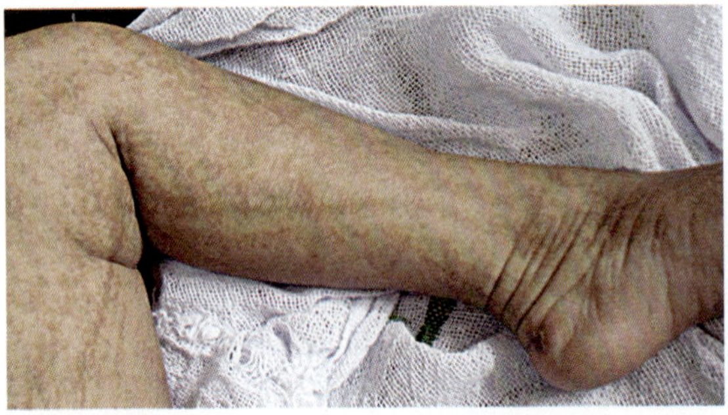

Fig.24.65 Change of skin lesions with growth of the child

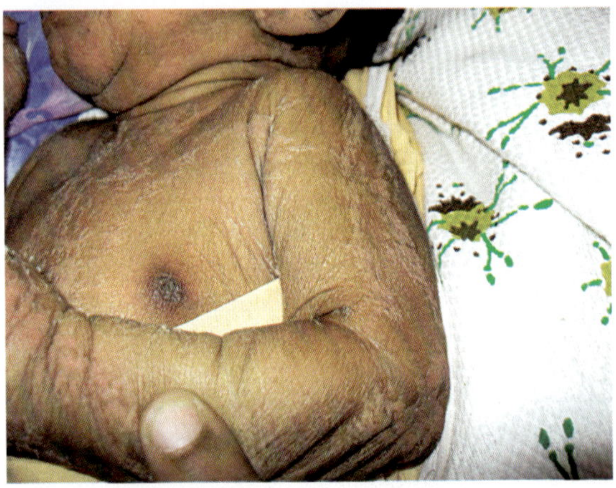

Fig.24.66 1st phase: Erythematous streak

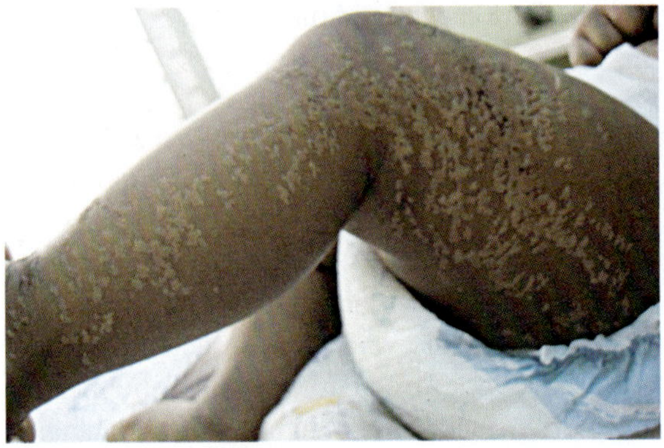

Fig.24.67 2nd phase: Verrucous plaques

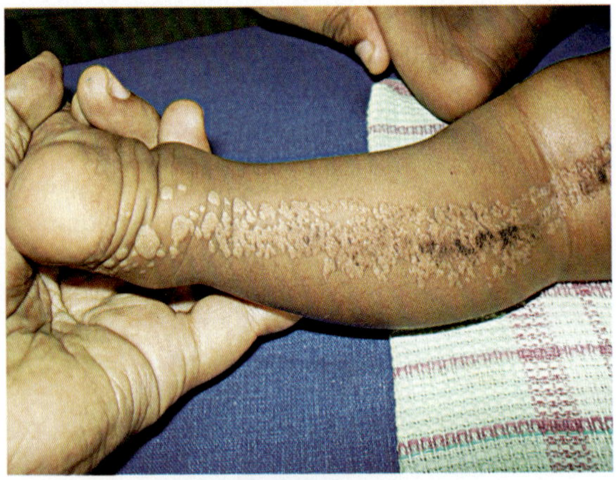

Fig.24.68 3rd phase: Hyperpigmentation

48.*This boy is sent for evaluation following multiple episodes of seizure. What is the diagnosis?

A: Sturge-Weber syndrome. The cutaneous lesions in Sturge-Weber syndrome is a non-elevated reddish one (port-wine stain) and is usually confined to the distribution of one or more branches of the trigeminal nerve. Thus, the port wine stain stops at midline in the face (also see Fig. 6.161, p 140. The cutaneous lesion does not appear to be very flat in this picture. However, cutaneous haeman-gioma shown is more or less in the distribution of trigeminal nerve and is associated with seizures,

Hence, a diagnosis of Sturge-Weber syndrome is justified. A CT scan head is indicated to demonstrate calcification.

- Port-wine stain is usually seen within the cutaneous distribution of ophthalmic and/or maxillary divisions of the trigeminal nerve.

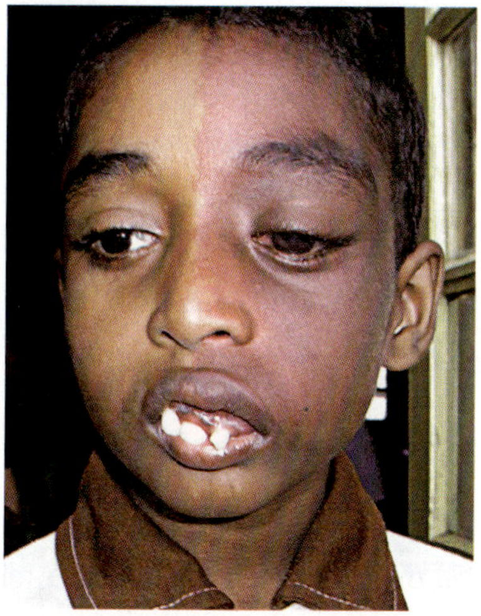

Fig.24.69 Haemangioma of face

Look for

- Contralateral hemiparesis
- Homonymuous hemianopic field deficit
- Ophthalmic manifestations occur if the port-wine stain involves the ophthalmic division of the trigeminal nerve. Telangiectasia of conjunctiva, ipsilateral exophthalmos, colobomata, buphthalmos or glaucoma.
- May have epilepsy and mental retardation.
- Occurrence is sporadic.
- CT scan and skull X-rays show rail road calcification (seldom visible in infancy) **(see Fig. 25.50)**.

49. *This child with seizures has the skin lesions shown below. Identify the skin lesions and the condition associated with it.

A: The skin lesions are ash leaf macules (Fig. 24.70), shagreen patch **(Fig. 24.71)** and adenoma sebaceum **(Fig. 24.72)**; the condition associated with it is tuberous sclerosis.

Tuberous Sclerosis

Skin:

- Ash leaf spot is the earliest evidence of the disease to become obvious **(Fig. 24.70)**.
- **Adenoma sebaceum**: Erythematous or flesh coloured papular lesions over nose and cheeks (rare under 2 years of age, but almost 100% by 35 years of age. So look for it in parents). The currently preferred terminology for adenoma sebaceum is angiofibroma. It is demonstrated in **Fig. 24.72**.
- Shagreen patch: See **(Fig. 24.71)**; it is elevated and orange peel like. Usual site is lumbosacral region.
- Subungual fibroma: Fleshy outgrowth of nail bed of fingers or toes (rare in childhood).
- Gingival fibromas

CNS:

- The sclerotic lesions of CNS are tuber like or potato like and hence the name tuberous sclerosis.
- Epilepsy in 95% (may present as infantile spasms or seizure may develop later), mental retardation in 50%.
- Retinal phakomata—raised mushroom-like lesion near the optic disc.

Other Organs:

- Cyst-like lesions in bones (especially in the phalanges) and irregular sclerosis.
- Palpable kidneys, polycystic kidneys or adenoma, fibroma, etc, of kidneys. Cardiac rhabdomyomata (usually in left ventricle, asymptomatic with no signs).
- Look for stigmata of disease in parents.

24

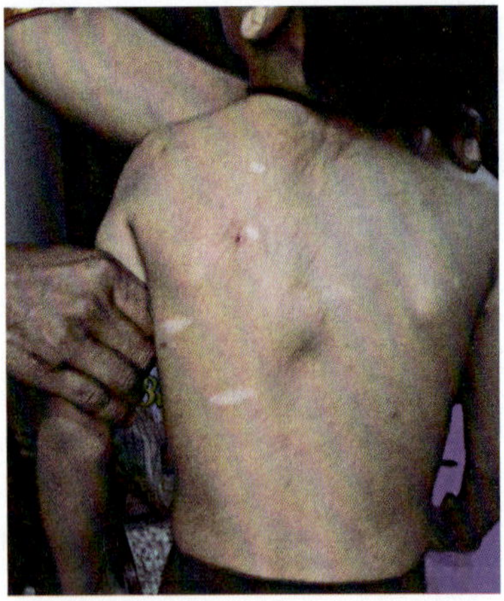

Fig.24.70 Ash leaf macules

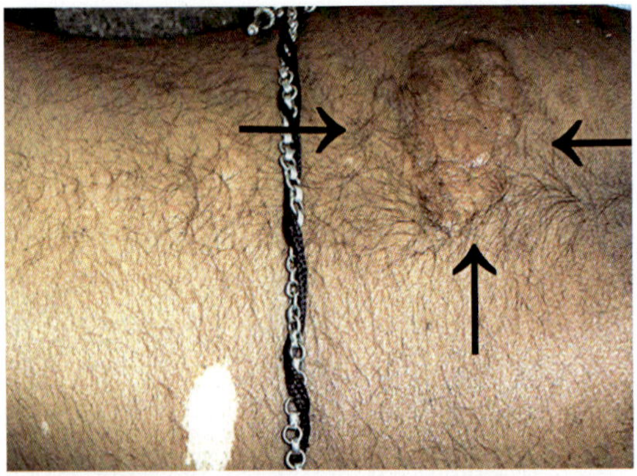

Fig.24.71 Shagreen patch

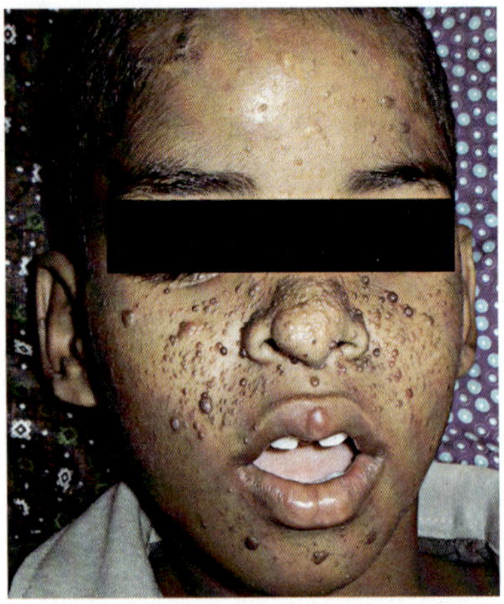

Fig.24.72 Adenoma sebaceum

- Autosomal dominant inheritance; about half the cases are sporadic due to new mutations. Gene is located on chromosome 9q34.

50.* What is the skin lesion shown? How is this related to CNS pathology?

A: The lesions shown are cafe-au-lait spots. The usual neurocutaneous syndrome associated with it is neurofibromatosis (von Reck linghausen disease). Cafe-au-lait spots can be there in many other diseases also and hence certain diagnostic criteria are put forward for the diagnosis of neurofibromatosis, as discussed below. Two distinct forms of neurofibromatosis exist: type 1 and type 2.

Type 1: Two or more of the following are needed to make the diagnosis.

- Six or more cafe-au-lait spots* greater than 5 mm in diameter pre-puberty or 15 mm post-puberty (present in almost all cases).
- Axillary or inguinal freckling, hyperpigmented spots about 2 mm in diameter.
- Two or more Lisch nodules (see Fig. 6.51 b, p 100). They are hamartomas of the iris (sometimes discovered only on slit-lamp examination).
- Two or more neurofibromas* or one plexiform neurofibroma.

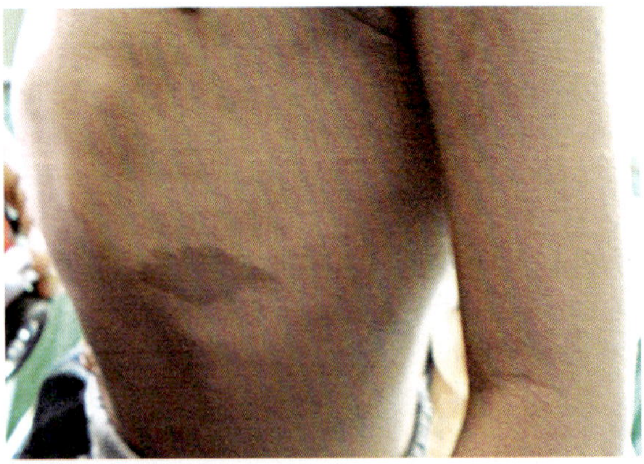

Fig.24.73

- Optic glioma, usually asymptomatic but may cause visual disturbance. Afferent pupillary defects, if present, may be detected by swinging flash light test (p 201).
- First-degree relative with neurofibromatosis type I.
- Typical bony lesions like sphenoid dysplasia (which may cause pulsating exophthalmos). Scoliosis is the most common bone abnormality but is not specific and hence not part of diagnostic criteria.
- Mental retardation, seizures, neurofibro-sarcoma arising in a neurofibroma, etc, are possible.
- 90% of cases of neurofibromatosis are type I.
- Autosomal dominant inheritance with high penetrance but variable expression.
- Gene located on chromosome 17q22.
- Management includes genetic counseling and treatment of complications.

Type 2: One of the following is needed to make a diagnosis:

- Bilateral acoustic neuromas. Acoustic neuromas may lead to hearing loss, facial weakness, dizziness and unsteadiness (signs of acoustic neuromas are often not present until the second or third decade).
- First-degree relative with neurofibromatosis type 2 and either eighth nerve masses or any two of the following: neurofibroma, schwannoma, glioma, meningioma or posterior subcapsular lenticular opacities.
- Cafe-au-lait spots and neurofibromas may be seen but are not part of diagnostic criteria of type 2.
- Autosomal dominant inheritance; gene is located on chromosome 22q.
- Management includes genetic counseling and treatment of acoustic neuromas and other tumours.

51. * This 10-year-old child was on treatment for "allergic conjunctivitis" because of constant redness in the eye. Now she is referred for gait abnormality. On examination, she is found to have ataxia. What is the diagnosis?

A: Ataxia telangiectasia. The picture shows many horizontal linear blood vessels on the bulbar conjunctiva.

- Telangiectasia* appear earliest on the bulbar conjunctiva (usually appears by 3–6 years). It may be seen on the bridge of the nose and auricles.
- Progressive ataxia* (usually over 2 years of age): Look for truncal ataxia when the child is quietly sitting and ataxic gait when the child is walking.
- Look for other cerebellar signs like intention tremor, nystagmus, etc.
- May have associated extrapyramidal manifestations in advanced disease like choreoathetosis.
- History of recurrent respiratory infection will be there, many times to the extent of producing clubbing due to bronchiectasis.
- Defective DNA repair leads to high incidence of lymphoreticular malignancy.

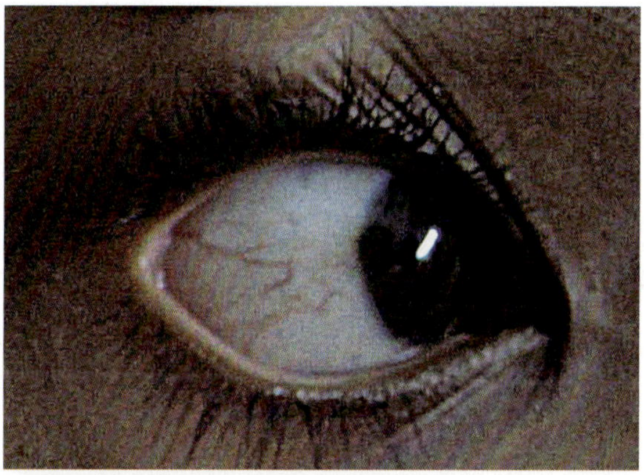

Fig.24.74 Telangiectasia

- Immune deficiency* with tonsil and thymus hypoplasia (lymphopenia), hypogamma globulinemia (low IgA). It is easy to remember as Ig**A** and **T** cell defect in **A**taxia **T**elangiectasia.
- Autosomal recessive: Gene defect on chromosome 11.
- Diagnosis is confirmed by chromosome fragility.
- No curative treatment is available.
- Management involves the treatment of infection and chemotherapy for malignancies.
- Ionizing radiation should be avoided (avoid X-ray tests whenever possible).
- Child is often wheelchair bound by 10–12 years.
- Life span is dependent on infections and neoplasia.

52. This erythematous flat non-pruritic rash was found in a child with fever and acute onset joint pains. What is this rash?

A: This rash with the given history could fit in with a diagnosis of erythema marginatum. This erythematous macular (i.e., not raised) non-pruritic rash has serpigineous borders and a central clearing, which are characteristic of erythema marginatum. The serpigineous borders are due to the fusing of borders of adjacent lesions. Erythema marginatum may become more obvious following a hot bath. Erythema marginatum and subcutaneous nodules (p 471) are rare, but when present, are strongly associated with the presence of carditis. Students must be familiar with the full details of rheumatic fever and it is recommended that the students see p 342. Read "Manual of Pediatric Practice" by the same author.

Fig.24.75 Note the serpiginous borders

53.* The drawing (Fig. 24.76) is of a child who is brought for evaluation of hypertrophy of one leg and a red cutaneous mark over the dorsum of foot. Examination revealed varicose veins. What may be the diagnosis?

A: Klippel-Trenaunay-Weber syndrome

- Asymmetrical hypertrophy of one or more limbs*
- Haemangiomas*
- Venous varicosities (these three form the diagnostic triad).
- Look for high-output cardiac failure and the occasional association of poly/syndactyly.

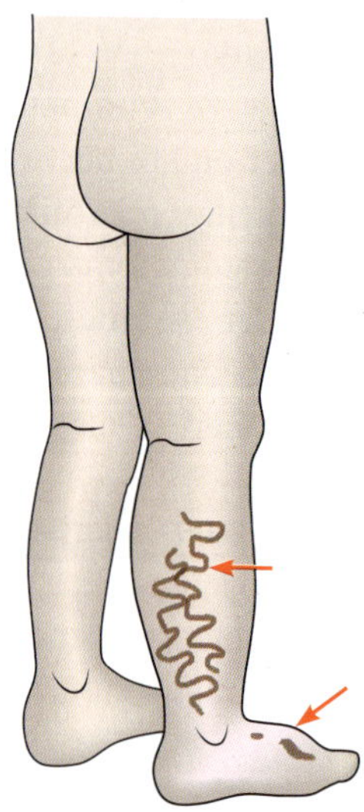

Fig.24.76 Note the serpiginous borders

- Inheritance is sporadic.
- Differential diagnosis: Milroy syndrome; hemihypertrophy syndrome.

54. This child was brought with complaints of being feverish and unwell for 2 days. Now he has the rash shown in the picture. What is the diagnosis?

A: Chickenpox. In herpes zoster, the rash is confined to a dermatome and is limited by the midline, which is the limit of the dermatome as well **(Fig.24.77 & 78).**

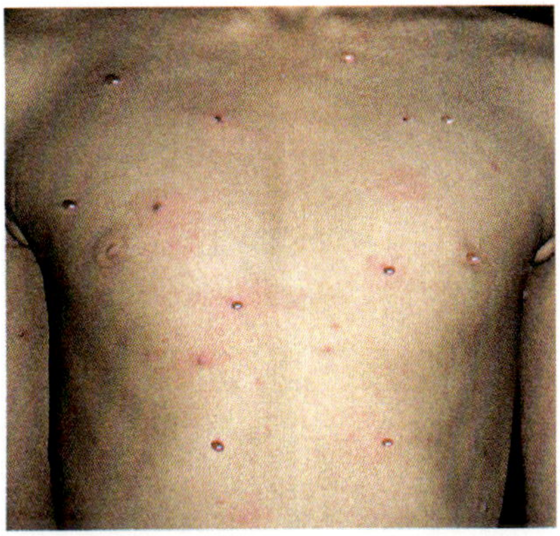

Fig.24.77 Varicella

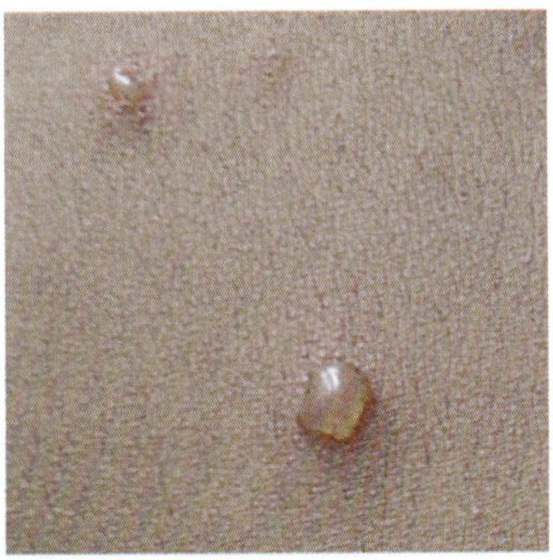

Fig.24.78 Note the dew drop vesicle

55. This child had history of fever, jaw pain, general malaise and the swelling shown below; he was diagnosed to have tonsillitis and treated for that. While on treatment he developed vomiting and neck stiffness. What is the diagnosis? (Fig.24.79)

A: Mumps with aseptic meningitis. It is common for the tonsils to get displaced to midline due to the swelling of mumps and that may have lead to the wrong diagnosis of tonsillitis by the first-contact physician. He must have taken the parotid swelling as the regional lymph node. The picture clearly shows the features of typical parotid swelling, filling up the depression at the angle of jaw and lifting up of ear lobe. One must look for pus from Stensen's duct, which could mean that it is infected secondarily with bacterial pathogens (parotid duct opens opposite second upper molar).

24

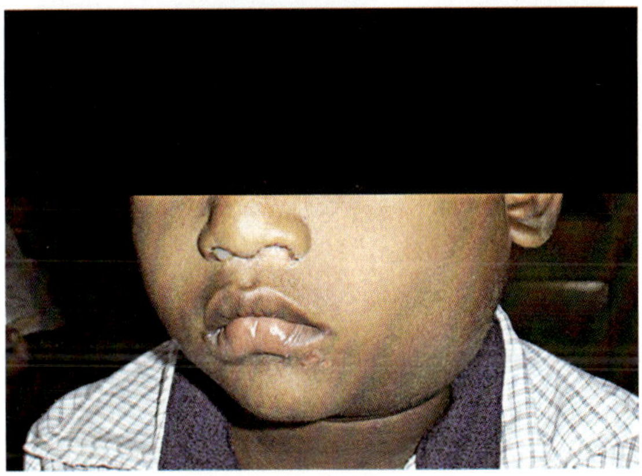

Fig.24.79 Parotid swelling

56. What is the abnormality demonstrated? Name three organisms that can cause this.

A: Whitish patch in the tonsil; group A streptococcus, diphtheria, Epstein-Barr virus. Tonsillar exudates are whitish in IMN, yellowish in streptococcus and gray in diphtheria (this is not an absolute rule).

There will be bleeding on attempted removal of diphtheritic membrane. In case of streptococcus, there will be no bleeding on attempted removal, because it is in reality an exudate and not a true membrane. Candidiasis looks milky white and there will be similar lesions over the tongue, throat, etc, not confined to tonsils.

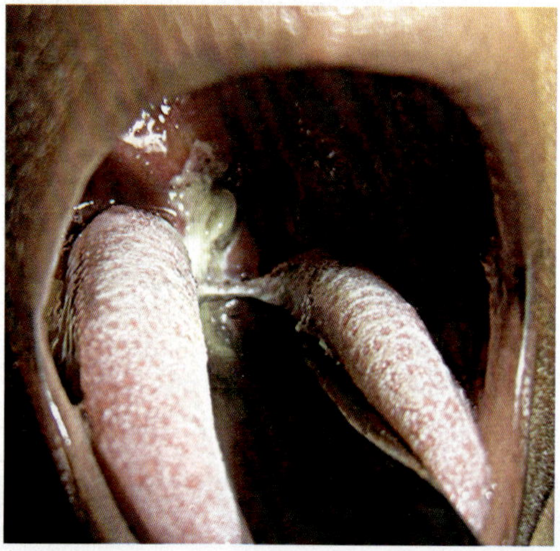

Fig.24.80 Patch on the tonsil

57. This child presented with haematuria. What is the lesion demonstrated?

A: Papular lesions of wrist and interdigital areas. Diagnosis is scabies. Scabies per se does not produce haematuria, but its secondary infection with streptococci can cause nephritis. In fact, it is the most common cause of nephritis in the underprivileged **(Fig.24.81 a & b, 24.82)**.

58.*This child presented with fever, diffuse erythema and crying while handling. Although the perioral lesions as seen in the picture were there, oral cavity was not involved. What is the diagnosis?

A: Staphylococcal scalded skin syndrome. The initiating lesion most often is a minor crack or pyoderma, which often goes unnoticed. The crying on handling is due to skin tenderness.

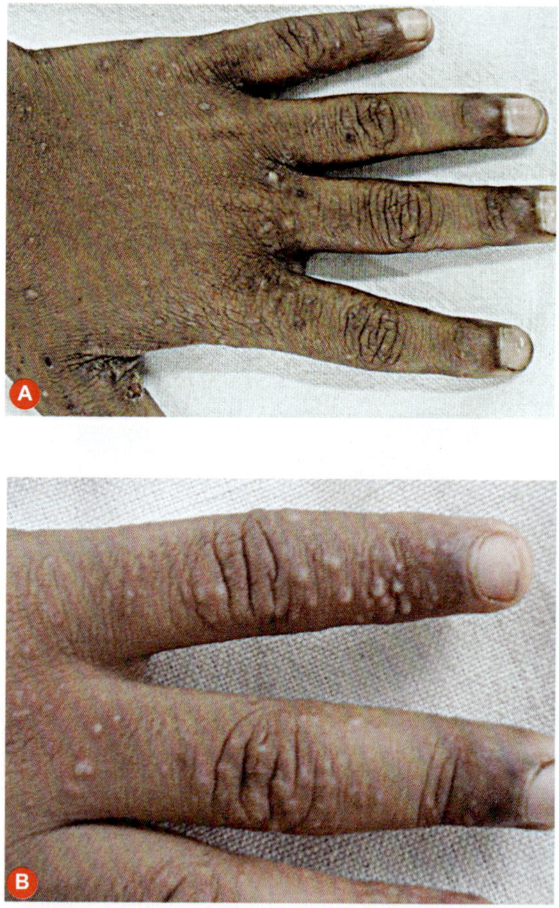

Fig.24.81

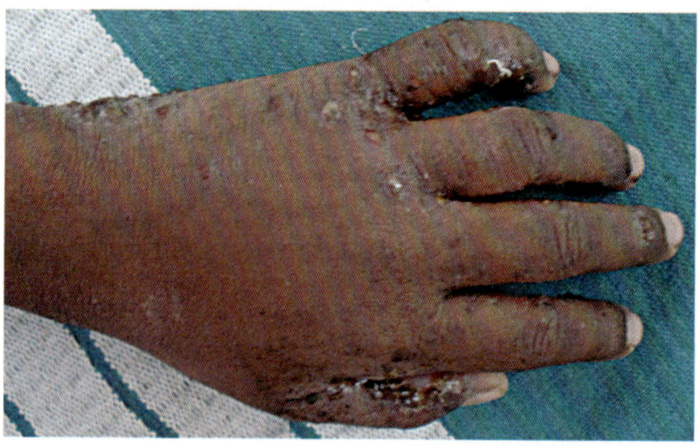

Fig.24.82 Scabies with secondary infection

Large sheets of skin peel off like a wet tissue paper to leave raw areas, which heal with no scarring **(Fig.24.83)**.

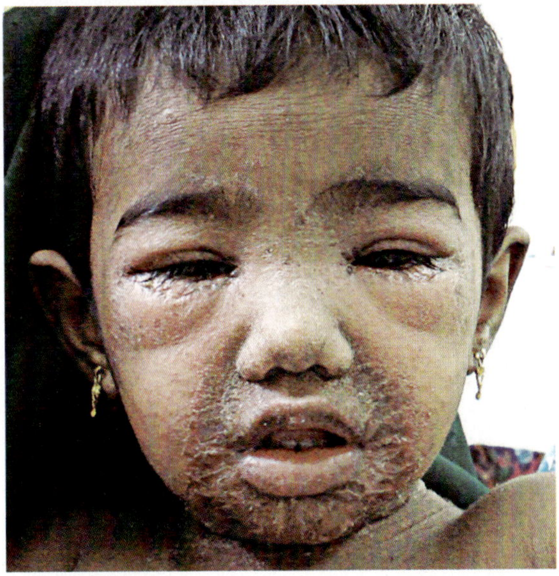

Fig.24.83

59. This test is done on a child who presented with altered sensorium, fever and seizures. The child had a history of fall following which he developed these symptoms over a few days. What is the diagnosis?

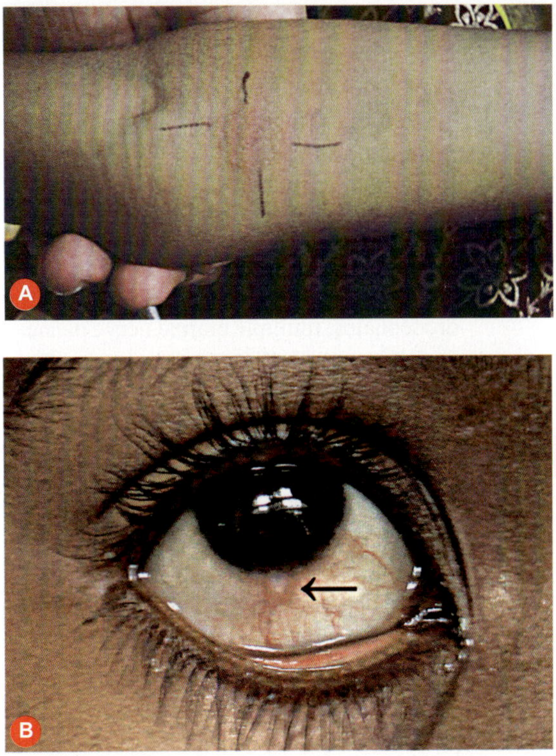

Fig.24.84 (A) Positive Mantoux text
(B) Phlyctenular conjunctivitis

A: The picture shows a positive Mantoux test and phlyctenular conjunctivitis. In a child with fever, seizure and altered sensorium, positive Mantoux test makes the diagnosis of tuberculous meningitis very likely.

Conjunctival phlycten is a small pinkish/grayish white elevated nodule situated in the midst of a localized hyperaemic area. The nodule is on the limbus, usually found near the *temporal border* of cornea (unlike that in **Fig 24.84 A & B)** with a leash of blood vessels running from it in a triangular fashion. In this picture, the phlycten is on the inferior border of cornea. See Fig. 6.50, p 99. Phlyctenular conjunctivitis is a type IV hypersensitivity reaction to a foreign antigen (examples include tuberculosis, streptococcus, staphylococcus, fungus, etc).

See p 274 for a long case discussion on TBM. Given below is a brief duscussion on TBM.

- History of recent measles or whooping cough; suggestive history of HIV; immunosuppressive therapy.
- Head injury: Many times, one may find a history of fall before the parents noticing the symptoms of TBM. It is possible that the fall possibly represents the first manifestation of the gradual development of drowsiness of TBM.
- PEM and lack of BCG vaccination can increase the chance of the child getting TBM.
- The history may show a slow evolution of symptoms rather than an abrupt onset of meningitis.

- Since the illness is likely to have been a long drawn one, look for bed sores.
- Look for allergic manifestations of TB, like phlyctenular conjunctivitis, erythema nodosum, etc.
- Fundus: Look for optic atrophy, papilloedema and choroid tubercles (see pp 189–192).
- The child can have features to suggest hydrocephalus; multiple cranial nerve palsies; various motor deficits; involuntary movements.
- Usually, there are features of encephalitis (altered sensorium and seizures) and meningitis (meningeal signs).
- Diagnosis is usually given as: Meningoencephalitis of insidious onset; with features of raised intracranial tension; with/without motor deficits in the form of———, cranial nerve palsies of———, abnormal movements in the form of————. The possible site of lesion is at ———, the probable aetiology being tuberculosis. The child has or has no PEM.

60. The child is being held by the axilla. What abnormality is being demonstrated? The child has average intelligence, has good manipulative skills of hands but has severe gait abnormality. Deep tendon reflexes are exaggerated, more so in the lower limbs and the plantar response is extensor. The child was delivered as a full-term baby. What is the diagnosis?

A: Cerebral palsy, possibly diplegia (see long case discussion p 252). Diagnosis is cerebral palsy with more involvement of lower limbs and good intellect. This fits in with a diplegic cerebral palsy. Diplegia does not mean that upper limbs will not be involved but only means it will be involved to a much lesser degree than lower limbs; hence the increased tendon jerks in upper limbs present here is explainable.

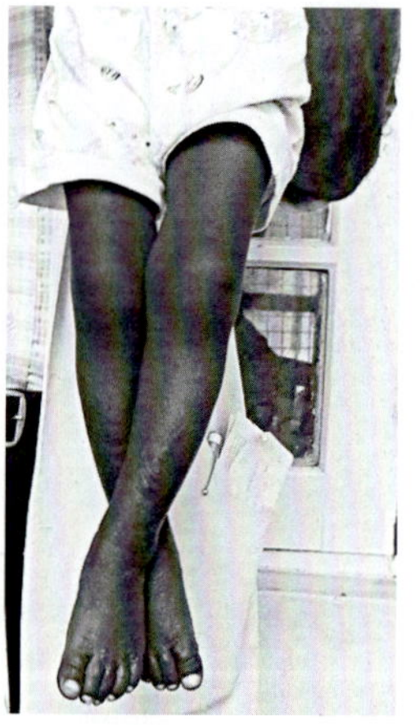

Fig.24.85 Scissoring

Cerebral diplegia is usually found in preterm deliveries because in premature babies, the periventricular area is the watershed area for vascular compromise and hence the lower limb fibres going via the periventricular area get involved. Once the baby is full term, this area is better vascularized and hence is no longer the watershed area. Hence, the odd point here for a diagnosis of diplegia is that the baby was a full-term delivery. It is explainable if we assume that the insults to brain in this child might have occurred during intrauterine life before the baby has become full term.

Tone may be elicited systematically following the scheme given under examination of nervous system. In a small infant, it may be difficult and a gross method is better suited. It is called "**180° flip**" where a supine infant is pulled to sit, held vertical, held in ventral suspension and finally put in prone position, completing the 180° flip.

- Supine: Assess any preferred positions, like external rotation of lower limb indicating weakness or floppiness on that side; "wind swept posture"; cortical fisting; abnormal movements; difference in size of two sides as in hemiplegia; dysmorphic features;

asymmetric tonic neck reflex; squint, etc. Floppy baby may have a frog leg posture.

- Pull to sit by hands: Assess grasp and head lag. When assessing head lag, support the head to avoid the apprehension of mother.
- Sitting: Assess sitting ability (with or without support; rounded or straight back; whether the child can balance if tilted to side, etc). Sitting can be graded if needed (see 'Manual of Pediatric Practice').
- Hold vertically under axilla: Detects tone, scissoring, any arching back due to excess extensor tone, can test automatic walking. Hypotonic baby will slip through the axillary grip.
- Ventral suspension: Hold the infant in ventral suspension with the examiner's hand supporting the chest and abdomen. It can detect excess extensor tone like arching back. If head is held up on ventral suspension, but there was no head control when pulled to sit, it means extensor hypertonia. Hypotonic baby remains limp, U shaped with head and limbs down.
- Parachute reflex: If the child is above 7 months, test parachute reflex on the way to placing the child on the bed. Note its presence and any asymmetry.
- Prone: Place the child prone in bed and look for any arching.
- Note: In assessing tone and reflexes, the head should be in midline; otherwise, asymmetric tonic neck reflex may act to give a difference of tone between the sides.
- The examination candidate must make sure he has checked the following: detailed antenatal, natal and postnatal history; head circumference; vision and hearing; back for kyphoscoliosis (very common); tooth decay (very common); evidence of pseudobulbar palsy (e.g., drooling); palpable mass in abdomen (constipation is so very common and hence palpable faecal mass is likely); dislocation of hip; assessment of nutrition (most often growth retarded); feeding problems; bladder and bowel; gait; bed sores; contractures; vasomotor changes (affected limbs may be cool with peripheral cyanosis); other associations (cataract, squint, mental subnormality, seizure, speech, abnormal movements, etc).

Quadriplegic CP is the severest form of spastic CP. In addition to involvement of all the four limbs, there is pseudobulbar palsy (since swallowing is a problem, tube feeding may be needed), mental retardation and difficult to control seizures. Speech and visual abnormalities may be associated.

24

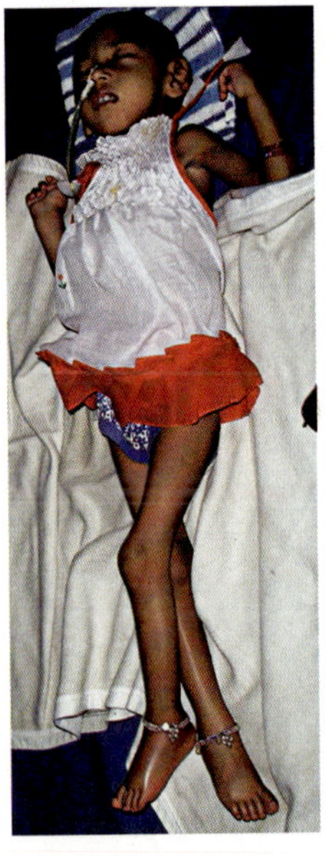

Fig.24.86 Quadriplegia

61.* What is the diagnosis? How will you clinically assess the possible level of lesion? What are the complications?

A: Meningomyelocele. Figure also shows patulous anus (see p 272).

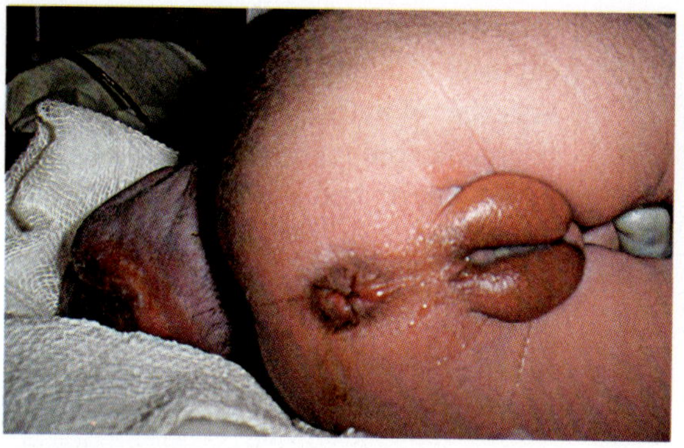

Fig.24.87

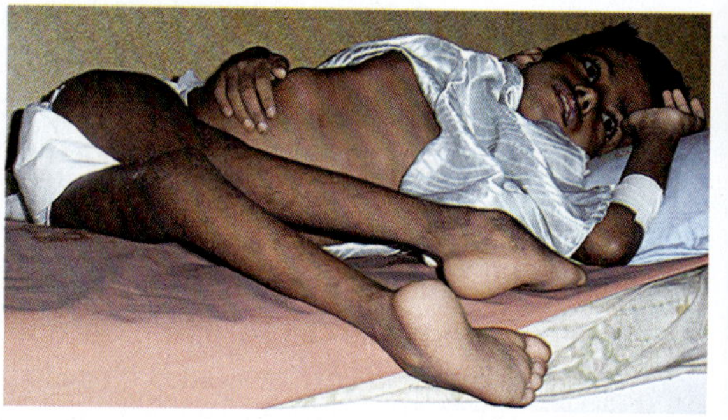

Fig.24.88 Typical position in meningomyelocele

The task will be to determine the level of lesion, functional assessment and to look for complications.

- At level of T8, there will be flaccid paralysis of whole of lower limb (frog leg position) and abdominal wall. If the level is below L4, hip flexors, hip adductors and quadriceps are strong (L1–L3), whereas hip extensors are weak (S1–S2). Strong hip adduction may produce posterior dislocation of hip. The position of limb will be flexed hip, extended knee (sometimes genu recurvatum) and equinovarus foot.

  If the lesion is a bit lower (say L5), tibialis anterior may remain active as a dorsiflexor (L4), so that it will overcome the weak plantar flexion (S1–S2); hence the foot will be dorsiflexed and inverted. The paralysis is flaccid, has sensory loss and the bladder function is affected (neurogenic bladder). Hence, repeated urinary infection is a big problem.
- If the lesion is at L3 or below, most of the lower limb function is preserved, but there is paralysis of bladder and anal sphincters and saddle anaesthesia. Sacral lesions may cause bladder/bowel symptoms in the absence of lower limb motor signs.
- It is important to recognize that the paralysis is flaccid although the lesion is in the cord. It is because the loss of neural tissue results in total cutting off of any connection of LMN with the cord.
- If there is asymmetry of involvement of both legs, it could mean that only ½ of the cord is involved.
- Look for reflexes to localize: Cremasteric (L1), knee (L3), ankle (S1) and anal (S4).
- Periconceptional folic acid supplementation will reduce the incidence of neural tube defects (meningomyelocele, spina bifida, encephalocele and anencephaly).
- In open neural tube defects, maternal amniotic fluid α-fetoprotein will be elevated.
- Most important complications to look for are renal infections (chronic renal failure, hydronephrosis, etc), CNS infections (due to ruptured meningomyelocele) and hydrocephalus. Measurement of BP is important as it may be elevated in chronic renal failure, which may occur due to repeated renal infections.
- The student should not forget to mention the obvious things like a feeding tube or VP shunt. Hydrocephalus is a common association. Bed-sores are likely and hence must be looked for.
- Tone, power, reflexes and sensation should be tested to establish level of

lesion. Sometimes below the level of myelocele, there may be an isolated segment of spinal cord to which nerves are connected. In such cases, pin prick will produce withdrawal of leg. But it is not a cerebral action, but a local spinal reflex. The fact that the child is withdrawing the leg to pain without appreciating the pain or knowledge that the leg is withdrawn, should help the student to interpret this reflex movement correctly.

62.* What is the lesion shown?

A: Encephalocele. It is midline in location and is in connection with the skull. There may be an impulse on crying. Meckel-Gruber syndrome is occipital encephalocele with polydactyly, renal anomaly and cleft lip/palate **(ref. 5)**.

Cranial meningocele contains CSF-filled meningeal sac only, whereas the encephalocele contains the sac plus cerebral cortex **(ref. 5)**. Clinically, transillumination will give a clue as to whether sac contains only fluid or has brain matter as well.

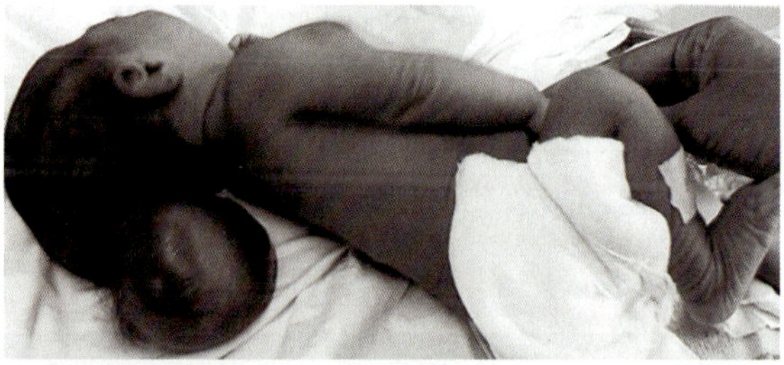

Fig.24.89

63.* A 10-year-old child was referred for assessment of scoliosis. On examination, the child was found to have ataxia, extensor plantar response but absent ankle jerk. What is the diagnosis?

A: Friedreich ataxia. The diagnosis has got to be an ataxia with pyramidal signs and neuropathy and hence Friedreich ataxia.

- Progressive gait disturbance due to ataxia from about 8–10 years of age.
- Extensor plantar response
- Absent ankle reflex
- Cerebellar and posterior column functions must be assessed (abnormal findings are expected); also assess hearing and vision.
- Speech: Usually explosive dysarthria (cerebellar).
- Tone may be reduced in the affected parts.
- Lower limbs are affected more than upper limbs, distal parts are affected more than proximal.
- Look for hammer toe; pes cavus; kyphoscoliosis.
- Look for clinical evidence of cardiomyopathy, arrhythmia, etc. ECG may show T wave changes.

24

64. Seven-year-old child presents with acute onset inability to move the lower limbs. There is no history of trauma and no spinal tenderness. There is hypotonia and absent reflexes in lower limbs. Plantar response is normal. There is no demonstrable sensory deficits. The sensorium of the child is normal.

A: The description fits in for a diagnosis of acute flaccid paralysis (see p 269). The usual differential diagnosis of acute flaccid paralysis are Guillain-Barre syndrome, poliomyelitis, traumatic neuritis and transverse myelitis. In acute stage of transverse myelitis, the reflexes may be depressed because of spinal shock but plantar must be up-going. In addition, in this case there is no sensory level as is expected in transverse myelitis.

The following is a brief discussion on GBS:

- Non-specific respiratory or GIT illness in preceding 2-4 weeks (Campylobacter). Also ask for any vaccines preceding the illness.

- *Symmetrical* lower motor neuron type of weakness, usually starting in lower extremities (in polio, the involvement is asymmetrical and patchy).
- Hypotonia and hyporeflexia or areflexia.
- Careful examination may bring out slightly more involvement of proximal compared to distal.
- Trunk and bulbar musculature may be affected in established cases.
- Fever is unlikely with the onset of paralysis (in poliomyelitis there will be fever).
- Insidious symptoms of sensory deficit, pain or paraesthesia may precede motor weakness but unlikely *after* the motor weakness is well established.
- Cranial nerve palsies may be present, facial nerve involvement is most common, 9th and 10th nerves being the next common. Look for dysphagia and facial nerve palsy, especially note that facial nerve palsy can be bilateral.
- If there is extraocular muscle involvement, think of Miller-Fisher syndrome (ataxia, external ophthalmoplegia and areflexia).
- Comment on sweating or flushing and measure BP for orthostatic hypotension (autonomic dysfunction).
- Do a single breath count test daily, to see if respiratory muscles are failing.
- Nerve conduction velocity is reduced and EMG will be consistent with lower motor neuron deficit.
- CSF may show albuminocytologic dissociation. Fewer than 10 cells but high protein in CSF. In poliomyelitis, there will be a lot more of cells.
- Treatment with plasmapheresis or immunoglobulins may be beneficial. Steroids controversial.
- Mechanical ventilation is indicated for respiratory failure and if progression to dysphagia, shoulder paresis, etc.
- Stool samples must be sent for culture as per AFP surveillance program.

65.* What is the sign shown and what is the diagnosis? Mention a few other signs that may be there in this condition.

A: Setting sun sign. The diagnosis is hydrocephalus (see p 262). Other signs are full fontanelle, separation of sutures, optic atrophy (papilloedema and not optic atrophy if recent onset), stridor, dilated scalp veins, exaggerated lower limb reflexes, etc.

- Measure and plot occipital-frontal circumference (OFC) if charts are provided in exam.

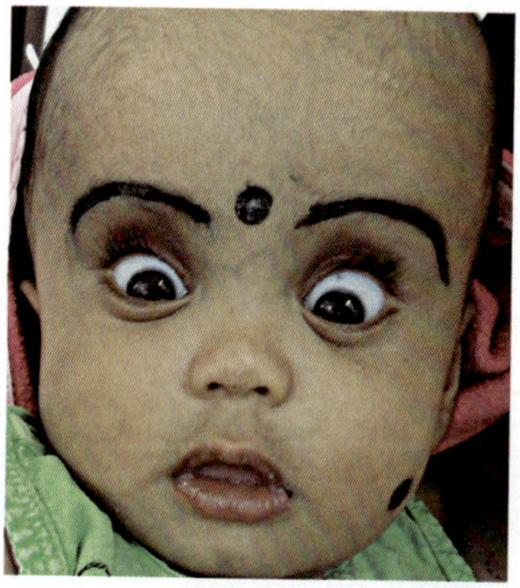

Fig.24.90 Hydrocephalus

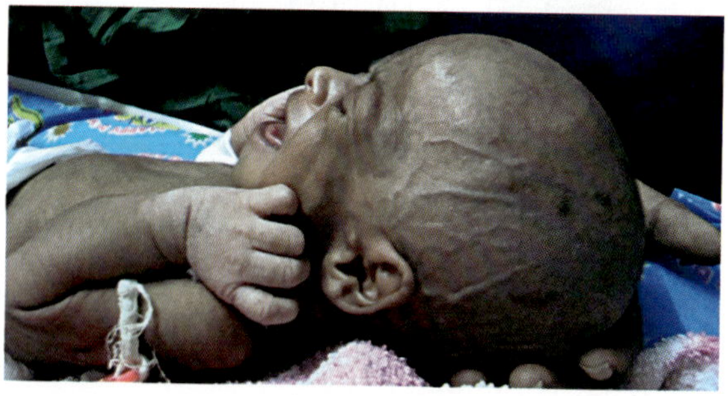

Fig.24.91 Dilated veins in hydrocephalus

- Look for ventriculoperitoneal shunt/surgical scars.
- Look for signs of raised intracranial pressure.
- Look for cranial bruit—vein of Galen malformations.
- Look for evidence of spina bifida.
- Check vision/eye movements/fundi.
- In neonate or infant, comment on full fontanelle, widened sutures, etc.
- In older children, look for "cracked-pot sound" on percussion of skull.

66.* What is the diagnosis?

A: The abnormal eye is held open by hand, which means there is ptosis. In addition, that eye is turned slightly down and out. Pupil on the affected side is dilated. Hence, it is a case of third nerve palsy. The features of third nerve palsy are:

- Ptosis (complete or partial).
- Eye is deviated down and out (elevate the lid to visualize it).
- Pupil may be dilated.
- Note that third nerve palsy need not always be complete.
- The usual aetiologies are: meningitis (especially tuberculous); brain stem encephalitis; Miller-Fisher variant of Guillain-Barre syndrome (ataxia, areflexia and external ophthalmoplegia); tumours (e.g., brainstem glioma).

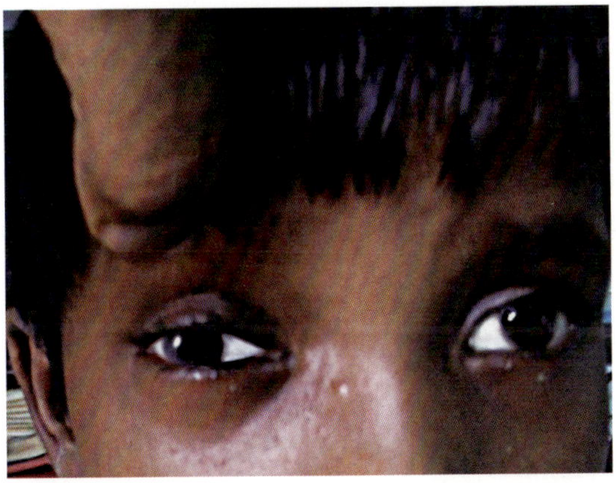

Fig.24.92 III Nerve palsy

67.* This child is trying to look to the left (Fig. 24.93). What abnormality is found?

A: The left eye is not abducting despite of full adduction of the right eye. It is left 6th nerve palsy. The features of abducent nerve palsy are:

- Failure of abduction of the affected eye.
- Maximal diplopia on looking to affected side, images being parallel and separated horizontally.
- Aetiologies include those mentioned under 3rd nerve palsy. However, 6th nerve may also be involved as a false localizing sign in raised intracranial pressure (due to the long course of the nerve).

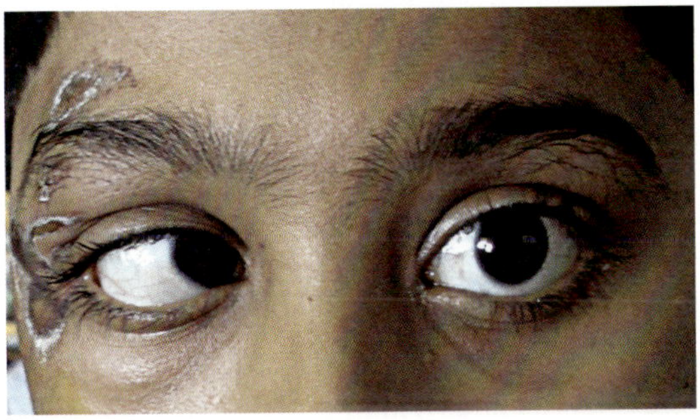

Fig.24.93 VI nerve palsy

68. What abnormality is demonstrated?

A: Facial nerve palsy. The most common cause of facial palsy in a child is Bell's palsy (isolated LMN VII nerve palsy of uncertain aetiology). See p 204 to differentiate between LMN and UMN. Facial nerve palsy in a newborn is usually LMN, due to pressure in utero, efforts during delivery or use of forceps for delivery. Rarely, it may result from congenital nuclear agenesis of VII nerve (Moebius syndrome).

24

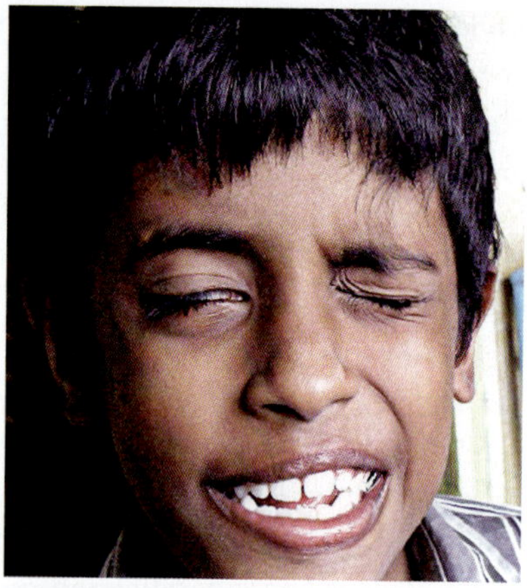

Fig.24.94 Facial palsy

The features of facial nerve palsy:

- Deviation of angle of mouth (deviates to the normal side).
- Difficulty in blowing out cheeks.
- Incomplete closure of eyes (the eye on the affected side cannot be closed completely).
- Wrinkling forehead is relatively preserved in upper motor neuron lesion, but in lower motor neuron lesion the upper and lower face is equally affected.
- Pouting of lips (e.g., to kiss a pencil held in front of lips) is defective.
- Associated features vary with site of lesion and include loss of taste on anterior two-third of tongue or hyperacusis.

Causes:

- Birth injury (usually resolves in weeks to months)
- Guillain-Barre syndrome
- Space-occupying lesion
- Bell palsy: Acute isolated unilateral facial palsy of undetermined cause (idiopathic or post viral). 80% make complete recovery in 3 months. Treatment is to protect eye and a short course of prednisolone 2 mg/kg/day.

69.* The child complains of nasal regurgitation of fluids. What abnormality is shown?

A: Right sided palatal palsy. The uvula is to the left; the U curve formed by the left half of the palate is narrower, showing that there is active contraction on the left side, which draws the uvula also to the left side. The most common cause of isolated palatal palsy in yesteryears was diphtheria. Nowadays demyelination is the most common cause.

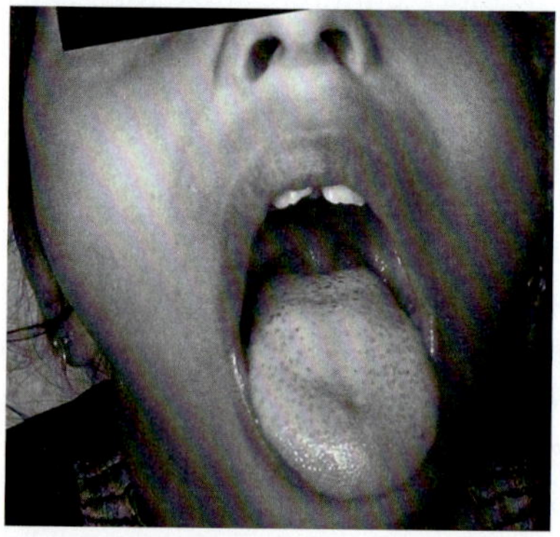

Fig.24.95 Note the soft palate and uvula

70.* What abnormality is seen when the tongue is put out?

A: The tongue is deviated to the left. The left half of the tongue is atrophic compared to the right half. Diagnosis is left sided hypoglossal palsy.

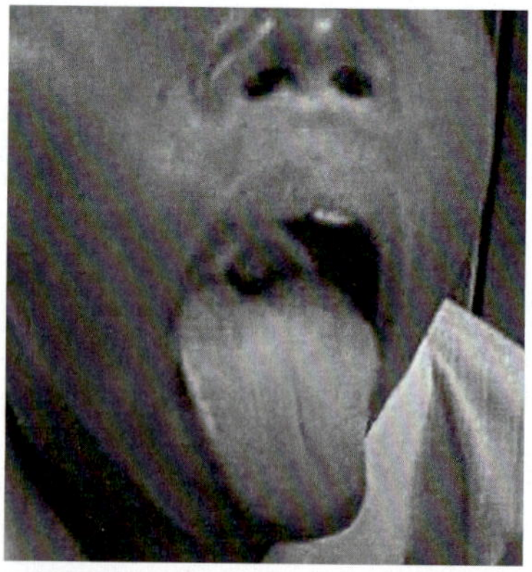

Fig.24.96 This picture is edited for clarity

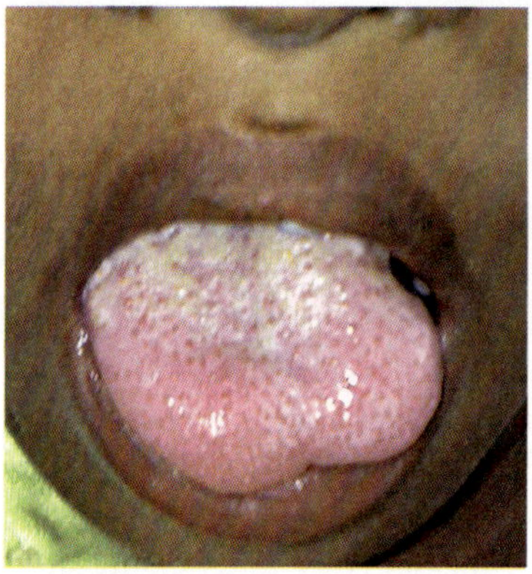

Fig.24.97 XII nerve palsy

71.* This newborn has paucity of movement of one limb. What is the abnormality?

A: All limbs except one are in a state of good flexion. The abnormal limb lacks flexion, remains adducted and internally rotated at shoulder and forearm remains pronated (waiter's tip position). The chance of spontaneous recovery is fairly good, especially if hand grasp is preserved. Often, Erb's palsy is due to the shoulder traction during delivery.

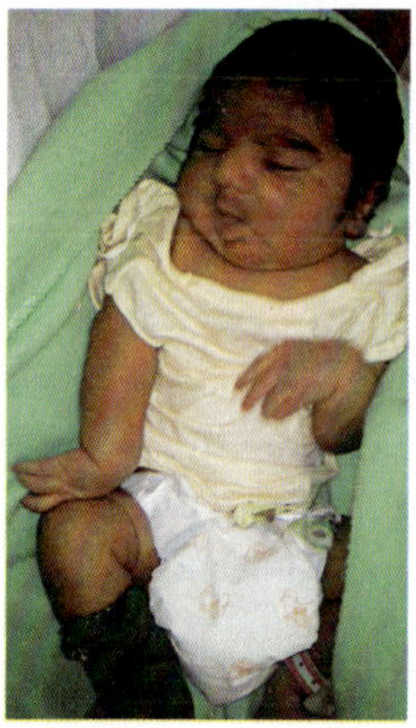

Fig.24.98 Erb plasy in newborn

72. * This child is sent for evaluation of difficulty in getting up from sitting position and frequent falls during walking. What abnormality is demonstrated? What is the diagnosis?

A: Calf muscle hypertrophy. Duchenne muscular dystrophy. See p 279 for long case discussion.

- Onset is usually within 3 years. Difficulty in getting up from floor (Gower's manoeuvre, see p 186), climbing stairs and prominent lumbar lordosis are the initial signs. Weakness is most marked in proximal muscles. Gower's manoevure: The boy is asked to lie supine and then to get up. He rolls over to prone, then on to the knees, then on "all fours," and then "climbs up" the legs to stand.
- Hypertrophy of calf muscles, deltoid and a few others, but these muscles are weak (pseudohypertrophy).
- Selective hypertrophy and wasting of different muscles in the same region results in Valleys sign: ask the child to abduct arm to 90°, with elbow flexed at 90° and hands preferably facing upwards: viewed from the back there is an oval depression (due to wasting) at posterior axillary fold with hypertrophied muscles at its two borders, deltoid superolaterally and infraspinatous inferomedially.

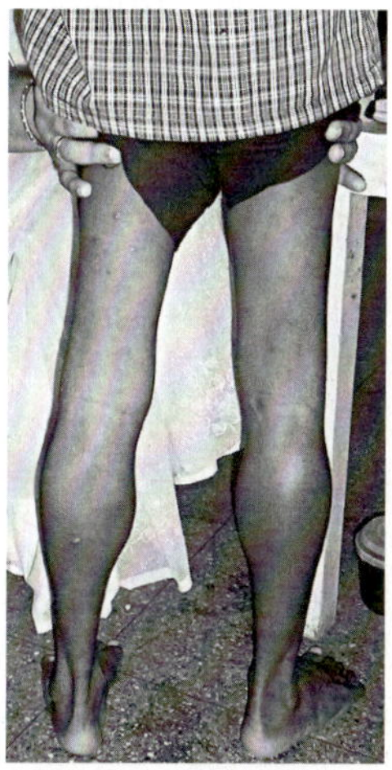

Fig.24.99

24

- Tendon reflexes may become depressed in proportion to muscle weakness.
- Wasting of pelvic girdle muscles.
- Contractures of the Achilles tendon occur early. Toe walking with frequent falls results.
- Waddling gait (Trendelenburg sign is positive, i.e., the hip drops down when the ipsilateral foot is raised).
- Cardiomyopathy may occur late in the course of illness (look for arrhythmia and cardiac failure).
- Scoliosis.
- X-linked recessive inheritance or new mutations (one-third have new mutations).
- Female carrier is non-symptomatic but may have pseudohypertrophy and weakness of pelvic girdle.
- Diagnosis is made on elevated CPK, myopathic EMG (brief small amplitude polyphasic potentials characteristic of muscle disease) and characteristic findings on muscle biopsy.
- Despite the supportive treatment, death occurs in the second decade.
- Calf hypertrophy may be occasionally present in Kugelberg-Welander disease (spinal muscular atrophy type III).

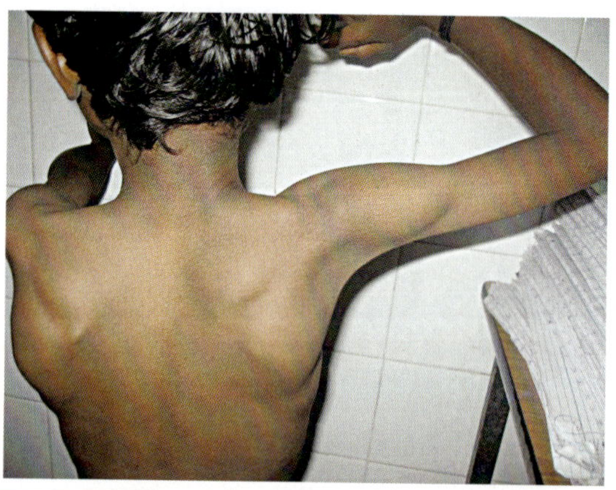

Fig.24.100 Valley sign *(Courtesy: Dr Indu Priya)*

Fasciculation (if present) and absent knee jerks may help in differentiation.

73.* An infant is brought for assessment of floppiness. How will you proceed?

A: The following is an examination oriented brief discussion on floppy infant (also see p 177 & 265 for long case discussion).

Assess tone by feeling the muscle (soft and flabby), resistance to passive movements (may have excessive range of movements at joints), assessing range of movements and shaking limbs. Hypotonic infant may remain in frog leg position when supine. Look for joint contractures, which may be there in long-standing cases. Hold the child by axilla and look for any falling through, indicating poor tone. Head lag may be demonstrated by pulling to sitting position holding on the shoulders (make sure you support the head from falling back). Poor trunk tone can be demonstrated holding by ventral suspension. Decreased tone can also be demonstrated by testing various angles like hip adduction, popliteal angle, ankle flexion, scarf sign, etc. See p 528 for 180° flip manoeuvre.

- Hypotonia + Mental retardation + Brisk reflexes: CNS cause. There may be associated seizures. Students must note that hypotonic cerebral palsy presents with hypotonia and *brisk* reflexes.
- Hypotonia + Dysmorphic features: Chromosomal. Look for dysmorphic features. Hypotonia in Down's syndrome is of doubtful origin, but generally thought to be "central" in origin but do not have increased reflexes. Seizure is also not part of Down's syndrome. One diagnoses Down's syndrome by typical facies and other features and not by work-up of a case of hypotonia. Prader-Willi syndrome is another example of chromosomal anomaly causing hypotonia.

- Hypotonia + Upgoing plantar reflex + Demonstrable level of sensory deficit: Spinal cord level (transverse myelitis). During the acute stage, one may get hypotonia and reflexes that are variable.
- Hypotonia + Alert child + Absent DTR: Anterior horn cell disease. In Werdnig-Hoffman disease, there may be history of decreased fetal movements. Fasciculation of tongue may be demonstrable.
- Hypotonia + Normal DTR + Progressive deterioration as the day advances: Neuromuscular junction (myasthenia). Infantile botulism is another example.
- Hypotonia + Decreased muscle mass/wasting, DTR sluggish, in proportion with muscle weakness: Muscle disease, e.g., congenital myopathies (hypertrophy muscles in case of Duchenne muscular dystrophy). There may be waddling gait and rising from sitting position is difficult and may bring out Gower's sign.
- Hypotonia + Decreased muscle mass/wasting, DTR sluggish, deep reflexes being more sluggish than what is expected for the muscle weakness: Neuropathy (e.g., GBS. In GBS, the weakness is symmetrical, proximal weakness more pronounced). In fact, decreased reflexes may precede actual muscle weakness. Note that in other neuropathies, the weakness is distal more than proximal and there may be sensation of "pins and needles."
- Hypotonia + Otherwise normal child: Congenital benign hypotonia. Tone normalizes, as the child grows older.

Aetiology (See p 177)

Following is a brief discussion on spinal muscular atrophy type I (Werdnig-Hoffmann disease):

- Presents soon after birth
- Marked hypotonia
- Areflexia
- Characteristic 'pithed frog's leg posture'—abducted hips and flexed knees
- Alert facies with intact eye movements
- Weak cry
- Tongue fasiculations
- Thorax flattened laterally due to intercostal weakness

74.* This child has a pulmonary ejection murmur, multiple black spots and mild degree of deafness. What is the diagnosis?

A: Multiple lentigines syndrome or LEOPARD syndrome. The picture shows multiple dark 1–5 mm lentigines of face and neck.

- **L**entigines
- **E**CG abnormalities
- **O**cular hypertelorism
- **P**ulmonary stenosis
- **A**bnormalities of genitalia
- **R**etardation of growth
- **D**eafness

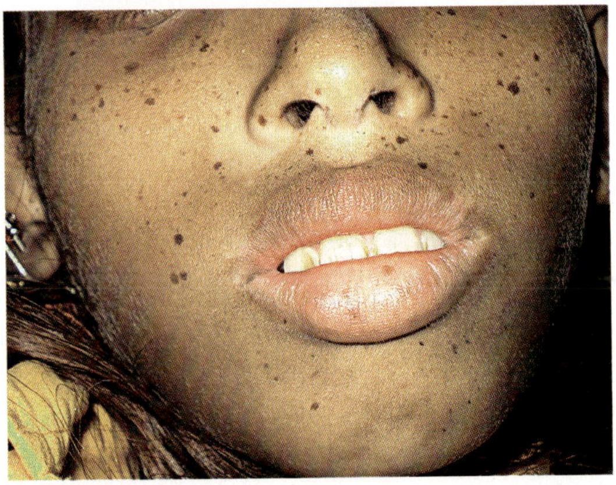

Fig.24.101

75.* Spot the diagnosis (Fig. 24.102).

A: Horner's syndrome. The picture shows one-sided partial ptosis, miosis and decreased sweating.

The features of Horner's sydrome:

- Partial ptosis*

24

- Miosis*, best looked for in dim light where normal pupil dilates
- Anhidrosis of ipsilateral side of face* (Note the decreased sweating of the affected side)
- Enophthalmos*
- Congenital cases may show heterochromia of iris.
- Sympathetic denervation of the eye causes Horner's syndrome. It may be because of: brachial plexus damage at birth; neuroblastoma or other tumours in the mediastinum or cervical region; injury to superior cervical ganglion or sympathetic trunk (e.g., post-surgical); rarely, it is congenital (autosomal dominant).

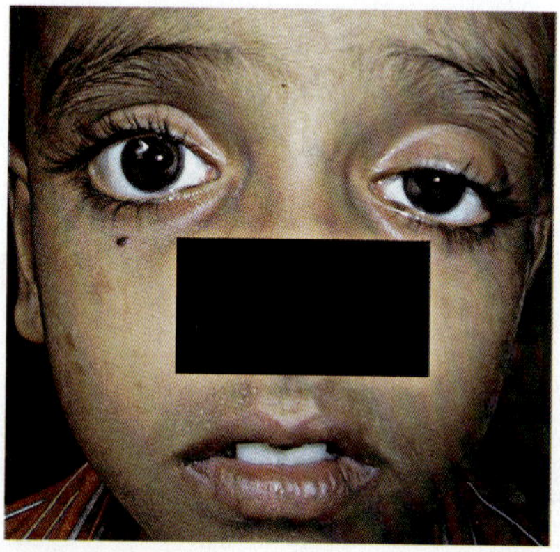

Fig.24.102 Note the eyes and sweating

76. This child was earlier evaluated for the need for surgical intervention for craniosynostosis. The most striking feature of this child is the very protruding eyeballs. He has no abnormalities of digits of hands and feet and has no syndactyly or polydactyly. What diagnosis is probable?

A: Crouzon's syndrome (Fig. 24.103): Protruding eyeballs is the hallmark of Crouzon syndrome. The other conditions associated with craniosynostosis are Apert and Carpenter. The absence of syn/polydactyly rules out both.

The still rarer Pefiffer syndrome has broad thumb and first toe and syndactyly may be there.

- Craniosynostosis*: Coronal, metopic and sagittal sutures. The shape of skull depends on which sutures fuse in which order. These children must be followed up for raised intracranial pressure and subsequent optic atrophy.
- Proptosis due to shallow orbits*
- Hypertelorism
- Midfacial hypoplasia (hypoplasia of maxilla)
- Conductive hearing loss
- Normal intelligence
- Inheritance is autosomal dominant with variable expression **(Fig.24.103)**.

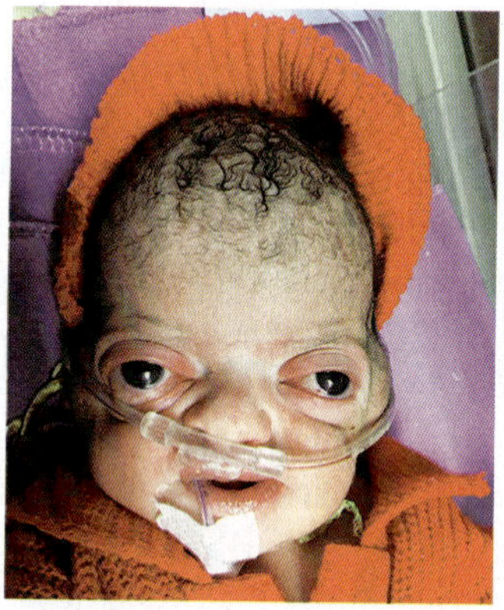

Fig.24.103 Crouzon

77.* Face and hand of a child are shown in the Figs. 24.104–24.106. What is the diagnosis?

A: Apert syndrome. In fact, it is easier to make the diagnosis by viewing the face from the side, which makes it easier to appreciate the high head and brachycephaly (see the drawing).

- Downslanting palpebral fissure, small nose, maxillary hypoplasia, shallow orbits (hence proptosis).
- Head: Short anterior-posterior diameter of skull (look at the side profile) due to craniosynostosis*, especially the coronal

suture. Curiously, fontanels may remain large and may close late.

- Syndactyly*
- Narrow palate
- Mental deficiency may be present but not gross.
- Differential diagnosis: In Carpenter syndrome, there is polysyndactyly. In Crouzon syndrome, there is no syndactyly or polydactyly. The most striking feature in Crouzon is marked proptosis

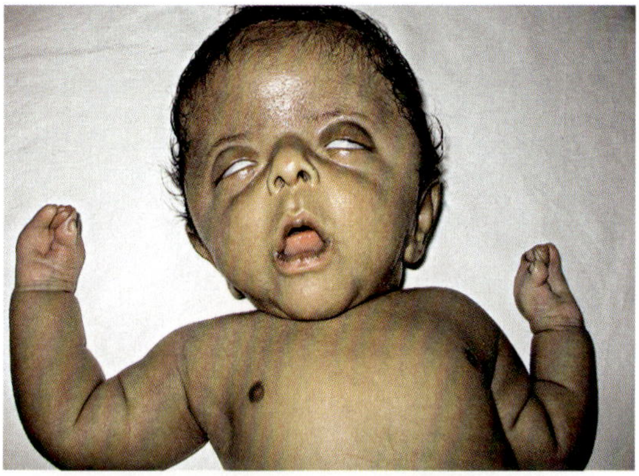

Fig.24.104

78.*Below is shown the most common heritable form of mental retardation in males. Describe the features and give the diagnosis.

A: Fragile X syndrome. Long face, large ears and prominent jaws are obvious in the drawing. Listed below are the usual features:

- Large head with prominent forehead
- Normal height
- Long thin face
- Prominent jaw
- Large posteriorly rotated ears
- Large testes (macro-orchidism, usually not obvious till 6 years).
- Hyperkinetic behaviour
- Mental retardation (it is the most common heritable form of mental retardation in males; however, it is to be noted that fragile X syndrome can occur in girls as well. It is X-linked dominant and hence female carriers may be affected, of course mildly).
- Constriction in X chromosome is demonstrable when the cells are grown in folate-deficient media.

24

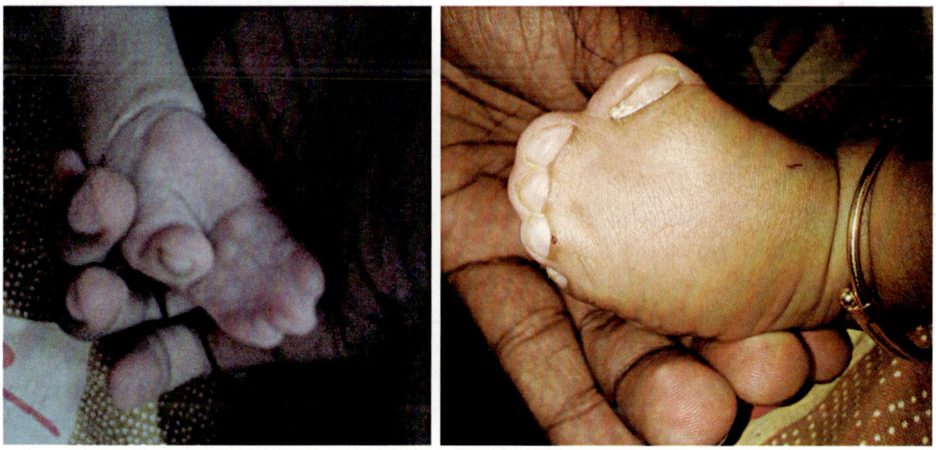

Fig.24.105 Apert syndrome

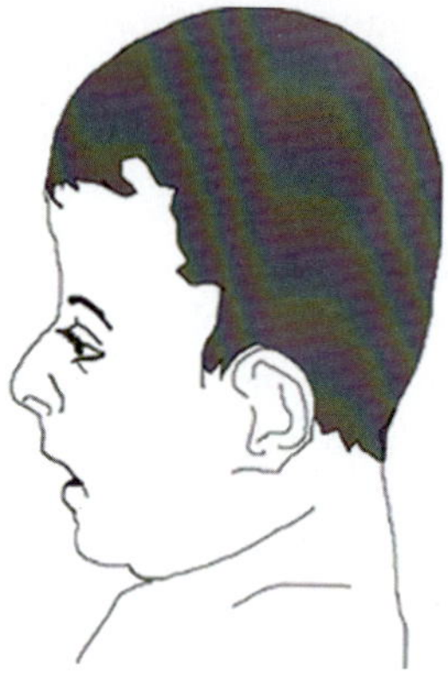

Fig.24.106

- The abnormality is caused by familial mental retardation *(FMRI)* gene expansion at Xp27.3. Gene normally contains less than 50 CGG repeats. When this repeat length has expanded to more than 200, the fragile X syndrome results. The trinucleotide expansion increases with each generation. An increasing severity of clinical manifestation is seen with increasing expansion of trinucleotide repeat sequence and thus an increasing severity may be observed over generations **(Fig.24.107 A & B)**.

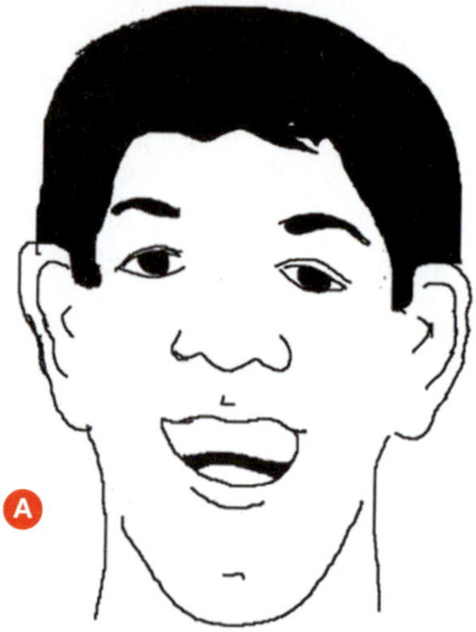

A

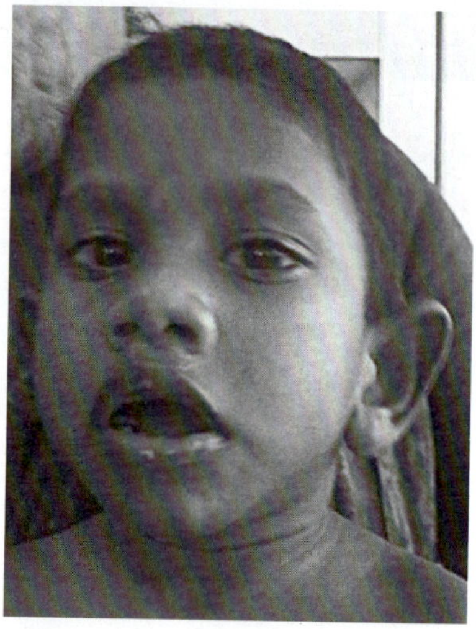

B

Fig.24.107

79.* This child was sent for evaluation of distressing obesity. What is the diagnosis?

A: Cushing syndrome. Most often, it is due to steroid use.

- Rounded face with prominent cheek (moon face), double chin, buffalo hump, generalized obesity and short stature. The most common organic cause is a functioning adrenocortical tumour. Many times, tumour may secrete some androgens also and hence there may be some virilization.

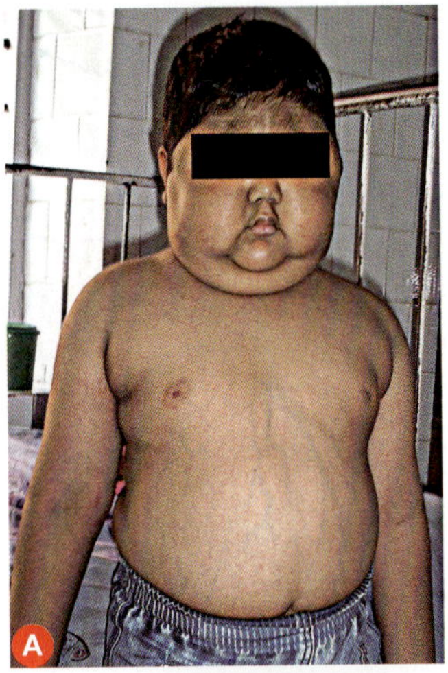

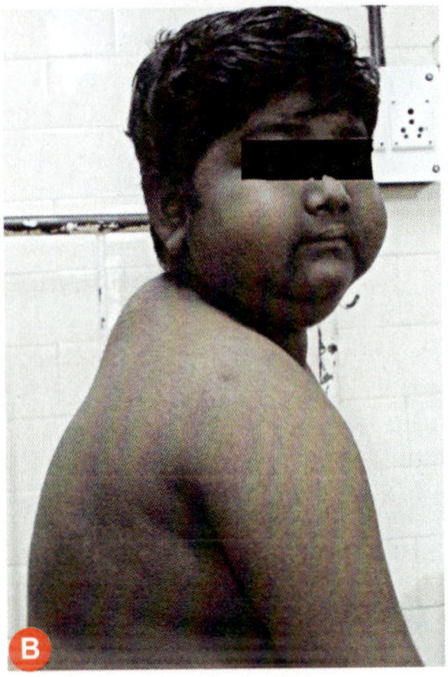

Fig.24.108 Cushing syndrome

80. * A school going child is brought for evaluation of short stature. His teachers considered him good at studies and rated him as a well-behaved child. Spot the diagnosis from this picture. What abnormality is shown in the leg?

A: Hypothyroidism. The picture shows a child with rounded face, periorbital oedema, protruding tongue and a dull expression. Hypothyroidism of late onset (after the critical period of brain development) may not lead to mental retardation and hence may present just as short stature; that may be the reason why the school-going child was not considered bad at school. However, at least some poor interest in studies is expected. May be the teacher equated his placidity with good behaviour!

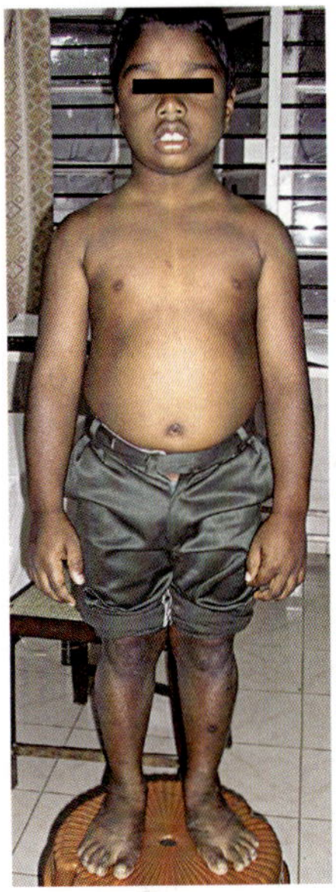

Fig.24.109 Hypothyroid

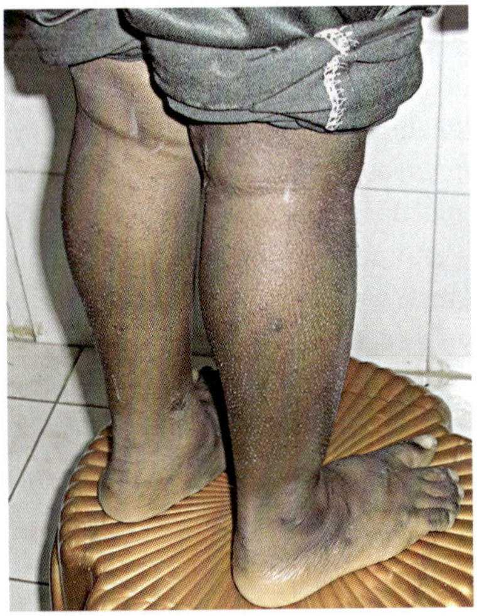

Fig.24.110 Note the calf muscle hypertrophy

Complaints may be intellectual retardation, short stature, etc; in very small infants, constipation, prolongation of jaundice, delayed passage of meconium, poor feeding, sleepiness, etc, may be the complaints. Drug history of child and mother must be looked into (e.g., iodine, antithyroid drugs).

- Pallor
- Hoarse cry
- Dry, rough and cool skin
- Sparse and brittle hair
- Delayed closure of fontanels
- Intellectual retardation (delayed milestones of development)
- Short stature and overweight
- Pulse rate is slow; may have reduced BP
- Hypotonia, muscle weakness and protuberant abdomen
- Delayed relaxation phase of the ankle jerk
- Upper segment–lower segment may be of infantile proportions.
- Delayed eruption of tooth.
- Diffusely enlarged, firm, non-tender goitre may be present in rare cases of congenital enzyme deficiency or iodine deficiency. In children, the most common cause is dysgenesis of thyroid gland and hence no goitre will be found.
- Hashimoto's thyroiditis is the most common cause of goiterous hypothyroidism in grown-up children; diagnosed by biochemical evidence of hypothyroidism and presence of antibodies to thyroid microsomal antigen and thyroglobulin.
- Pendred syndrome is sensorineural deafness, hypothyroidism and goitre; autosomal recessive in inheritance.
- Kocher-Debre-Semelaigne syndrome: Calf muscle pseudohypertrophy in hypothyroidism (very rare) (Fig.24.110). Also see p 452.

81.* This male child was brought with the complaint of his urine not coming through his penis but from the cleft below. Describe the findings and what is the diagnosis?

A: It seems the child has got a penis. A fold of skin above its base, if present, is common with clitoris and not penis. It seems his urethral opening is not in his "penis". A penis-like structure without urinary opening can be clitoris. The scrotum appears bifid or split, so it can be labia or an abnormal scrotum. The probable labia show some prominence, which must be palpated to see if it is a mass (testes). Diagnosis is ambiguous genitalia.

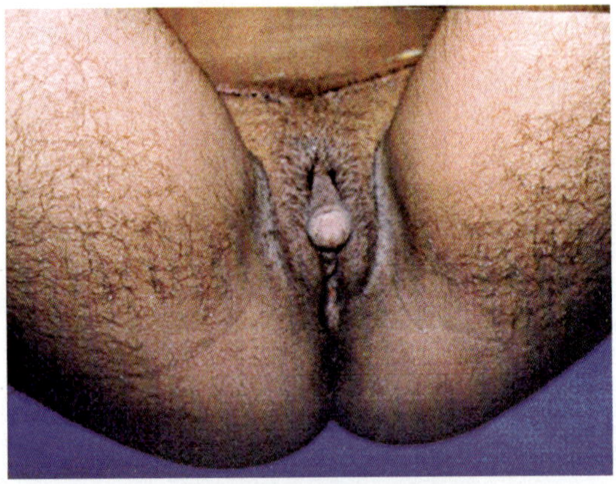

Fig.24.111 Ambiguous genitalia

The clinical discussion will depend on whether the testes are palpable or not. See p 454

If the testes are palpable (palpable gonad in genital area is usually testes), then this child is a male pseudohermaphrodite, meaning he is an under virilized male. There is a defect in synthesis of androgens or defect in conversion of testosterone to dihydrotestosterone or insensitivity of tissues to the action of testosterone. If testes are not palpable, the child may be considered as a virilized female (female pseudohermaphroditism). Congenital adrenal hyperplasia due to 21-hydroxylase deficiency is the most common cause (See p 454).

82. * A 4 ½-year-old girl presented with precocious puberty and hyperpigmented spots over the chest. X-ray was taken for assessment of bone age; bone age was normal but some other abnormality was detected in the bone. What is the probable diagnosis?

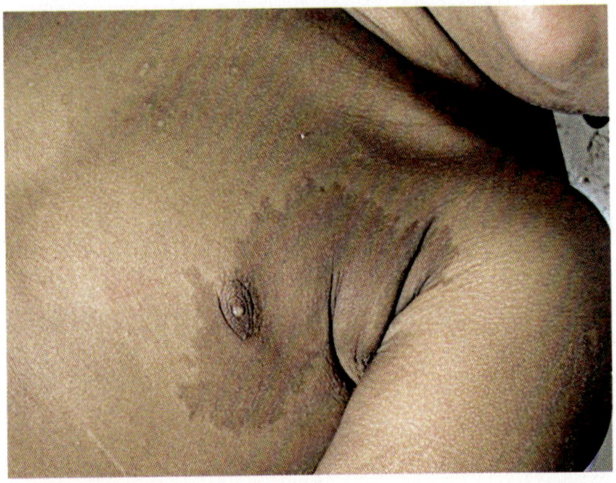

Fig.24.112 Note the ragged edges of cafe au lait spot ("Coast of Maine")

A: McCune-Albright syndrome (polyostotic fibrous dysplasia). Cafe-au-lait spots, bone lesions along with precocious puberty are the typical diagnostic features of McCune-Albright syndrome.

- It is a syndrome of patchy cutaneous pigmentation* and fibrous dysplasia of bone*.
- Precocious puberty* (commoner in girls than boys, usually evident in toddler age).
- Caf-au-lait spots *with characteristic ragged edges.*
- May develop fractures, due to thinning of bones. Asymptomatic bone lesions require no therapy.
- There may be manifestations of *hyper*secretion of other endocrine glands. It seems the defect is with cyclic AMP through which all these hormones act.
- Sporadic in occurrence.
- *Note*: This entity should not be confused with pseudohypoparathyroidism (see p 504).

83.* A 10-year-old female who was on medications for a febrile illness, has now presented with violacious red, raised, tender lesions shown in the picture. What is it?

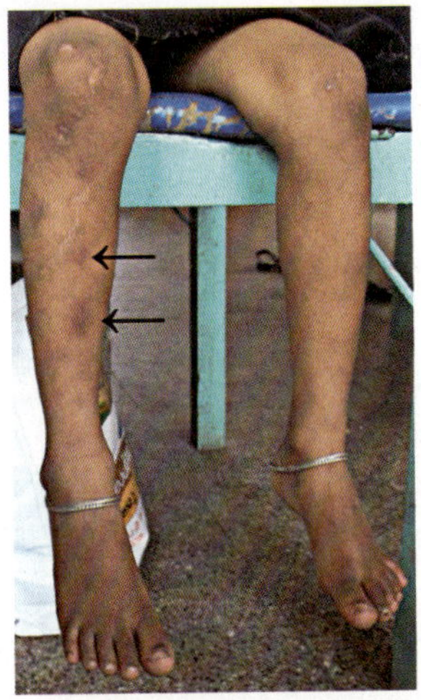

Fig.24.113

A: Erythema nodosum

Erythema nodosum is a raised, shiny, bluish red, tender lesion with indistinct margin, usually seen over the shin. It can be secondary to many aetiologies like viral illness, bacterial illness (streptococcus), tuberculosis, drugs (like sulpha), inflammatory bowel disease, sarcoidosis, etc.

84.* This 2-year-old child has been unwell with fever for about 10 days, had extreme irritability, conjunctival congestion, red cracked lips erythematous rashes over the thigh and unilateral cervical lymphadenopathy. What is the likely diagnosis? What is the most serious complication? (Fig.24.114, 114a, 114b, 114c, 114d)

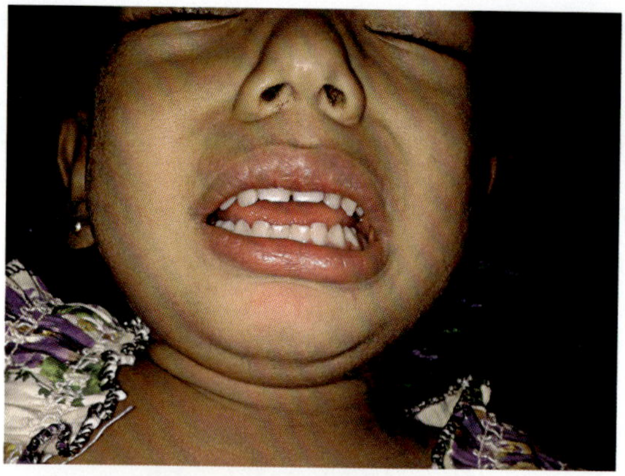

Fig.24.114 Cracked red lips

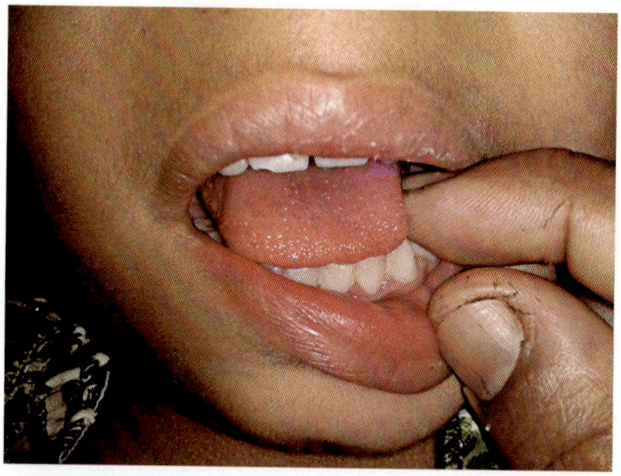

Fig.24.114a Strawberry tongue

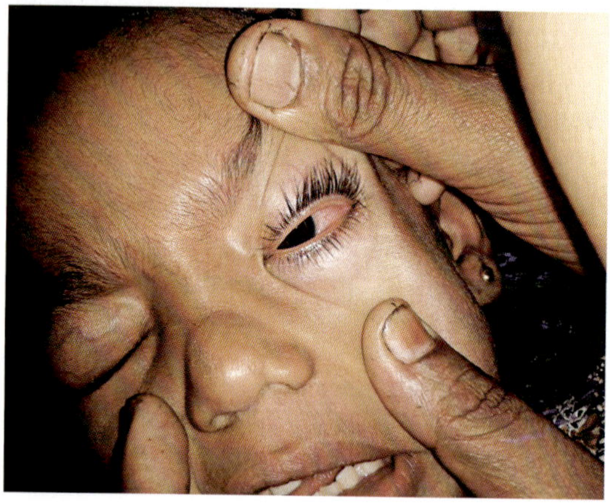

Fig.24.114b Nonpurulent conjunctivitis

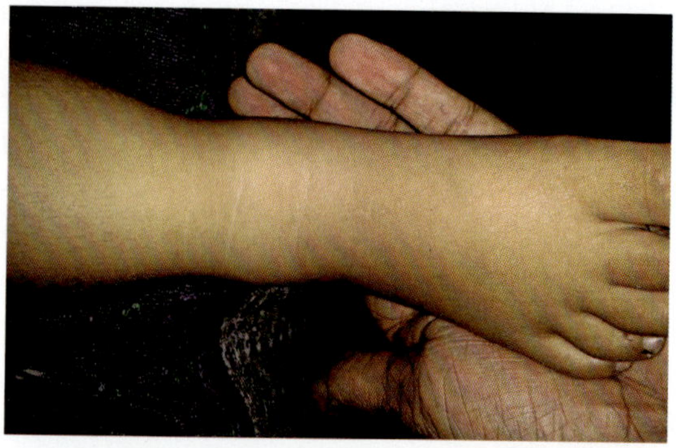

Fig.24.114c Edema of feet

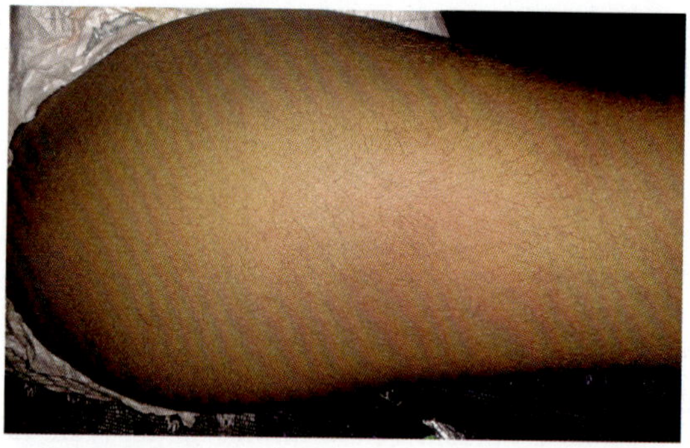

Fig.24.114d Rashes

A: Kawasaki disease. Development of coronary aneurysm is the most dreaded complication.

- It is a mucocutaneous lymph node syndrome.
- Age less than 5 years
- Fever of more than 5 days, for which no other cause could be found
- Cervical lymphadenopathy
- Non-purulent conjunctivitis
- Cracked red lips
- Rashes
- Arthritis
- Irritability
- Induration and oedema of hands and feet, which starts peeling after 10 days
- Treatment is IV gamma globulin

85. Examine the upper limb of this patient.

A: A question like this usually upsets the student. But actually it is simple. What is required is to examine the nervous system pertaining to the upper limb; make an examination of joints of upper limb (Ch.22); also make necessary nutritional assessment that is possible from upper limbs.

86.* In the picture of a short child given below, what are the salient features and what is the probable diagnosis?

A: The picture shows a large head, exaggerated lumbar lordosis and short arm compared to forearm. Thus, it is a rhizomelic short stature with large head: Achondroplasia.

- Disproportionately large head.
- Prominent forehead, depressed nasal bridge* and relatively prominent jaw.
- Disproprtionate short stature; Rhizomelic limb shortening* (proximal segments of limbs are relatively short).
- Short, broad hands and feet; lack of full adduction of fingers in extension, giving rise to the typical trident hand.
- Lumbar lordosis, thoracolumbar kyphosis and protuberant abdomen.

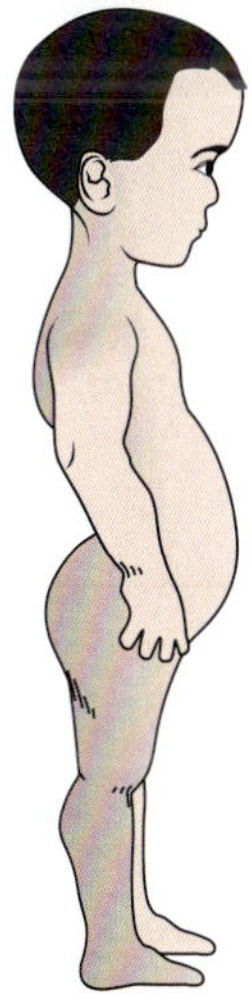

Fig.24.115

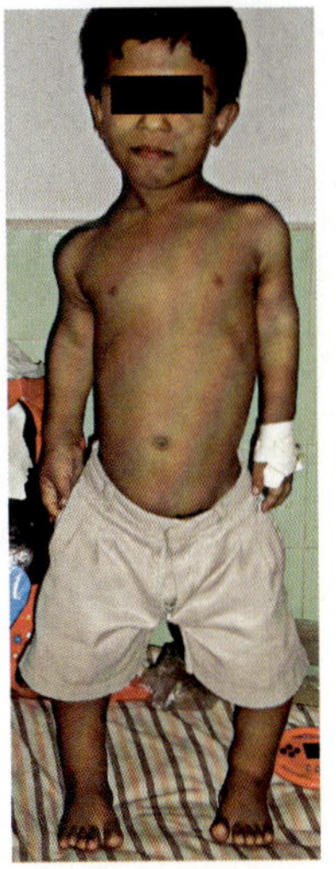

Fig.24.116 Achondroplasia

- Bowed legs and waddling gait.
- Trident hand: Fingers cannot oppose one another.
- Autosomal dominant inheritance; however, up to 90% of cases represent fresh mutation, all occurring in father's sperm; hence associated with advanced paternal age.
- Neurological complications: Hydrocephalus, spinal cord compression at the foramen magnum.
- No mental retardation.
- Mutation of fibroblast growth factor receptor 3 (*FGFR 3*) gene at chromosome 4p16.3.

87. *A 5-year-old child born of consanguinous marriage is brought with severe limitation of mobility, joint deformities and multiple nodular swellings over the joints. The elder sibling has the same problem. What is the diagnosis?

A: Farber's disease

The disease results from deficiency of a lysosomal enzyme ceramidase. Accumulation of ceramide in joints results in painful swollen joints and nodules/granulomas (thus juvenile

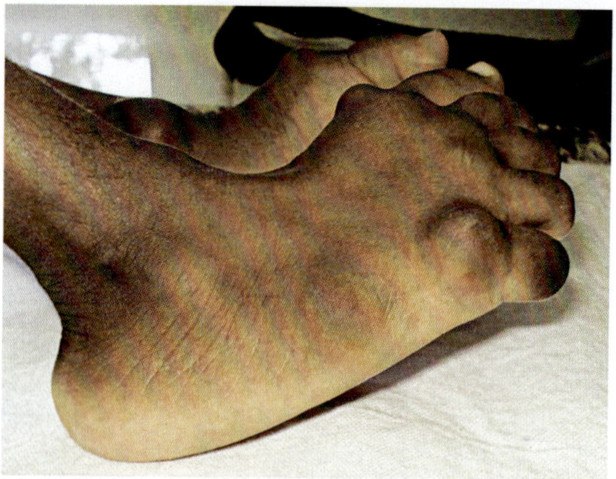

Fig.24.117

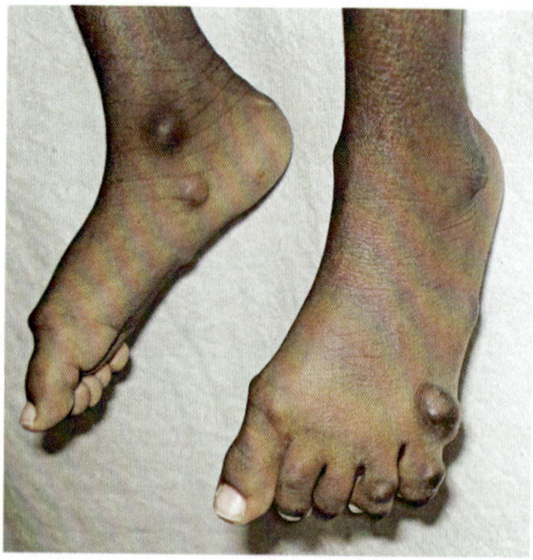

Fig.24.118

rheumatoid arthritis comes as a close differential diagnosis). Other clinical features include hoarseness of voice (due to vocal cord nodule/granuloma), failure to thrive, cardiac/CNS dysfunction, etc. The condition is autosomal recessive in inheritance.

88. *A 2-year-old child born of consanguineous marriage is brought with history of growth and developmental retardation. The parents felt that the child had been rather floppy compared to other children. The child underwent surgery for cataract a few months ago and is now wearing spectacles. The arrows in the picture points towards a few clinical signs. What is the diagnosis?

A: Lowe syndrome

Lowe syndrome is oculocerebrorenal syndrome. The transmission is X linked. The symptoms are detectable during infancy itself and consist of progressive growth failure, hypotonia, mental retardation, behavioural abnormalities, renal tubular manifestations of Fanconi syndrome and rickets. No specific treatment is available; surgery for cataract may be considered.

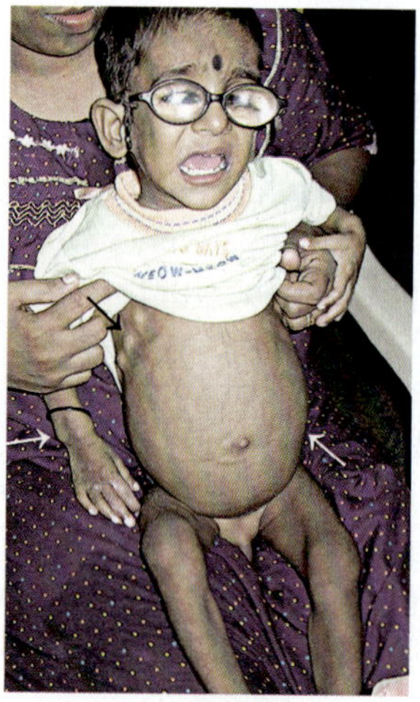

Fig.24.119

89. * A 9-year-old boy was brought with complaints of on and off fever and myalgia of 3 months duration. Two days ago, he developed nasal regurgitation and nasal twang of voice. He had violaceous erythema in the periorbital area, tender swelling over both shoulders and weakness of proximal muscles. His deep tendon reflexes were sluggish. What is the diagnosis?

A: Juvenile dermatomyositis (see p 479). Heliotrope rash (periorbital violaceous erythema) often with periorbital oedema, symmetrical proximal muscle weakness (sparing extraocular and facial muscles) and tender swelling of muscles (with elevated muscle enzymes) makes the diagnostic triad. Gottron's papules (erythematous scaling) may be seen over the dorsal aspects of metacarpophalangeal and proximal interphalangeal joints.

90. *This child was having skin lesions since about 1 year of age. Lesions consist of erythema followed by bullae and crusting. Lesions are maximal over the face, hands and forearm. There are both hyper- and hypopigmented lessions. As seen in Fig. 24.120, the upper arm and chest are spared. He is below average in studies. He has some intolerance of bright light. There is history of recurrent keratitis.

A: Xeroderma pigmentosum. This is an autosomal recessive disorder with a defect in nucleotide repair. Wavelength of light that produces DNA damage is around 280–340 nm. The areas involved in this child are all sun-exposed areas. Skin changes are first noted during early childhood when the child gets exposed to sun. However, light from unshielded fluorescent bulbs and sunlight passing through glass windows are also considered harmful and may explain lesions appearing during infancy.

Mental subnormality and sensorneural hearing loss occur in 30% patients.

Combination of microcephaly, mental retardation, deafness and depressed deep tendon reflexes due to peripheral neuropathy is De Sanctis Cacchione syndrome.

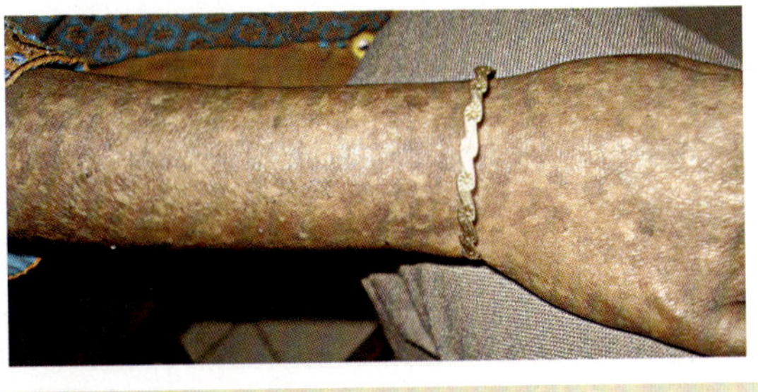

Fig.24.120 Xeroderma pigmentosa

Affected children should be protected totally from sun exposure; protective clothing, eyeglasses and opaque broad-spectrum sunscreen creams should be used. Early detection and removal of malignancies is mandatory (malignancies are basal cell carcinoma, squamous cell carcinoma and malignant melanoma). Affected families should have genetic counseling (25% chance of recurrence in siblings). Prenatal diagnosis is possible via amniocentesis. Megadose vit A is on trial to prevent skin malignancies. Since the child cannot be exposed to sunlight, supplementation of vit D is essential.

24

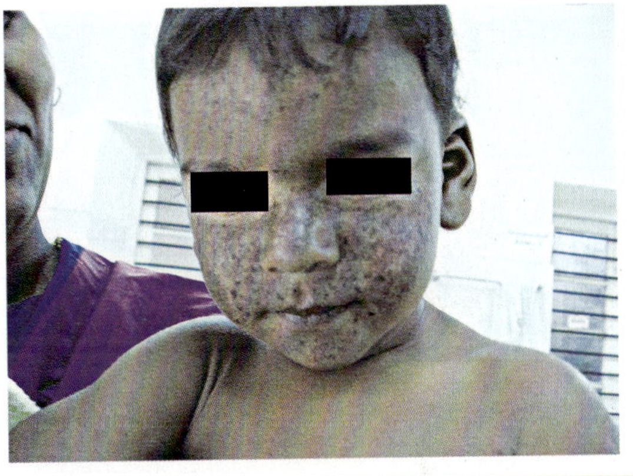

Fig.24.121 Xeroderma pigmentosa

91. 1-year-old child, was brought with fever of 5 days duration and distressing cough. He had excessive lacrimation the previous day, which gave way to red eye today and there is generalized rash (Fig. 24.122–24.124). He had been in hospital for diarrhoea 2 weeks ago. On examination, child is febrile, irritable, has conjuctival congestion and generalized erythematous maculopapular rash, which involved palms also. Auscultation revealed bilateral crepitations. What is the most probable diagnosis?

A: Measles

Measles is a highly contagious disease (caused

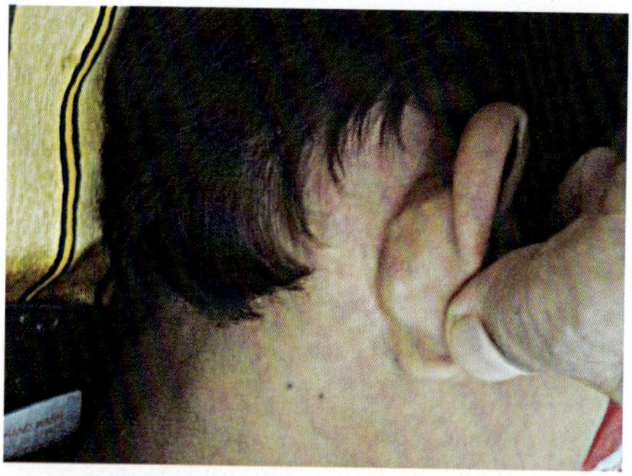

Fig.24.122 Measles rash behind the ear, usually the first place for rashes to appear

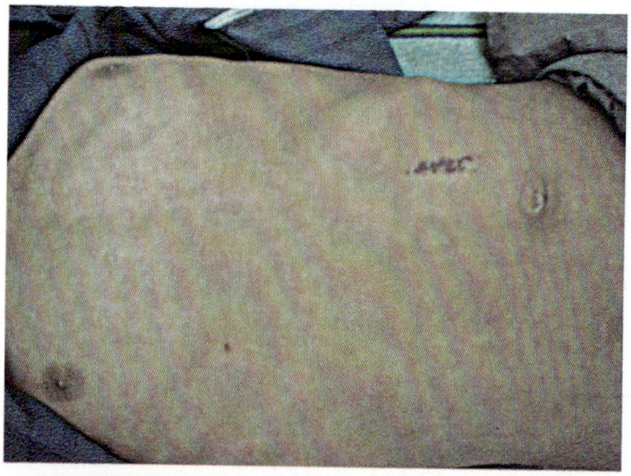

Fig.24.123 Measles rash

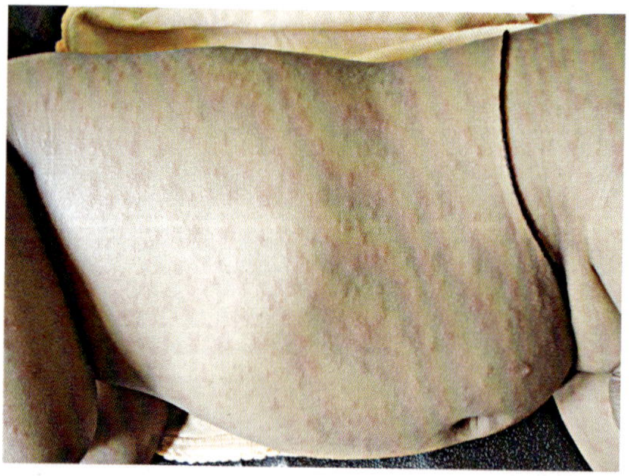

Fig.24.124 Measles rash: Note the maculo-papular nature

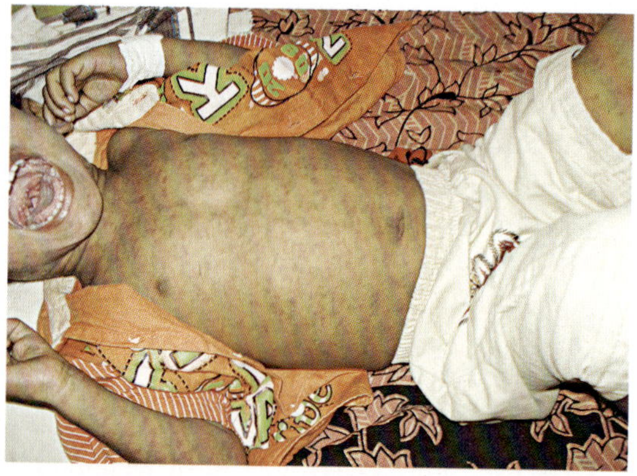

Fig.24.125 Brownish desquamation of measles rash

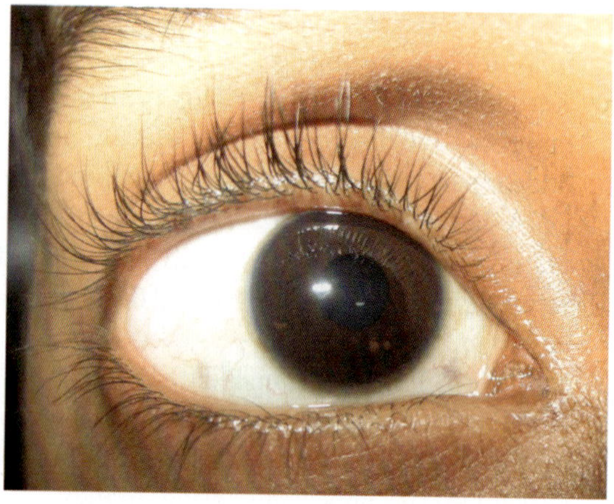

Fig.24.126 Lisch nodule (see page 522) *Courtesy: Dr Sheela Nampoothiri.*

by an RNA virus). It is quite possible that the child had a contact with measles during his hospital stay 2 weeks back (Incubation period is 10–12 days).

Clinical features: Prodromal phase lasts for 3 days. Fever, dry hacking cough, running nose, redness of eyes and excessive lacrimation are the usual features. On the 3rd or 4th day, Koplik spots appear (greyish white spots surrounded by erythema over the buccal mucosa opposite to 2nd molar tooth) Fig. 17.7, p 392.

The rash appears typically on the 5th day of fever. Erythematous maculopapular rash, which starts behind the ear, spreads to forehead, face, neck, trunk, extremities, palms and soles within 48 hrs. With the appearance of rash, there is abrupt increase in fever which remains high for 48 hrs. Rash disappears with brownish desquamation in the next 4–5 days.

Complications: Think of involvement of mucous membranes and you can enumerate the common complications; i.e., bronchopneumonia (secondary bacterial), interstitial pneumonia due to measles virus (Hecht cell pneumonia), otitis media, diarrhoea.

CNS: Rarely encephalomyelitis; as a late complication, SSPE (subacute sclerosing panencephalitis)

Precipitation of malnutrition; reduced cell mediated immunity (hence reactivation of latent tuberculosis); anergy (e.g., false negative Mantoux reaction).

92. What is the skin abnormality in this newborn (Fig 24.127)? What are the complications? What is the management?

A: Aplasia Cutis Congenita

It is a developmental absence of skin, usually noted on the scalp as multiple or solitary (70%), non-inflammatory, well-demarcated, oval or circular 1-2 cm ulcers. The appearance of lesions varies, depending on when they occurred during intrauterine development.Those that form early in gestation may heal before delivery and appear as atrophic, fibrotic scars with associated alopecia, whereas more recent defects may manifest as ulcers. Only the epidermis and upper dermis may be involved, resulting in minimal scarring or hair loss but may extend to the deep dermis, to the subcutaneous tissue, and, rarely, to the periosteum, skull, and dura.

Associated with meningomyelocele, gastroschisis, omphalocele, orspinal dysraphism. Aplasia cutis congenita in association with

24

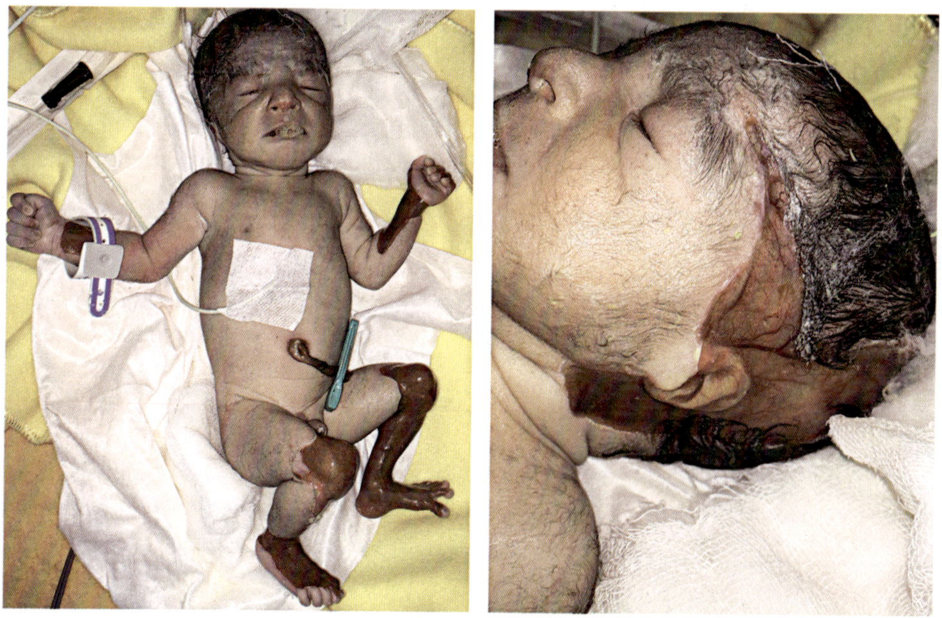

Fig.24.127 Aplasia

fetus papyraceus is apparently caused by ischemic or thrombotic events in the placenta and fetus.

Complications: Hemorrhage, secondary local infection, meningitis.

Management: If the defect is small, recovery is uneventful, with gradual epithelialization and formation of a hairless atrophic scar over a period of several weeks. Small bony defects usually close spontaneously in the 1st year of life. Large or numerous scalp defects may require repair. Truncal and limb defects, despite being large, usually epithelialize and form atrophic scars, which can later be revised.

93. Identify the skin abnormality (Fig. 24.128). In what condition are they seen?

A: **Blue Berry Muffin spots**

They are generalized(more often on the trunk, head, and neck) hemorrhagic purpuric eruptions that on histopathology shows dermal erythropoiesis. Congenital infections (Cytomegalovirus and Rubella), haemolytic disease of newborn, Hereditary spherocytosis, Neuroblastoma, AML, LCH, Neonatal Lupus, vascular lesions like Multiple hemangiomas of infancy, multifocal lymphangioendotheliomatosis, blue rubber bleb nevus syndrome and multiple glomangiomas are conditions that should be considered in the differential diagnosis of an infant with a blueberry muffin appearance. It was initially described for Congenital Rubella Syndrome.

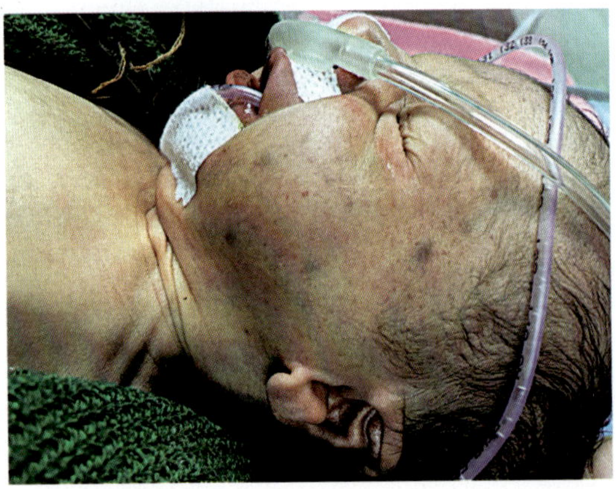

Fig.24.128 Blueberry

94. 9 month old infant presented to the casualty with complaints of fever and rhinitis, became irritable from today afternoon. On examination the child had disproportionate regular tachycardia and an ECG was taken (Fig 24.129). Identify the ECG abnormality? What is the management?

A: **Supraventricular Tachycardia**

Lead II ECG shows narrow QRS complex tachycardia (rate=214) with an absent p-wave. Compared to sinus tachycardia SVT has an unvarying heart rate of >200 in infants and >180 in older children. SVT is a general term that includes all forms of paroxysmal tachycardia except VT. There are 3 major sub categories: Re-entrant tachycardia with an accessory pathway, without an accessory pathway, ectopic tachycardia. It has usually an abrupt onset and the only complaint in older children might be palpitation. SVT in young infants may be precipitated by acute infections like URI or drugs (decongestants, bronchodilators) and may present in heart failure as the SVT may go unrecognized.

Management is emergency reversal to the sinus rhythm. Vagal manouvers(ice water application over the face for 10-15 sec/ Valsalva manouvre) may be attempted but Adenosine by rapid iv push via a proximal vein (100mcg/kg upto 300mcg/kg) followed by saline flush is the treatment of choice in stable patients. In unstable patients DC version (0.5J/kg) is recommended. Once the child has been reverted to sinus rhythm repeat ECG to see for features of WPW(short PR, deltawaves). Add betablockers/ digoxin if no WPW and if there is WPW digoxin is contraindicated.

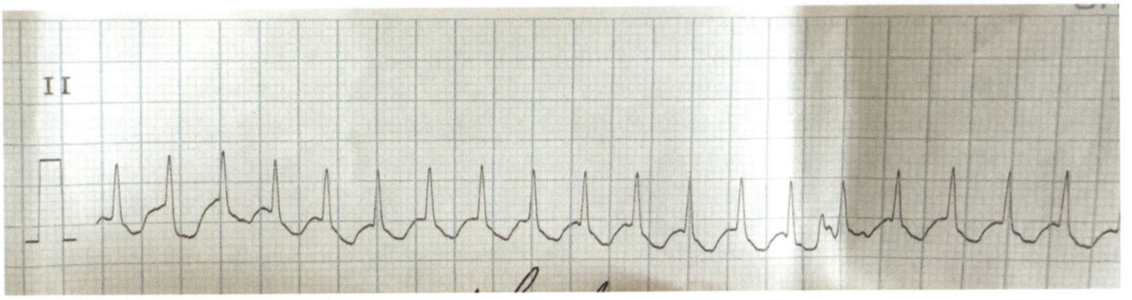

Fig.24.129 SVT

95. What is the diagnosis(Fig. 24.130)? What may be the probable risk factors for developing this condition?

A: **Follicular Hyperkeratosis or Phrynoderma.** It is characterized by excessive development of keratin in hair follicles, resulting in rough, cone-shaped, elevated papules. The openings are often closed with a white plug of encrusted sebum. It may be caused by multiple risk factors involving multiple nutrients(Vit-A, Vit-B complex, Vit-E, EFA), local factors like pressure and friction, and environmental factors in the setting of increased nutritional demand.

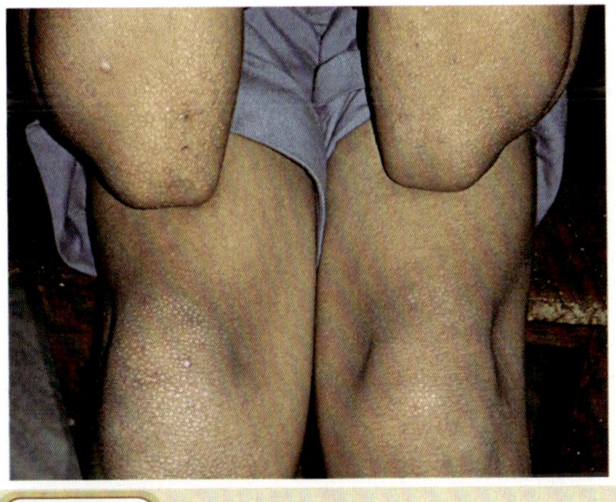

Fig.24.130 Phrynoderma

96. This term newborn was detected to have dew drop vesicles all over the body in crops on day 5 of life. The mother had similar lesions noted on day 1 (Fig 24.131). What could be the probable diagnosis? What is the treatment? What is its prevention?

A. **Neonatal varicella**

Treatment: Intravenous acyclovir, 60 mg/kg/day in divided doses every 8 hours, is recommended for minimum of 5-7 days, particularly for infants at the highest risk of adverse outcomes (the infant born to a woman who develops varicella from 5 days before until 2 days after delivery)

Prevention: Prevention is adviced for babies of women without evidence of immunity, Newborn infant whose mother developes chickenpox within 5 days before delivery or within 48 hours after delivery, Hospitalized premature infant (≥28 weeks' gestational age) whose motherhas no history for chickenpox or serologic evidence of prior infection,

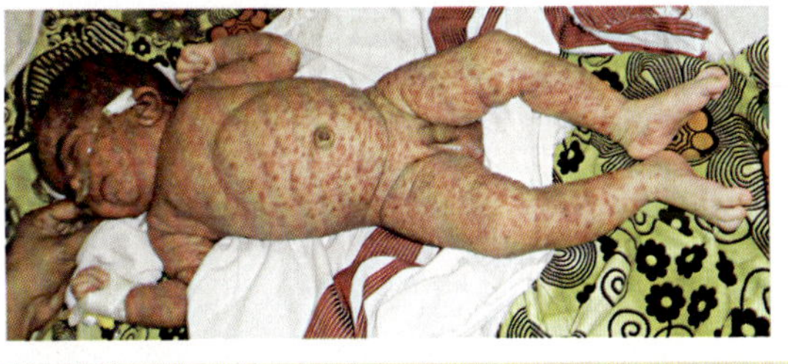

Fig.24.131 Varicella

24

Hospitalized preterm infants (<28 weeks' gestational age or birthweight ≤1000 g) regardless of the maternal history of varicella or varicella-zostervirus serostatus. Varicella Zoster Immunoglobulin (VZIG) is given intramuscularly at a recommended dose of 125 units per 10 kg bodyweight, up to a maximum of 625 units. If VZIG is unavailable, IVIG (400 mg/kg) can be substituted.

97. Identify the anomaly (Fig 24.132)? What embryonic defect causes this anomaly?

A. **Proboscis cyclopia**

It is caused by the failure of the embryonic prosencephalon to properly divide the orbits of the eye into two cavities.it is a rare form of holoprosencepahly. Typically, the nose is either missing/replaced with a non-functional nose (Proboscis). Proboscis usually forms above the single central eye (cyclopia)/on the back. Most such embryos are either naturally aborted or are stillborn upon delivery.

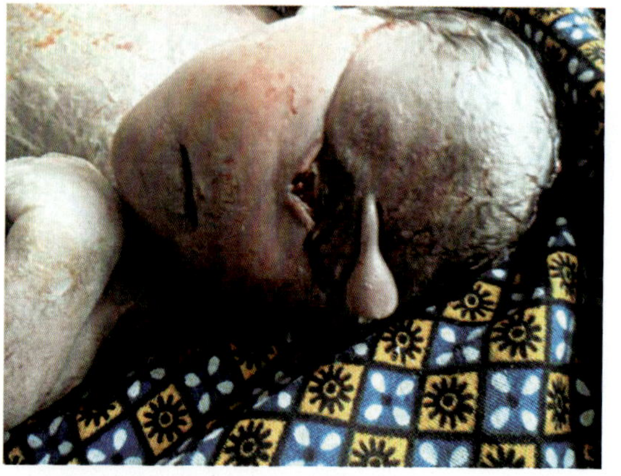

Fig.24.132 Proboscis cyclopia

98. 9-year-old boy presented with complaints of fever for 10 days, and pain, swelling and restricted movements of both the knee joints. He had a history of untreated sore throat 2 weeks back. What is the most probable diagnosis if the ECG of the boy is as shown (Fig 24.133)? What is the 2015 Revised Jones criteria?

A. **Acute Rheumatic Fever (1 major and 2 minor criteria are satisfied)**

ECG shows prolonged PR interval (≥ 200 msec)

Revised Jones criteria 2015

For all patient populations with evidence of preceding GAS infection initial ARF is diagnosed if there are 2 Major manifestations or 1 major plus 2 minor manifestations and recurrent ARF is diagnosed if there are 2 Major or 1 major and 2 minor or 3 minor criteria.

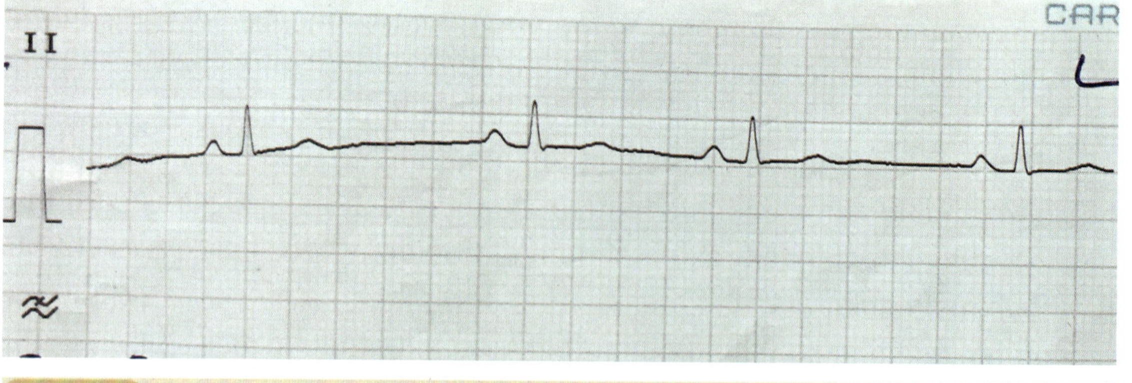

Fig.24.133 RHFever

Major criteria

1. Carditis (Clinical and/or subclinical)
2. Arthritis (Monoarthritis or polyarthritis, Polyarthralgia)
3. Chorea
4. Erythema marginatum
5. Subcutaneous nodules

Minor criteria

1. Monoarthralgia (If arthralgia/arthritis is not a major criterion)
2. Fever (≥38°C)
3. ESR ≥30 mm/h and/or CRP ≥3.0 mg/dL
4. Prolonged PR interval, after accounting for age variability (unless carditis is a major criterion)

99. Identify this skin lesion noted in this newborn (Fig. 24.134). Initial lesions were pustular which ruptured to leave these lesions.

A. **Benign pustular melanosis**

It is a transient, benign, self-limited dermatosis of unknown etiology that is characterized by 3 types of lesions: (1) evanescent superficial pustules, (2) ruptured pustules with a collarette of fine scale, at times with a central hyperpigmented macule, and (3) hyperpig mented macules. Lesions are present at birth, and 1 or all types of lesions may be found in a profuse or sparse distribution. Pustules represent the early phase of the disorder, and macules, the late phase. The pustular phase rarely lasts more than 2-3 days; hyperpigmented macules may persist for as long as 3 mo. Sites of predilection are the anterior neck, forehead, and lower back, although the scalp, trunk, limbs, palms, and soles may be affected.

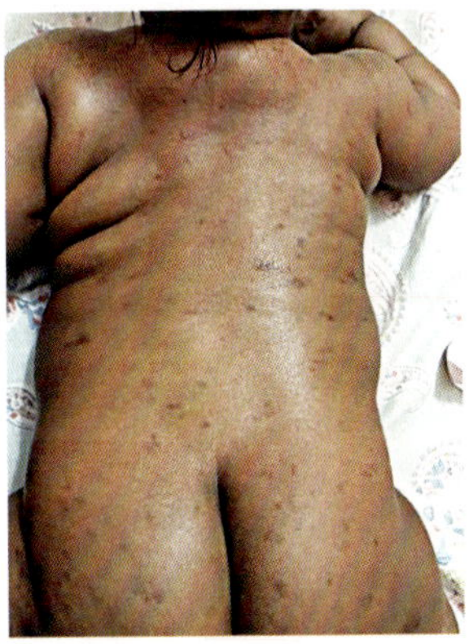

Fig.24.134 BPM

100. Note the skin lesions noted in this child (Fig. 24.135). What are they? When do you find these?

A. **Striae or Stretch marks**

Stretch marks appear as parallel streaks of red, thinned, glossy skin that over time become whitish and scar-like in appearance. Causes include Cushing syndrome, Ehlers-Danlos syndrome, Pregnancy, Puberty, Obesity, Overuse of cortisone skin creams. The stretch marks may be slightly depressed and have a different texture than normal skin.

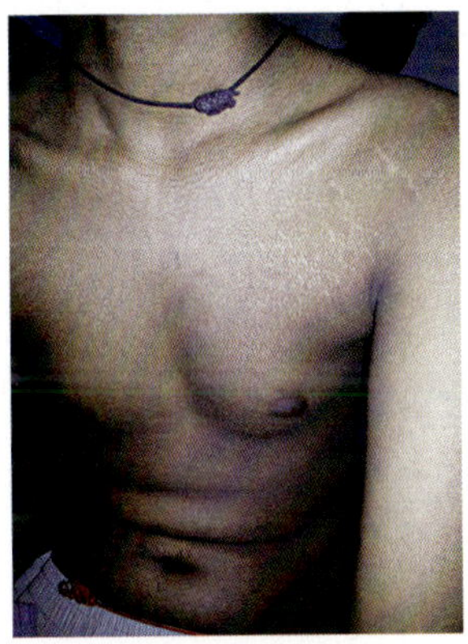

Fig.24.135 Stretch marks

101.Read the ECG of this newborn and comment (Fig 24.136).

A. **Congenital complete heart block (type 3 AV block)**

There is no constant relation between the P waves and the QRS complex.QRS duration may be prolonged, or it may be normal if the heartbeat is initiated high in the AV node or bundle of His.The atria and the ventricles are contracting at different rates.Congenital complete AVblock is presumed to be caused by autoimmune injury of the fetal conduction system by maternally derived immunoglobulin G antibodies (anti-SSA/Ro, anti-SSB/La) in a mother with overt or, more often, asymptomatic systemic lupus erythematosus or Sjögren syndrome.Cardiac pacing is recommended in neonates with low ventricular rates (≤50 beats/min), evidence of heart failure, wide complex rhythms, or congenital heart disease. Isoproterenol, atropine, or epinephrine may be used to try to increase the heart rate temporarily until pacemaker placement can be arranged.

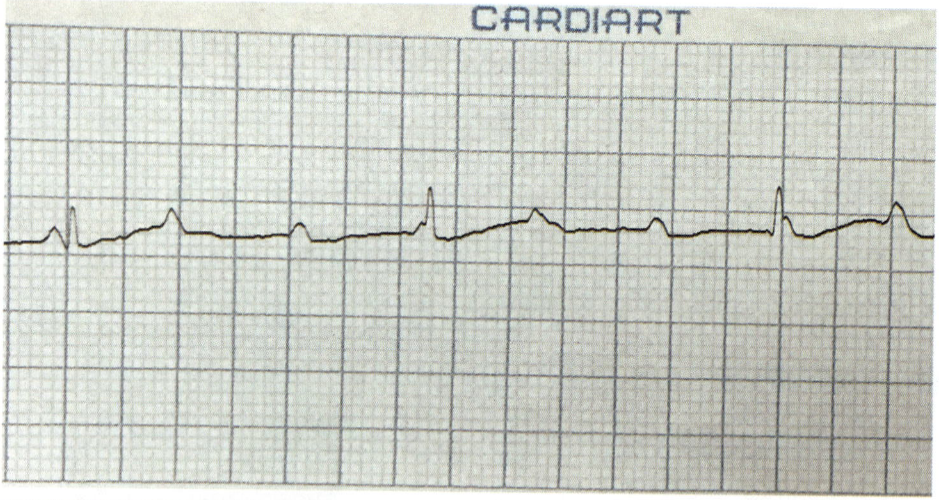

Fig.24.136 Complete Heart Block

CHAPTER 25

Image Gallery II : X-Rays and CT & MRI

In this section, the X-rays that are usually kept in examination are discussed. Questions with * mark are generally meant for postgraduate students and hence the undergraduates can skip them.

List of images in this section.

X-rays (List in alphabetical order)

CT Scans (List in alphabetical order)

11. Tuberculoma (p 578)
12. Tuberous sclerosis ("Candle dripping") (p 574)

MRI Scans
1. Multiple tuberculoma (p 578)
2. Meningomyelocoele (p 579)

1. What is the X-ray diagnosis?

A: Lung abscess. There is no tracheal or mediastinal shift. There is a rounded shadow and inside it is opacity with a horizontal upper level. Lung marking can be seen through the lucent area in the cavity. Thus, it is a cavity with a fluid level within the lung and hence it is a lung abscess. Lung abscess can be primary when it occurs in a normal host. It is secondary when it occurs in a pre-existing disease state like neuromuscular problems. Thus, secondary lung abscesses have aspiration and hence anaerobes as the organism. Primary lung abscess may be because of staphylococci.

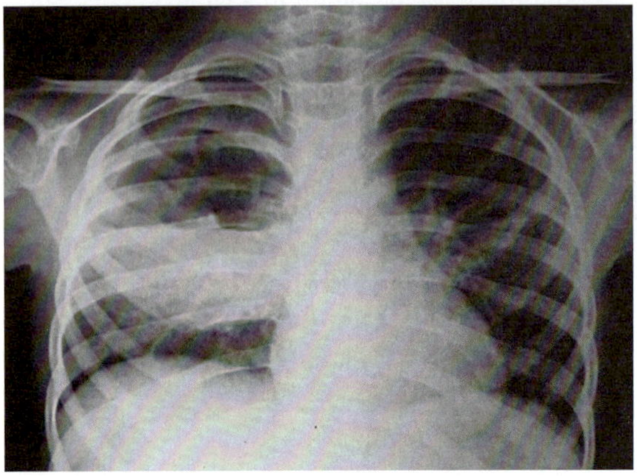

Fig.25.1

2. What is the X-ray diagnosis (Fig.25.2)?

A: Collapse involving segments of right lower lobe. There is mediastinal shift to right. There is a triangular shadow on the right side in touch with the cardiac shadow, but the cardiac shadow is seen very well through the opacity. Hence, the opacity is at a different plane from that of the heart, i.e., it is not the middle lobe, but lower lobe that is involved. There is blurring of diaphragm as the shadow is in touch with the diaphragm, again proving that the opacity is in the lower lobe. Collapse of lower lobe basal segments can occur because of aspiration in an upright child. Other findings that may be there in collapse are crowding of ribs, elevation of diaphragm of the same side, etc.

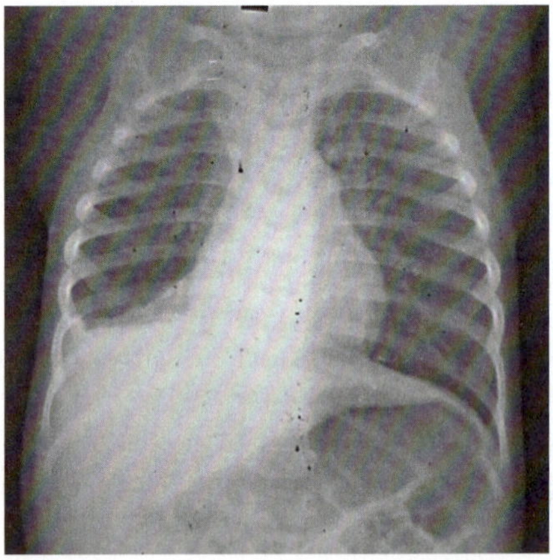

Fig.25.2

3. *This apparently well child with no fever suddenly developed paroxysmal cough and hence is brought to the casualty service. What is the finding in this X-ray?

A: There is shift of mediastinum to the right (in the X-ray shown, more than ½ of cardiac shadow is to the right of spine). There is a dark lung on the left and comparatively less dark lung on the right. It could be obstructive emphysema due to foreign body obstructing one of the major airways on the left side. Sudden onset and absence of fever argues against an infection. Since lung markings are well seen in the dark lung on the left side, it is not pneumothorax. Unless the caretaker witnesses a choking episode, many a time, history of aspiration may not be obtainable.

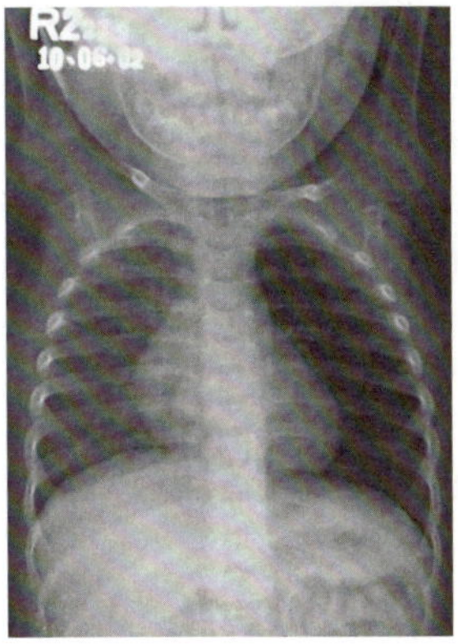

Fig.25.3

4.* What abnormality is seen in this X-ray? Name two most important investigations that must be considered in this case.

A: Numerous rounded shadows are seen. The diagnosis may be miliary TB though X-ray appearance is not classical. The rounded shadows are much bigger than the classic miliary mottling, possibly because the miliary nodules have started to spread out to coalesce. Note the hilar shadow. Gastric lavage for AFB staining and Mantoux test are the two investigations of choice. Although the Mantoux may be negative, it is still more useful than many modern investigations.

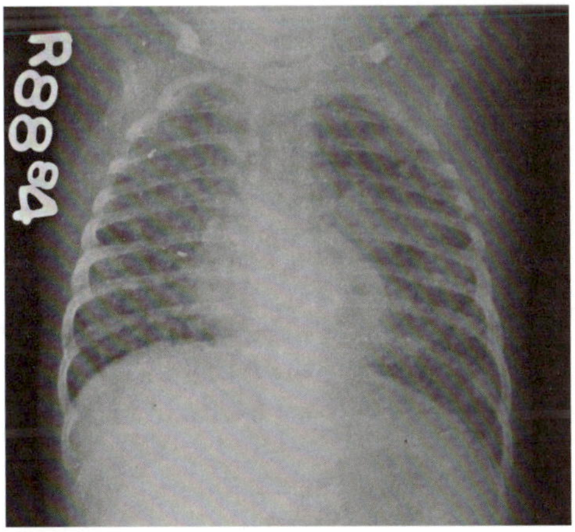

Fig.25.4

5.* This child is brought for evaluation of recurrent respiratory infections and weight loss. What do you find in the X-ray (Fig. 25.5)? What one history and one investigation will help to diagnose this condition?

A: The X-ray shows hilar glands bilaterally. Probable diagnosis is primary complex. History of contact with an adult case of TB and Mantoux test will help to strengthen the suspicion. It is to be noted that hilar gland per se will not be diagnostic of TB.

Hilar enlargement is difficult to interpret. First make sure the film is not a rotated one, in which case one hilum may appear spuriously enlarged (in a properly positioned X-ray, the medial ends of clavicles must be equidistant from spinous process). Now look at the outer edge of hilum. Normally, it is a bit concave; if it appears convex, it is enlarged. Lymphadenopathy gives a smooth lobular appearance to the hilar shadow. Presence of calcium inside shadow tells it is almost certainly a lymph node.

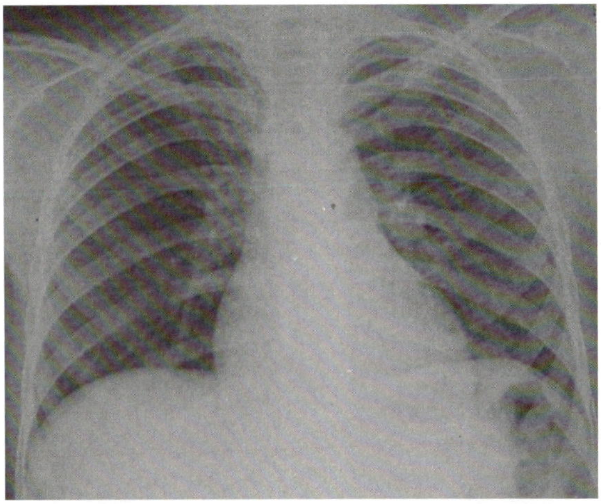

Fig.25.5

6. **What is the X-ray diagnosis? How can you make a clinical diagnosis of this condition?**

A: Hydropneumothorax. Trachea and mediastinum are shifted to the opposite side. On the right side is a uniform opacity with a horizontal upper level, above which there are no lung markings. Clinical diagnosis is possible by demonstrating a horizontal upper level above, which can be made to shift (shifting dullness).

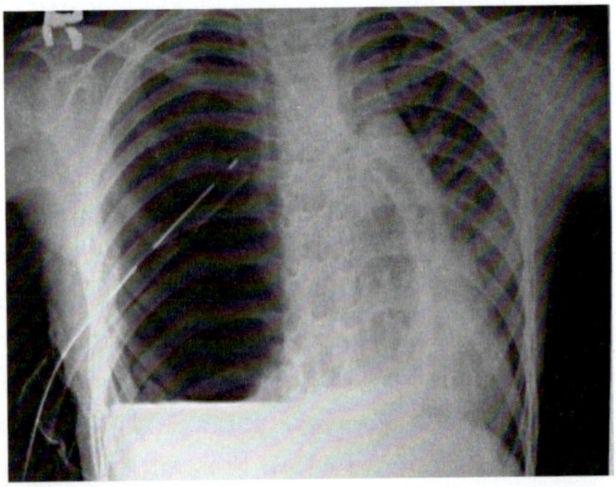

Fig.25.6

7.* **What is the X-ray diagnosis?**

A: Right upper lobe consolidation. The horizontal fissure appears bulging out, which could mean the aetiology to be Klebsiella. Within the area of consolidation there are lucencies that could mean a necrotizing pneumonia, which again could be Klebsiella. Staphylococcal pneumonia and lung abscess are close differential diagnosis.

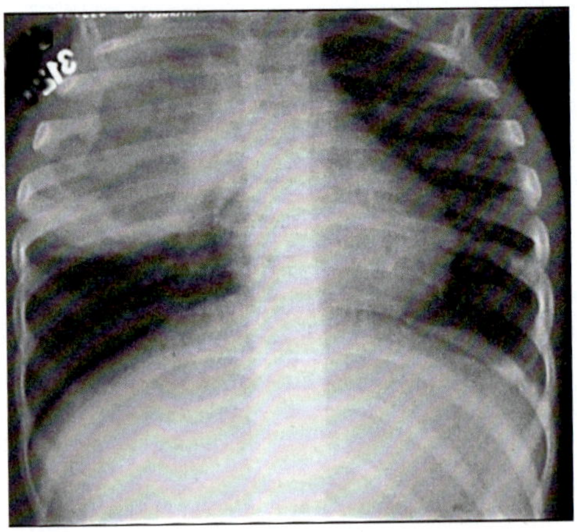

Fig.25.7

8. **Read this X-ray (Fig.25.8).**

A: There is a uniform white shadow on the right, which appears to stop sharply at a level, possibly at horizontal fissure. There is no shift of trachea or mediastinum. It is consolidation of right upper lobe (lobar pneumonia).

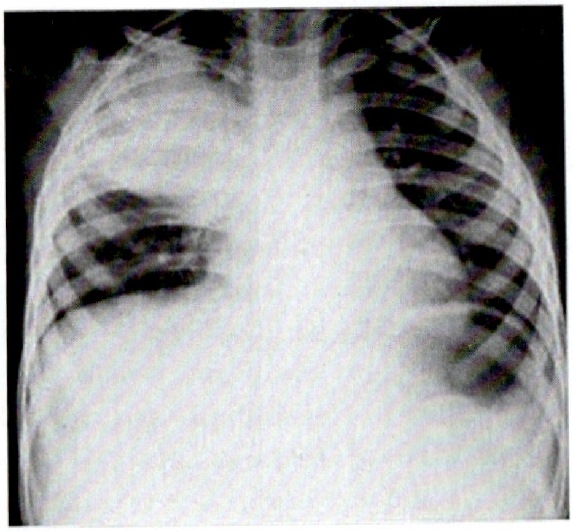

Fig.25.8

Lobar Pneumonia

- Comment on respiratory distress and cyanosis; also mention if any danger signs are present or not (danger signs are: altered sensorium, inability to drink, seizures, cyanosis, severe PEM, grunt, stridor in a calm child, etc).
- Increased respiratory rate.
- Use of accessory muscles of respiration/lower chest in-drawing (it should be persistent to be taken as significant).
- Trachea is central.
- Reduced expansion on the affected side.

- Dull or impaired precussion note over the area of consolidation.
- Bronchial breath sounds over the area of consolidation.
- Vocal resonance is increased over the affected area.
- In older child, test for whispering pectoriloquy.
- Most common bacterial pathogen is *Streptococcus pneumoniae*. In areas where Hib immunization is not being practiced, *H. influenzae* is the most common organism below 4 years of age. If the child has coexisting pyoderma, staphylococcal pneumonia is a possibility although lobar pneumonia is not the presentation of staphylococcal pneumonia.

9. Read this X-ray and give a diagnosis.

A: Trachea and mediastinum are shifted to the opposite side. There is a uniform white shadow with a higher level in the axilla. The costophrenic and cardiophrenic angles are obliterated. The margin of right diaphragm is not well made out. The diagnosis is pleural effusion.

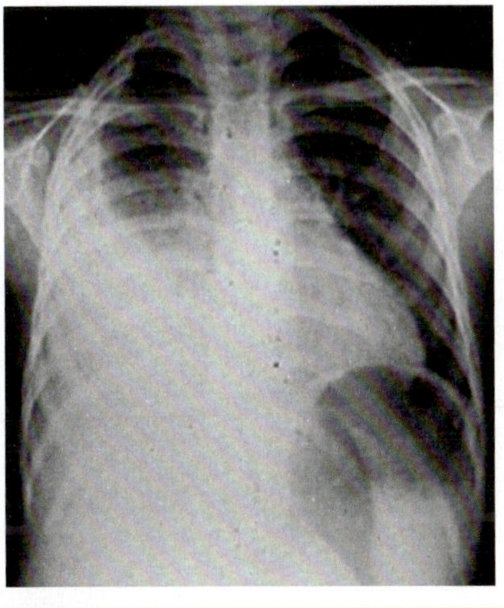

Fig.25.9

Clinical Points on Pleural Effusion

- Tachypnoea
- Clinically, the trachea and apex beat are displaced away from the side of the effusion.
- There is reduced expansion on the affected side.
- Percussion note is stony dull over effusion.
- Reduced or absent breath sounds over the area of effusion; bronchial breath sounds are sometimes heard just above the upper effusion level (see Respiratory System for explanation).
- Decreased vocal resonance over the effusion (in younger children, crying may be made use of to assess VR).
- The student should note if a drain is in situ or if there is aspiration mark on the chest.
- Pleural fluid could be transudate (e.g., nephrotic syndrome, CCF, etc) or exudates (bacterial infections including tuberculosis). Blood-stained fluid may be because of a traumatic tap, tuberculosis or malignancy. Chylothorax can arise from lymphatic drainage problem, e.g., post-cardiac surgery. Empyema results from bacterial infections like *Streptococcus pneumoniae, Staphylococcus aureus*, etc. Bulging of intercostal spaces and clubbing may point towards empyema.

10. This child on treatment for pneumonia suddenly deteriorated and the X-ray is shown here. What is the diagnosis? (Fig. 25.10)

A: Pneumothorax. The trachea and mediastinum are shifted to the opposite side. The diaphragm is pushed down. The lung area is very dark without any vascular markings. The shadow of collapsed lung is clearly seen through the heart shadow.

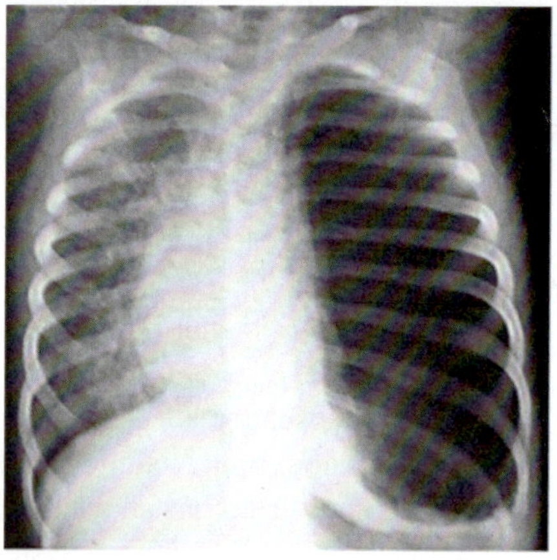

Fig.25.10

11.* Discuss this X-ray (Fig. 25.11) and give a possible diagnosis.

A: The X-ray shows gross shift of trachea and mediastinum to the opposite side. There is flattening of the diaphragm on left side. From this picture it is not clear if lung markings are visible on the left side. If no lung markings are visible, the diagnosis is tension pneumothorax. Absence of lung markings and shadow of collapsed lung margins are the two most important pointers to the diagnosis of pneumothorax. A probable margin of collapsed lung is visible on the left side with the heart shadow.

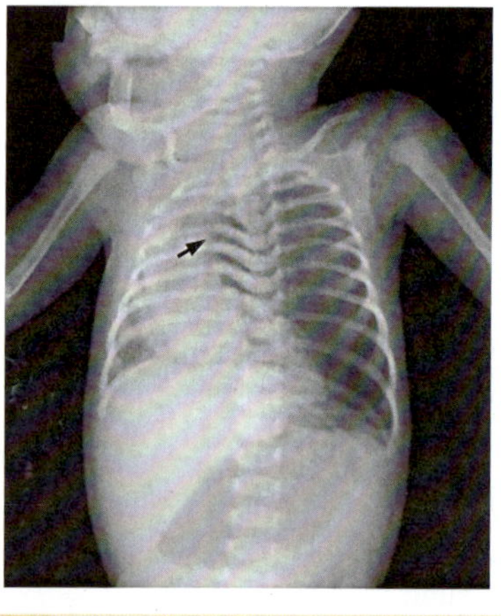

Fig.25.11

However, there is herniation of lung to the right side. Herniation to the opposite side is very much suggestive of congenital lobar emphysema. Hence, the first possibility is tension pneumothorax and the closest differential diagnosis is congenital lobar emphysema. Some more points in history or physical examination are required before deciding on the diagnosis from this X-ray.

Left upper lobe is the most common site for congenital lobar emphysema. The emphysematous lung herniates into the right hemithorax (generally demonstrable in X-ray); the X-ray also shows mediastinal shift to the opposite side. The baby generally presents as severe respiratory distress in early infancy.

12. *What is the diagnosis? What is the most probable cause for this? (Fig. 25.12)

A: The X-ray shows an opacity that blurs the cardiac margin it touches and having a straight upper margin. Anatomically, the upper straight margin has to be the horizontal fissure. Hence, the part below that is the middle lobe. Middle lobe opacity obliterates the cardiac margin it is in touch with (silhouette sign), which is true in this picture. Therefore, it is a middle lobe

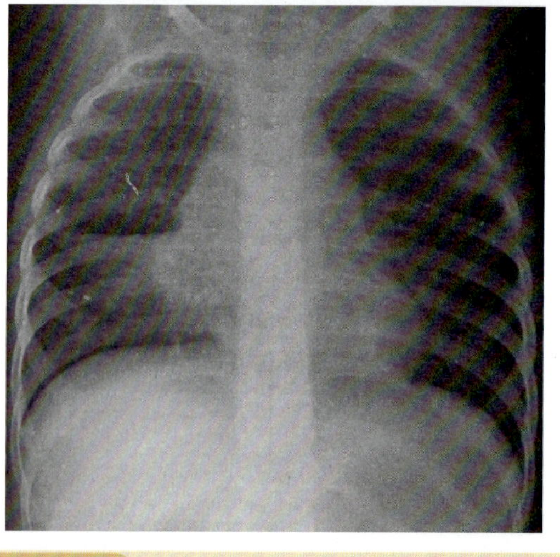

Fig.25.12

consolidation. There is not enough evidence to say collapse. The probable cause is obstruction of the bronchus aerating the middle lobe by lymph node (tuberculosis) or mucous plug (asthma). Foreign body obstruction is very unlikely in middle lobe.

13. *What abnormality is seen? This X-ray belongs to an asthma patient. (Fig. 25.13)

A: Subcutaneous emphysema (surgical emphysema) and patchy areas of alveolar consolidation. Asthma is the most common cause in a child, but trauma and air leak following chest tube insertion are other causes. Here, there is air in the neck region but not much air in the chest wall. There is air shadow in the mediastinum as well, showing that the air has leaked up through the mediastinum.

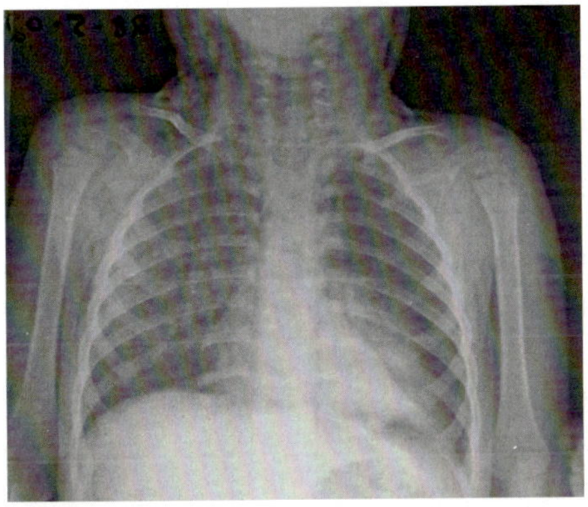

Fig.25.13

14. This X-ray is from a patient with pneumonia. Can you comment on the aetiology? (Fig. 25.14)

A: The X-ray shows multiple abscess cavities. Staphylococcal pneumonia.

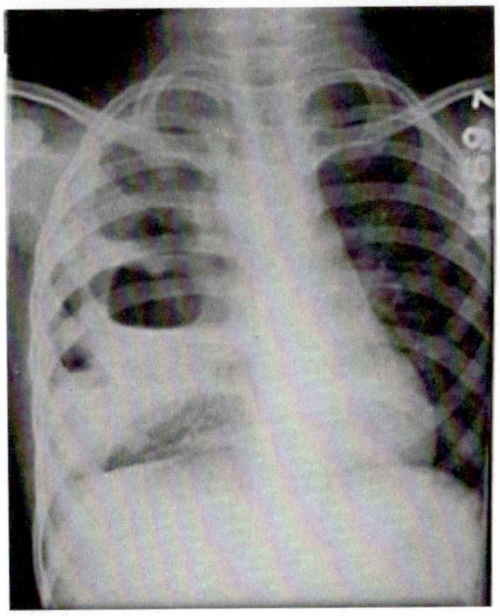

Fig.25.14

15. *This X-ray (Fig.25.15) belongs to a preterm baby who developed respiratory distress within 4 hrs of birth. What is the diagnosis?

A: HMD or hyaline membrane disease. There is uniform ground glass appearance in X-ray. Also note the "low-volume lung" due to failure of the lung to expand fully.

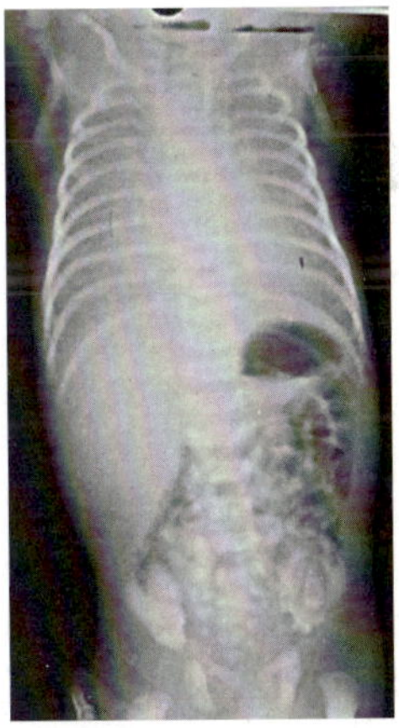

Fig.25.15

16. This child presented with acute onset dyspnoea. What does the X-ray show? (Fig. 25.16)

A: The X-ray shows hyperexpansion with flattened and pushed down diaphragm and relatively vertically placed heart. It fits in well with a diagnosis of asthma. A few parenchymal shadows are there, which may indicate small areas of atelectasis due to bronchospasm or secondary infection following prolonged bronchospasm.

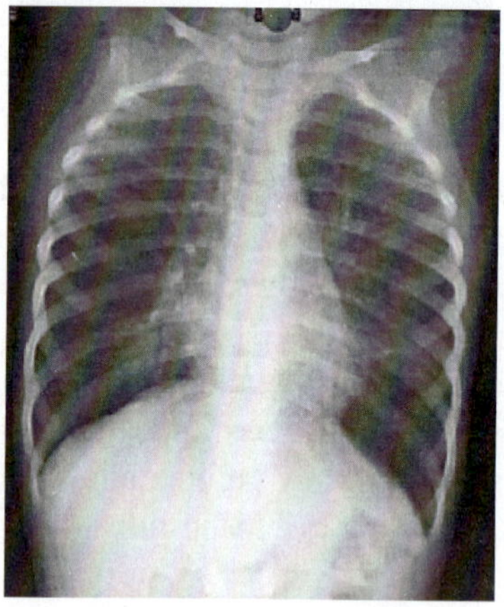

Fig.25.16

17.* This X-ray belongs to a 12-year-old girl who has had 16 hospitalizations for respiratory complaints. What is the X-ray diagnosis? Which single clinical sign will clinch the diagnosis? (Fig. 25.17)

A: The X-ray shows honeycomb shadows bilaterally and a cavity in the left upper zone. The X-ray diagnosis is bronchiectasis. The cavity could be tuberculous and that could be the reason for the bronchiectasis; that is what can be inferred from this X-ray. As a single clinical sign to clinch the diagnosis, clubbing seems to be the most appropriate one **(see Fig. 25.51)**.

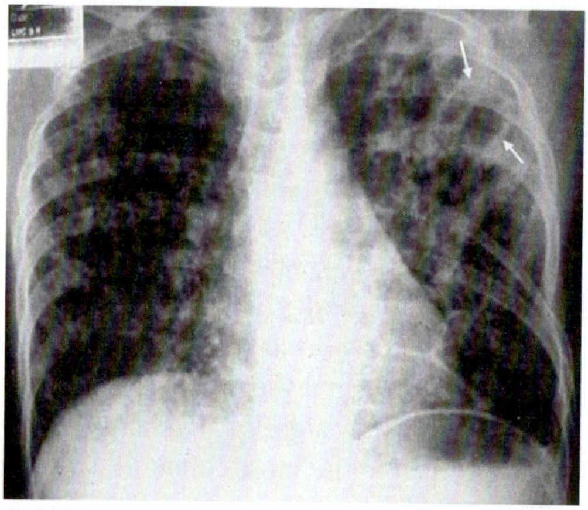

Fig.25.17

Clinical Points on Bronchiectasis

- Productive cough with copious expectoration.
- There may be history of haemoptysis.
- Often, there is growth retardation because of the chronic problem.
- Cyanosis may be present in severe cases. So look carefully for it. Early cyanosis will look like a plethoric nail.
- Clubbing.
- Chest deformity may be present, e.g., Harrison's sulci.
- There may be palpable sounds like crepitations or rhonchi.
- Coarse bubbly crackles and wheeze may be found on auscultation.
- Kartagener's syndrome may be associated, so look for dextrocardia.
- Investigate for cystic fibrosis, α-one antitrypsin deficiency, hypogammaglobulinaemia, etc.
- Acquired bronchiectasis can occur after measles, whooping cough, tuberculosis and neglected foreign body aspiration (hence ask for suggestive history). Bronchiectasis changes following measles and whooping cough may get reversed.

- Bronchiectasis may follow prolonged obstruction due to foreign body. Hence, history of aspiration and seizures are important.
- Management includes treatment of any underlying disorder, postural drainage, chest physiotherapy and antibiotics (during infective exacerbations). Surgical removal of the affected area is an option in localized involvement if rest of the lung function is good.

18. *What is the diagnosis? (Fig. 25.18)

A: There is a sail shadow on the right side and wavy margins of the heart on the left side. Therefore, it is a thymus shadow. Since thymus is anterior structure, the indentations of ribs are seen in it, and that produces the wavy margin.

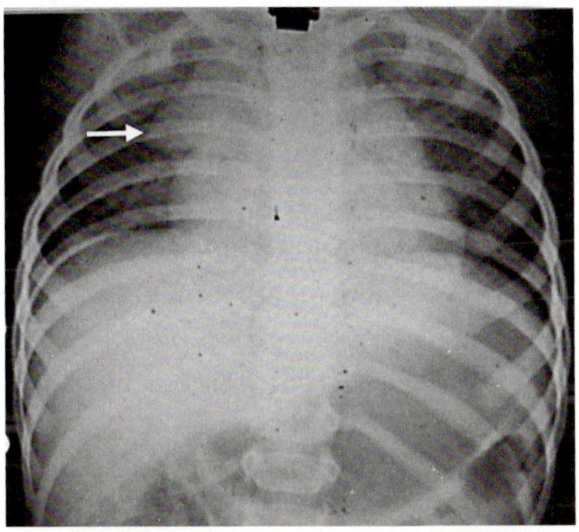

Fig.25.18

19.* This child with acute glomerulonephritis developed acute respiratory distress. There is no fever. What does the X-ray show? (Fig. 25.19)

A: The X-ray shows spreading out opacity from hilum. Infection is unlikely in the absence of fever. Given the clinical scenario, the most likely diagnosis is pulmonary oedema (circulatory overload and hence cardiac failure are likely in acute nephritis). If you have some imagination, you can even visualize bat's wing in this X-ray.

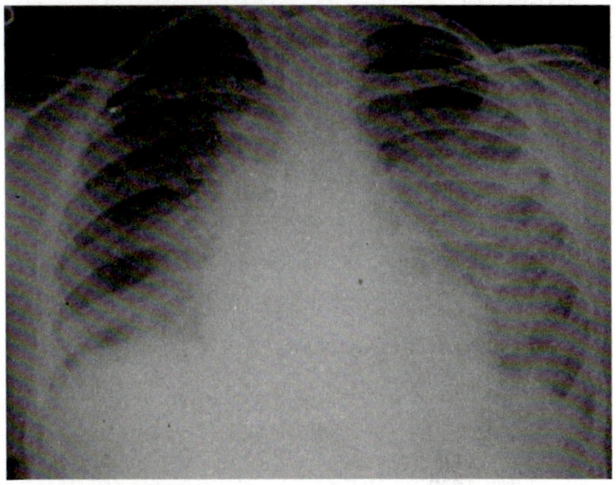

Fig.25.19

20. This child was admitted with history of nocturnal dyspnoea and haemoptysis. Interpret the X-ray (Fig. 25.20).

A: Mitral stenosis. There is cardiomegaly, dilatation of main pulmonary artery, visible bulge of left atrial appendage and prominent vascular shadows in the medial third of lung field. Pulmonary artery segment, left atrial appendage and a right ventricular type of apical contour together gives the appearance of straight-

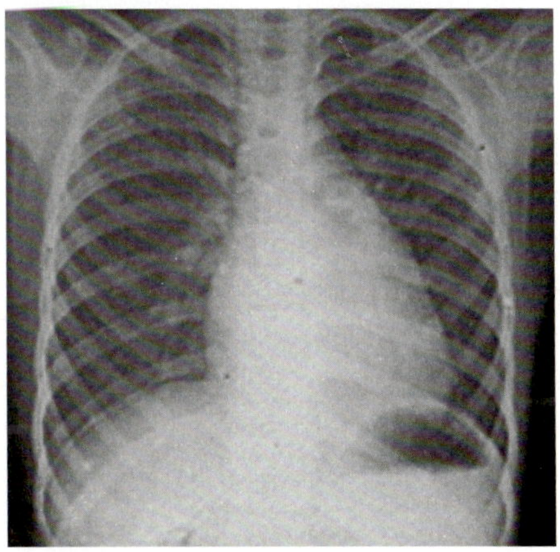

Fig.25.20

25

ening of left heart border (typical RV type of apex is not very obvious in this film. Typical RV apex is seen in **Fig.25.22**).

21. Interpret the X-ray that belongs to a child with congenital heart disease. (Fig. 25.21)

A: The X-ray shows cardiomegaly, pulmonary plethora (lung markings extending to the periphery of the lung field) and a prominent main pulmonary artery segment. The right heart border appears rounded and fuller, pointing towards a right atrial enlargement. Cardiothoracic ratio (ratio of thoracic width and cardiac width) is increased. Apex appears to dip into the diaphragm, possibly a left ventricular type of apex. Thus, it appears to be an X-ray of a left-to-right shunt lesion. Points to differentiate various left-to-right shunts: dilated ascending aorta in PDA; absence of left atrial enlargement in ASD. Left atrial enlargement is seen as shadow-in-shadow on the right cardiac border (likely to be present in VSD and PDA).

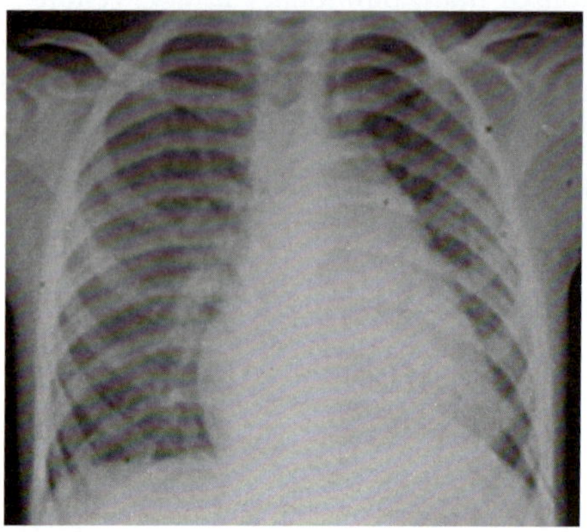

Fig.25.21

22. This X-ray belongs to a child with congenital heart disease. Interpret the X-ray.

A: Tetralogy of Fallot. Cardiothoracic ratio is near normal, there is decreased lung vascularity (lung fields are black), absence of shadow of main pulmonary artery segment and the apex is lifted up (boot shaped). Right aortic arch, if present, supports the diagnosis of TOF (aortic arch is identified by the indentation of tracheal shadow). **(Fig. 25.22)**

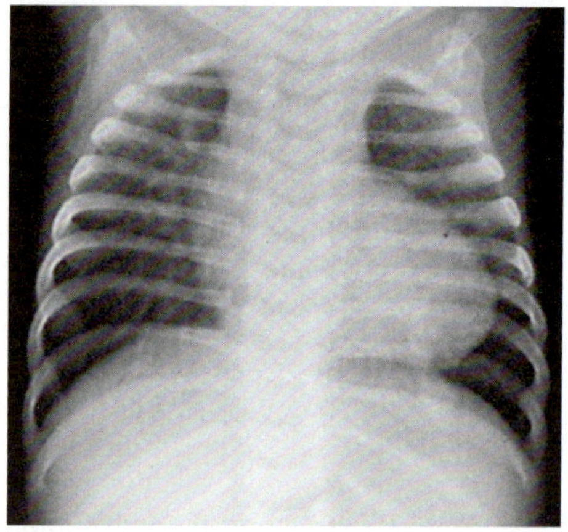

Fig.25.22

23.* What is the diagnosis? (Fig. 25.23)

A: The X-ray shows enlarged globular heart. The cardiac margins are clear cut (normally there is minimal blurring of cardiac margins due to contractions of heart). Diagnosis is pericardial effusion. Usual causes are TB, staphylococcal pyopericardium, etc. Effusion in other situations like collagen vascular diseases, myxoedema, cardiac failure, etc, are small in quantity. A close differential diagnosis for this film is dilated cardiomyopathy.

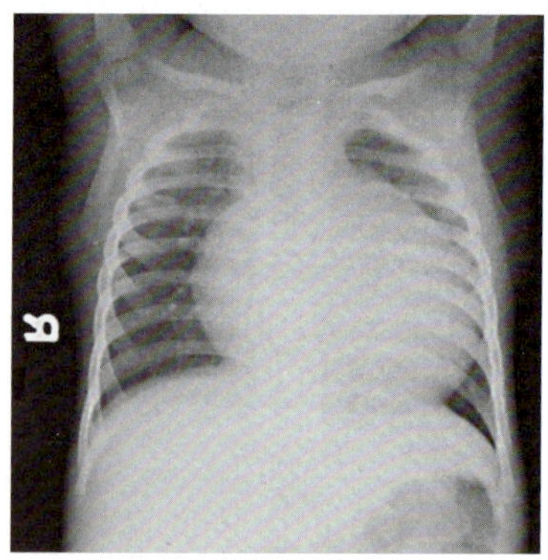

Fig.25.23

24. This child has history of recurrent ear and lung infections. The X-ray is shown here. What is the diagnosis? (Fig. 25.24)

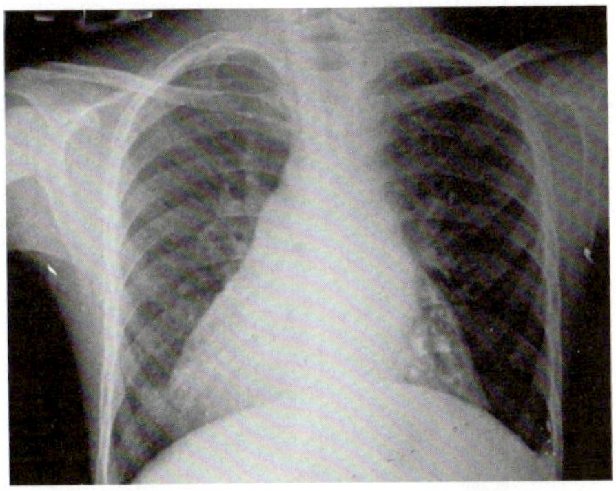

Fig.25.24

A: Kartagener syndrome (primary ciliary dyskinesia). The X-ray shows dextrocardia and bronchiectasis. The situs is not clear from this film (from this film, cannot say where the liver is). Features of Kartagener syndrome are:

- Dextrocardia
- Situs inversus
- Bronchiectasis
- Chronic sinusitis; Otitis media (conductive hearing loss)
- Anosmia
- Sterility in males due to sperm immotility

25. *This child is referred for evaluation of respiratory distress. What is the diagnosis? Which pulmonary problem is the most serious one in this scenario? (Fig. 25.25)

A: Diaphragmatic hernia. The left lung is filled with bubbly shadows; left diaphragm is not seen well because the abdominal contents are coming to thorax through the defect in diaphragm. There is continuity of bowel gas shadows from abdomen to the chest (not well seen here). It is not multiple pneumatoceles of staphylococcal pneumonia, because such a gross mediastinal shift is unlikely without pneumothorax in staphylococcal pneumonia.

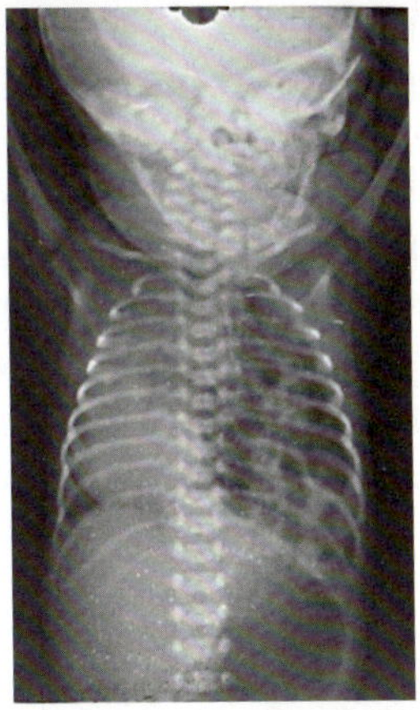

Fig.25.25

The abdomen of the neonate will look scaphoid, as the contents have all gone into the chest. Since the bowel fills the chest, the lung does not develop properly on this side; the most common cause of mortality is pulmonary hypoplasia.

26. *What is the diagnosis? (Fig. 25.26)

A: Eventration of diaphragm. Trachea and mediastinum are shifted to the opposite side; diaphragm is seen high up with loops of intestine below. Since intestine has not gone past the diaphragm, it is not diaphragmatic hernia. Note that eventration need not necessarily produce shift of mediastinum.

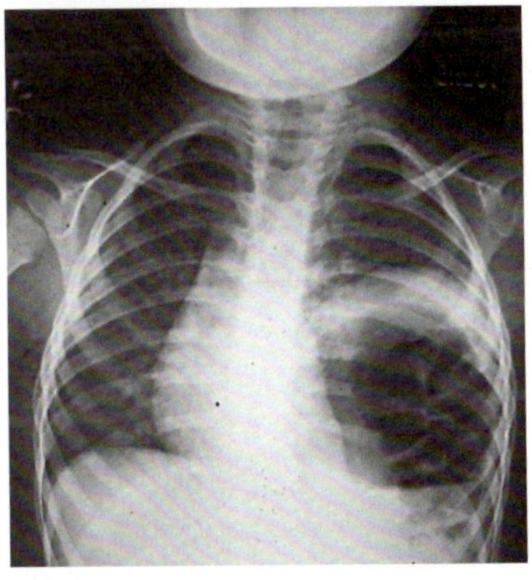

Fig.25.26

25

27. *What is the classical finding demonstrated in this X-ray of newborn? What syndrome is it associated with?

A: Abdomen shows double bubble appearance and absence of gas shadows distal to that. Diagnosis is duodenal atresia. It has strong association with Down's syndrome. Single bubble shadow occurs in pyloric obstruction and triple bubble shadow occurs in jejunal obstruction. Many bubbles occur in ileal/colonic obstruction (multiple fluid levels).

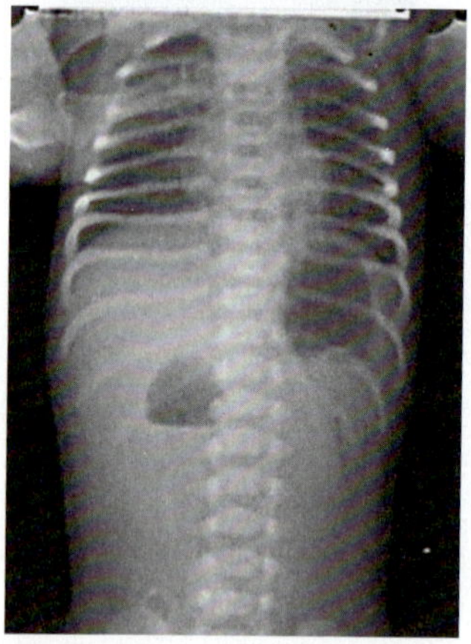

Fig.25.27 Double bubble

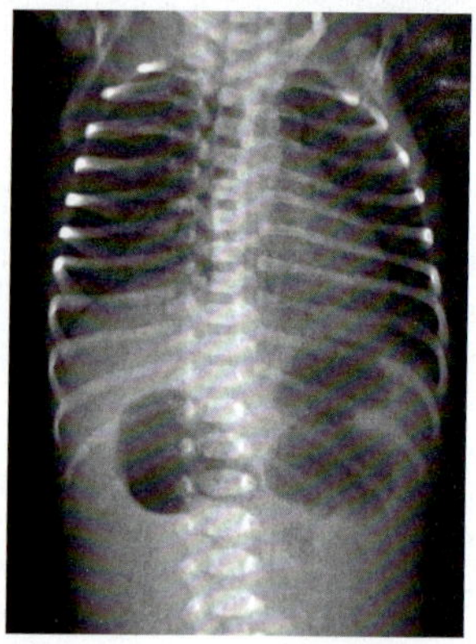

Fig.25.28 Triple bubble appearance

28. What is the diagnosis?

A: There are many air–fluid levels and lower abdomen is without any gas shadow. It is intestinal obstruction; most probably mechanical obstruction, beyond which there are no gas shadows.

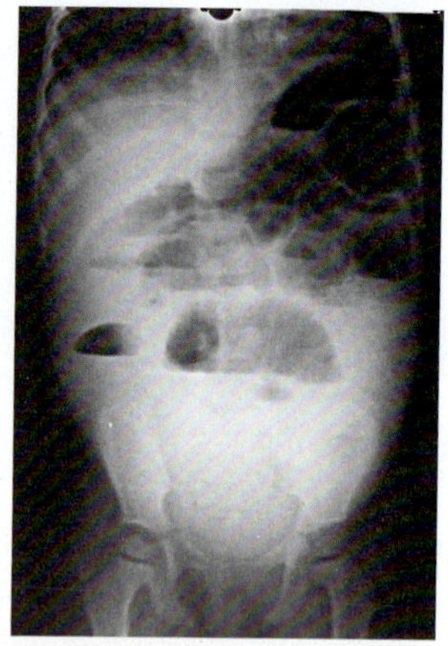

Fig.25.29 Multiple air fluid levels

29. * This investigation was done for an abnormality detected by the mid wife. What is this investigation and what is the abnormality?

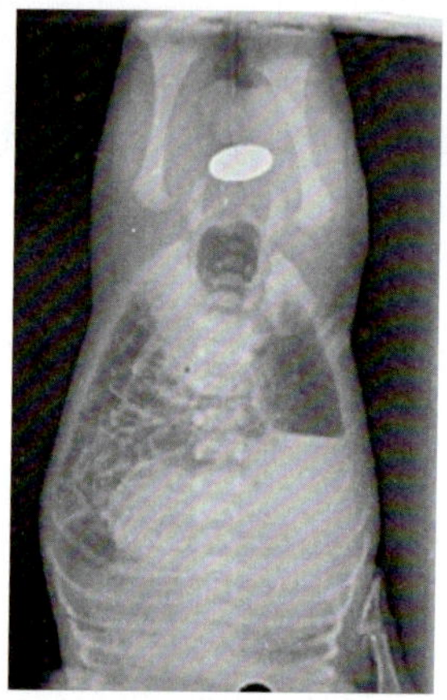

Fig.25.30 Invertogram

A: Invertogram. It is done in cases of imperforate anus to know to which level the intestinal gas reaches. It is usually done after 18 hrs of birth to give time for bowel gas to reach down. A radiopaque coin is pasted and the child is inverted and the X-ray taken. It is quite common for the midwife to detect the abnormality for the first time during routine cleaning of perineum.

30. Spot the diagnosis. (Fig. 25.31)

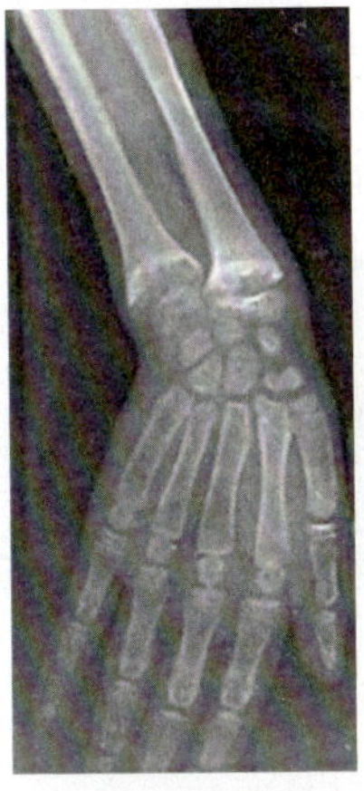

Fig.25.31

A: Rickets. Normally, the ends of long bones must be slightly convex. Here, the ends of radius and ulna are concave (cupping) with breaks in continuity (fraying). The ends of bones are widened (splaying). Usually, there will be an increase in distance between the ends of radius/ulna and metacarpals due to uncalcified osteoid. Rickets is discussed in detail elsewhere (see p 77 and 490).

31. *Give the diagnosis and discuss this X-ray.

A: Scurvy. The X-ray shows sharp pencil thin cortex; epiphysis have sharp ring-shaped outline with ground glass appearance inside; thickened white line at metaphysis (white line of Fraenkel). There is a linear zone of destruction (arrow). No subperiosteal haemorrhages are visible here (they may become visible during healing due to calcification).

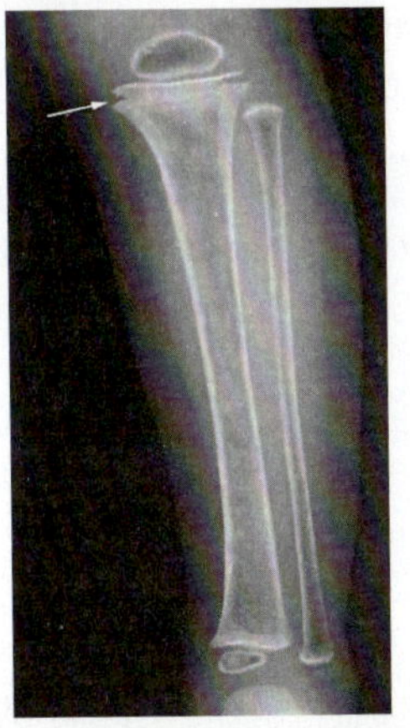

Fig.25.32a Scurvy

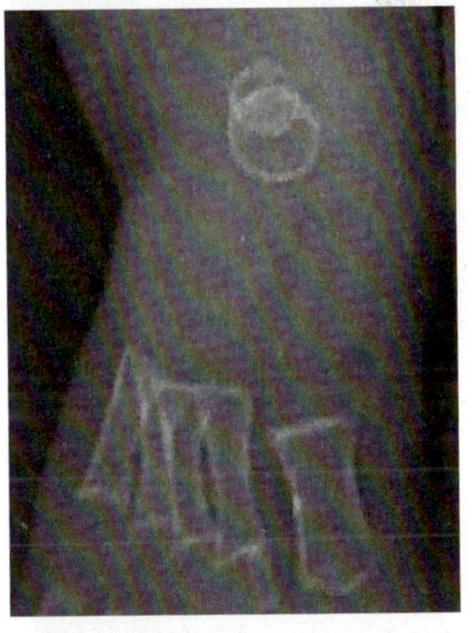

Fig.25.32b Scurvy

32. *This child is being evaluated for refusal to move the limbs. What is the X-ray diagnosis? (Fig. 25.33)

A: Congenital syphilis. There is periosteal elevation of both femurs. There is loss of continuity of medial upper border of one tibia, an early evidence of destruction (Wimberger sign: radiolucency at medial tibial metaphysis). Painful limbs with periosteal elevation is possible in osteomyelitis also, but it is ridiculous to assume that osteomyelitis affected so many bones simultaneously. The X-ray findings are unlike scurvy, a close differential diagnosis of painful limb in an infant.

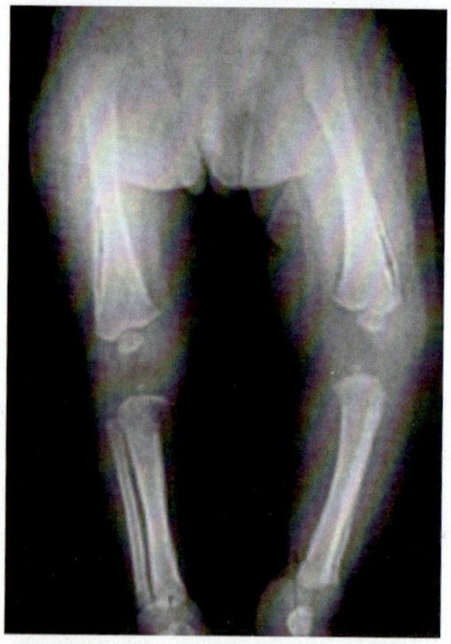

Fig.25.33

33. *This X-ray belongs to a child with transfusion-requiring anaemia and hepatosplenomegaly. What is the diagnosis?

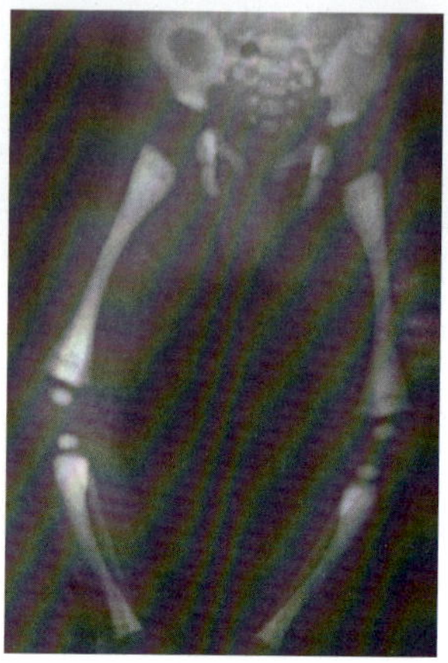

Fig.25.34 Osteopetrosis

A: The bones are uniformly chalky white with no differentiation of medullary cavity. The diagnosis is osteopetrosis. Hardly any other condition has a similar X-ray picture.

34. *What is the diagnosis? (Fig. 25.35, 25.36)

A: Mucopolysaccharidoses. The metaphysis of radius and ulna appear irregular; the radius and ulna may face each other forming a V shape (not obvious in this patient); the metacarpals are conical or pointed or pinched out proximally (the changes are seen in a few metacarpals here). The lumbar spine shows anterosuperior hypoplasia resulting in apparent beak-like projection on the anterior lower margins. Mucopolysaccharidoses is discussed in detail elsewhere (see p 499).

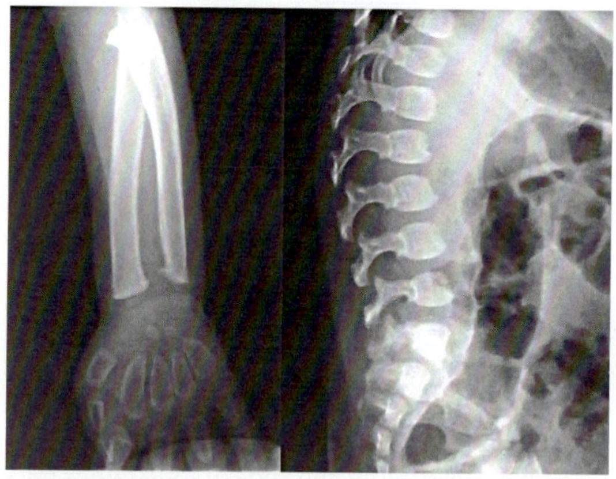

Fig.25.35

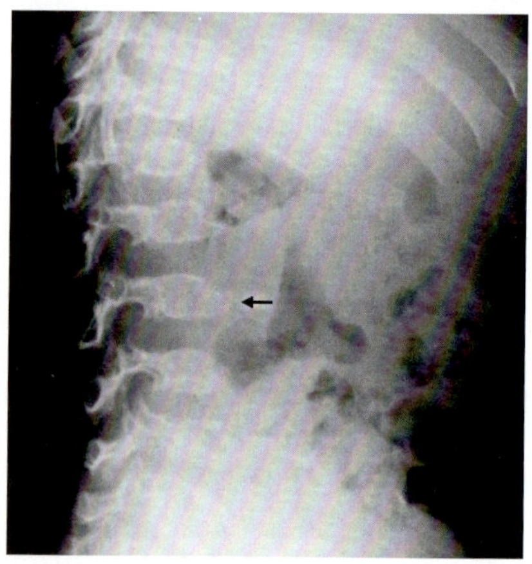

Fig.25.36

Anterior beaking of lumbar vertebrae (well seen in L4, L5) may be seen in MPS. However, in Morquio syndrome all vertebrae can be affected. In hypothyroidism, the anterior beaking usually involves T12, L1.

35. *What abnormality is demonstrated?

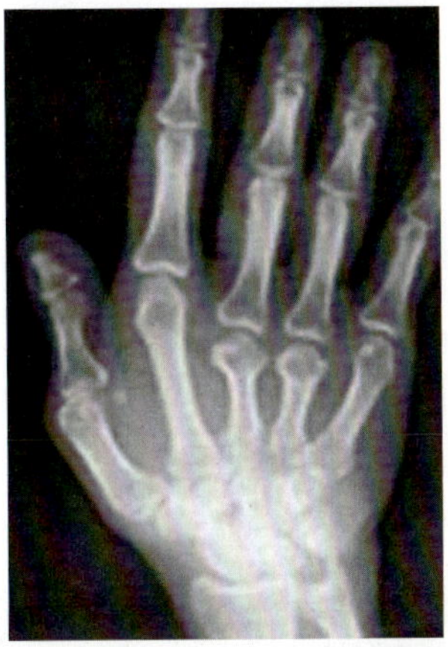

Fig.25.37 Short metacarpals (3rd, 4th)

A: Short metacarpals, especially third and fourth. It may be found in Albright hereditary osteodystrophy (pseudohypoparathyroidism), which is discussed elsewhere (see p 504).

36.* What does the X-ray skull show?

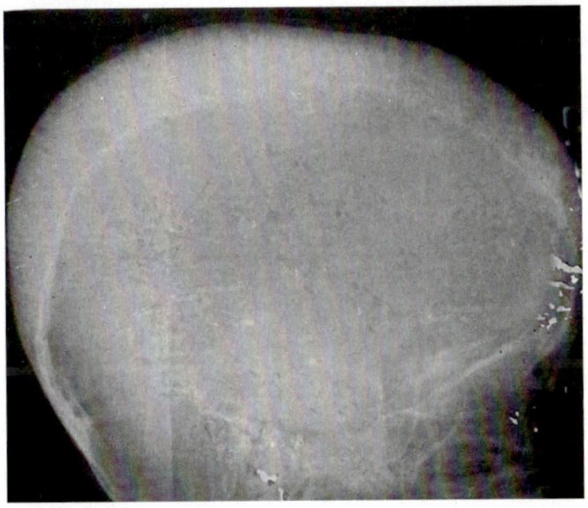

Fig.25.38 "Hair-on-end"

A: It shows hair-on-end appearance. It is seen in severe congenital haemolytic anaemia like thalassaemia if they are not adequately transfused. The salient points regarding examination of a case of thalassaemia are liste below.

- Note the ethnic origin and consanguinity of marriage. Enquire about deaths in family.
- Frontal and parietal bossing, maxillary overgrowth, prominent malar eminence, broad nasal bridge and malocclusion of teeth.
- Anaemia, jaundice (secondary to haemolysis) and skin pigmentation.
- Short stature and delayed puberty.
- Periungual and palmar crease pigmentation.
- Congestive cardiac failure, murmurs (due to anaemia).
- Look for hepatosplenomegaly and ascites.
- Peripheral oedema, if present, may be secondary to liver disease or congestive cardiac failure.
- Test vision and hearing (impairment due to desferrioxamine therapy).
- Enquire if the child is given additional vaccines like *H. influenzae*, pneumococcal, hepatitis B, etc.
- Hypothyroidism and diabetes mellitus may develop due to iron overload.
- Bone marrow transplantation may offer cure.

Given below are some salient features of sickle cell anaemia.

- Pallor and jaundice.
- Recurrent episodes of musculoskeletal or abdominal pain.
- Splenomegaly may be present in small children, but often absent in the grown-ups (repeated splenic infarction leads to a small fibrotic non-palpable spleen).
- Look for ejection systolic murmur and signs of cardiac failure due to anaemia.

25

- Examine joints: There may be swelling and/or effusions or chronic joint disease. Previous aseptic necrosis of femoral heads may cause a limp. Digits may have become short secondary to dactylitis.
- Look for evidence of old cerebrovascular accidents including hemiplegia.
- Look for leg ulcers, especially around ankles (rare in the first decade but commoner with advancing years).
- Overwhelming sepsis with *Streptococcus pneumoniae*, *Haemophilus* and *Meningococcus* are likely.
- Diagnosis made by haemoglobin electrophoresis.
- Management includes regular folic acid, prophylactic pencillin, vaccination (pneumococcal and Hib), transfusion programmes and psychosocial support.
- Bone marrow transplantation may offer cure.

Given below are some salient features of hereditary spherocytosis:

- Anaemia and jaundice, but usually not transfusion dependant.
- There may be a history of neonatal hyperbilirubinaemia.
- There may be a positive family history of anaemia, jaundice, splenectomy or gallstones.
- Child will have splenomegaly.
- Autosomal dominant. So one of the parents may have splenomegaly (examine parents).
- Investigation: Spherocytosis, reticulocytosis, increased osmotic fragility and negative Coombs test.

37. * What is the diagnosis?

A: There is narrowing of the intervertebral spaces and collapse of the vertebra. Diagnosis is TB spine (Pott's spine).

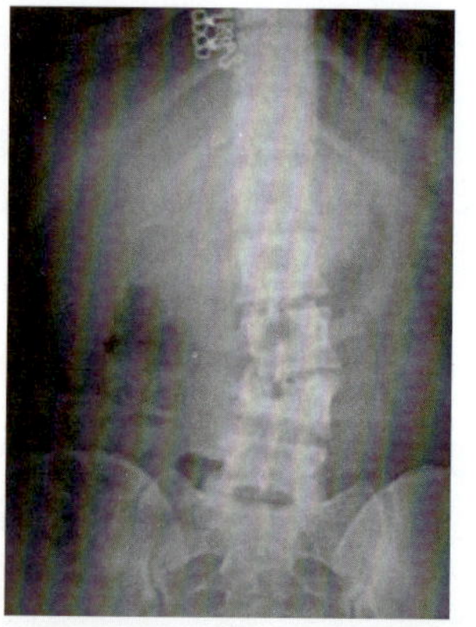

Fig.25.39 Pott's spine

38. *This X-ray belongs to a patient who is being planned a surgical procedure for a congenital heart disease. What is the diagnosis? (Fig. 25.40)

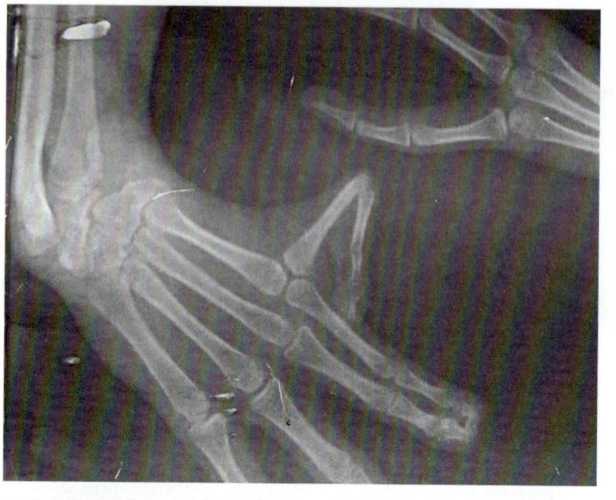

Fig.25.40

A: Holt-Oram syndrome. The X-ray shows radial anglulation, syndactyly and abnormal thumbs. In fact, the first metacarpal is missing in its normal position. Also see p 485.

- Upper limb defects*: Limb reduction defects of variable severity—May vary from thumb hypoplasia to phocomelia. Sometimes, thumb is finger like (triphalangeal thumb).

- ASD is the heart disease associated*. Less commonly VSD.
- Inheritance is autosomal dominant with variable expression.
- Absent pectoralis major may be an association.

39. *This child was treated with high dose of activated vitamin D and phosphates. This X-ray shows hardly any improvement. What has gone wrong? (Fig. 25.41)

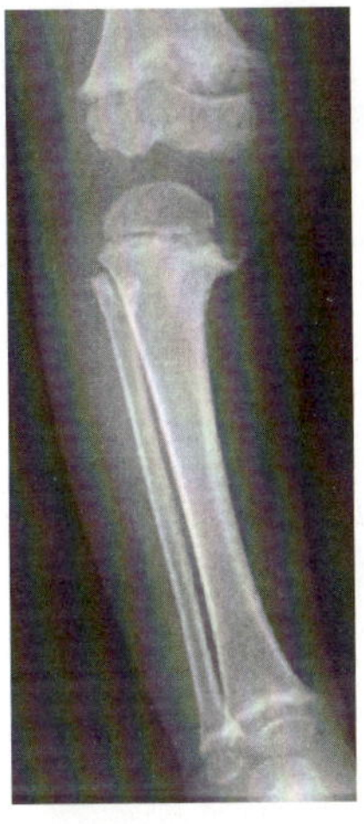

Fig.25.41

A: Nothing has gone wrong except that the diagnosis of rickets was wrong! The X-ray is suggestive of metaphyseal dysplasia. The X-ray is typical of rickets with cupping and fraying. However, since the child did not respond to active vitamin D and phosphate, one has to think of alternate diagnosis. A close look at the X-ray shows that unlike rickets, here the epiphysis is spared. Therefore, it fits in with a diagnosis of metaphyseal dysplasia.

40. *The X-ray shown belongs to a 9-year-old child with limping. What finding in this X-ray may explain the limp? (Fig. 25.42)

A: The right head of femur appears smaller and deformed. The X-ray is suggestive of Perthes disease.

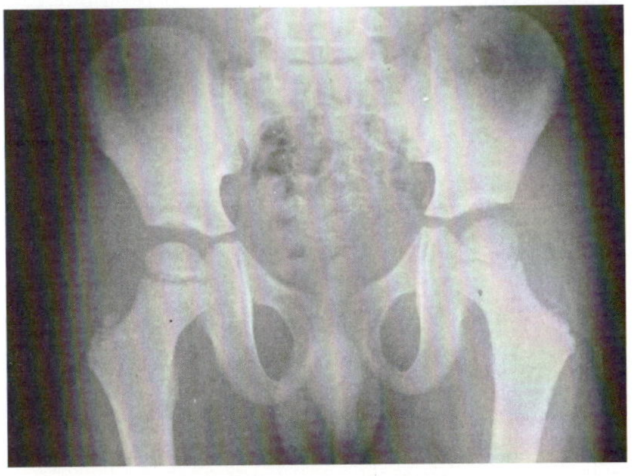

Fig.25.42

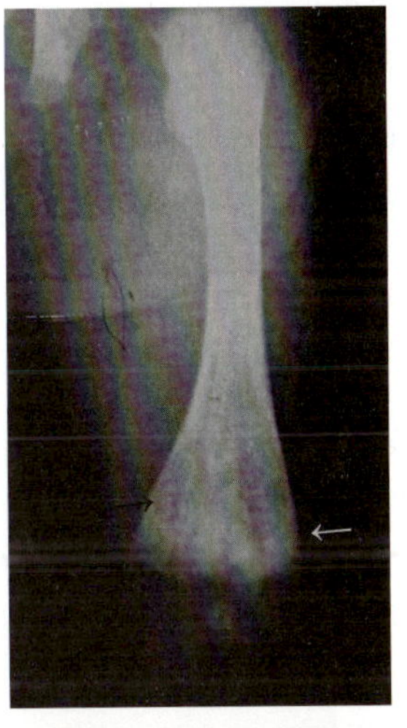

Fig.25.43 Celery stalk appearance. Celery is a vegetable with long stalk that we do not see in our place; but do not worry, just visualize the paddy plants plucked and stalked together in a container. It looks like many vertical lines. Hence, the vertical linear lucenies at the end of long bones seen in osteitis of congenital rubella is simulated to celery stalk. Note the linear lucencies at the lower end of femur

25

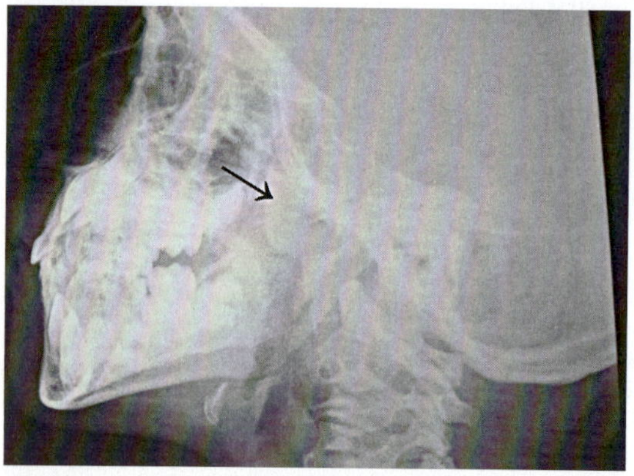

Fig.25.44 X-ray showing adenoid

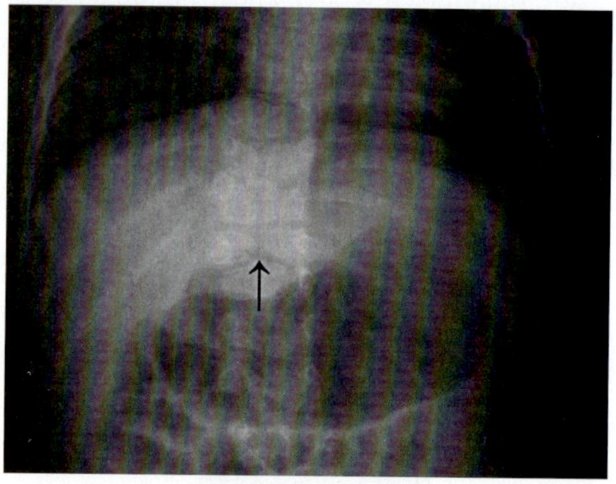

Fig.25.45 Hemivertebra. May be found in Noonan syndrome, Alagille syndrome, Aicardi syndrome etc.

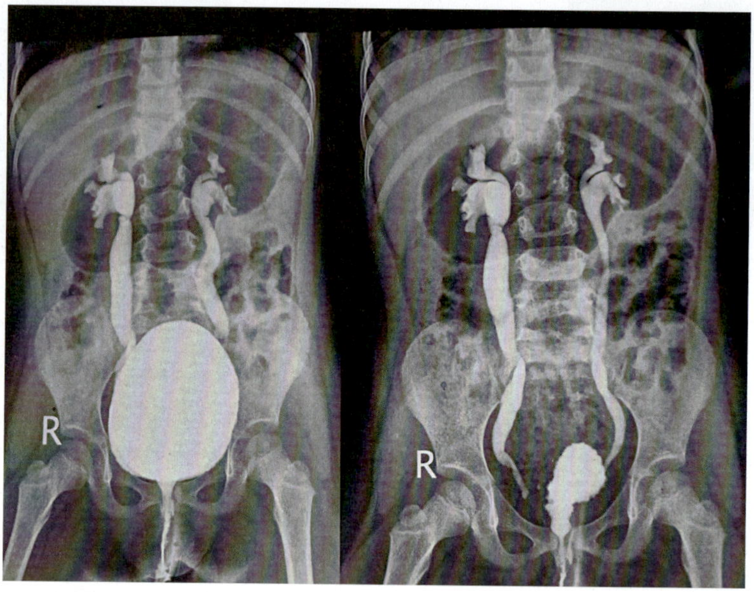

Fig.25.46 MCU showing reflux. This is a MCU picture showing bilateral reflux up the ureter, reaching the kidneys while the child is micturating. Thus, an obstruction to bladder emptying is likely. Posterior urethral valve is the most common cause in a male child.

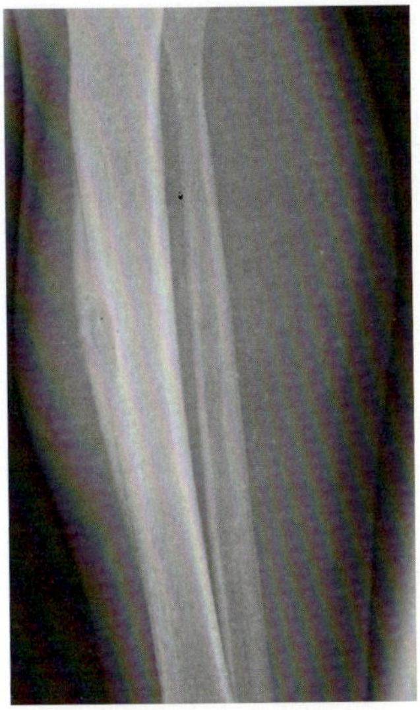

Fig.25.47 Osteomyelitis. Periosteal elevation with new bone formation is seen in tibia. There is surrounding soft tissue swelling.

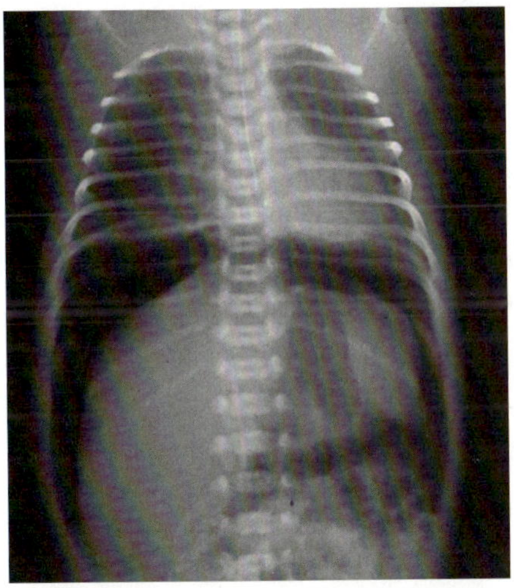

Fig.25.48 Pneumoperitoneum. Note the gas under the diaphragm.

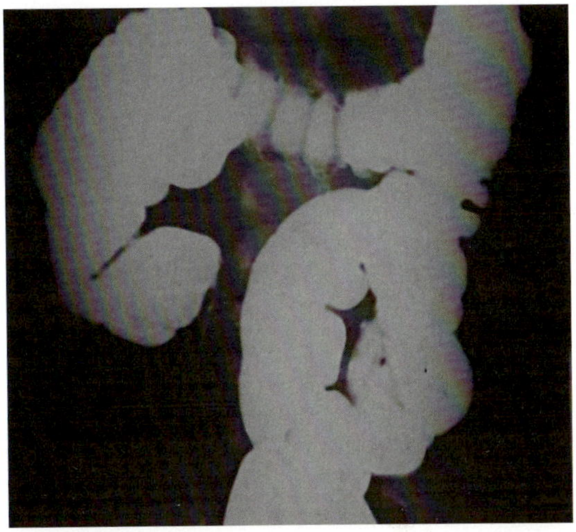

Fig.25.49 Pulled-up caecum. Cecum is seen pulled up in this barium enema; ileocaecal tuberculosis and intussusception are the possibilities.

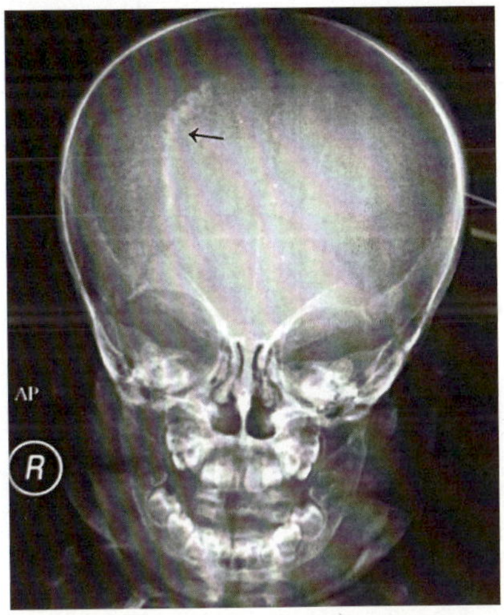

Fig.25.50 Note the rail road calcification; typically described in Sturge-Weber syndrome (due to calcification of the haemangiomatous vasculature); See p 492

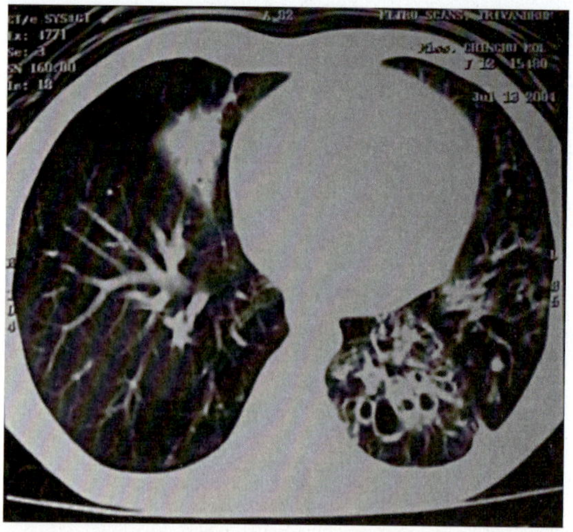

Fig.25.51 Bronchiectasis of posterior segments of the left lower lobe.

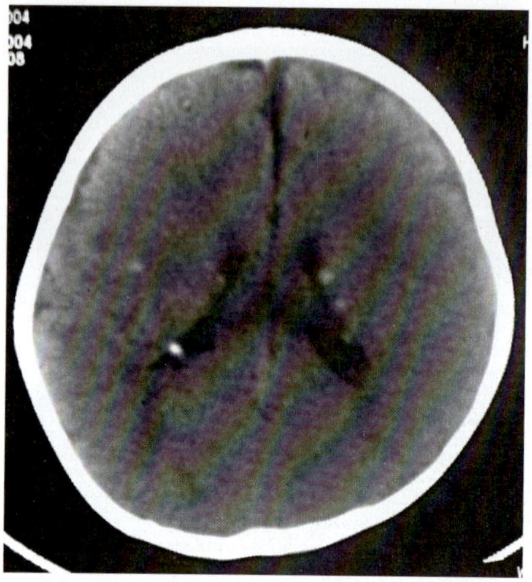

Fig.25.52 "Candle dripping". Note the calcific densities jutting into the ventricle; these are the tubers of tuberous sclerosis. The calcification of CMV is periventricular but does not jut into the ventricle.

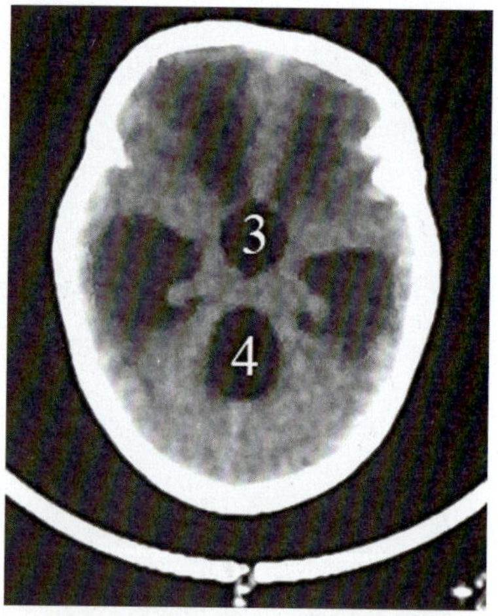

Fig.25.53 Communicating hydrocephalus: All the four ventricles are dilated, which means the obstruction is beyond the fourth ventricle, i.e., in the arachinoid villi. The usual causes are pyogenic meningitis and subarachnoid bleed. Choroid plexus papilloma can produce similar picture due to excessive CSF production rather than obstruction.

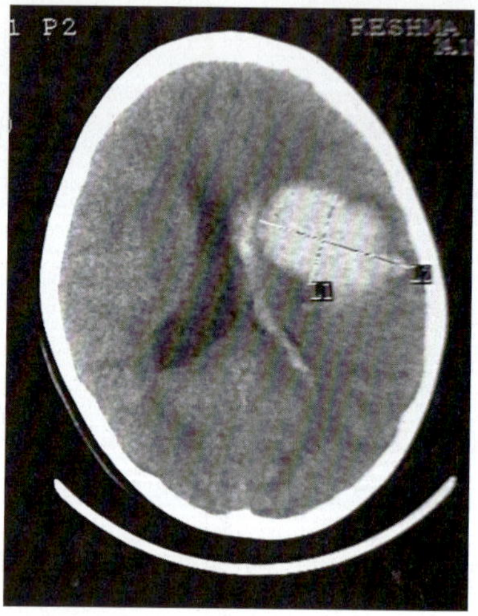

Fig.25.54 CT showing bleed. Hyperdense lesion with surrounding thin rim of hypodensity (oedema) compressing the lateral ventricle on that side. The parenchymal bleed has extended into the ventricle.

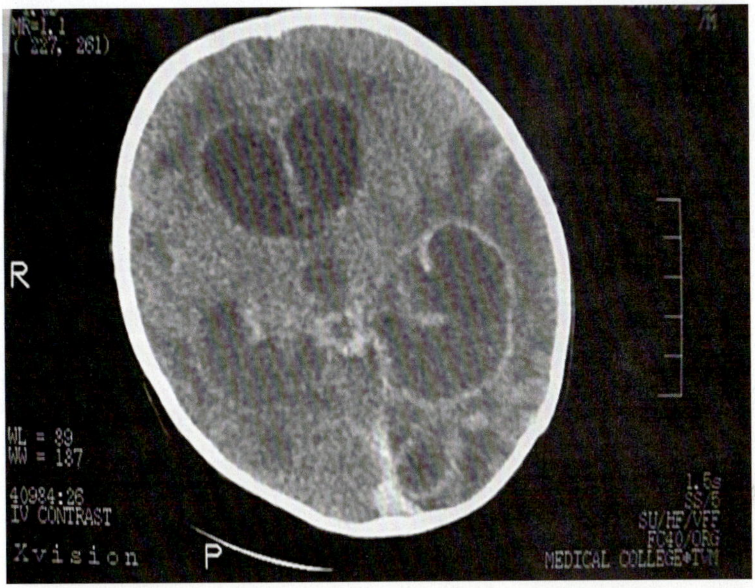

Fig.25.55 Brain abscess. Large hypodense lesion with contrast-enhancing peripheral rim suggestive of abscess. See description under ring-enhancing lesions (p 544).

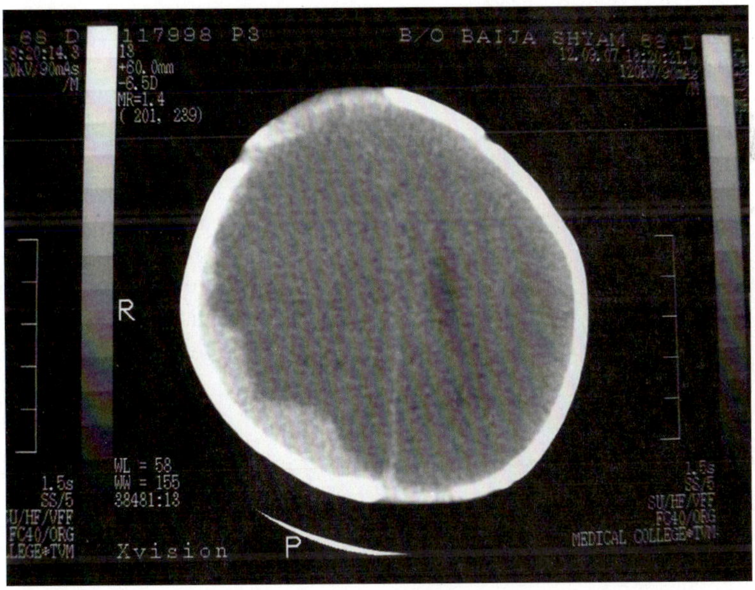

Fig.25.56 CT showing subdural bleed. Compare with Fig.25.61.

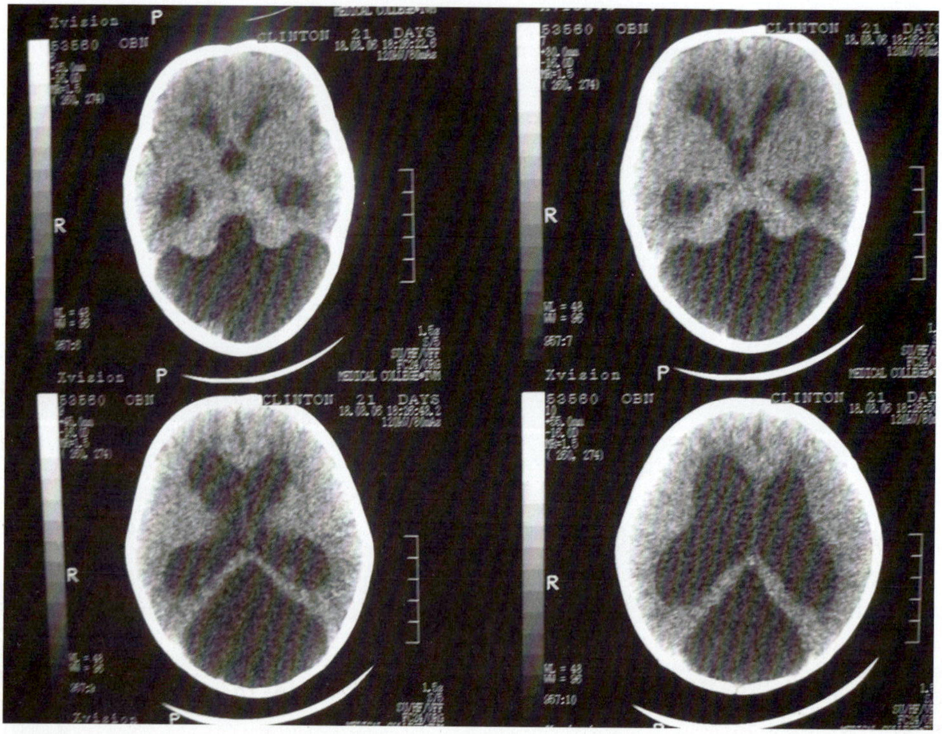

Fig.25.57 Dandy-Walker malformation

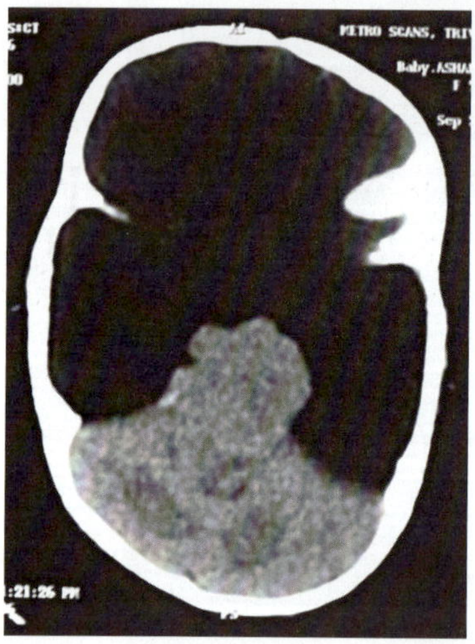

Fig.25.58 Hydranencephaly

- Fig.25.57 shows cystic expansion of the 4th ventricle, in the posterior fossa; associated anomalies include agenesis of posterior cerebellar vermis and corpus callosum.
- Clinical features include prominent occiput, rapid increase in head size (hydrocephalus), pyramidal tract signs, cerebellar ataxia and delayed motor and cognitive development.

CT shows that the whole of cortex is replaced with a bag of water. Diagnosis is hydranencephaly (Fig. 25.58)

- Vascular insults, injuries, infections or traumatic disorders after the 12th week of gestation may result in this extreme form of porencephaly.
- Obstruction to the blood flow to the territory supplied by the internal carotid artery, sparing those supplied by the vertebral arteries (basal part of temporal and occipital lobes, hippocampus, amygdaloid nucleus, cerebellum & brainstem) results in hydranencephaly.
- Head size may be normal at birth; because the enormous amount of fluid seen in the CT is at a place where normal brain should have been and hence the enlargement of head need not be a presenting feature.
- Spontaneous reflexes may be normal (controlled by the lower parts of the brain) but with almost absent cortex, no meaningful life is possible. Severe mental retardation with spastic quadriplegia results.

Transillumination test may be positive (p 211) and is a useful bedside diagnostic tool before CT scan.

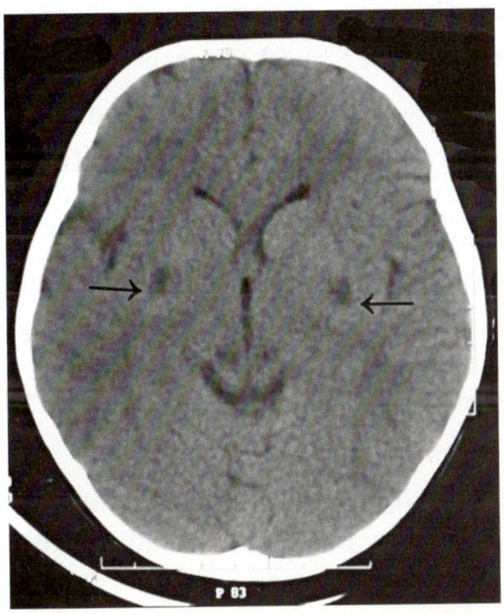

Fig.25.59 Leigh disease (bilateral basal ganglia hypodensity). Hyperdensity in basal ganglia (calcification) may be seen in hypoparathyroidism; pseudohypoparathyroidism; pseudopseudohypoparathyroidism; hyperparathyroidism; Fahr disease etc.

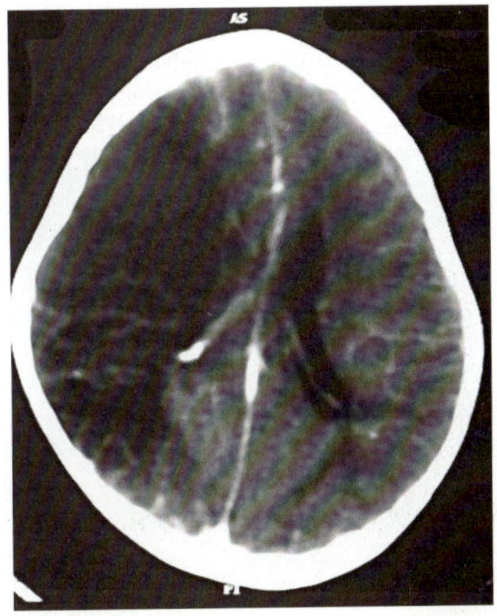

Fig.25.60 MCA territory infarct. Hypodensity of the left hemisphere sparing parts of frontal and occipital lobes. Thus, it is an infarct involving the territory of middle cerebral artery.

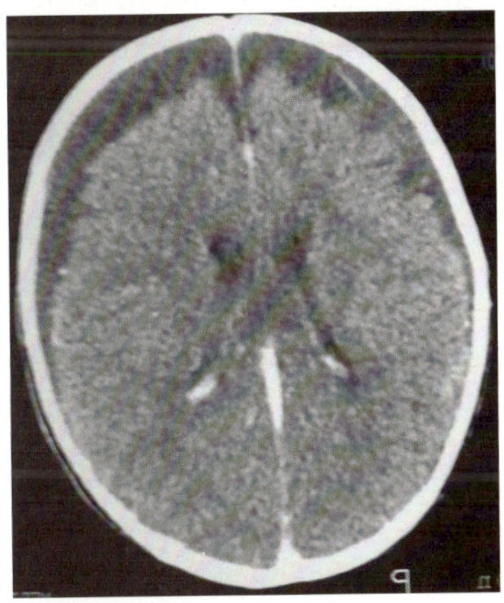

Fig.25.61 Subdural effusion. Compare with Fig. 25.56.

Subdural effusion

- Most commonly occurs as a complication of pyogenic meningitis.
- Subdural effusion is suspected when there is:
  - Persistence of fever or reappearance of fever after an afebrile period
  - Bulging fontanel
  - Persistent vomiting or persisting seizures
- Symptomatic subdural effusions must be drained; both sides have to be tapped in the same sitting.

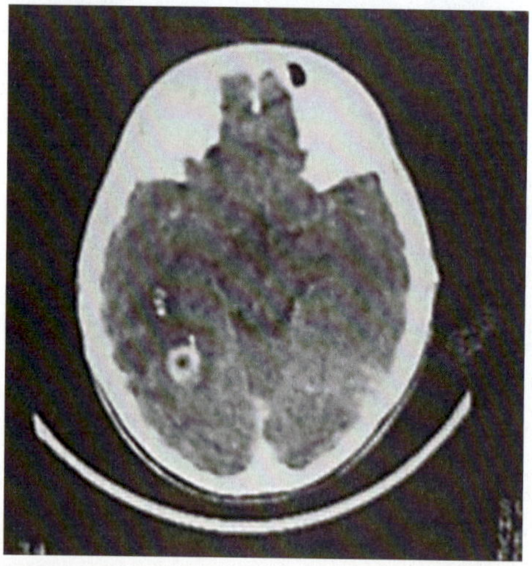

Fig.25.62 Tuberculoma

The CT (Fig. 25.62) shows Ring-enhancing Lesion

The MRI (Fig 25.63) shows Multiple Ring-enhancing Lesions

Differential diagnosis for ring enhancing lesions are neurocysticercusis, tuberculomas, HIV/AIDS, toxoplasmosis, fungal infections such as cryptococcosis or histoplasmosis, primary brain tumors, metastasis, brain abscesses, granulomas, resolving hematomas, and infarcts.

Neurocysticercosis

- May be single but often multiple small rings, 20 mm (or smaller) in size are found; multiple rings gives a "stary sky appearance."

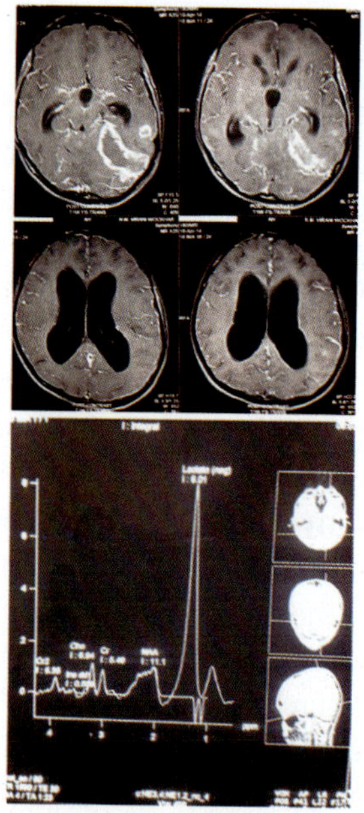

Fig.25.63 Multiple ring enhancing lesions

- Usually supratentorial in location.
- Scolex may be found within the ring, a finding more likely to be brought out by MRI scan (hyperintense on T2W).
- Perilesional oedema may or may not be there; even when present, midline shift is unlikely.
- Most common at the gray-white junction

Tuberculoma

- May be single or multiple conglomerate irregularly shaped; even when multiple, only a few lesions will be there.
- Rings are larger than that of cysticercosis (greater than 20 mm in size) and have thicker walls
- They are hypointense on T2 weighted MRI.
- Peri lesional oedema may be quite significant and may cause midline shiftwith focal neurological deficits.
- There may be basal exudatesand hydrocephalus.

- Tuberculomas are more common in posterior fossa
- A history of contact with a case, positive PPD reaction and X -ray findings may help in the diagnosis of tuberculoma.
- An MRS of brain tuberculomas commonly detects peaks of lipid lactate attributable to large lipid fractions in tuberculosis bacillus. It will also have increased choline levels and decreased N acetyl aspartate and creatine levels. There will be multiple aminoacid peaks in MRS of NCC. The Proton-MRS allows for non-invasive identification of tuberculoma with high specificity
- Brain abscess is an enhancing ring, but is quite large and rarely causes confusion with cysticercosis (see p 575).

The MRI (Fig No: 25.64) shows Meningomy elocoele

- The lumbosacral spine in the posterior aspect shows a moderate to large meningomyelocoele sac with terminal end of spinal cord tethered to it, roots are not clearly defined though.
- There is no associated lipoma. The sac is filled with CSF.
- Overlying skin and subcutaneous tissue are also seen.

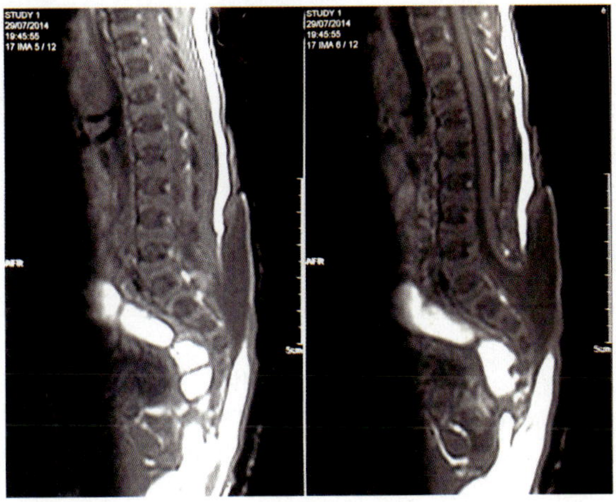

Fig.25.64 Meningomyelocoele

CHAPTER 26

Viva and OSCE

VIVA

Oral examination usually is structured to contain a few stations. The usual stations are:

- **X-ray**: X-ray has been dealt with in the previous chapter.
- **Nutrition**: Here, different food articles are kept and the student is expected to be able to discuss its nutritional aspects. The usual materials kept are cereals (rice, wheat, ragi, etc), pulses (green gram, black gram, bengal gram, nuts, etc), green leafy vegetables, other vegetables, milk, egg and other common items used for infant feeding (Fig. 26.1). A brief account can be found in the chapter on growth, development and nutrition.
- **Instruments and practical procedures**: It is best to read the procedures from **ref. 10 or 11**; both books are by the same author. The student should be able to identify and assemble laryngoscope and ambu bag; they must know how to use these **(ref. 11)**. Other instruments that are usually kept for table viva are (Fig. 26.2): LP needle, bone marrow aspiration needle, bone marrow trephine needle, liver biopsy needle (Menghini and Vim Silverman), IV needle, feeding tube, red rubber catheter, flatus tube, tuberculin syringe, insulin syringe, oral thermometer, rectal thermometer, tongue depressor, scalp vein set, intraosseous needle, IV infusion set, etc.

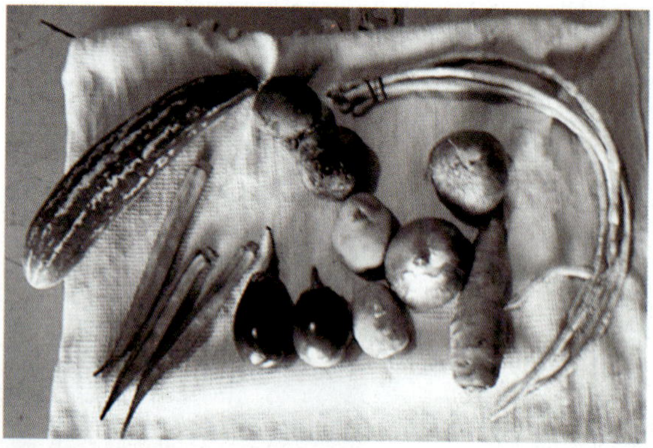

Fig. 26.1 Vegetables

- **Drugs**: The usual drugs kept are drugs in emergency kit (adrenaline, atropine, sodium bicarbonate, calcium gluconate, potassium chloride, 25% glucose, mannitol, etc); IV fluids (multiple electrolyte solution, normal saline, Ringer's lactate, 5% glucose, etc); drugs used in asthma (metered dose inhalers, salbutamol, aminophylline, magnesium sulphate, etc); steroids (hydrocortisone, methyl prednisolone, prednisolone, dexamethasone, etc); vitamins; commonly used antibiotics; anti-TB drugs; anticonvulsants (diazepam, phenytoin, phenobarbitone, etc); cardiac drugs (furosemide, digoxin, etc); analgesic/antipyretics, etc. The student can use "Pediatric Prescriber" by the same author and publisher to gather information on relevant drugs.

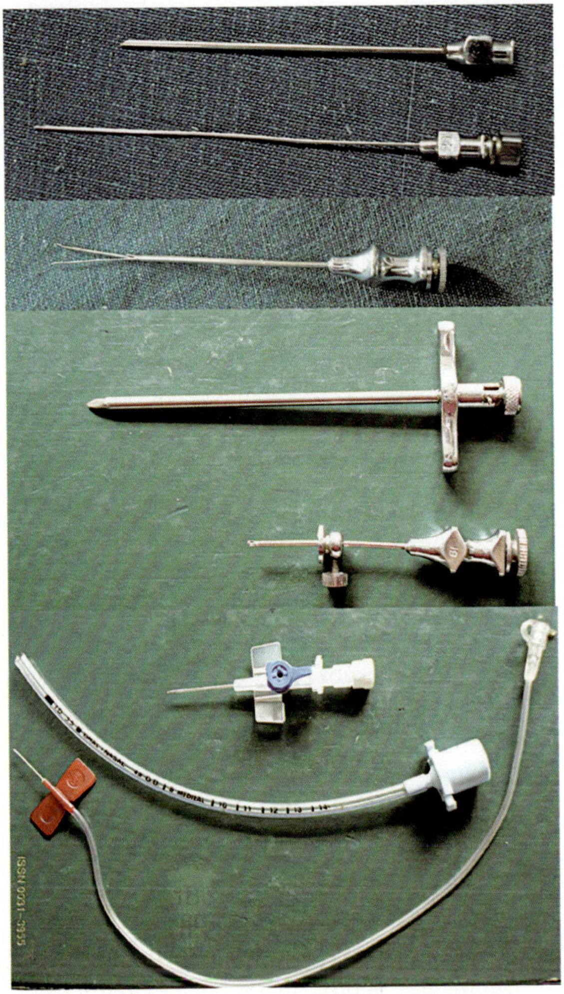

Fig.26.2 Instruments. Figure shows from above downwards, pleural fluid aspiration needle, LP needle (LP needle has a stylet, whereas pleural aspiration needle doesn't), Vim Silverman needle (note the bifid split stylet), bone marrow trephine needle (quite thick needle with a thick inner trochar for piercing the bone), bone marrow aspiration needle (note the guard, stylet and shorter and less stouter appearance), IV cannula, un-cuffed enotracheal tube and scalp vein needle set ("butterfly needle").

- Immunization: A brief account is given along with general examination (see p 32). For more details, the student can consult **ref. 10 or 11**. The student must be thorough with the national schedule (the proper time of vaccination, side effects, dose, storage conditions, simultaneous use with other vaccines, special national drives like pulse polio, etc). In addition, reasonable knowledge on newer vaccines and combination vaccines is expected.
- Paediatric emergencies: Undergraduate students can consult "Pediatric Prescriber" by the same author and publisher as it gives the most compact account of emergencies. Postgraduate students can consult "Manual of Pediatric Practice," again by the same author and publisher for a more detailed discussion on the management of paediatric emergencies.
- Interpretation of charts: Here, charts showing laboratory investigations will be kept for the student to interpret. Usually, simple charts are kept like haemolytic/obstructive jaundice; TB/pyogenic meningitis, etc. It is generally not different from what the student may have done during their pathology classes.
- Slides and specimens: Very unusually common slides (e.g., spherocytosis, sickle cell anaemia, leukaemia) and common specimens (e.g., Wilms tumour, cirrhosis, etc) may be kept. Presently, slides and specimens are not part of MD examinations in most universities; however, there were occasions when these were kept for DNB exams. Hence, it is advisable for DNB candidates to spend an hour in pathology department to see the slides and specimens before going for examination.

OSCE

Objective structured clinical examination (OSCE) has become part of assessment of candidate in most universities. It is generally used to assess the skill of the candidate in eliciting clinical findings. As the candidate is performing the required task, the examiner will observe and put marks depending on the checklist of various steps. Sometime a couple of related questions also will be pasted in station, which have to be answered. OSCE is potentially high mark yielding and may even help the candidate to get through exams even when the clinical case discussion has not been up to the mark. Hence OSCE is a very important part of examination for any candidate.

I. Clinical Skill Station

Basic Steps

- Always examine the child standing on the right side of the patient (conventional).
- Always seek permission for examination and explain the procedure to the patient/parent.
- For examination of newborn, wash hands before touching the child. Then dry and warm the hand and stethoscope before touching the newborn.
- Never produce discomfort or pain to the child because of wrong methods.
- These steps will not fetch marks for candidate, but failure to observe these steps may result in negative marks.

Elicitation of any clinical finding may become part of OSCE and hence it is not possible to give exhaustive discussion here. It may be found in the sections of general examination and system examination. A few OSCE stations will be discussed below for the student to get the feel of how it is. A sample OSCE station with the mark allotment is given below.

Examine for Icterus (Total 1 mark)

- Take the child to the window to examine in adequate daylight (1/4 mark).
- Examine the posterio-lateral sclera when the patient looks down (1/4 mark).
- Examine the soft palate, palms and skin (1/4 mark).
- One question to be answered (1/4 mark). Example of a question is given below:
  Why is icterus looked for in sclera?
  As sclera is rich in elastin tissue, which has a high affinity for bilirubin.

Examine for Clubbing

- Look at the nails tangentially. Loss of angle between nail bed and skin on the dorsal surface of digit.
- Palpate the nail bed for fluctuation.
- Do Schamroth sign: Oppose both thumbs on their dorsal aspect.
- Look for widening and tenderness of the ends of long bones if clubbing is gross (hypertrophic pulmonary osteoarthropathy).
- Compare nails of fingers and toes, preferably keeping them side-by-side for comparison.
- Check parents for clubbing.
- A sample question: What are the grades of clubbing (see p 126)

Lymphadenopathy

- To palpate the cervical lymph nodes, approach from behind is the classical teaching.
- Flex the patient's neck forwards and tilt the neck to the side of examination.
- Palpate for cervical (superficial and deep), submental, submaxillary, preauricular, posterior auricular, occipital nodes, etc.
- Palpate between the two heads of sternomastoid for scalene nodes (important in adults).
- Comment on location, size, number, tenderness, matting, consistency, etc.
- Examine for axillary, inguinal, epitrochlear, popliteal nodes, etc. For examination of axillary gland, keep child's arm on the examiner's forearm and palpate against chest wall, lateral axillary wall, anterior axillary fold, posterior axillary fold and deep into the apex of axilla for nodes there.

Oedema

- Apply pressure over a bony point for a few seconds, but up to 1 min is required for minimal oedema. Use thumb for applying pressure (may be because it is a large digit to leave a large pit or it is a stronger finger or just a convention). The pressure should be just right to detect oedema but not to give pain. If the examiner feels that the child is made to yell because of undue pressure, negative marks will be awarded.
- Examine above the medial malleolus over the tibia (in an ambulant patient). Examine other areas like sacral area (in a bed-ridden patient), puffy lids, etc.
- If present, comment as: uni/bilateral; pitting/non-pitting.
- Examine both sides.

Examine the Pulse

- To palpate the radial pulse, semipronate the forearm, flex the wrist and feel the pulse.
- To palpate the brachial pulse, flex the arm, palpate medial to the biceps tendon.
- Palpate all peripheral pulses. Always compare both sides.
- NEVER palpate both carotids simultaneously. This may lead to cerebral hypoxia and hence may fetch negative marks.
- Look for rate, rhythm, character, volume, character of the vessel wall and radiofemoral delay. Refer to section on cardiovascular system for details.

Record BP

- Tie an adequately sized cuff (should cover 2/3rd of the length of the arm).
- Determine the systolic pressure by palpatory method.
- Record the BP by auscultatory method.
- Record the BP in all four limbs. Record BP supine and standing.

Locate the Apex Beat

- Expose the precordium well.
- Make the patient lie supine.
- Locate by inspection.
- First locate by palpating with the palm.
- Then locate to an intercostal space by the pulp of index finger.
- After locating the site of the apex, patient may be turned to the left side for better appreciation of the character—tapping or heaving.
- Comment on: site, character (normal/tapping/heaving), palpable sounds and thrills at the apex.

26

Look for Left Parasternal Heave

- Expose the precordium well.
- With the patient on supine position, look for parasternal heave with the ulnar aspect of the palm.
- A pencil placed over the parasternal area will act as an amplifier of the parasternal movement and may help detect subtle movements.

Murmur of Mitral Stenosis

- Auscultate in supine position.
- Auscultate over the apex, with the bell.
- Time with carotid pulse, if needed.
- Comment about the nature of the murmur, pitch, duration, character, presystolic accentuation, loudness of S_1.
- Turn the patient to left lateral position or ask the patient to hold his breath in expiration or to briefly exert himself to bring on the subtle murmur. These may have to be done as a patient without any murmur may be kept (because it is only the method of examination that is assessed).

Palpation of Spleen

- Ask the patient to lie down supine with the abdomen well exposed.
- Ask the patient to flex both hips and knees.
- Ask the patient to breathe deeply and relax.

- Begin palpation from the right iliac fossa.
- Palpate towards the left hypochondrium.
- If spleen is palpable measure it from costal margin.
- Look for splenic notch.
- To look for minimal enlargement, turn the patient to right lateral position, extend the right leg, flex the left leg and palpate just below the left costal margin for spleen tip (left hand pushing the left chest wall medially).

Examine the Knee Jerk

- Patient can be supine or sitting up.
- Explain the procedure to the child and win his confidence.
- Hold the knee hammer loose to produce a good swing as the tendon is struck.
- Expose the contracting muscle belly to observe for contraction. For knee jerk, it is quadriceps, so expose the thigh.
- Compare both sides.
- If reflex cannot be elicited, try reinforcement.
- Elicitation of knee jerk should not cause pain. If it does, usually the method is wrong and negative marks are likely.

Examine the eye

- Position (E.g. slant, hypertelorism) epicanthic fold
- Lid- Ptosis, oedema, diurnal variation.
- Squint- paralytic, concomitant (Pg. 197), cover uncover test (Pg. 198)
- Nystagmus
- Iris- Coloboma, aniridia (aniridia is often hypoplasia and not absence)
- Lens- cataract, dislocation.
- Fundus- optic disc, retina.
- Test vision (Pg. 187)
- Test extraocular movements (Pg. 193)
- Pupillary reflex
- Conjunctival reflex (corneal reflex best avoided)
- Bruit over the eye.

Examine the Gait

- Ask to walk and observe (Pg. 183)
- Heel and toe walking (cerebellar)
- Walk on toe (S1)
- Walk on heel (L5)- not possible in CP, DMD
- Walk on outside of feet- brings out subtle hemiplegia as child walks with typical hemiplegic gait (Caution- do not overinterpret, this being unusual position, child may walk bizarre)
- Run
- Stand on each foot
- Rhomberg test
- Stooping to touch the toe (look for scoliosis)
- Lying on the floor and getting up (Gower sign)
- Squat and get up
- After examination, give your opinion and tell what more clinical examination (general or systemic) needed to substantiate or rule out your diagnosis.

II. History Station

Take Immunization History

- BCG, also enquire about scar
- DPT, OPV whether taken and if so at the right time or not
- Measles, if taken, when
- Boosters
- Optional vaccines
- Pulse polio
- Negative mark if BCG scar is looked for on the right arm!

III. Newborn Station

Please refer to the basic steps (see above). Usual tasks are assessment of gestational age, assessment of jaundice, spot the diagnosis like erythema toxicum, cephalhaematoma, etc.

IV. Measurement Station

The candidate is required to make one measurement like height, weight, mid-arm circumference, head circumference, etc, and answer related questions (like comment on the nutritional status of this child).

Sample question: Measure the mid-arm circumference of this child (one mark for the correct method of measurement). To which colour code of Shakir's tape will this measured value correspond to (½ mark)? Name the age-independent anthropometric measurement ratio that incorporates the mid-arm circumference and the height (½ mark).

V. Heath Education (Counseling) Station

The candidate is required to give health education to the mother regarding any specific aspect; e.g., feeding of a preterm child, advice on breast-feeding, treatment in case of diarrhoea, nutrition advice for a PEM child, etc. Also included in this session are discharge advises to be given to mothers for their children with diseases like febrile fits, rheumatic fever, ITP, urinary infection, nephritic syndrome, etc.

VI. Charts

Charts containing lab reports on urine, CSF, blood, pleural fluid, etc, will be kept for interpretation. Rarely, X-rays may be kept although it is not the usual practice as X-ray forms part of viva session.

Sample question: A 5-year-old child with fever, vomiting and yellowish discolouration of urine has the following laboratory report:

Serum bilirubin 20 mg% (indirect fraction 6 mg%), SGOT 2145 IU, SGPT (ALT) 2550 IU, alkaline phosphatase 455 IU, prothrombin time 32 sec (control 13 sec).

1. What is the most probable diagnosis?
2. From the laboratory report, what immediate complication do you anticipate?
3. What drugs will you use to prevent or limit this anticipated complication?
4. What is the first-line intervention for fever in this child?

For each question, ½ marks each will be allotted out of a total of 2 marks from this OSCE station. Obviously, it is viral hepatitis and the prothrombin time that makes one anticipate bleeding as a complication. Vitamin K and fresh frozen plasma are interventions that may prevent or limit this complication. All antipyretics are hepatotoxic to variable degrees and hence the first-line intervention is tepid sponging.

VII. Clinical Scenario Station

A clinical scenario (clinical case history) will be given for the student to formulate a diagnosis and answer related questions. The student can refer to short cases section of this book (the undergraduates can skip the cases marked for postgraduates).

Sample question: A 6-year-old boy running a fever develops a crop of 5–6 papular rashes over the upper chest, which became clear fluid-containing vesicles by evening. The next morning new crops of lesions were noticed over the abdomen and the thigh and the already existing clear vesicles turned cloudy and some of them have already ruptured due to the child scratching it.

1. What is your diagnosis?
2. What is the most common complication?
3. Name the specific drug for treatment?
4. How can you prevent this disease in child population?

The clinical history is typical of chickenpox. Although so many complications are possible, the most common one is the secondary infection of the skin lesions. The specific drug is acyclovir and prevention is by immunization.

VIII. Draw and Label Station

The student is required to make simple drawings with correct labeling. Usual tasks are to draw blood cells (normal and abnormal, LE cells, etc), parasites (helminths, malaria, etc), urinary sediments, growth curves (growth pattern of brain, lymphoid tissue, genitals, etc), cardiac murmurs, respiratory sounds, etc.

OSCE FOR POSTGRADUATE EXAMINATIONS

Postgraduate OSCE is more elaborate one assessing various clinical as well as a few non-clinical skills. Like undergraduate OSCE, there will be manned and unmanned stations.

Newborn Resuscitation

The candidate must know how to respond to the specific situation given in the question (e.g., you are called to attend the delivery where there is meconium-stained amniotic fluid). The candidate must be thorough with the newborn resuscitation protocols. The student may consider referring to the Ch.1 of *Manual of Newborn Care* by A Santhosh Kumar (Paras Medical Publisher).

Procedures and Instruments

The usual ones are lumbar puncture, ascitic tap, pleural tap, liver biopsy, renal biopsy, bone marrow aspiration, bone marrow trephine biopsy, endotracheal intubation, surfactant administration, intraosseous line, etc. Sometimes, the students may be required to demonstrate the procedure in mannequins.

Counseling

In addition to what is described under the undergraduate OSCE, genetic counseling, counseling in HIV, etc, may figure.

Demonstration of Clinical Signs

Any clinical signs may figure in this section. Refer to the relevant sections in this book.

Assessment of Development

Here, the student must assess development from history as well as his own interaction with the child.

Spotters (actual clinical cases or photos)

Readily obvious clinical material may be kept. For example, Apert syndrome; cataract, etc. Relevant questions also will figure in the discussion.

Slides

Usual ones are haematology slides (e.g., sickle cell anaemia, leukaemia, spherocytosis, malaria, etc); rarely microbiology preparations may figure (e.g., acid-fast bacilli, *Vibrio cholerae,* etc). (The following slides are provided by Dr CP Muthukrishnan).

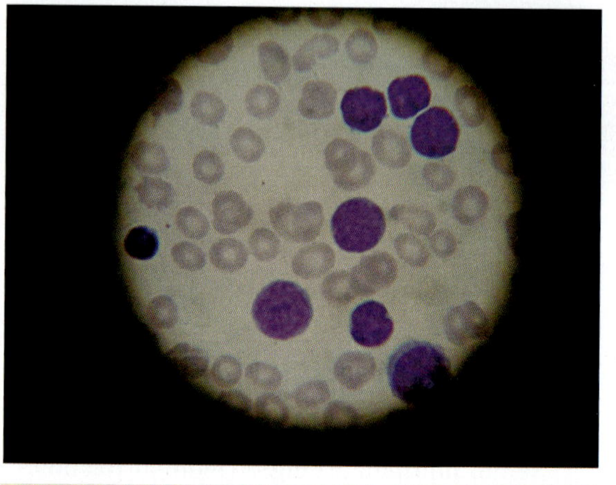

Fig.26.3 Acute lymphoblastic leukaemia. Lymphoblasts have scanty cytoplasm and inconspicuous nucleoli (nucleoli not more than one or two); compare with myeloblast.

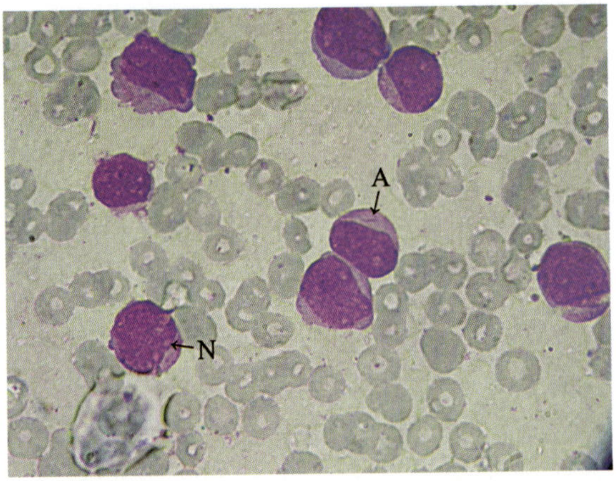

Fig.26.4 Acute myeloblastic leukaemia. Myeloblasts are showing Auer rods. N = nucleolus; A = Auer rods. Even if the Auer rods are not made out, myeloblast may be identified by the relatively more cytoplasm (compared to lymphoblast) and many nucleoli.

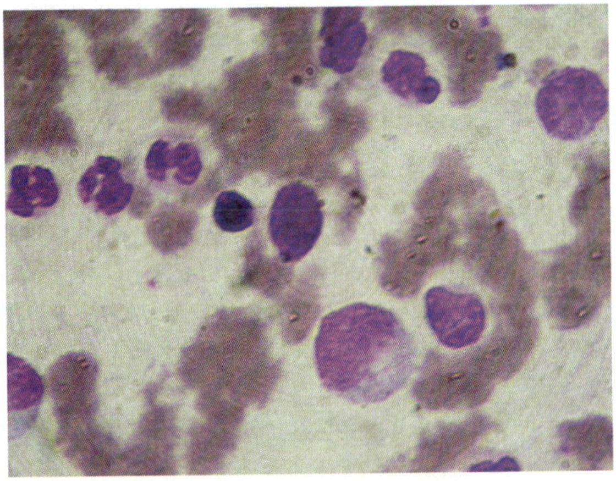

Fig.26.5 Chronic myeloid leukaemia. Both the mature granulocytes and the blasts in varying stages of maturation are seen in the same field. Tip: Blasts in acute leukaemia are like school children in uniform, all blasts looking alike; chronic leukaemia is like college girls in different dresses, the immature cells of various sizes and stages of maturation are seen.

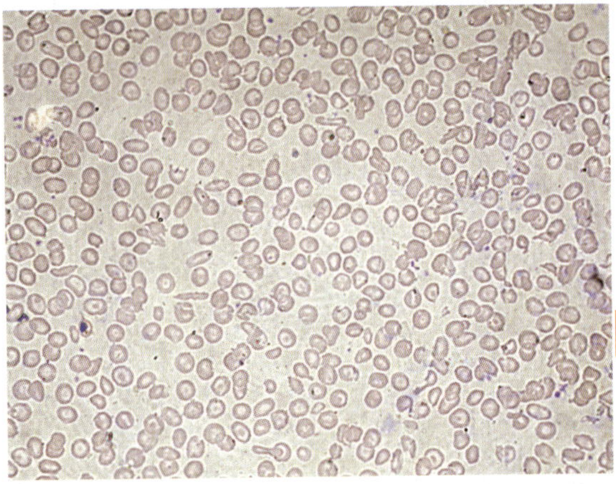

Fig.26.6 Hypochromic microcytic anaemia; the cells show central pallor occupying more than 1/3rd of the cell size. Note the pencil-shaped cells, the ovalocytes and the microcytes.

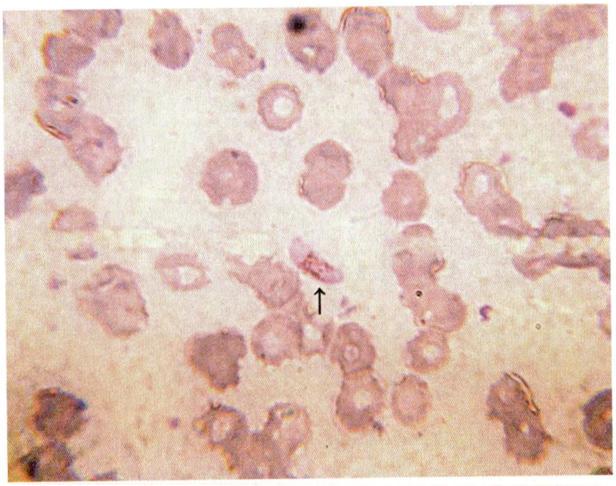

Fig.26.7 Note the banana (cresent) shaped gametocyte of falciparum malaria.

26

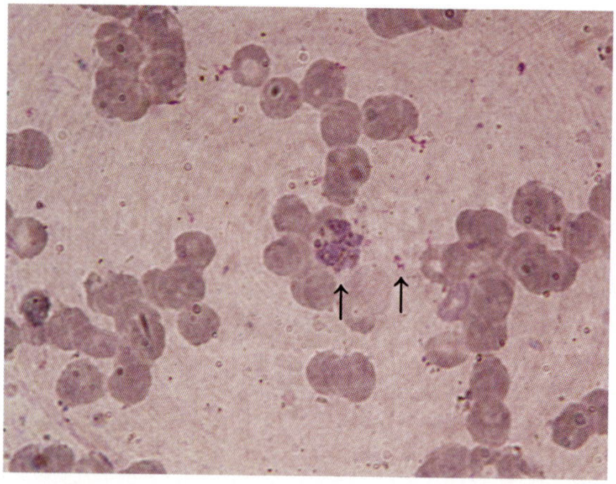

Fig.26.8 Trophozoits of malarial parasites are seen within a damaged RBC; malarial pigments are seen outside the RBCs as well.

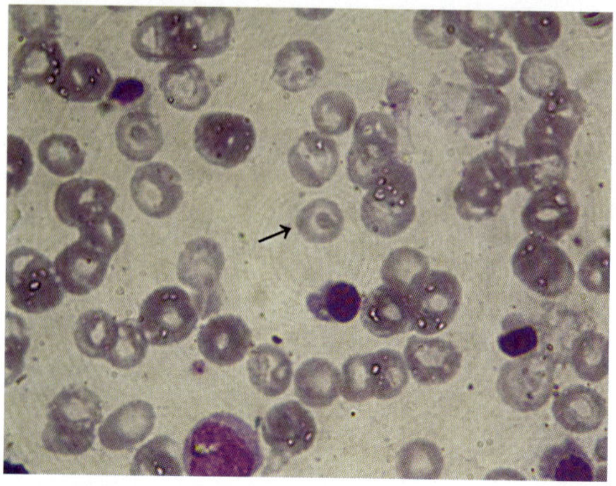

Fig.26.9 Thalassaemia. The slide shows hypochromic microcytic anaemia. Large intensely staining nucleated cells seen are the normoblasts. The arrow shows a target cell.

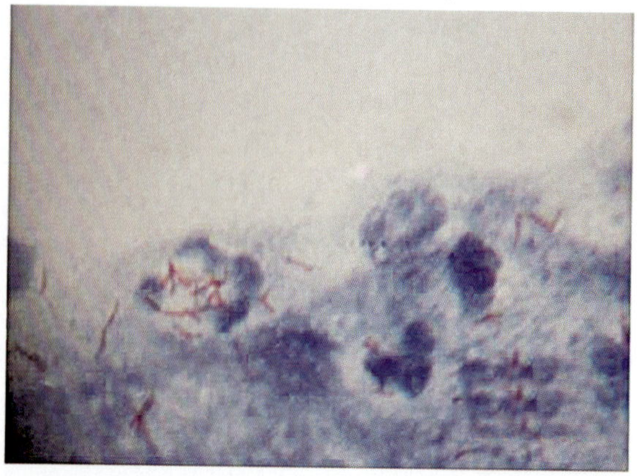

Fig.26.10 Acid-fast bacillus

Statistical Problem

This has become routine in PG exams and hence the student must read about this.

Given below are a few examples of statistical questions related to tests of significance (*Courtesy*: Dr S Geetha).

I. Specify the test of significance you would apply to find out whether differences between samples are significant or not in each of the following situations:
   1. Comparison of means of haemoglobin before and after iron supplementation in ten children. Distribution of haemoglobin levels is non-Gaussian. ***Ans***: Wilcoxon signed rank test. If the distribution were Gaussian, paired *t* test is used.
   2. Comparison of proportions of ten patients of lung cancer between smokers (8/12) and non-smokers (2/13). ***Ans***: Fischer's exact test. You should be familiar with drawing 2 x 2 (two by two) tables. Because if the question was to calculate the risk, then odds ratio may have to be calculated.
3. Comparison of means of serum bilirubin levels in two groups of neonates treated with phenobarbitone (n=20) and without phenobarbitone (n=20), respectively. Distribution of outcome variable is Gaussian. ***Ans***: Student's *t*

test. If distribution were non-Gaussian, the test to be used is Mann-Whitney *U* test.

4. Comparison of means of PEFR in four groups of children aged 8–10, 10–12, 12–14 and 14–16 years of age, respectively. The means are distributed in a Gaussian manner. ***Ans***: analysis of variance (ANOVA).

The student is advised to be familiar with the terms like sensitivity, specificity, positive and negative predictive values, odds ratio, student's *t* test, incidence, prevalence, etc. The student may be required to calculate vital statistics from the given data.

Karyotype

Usual ones kept are Down, Turner, Klinefelter, etc.

(The karyotype pictures are provided by Dr VH Sankar.)

	Lung cancer +	Lung cancer -	Total
Smoker	a (8)	b (4)	12
Non-smoker	c (2)	d (11)	13
Total	10	15	
Odds ratio = ad/bc = (8 x 11) ÷ (2 x 4) = 11 (smoker has higher odds for getting cancer)			

	Distribution	Test used
Comparison of **means** in a **single population** before and after intervention	Gaussian	Paired *t* test
	Non-Gaussian	Wilcoxon signed-rank test
Comparison of **means** in **two different populations**	Gaussian	Student's *t* test (when n is less than 30) Z test when n is more than 30
	Non-Gaussian	Mann-Whitney *U* test
Comparison of **proportions**		Chi-square test; if any variable is less than 5, Fisher's exact test is used
Parametric tests are *t* test and *Z* test. Non-parametric tests are chi-square test, Mann Whitney *U* test, Wilcoxon signed rank test, etc.		

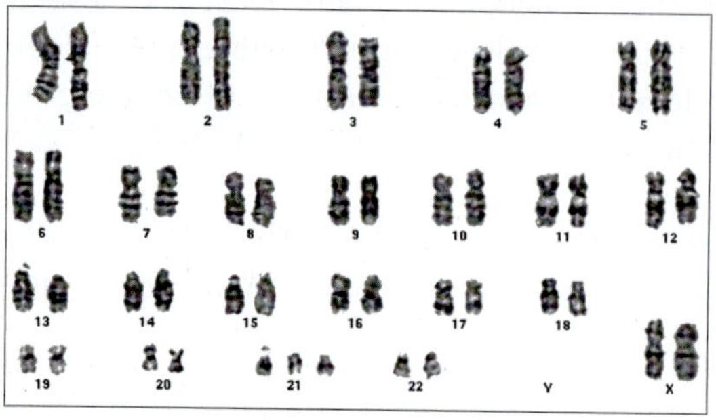

Fig.26.11 Note that the 21 group consists of three instead of the normally expected two chromosomes. Thus, it is trisomy 21.

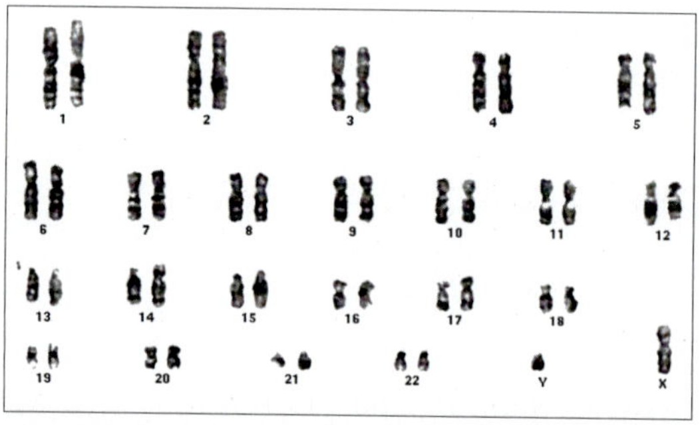

Fig.26.12 Part of one of chromosome 21 is translocated to chromosome 14. Note the missing part in one 21st chromosome and corresponding lengthening of the 14th chromosome.

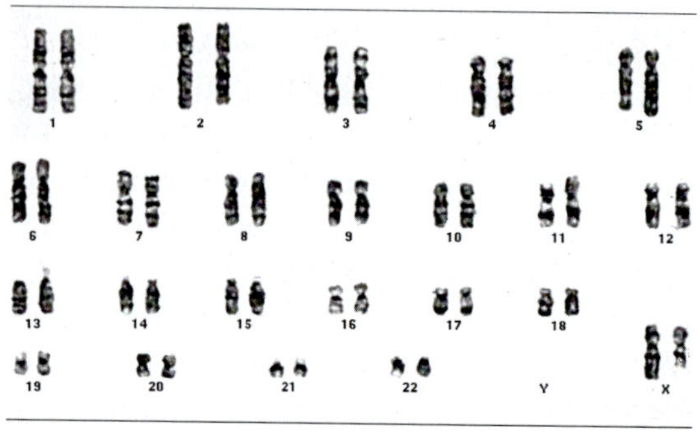

Fig.26.13 Note that a part of one X chromosome is missing. So it is a Turner (although typically one X chromosome altogether must be missing in classical Turner).

X-rays

CT and MRI may also be rarely kept. Please refer to the relevant section in this book.

ABG and Ventilator Settings

The student may consider reading Ch.3 of *Manual of Paediatric Practice* by A Santhosh Kumar (Paras Medical Publisher).

ECG

The usual ECGs kept are early transition of tetralogy of Fallot, left axis deviation of endocardial cushion defect, rSR pattern of ASD, huge P waves of Ebstein anomaly, supraventricular tachycardia, atrial flutter, complete heart block, long QT syndrome, hyperkalaemia, etc. The student may consider reading *Pediatric ECG* by A Santhosh Kumar (Paras Medical Publisher).

Drugs

Others: The student can expect questions from immunization, waste management, etc.

The given picture is an investigation done on a 50-day-old baby with cholestatic jaundice. Identify the investigation.

The investigation shown is hepatobiliary scintigraphy.

1. What is the finding shown — The isotope is not getting excreted into the gut; most probable diagnosis is biliary atresia.
2. What is the definitive treatment for this condition—Liver transplantation.

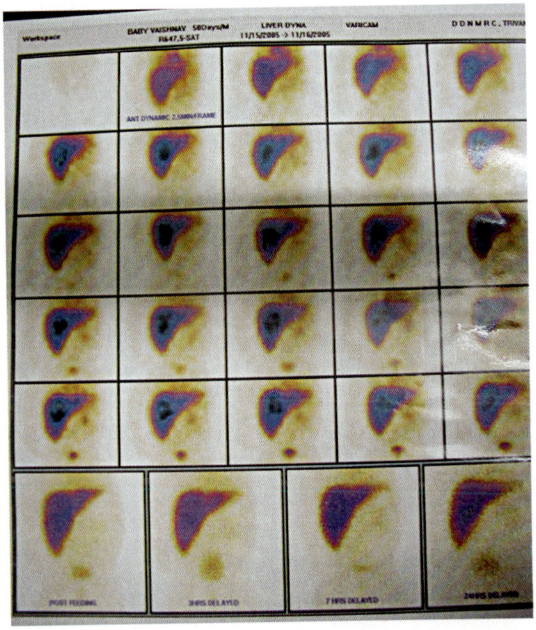

Fig.26.14

REFERENCES

1 Peter S Harper. *Practical Genetic Counseling*, 3rd ed. Butterworth & Co Publishers Ltd; 1988.
2. Parthasarathy A, Menon PSN, Nair MKC. *IAP Textbook of Pediatrics*, 2nd ed. Jaypee Publishers, New Delhi; 2002.
3. Campbell AGM, Mc Intosh N (eds). Forfar and Arneil's *Textbook of Pediatrics*, 5th ed. Churchill Livingston: Edinburgh.
4. Michael Swash. *Hutchison's Clinical Methods*, 20th ed. WB Saunders Company, London; 1999.
5. Behrman RE, Kliegman RM, Jenson HB (eds). *Nelson Textbook of Pediatrics*, 16th ed, WB Saunders Company, Philadelphia; 2000.
6. Smith DW. *Recognizable Patterns of Human Malformations*, 3rd and 6th ed. WB Saunders Company: Philadelphia.
7. Mc Millan JA, De Angelis CD, Feign RD, Warshaw JB. *Oski's Pediatrics*, 3rd ed. Lippincott Williams & Wilkins, Philadelphia; 1999.
8. Hay WW, Hayward AR, Levin MJ, Sondheimer JM (eds). *Current Pediatric Diagnosis and Treatment*, 16th ed. Lange/McGraw Hill, New York; 2003.
9. Ghai OP. *Essential Pediatrics*, 5th ed. Interprint, New Delhi; 2000.
10. Santhosh Kumar A. *Handbook of Pediatrics*, 5th ed. AIPD, Chennai; 2005.
11. Santhosh Kumar A. *Manual of Pediatric Practice*, 4th ed. Paras Medical Publisher, Hyderabad; 2014.
12. Santhosh Kumar A. *Pediatric Prescriber*, 7th ed. Paras Medical Publisher, Hyderabad; 2024.
13. Soma Raju B. *Clinical Methods in Cardiology*, 1st ed, Orient Longman, Hyderabad; 2004.
14. Harris W, Timms B, Choong R. *Examination Pediatrics*, 1st ed. Jaypee Brothers: New Delhi; 1993.
15. Silverman FM, Kuhn JP. *Essentials of Caffey's Pediatric X-ray Diagnosis*. Yearbook Medical Publisher: Chicago; 1990.
16. Volpe JJ. *Neurology of Newborn*, 3rd ed. WB Saunders Company: Philadelphia; 1995.
17. Sheila Sherlock, James Dooley. *Diseases of Liver and Biliary System*, 9th ed. Oxford Blackwell Scientific Publications, London; 1993.
18. Hardman JG, Limbird LE. *Goodman and Gilman's Pharmacological Basis of Therapeutics*, 9th ed. McGraw Hill: New York; 1996.
19. Elizabeth KE. *Nutrition and Child Development*, 7th ed. Paras Medical Publisher, Hyderabad; 2025.
20. Illingworth RS. *The Development of the Infant and Young Child*, 9th ed. Churchill Livingstone; 1999.
21. *Park*, 15th ed, p 507.
22. Markel H, Farrell MH, Oski AJ. *The Portable Pediatrician*, 2nd ed. Hanley & Belfus: Philadelphia; 2000.
23. Alagappan R. *Manual of Practical Medicine*, 2nd ed. Jaypee Publishers: New Delhi; 2002.
24. Krishnadas KV (ed). *Textbook of Medicine*. Jaypee Publishers: New Delhi.
25. RJ Vakil, AF Golwalla, SA Golwalla. *Physical Diagnosis*. MPP, Mumbai; 1999.
26. BH Athreya. *Clinical Methods in Pediatric Diagnosis*. CBS, New Delhi; 1990.
27. *Kendig's Disorders of Respiratory Tract in Children*. WB Saunders Co: Philadelphia; 1998.
28. A Santhosh Kumar. *Manual of Newborn Care*, 3rd ed. Paras Medical Publisher, Hyderabad; 2024.
29. Glaser AW, McIntyre J, Battin M. *Short Cases for Pediatric exams*, 1st ed. WB Saunders, Philadelphia; 2000.
30. Thomas R, Harvey D. *Neonatology*, 2nd ed, Churchill Livingstone, London; 1997.

Index

A

C

I

I

I

I

I

I

X

Y

Z